Physical Activity, Exercise Testing and Clinical Assessment in Sports Medicine

Physical Activity, Exercise Testing and Clinical Assessment in Sports Medicine

Editor

David Rodríguez-Sanz

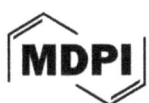

Basel • Beijing • Wuhan • Barcelona • Belgrade • Novi Sad • Cluj • Manchester

Editor
David Rodríguez-Sanz
Universidad Complutense de Madrid
Madrid, Spain

Editorial Office
MDPI
St. Alban-Anlage 66
4052 Basel, Switzerland

This is a reprint of articles from the Special Issue published online in the open access journal *Journal of Clinical Medicine* (ISSN 2077-0383) (available at: https://www.mdpi.com/journal/jcm/special_issues/Physical_Activity_Exercise_Testing).

For citation purposes, cite each article independently as indicated on the article page online and as indicated below:

Lastname, A.A.; Lastname, B.B. Article Title. *Journal Name* **Year**, *Volume Number*, Page Range.

ISBN 978-3-0365-9454-5 (Hbk)
ISBN 978-3-0365-9455-2 (PDF)
doi.org/10.3390/books978-3-0365-9455-2

© 2023 by the authors. Articles in this book are Open Access and distributed under the Creative Commons Attribution (CC BY) license. The book as a whole is distributed by MDPI under the terms and conditions of the Creative Commons Attribution-NonCommercial-NoDerivs (CC BY-NC-ND) license.

Contents

Wiesław Błach, Peter Smolders, Łukasz Rydzik, Georgios Bikos, Nicola Maffulli, Nikos Malliaropoulos, et al.
Judo Injuries Frequency in Europe's Top-Level Competitions in the Period 2005–2020
Reprinted from: *J. Clin. Med.* **2021**, *10*, 852, doi:10.3390/jcm10040852 1

Jorge Posada-Ordax, Julia Cosin-Matamoros, Marta Elena Losa-Iglesias, Ricardo Becerro-de-Bengoa-Vallejo, Laura Esteban-Gonzalo, Carlos Martin-Villa, et al.
Accuracy and Repeatability of Spatiotemporal Gait Parameters Measured with an Inertial Measurement Unit
Reprinted from: *J. Clin. Med.* **2021**, *10*, 1804, doi:10.3390/jcm10091804 9

Wen-Dien Chang, Shuya Chen and Yung-An Tsou
Effects of Whole-Body Vibration and Balance Training on Female Athletes with Chronic Ankle Instability
Reprinted from: *J. Clin. Med.* **2021**, *10*, 2380, doi:10.3390/jcm10112380 27

Yanfei Guan, Shannon S. D. Bredin, Jack Taunton, Qinxian Jiang, Nana Wu, Yongfeng Li and Darren E. R. Warburton
Risk Factors for Non-Contact Lower-Limb Injury: A Retrospective Survey in Pediatric-Age Athletes
Reprinted from: *J. Clin. Med.* **2021**, *10*, 3171, doi:10.3390/jcm10143171 41

Petr Bahenský, Václav Bunc, Renata Malátová, David Marko, Gregory J. Grosicki and Jan Schuster
Impact of a Breathing Intervention on Engagement of Abdominal, Thoracic, and Subclavian Musculature during Exercise, a Randomized Trial
Reprinted from: *J. Clin. Med.* **2021**, *10*, 3514, doi:10.3390/jcm10163514 51

Łukasz Oleksy, Anna Mika, Aleksandra Królikowska, Maciej Kuchciak, Magda Stolarczyk, Renata Kielnar, et al.
Composite Score of Readiness (CSR) as Holistic Profiling of Functional Deficits in Footballers Following ACL Reconstruction
Reprinted from: *J. Clin. Med.* **2021**, *10*, 3570, doi:10.3390/jcm10163570 63

Jose Castro-Piñero, Nuria Marin-Jimenez, Jorge R. Fernandez-Santos, Fatima Martin-Acosta, Victor Segura-Jimenez, Rocio Izquierdo-Gomez, et al.
Criterion-Related Validity of Field-Based Fitness Tests in Adults: A Systematic Review
Reprinted from: *J. Clin. Med.* **2021**, *10*, 3743, doi:10.3390/jcm10163743 73

Marta Pawłowska, Celestyna Mila-Kierzenkowska, Tomasz Boraczyński, Michał Boraczyński, Karolina Szewczyk-Golec, Paweł Sutkowy, et al.
The Effect of Submaximal Exercise Followed by Short-Term Cold-Water Immersion on the Inflammatory State in Healthy Recreational Athletes: A Cross-Over Study
Reprinted from: *J. Clin. Med.* **2021**, *10*, 4239, doi:10.3390/jcm10184239 93

Pamela Villavicencio, Cristina Bravo, Antoni Ibarz and Silvia Solé
Effects of Acute Psychological and Physiological Stress on Rock Climbers
Reprinted from: *J. Clin. Med.* **2021**, *10*, 5013, doi:10.3390/jcm10215013 107

Reza Mazaheri, Christian Schmied, David Niederseer and Marco Guazzi
Cardiopulmonary Exercise Test Parameters in Athletic Population: A Review
Reprinted from: *J. Clin. Med.* **2021**, *10*, 5073, doi:10.3390/jcm10215073 117

Filipe Manuel Clemente, Francisco Tomás González-Fernández, Halil Ibrahim Ceylan, Rui Silva, Saeid Younesi, Yung-Sheng Chen, et al.
Blood Biomarkers Variations across the Pre-Season and Interactions with Training Load: A Study in Professional Soccer Players
Reprinted from: *J. Clin. Med.* **2021**, *10*, 5576, doi:10.3390/jcm10235576 . . . . **129**

Nebojša Trajković, Darjan Smajla, Žiga Kozinc and Nejc Šarabon
Postural Stability in Single-Leg Quiet Stance in Highly Trained Athletes: Sex and Sport Differences
Reprinted from: *J. Clin. Med.* **2022**, *11*, 1009, doi:10.3390/jcm11041009 . . . . **149**

Marc Dauty, Vincent Crenn, Bastien Louguet, Jérôme Grondin, Pierre Menu and Alban Fouasson-Chailloux
Anatomical and Neuromuscular Factors Associated to Non-Contact Anterior Cruciate Ligament Injury
Reprinted from: *J. Clin. Med.* **2022**, *11*, 1402, doi:10.3390/jcm11051402 . . . . **159**

Daniel Pecos-Martín, Sergio Patiño-Núñez, Jessica Quintero-Pérez, Gema Cruz-Riesco, Cintia Quevedo-Socas, Tomás Gallego-Izquierdo, et al.
Mechanical Hyperalgesia but Not Forward Shoulder Posture Is Associated with Shoulder Pain in Volleyball Players: A Cross-Sectional Study
Reprinted from: *J. Clin. Med.* **2022**, *11*, 1472, doi:10.3390/jcm11061472 . . . . **169**

Arturo Pérez-Gosalvez, Francisco García-Muro San José, Ofelia Carrión-Otero, Tomás Pérez-Fernández and Luis Fernández-Rosa
Blood Pressure and Heart Rate Responses to an Isokinetic Testing Protocol in Professional Soccer Players
Reprinted from: *J. Clin. Med.* **2022**, *11*, 1539, doi:10.3390/jcm11061539 . . . . **179**

Anca Gabriela Stoianov, Jenel Marian Pătrașcu, Bogdan Gheorghe Hogea, Bogdan Andor, Liviu Coriolan Mișcă, Sorin Florescu, et al.
Dynamic Ultrasound Assessment of the Anterior Tibial Translation for Anterior Cruciate Ligament Tears Diagnostic
Reprinted from: *J. Clin. Med.* **2022**, *11*, 2152, doi:10.3390/jcm11082152 . . . . **195**

Iulia Iovanca Dragoi, Florina Georgeta Popescu, Teodor Petrita, Florin Alexa, Sorin Barac, Cosmina Ioana Bondor, et al.
Acute Effects of Sedentary Behavior on Ankle Torque Assessed with a Custom-Made Electronic Dynamometer
Reprinted from: *J. Clin. Med.* **2022**, *11*, 2474, doi:10.3390/jcm11092474 . . . . **203**

Alexandru-Dan Costache, Mihai Roca, Cezar Honceriu, Irina-Iuliana Costache, Maria-Magdalena Leon-Constantin, Ovidiu Mitu, et al.
Cardiopulmonary Exercise Testing and Cardiac Biomarker Measurements in Young Football Players: A Pilot Study
Reprinted from: *J. Clin. Med.* **2022**, *11*, 2772, doi:10.3390/jcm11102772 . . . . **223**

Nebojsa Cokorilo, Pedro Jesús Ruiz-Montero, Francisco Tomás González-Fernández and Ricardo Martín-Moya
An Intervention of 12 Weeks of Nordic Walking and Recreational Walking to Improve Cardiorespiratory Capacity and Fitness in Older Adult Women
Reprinted from: *J. Clin. Med.* **2022**, *11*, 2900, doi:10.3390/jcm11102900 . . . . **241**

Aleksandr N. Ovchinnikov, Antonio Paoli, Vladislav V. Seleznev and Anna V. Deryugina
Measurement of Lipid Peroxidation Products and Creatine Kinase in Blood Plasma and Saliva of Athletes at Rest and following Exercise
Reprinted from: *J. Clin. Med.* **2022**, *11*, 3098, doi:10.3390/jcm11113098 . . . . **257**

Ahmad Khiyami, Shibili Nuhmani, Royes Joseph, Turki Saeed Abualait and Qassim Muaidi
Efficacy of Core Training in Swimming Performance and Neuromuscular Parameters of Young Swimmers: A Randomised Control Trial
Reprinted from: *J. Clin. Med.* **2022**, *11*, 3198, doi:10.3390/jcm11113198 271

Ville Stenbäck, Juhani Leppäluoto, Rosanna Juustila, Laura Niiranen, Dominique Gagnon, Mikko Tulppo and Karl-Heinz Herzig
Step Detection Accuracy and Energy Expenditure Estimation at Different Speeds by Three Accelerometers in a Controlled Environment in Overweight/Obese Subjects
Reprinted from: *J. Clin. Med.* **2022**, *11*, 3267, doi:10.3390/jcm11123267 285

Maria Suhs, Andreas Stengel, Amelie Rudolph, Selina Schaper, Ellen Wölk, Peter Kobelt, et al.
Circulating Spexin Is Associated with Body Mass Index and Fat Mass but Not with Physical Activity and Psychological Parameters in Women across a Broad Body Weight Spectrum
Reprinted from: *J. Clin. Med.* **2022**, *11*, 5107, doi:10.3390/jcm11175107 295

Szczepan Wiecha, Przemysław Seweryn Kasiak, Igor Cieśliński, Marcin Maciejczyk, Artur Mamcarz and Daniel Śliż
Modeling Physiological Predictors of Running Velocity for Endurance Athletes
Reprinted from: *J. Clin. Med.* **2022**, *11*, 6688, doi:10.3390/jcm11226688 311

László Balogh, Krisztina Szabó, József Márton Pucsok, Ilona Jámbor, Ágnes Gyetvai, Marianna Mile, et al.
The Effect of Aerobic Exercise and Low-Impact Pilates Workout on the Adaptive Immune System
Reprinted from: *J. Clin. Med.* **2022**, *11*, 6814, doi:10.3390/jcm11226814 327

Jaak Jürimäe, Liina Remmel, Anna-Liisa Tamm, Priit Purge, Katre Maasalu and Vallo Tillmann
Associations of Circulating Irisin and Fibroblast Growth Factor-21 Levels with Measures of Energy Homeostasis in Highly Trained Adolescent Rhythmic Gymnasts
Reprinted from: *J. Clin. Med.* **2022**, *11*, 7450, doi:10.3390/jcm11247450 341

Rui Vilarinho, Ana Toledo, Carla Silva, Fábio Melo, Leila Tomaz, Luana Martins, et al.
Reference Equation of a New Incremental Step Test to Assess Exercise Capacity in the Portuguese Adult Population
Reprinted from: *J. Clin. Med.* **2023**, *12*, 271, doi:10.3390/jcm12010271 351

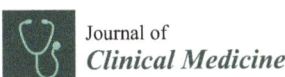

Article

Judo Injuries Frequency in Europe's Top-Level Competitions in the Period 2005–2020

Wiesław Błach [1,2], Peter Smolders [2], Łukasz Rydzik [3,*], Georgios Bikos [4], Nicola Maffulli [5,6,7], Nikos Malliaropoulos [6,8,9], Władysław Jagiełło [10], Krzysztof Maćkała [1] and Tadeusz Ambroży [3]

1. Faculty of Physical Education & Sport, University School of Physical Education, 51-612 Wroclaw, Poland; wieslaw.judo@wp.pl (W.B.); krzysztof.mackala@awf.wroc.pl (K.M.)
2. European Judo Union, 1200 Vienna, Austria; smolderspeter@skynet.be
3. Institute of Sports Sciences, University of Physical Education, 31-571 Krakow, Poland; tadek@ambrozy.pl
4. Euromedica-Arogi Rehabilitation Clinic, 54301 Thessaloniki, Greece; bikosg77@yahoo.gr
5. Department of Orthopaedics, School of Medicine, Surgery and Dentistry, 89100 Salerno, Italy; n.maffulli@qmul.ac.uk
6. Centre for Sports and Exercise Medicine, Queen Mary, University of London, London E1 4DG, UK; contact@sportsmed.gr
7. Institute of Science and Technology in Medicine, Keele University School of Medicine, Stoke on Trent E1 4DG, UK
8. Sports and Exercise Medicine Clinic, 54639 Thessaloniki, Greece
9. Sports Clinic, Rheumatology Department, Barts Health NHS Trust, London E1 4DG, UK
10. Department of Sport, Gdansk University of Physical Education and Sports, 80-336 Gdansk, Poland; wjagiello1@wp.pl
* Correspondence: lukasz.gne@op.pl; Tel.: +48-730-696-377

Abstract: Background: The present study assesses the frequency of injury in Europe's top-level judokas, during top-level competitions, and defines risk factors. Methods: The members of the EJU Medical Commission collected injury data over the period of 2005 to 2020 using the EJU Injury Registration Form at Europe's top judoka tournaments. Results: Over the 15 years of the study, 128 top-level competitions with 28,297 competitors were included; 699 injuries were registered. Of all competitors, 2.5% needed medical treatment. The knee (17.4%), shoulder (15.7%), and elbow (14.2%) were the most common anatomical locations of injury. Sprains (42.2%) were by far the most frequent injury type, followed by contusions (23.1%). Of all contestants, 0.48% suffered an injury which needed transportation to hospital. There was a statistically significant higher frequency of elbow injuries in female athletes ($p < 0.01$). Heavy-weight judokas suffered a remarkably low number of elbow injuries, with more knee and shoulder injuries. Light-weight judokas were more prone to elbow injuries. Conclusions: We found there was a low injury rate in top-level competitors, with a greater frequency of elbow injuries in female judokas. During the 15 years of injury collection data, an injury incidence of 2.5% was found, with a remarkable high injury rate in the women's −52 kg category, and statistically significantly more elbow injuries in women overall.

Keywords: sports injuries; judo; frequency; prevalence; type

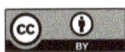

1. Introduction

Judo is a highly technical sport based on the principle of "maximum efficiency with minimum effort" [1]. A judo fight starts with the opponents both standing, attempting to throw each other off balance. After a throw, judokas transition to ground-fighting, the so-called "ne-waza" [2].

The fighting environment consists of constant changes of actions with applications of different movement structures [3]. The more athletes train and compete, the greater the range of powerful throwing techniques they are exposed to, and the chance of injury [4–8]. The frequency and number of injuries, as well as the severity of the injury, influences further training and competitions [9].

Recent studies analysing the frequency and type of injury in judo are available [10–15]. The rate of injury ranges between 12.3% and 30% [16,17]. Data on a large population (all ages and levels of performance) of French judokas during contests showed an injury incidence slightly above 1.1% [18].

The aim of the present investigation was to assess the frequency of injury in Europe's top-level judokas during high-level contests.

2. Materials and Methods

2.1. Subjects

Data were collected from a group of 26,862 high-performance judokas (15,571 men and 11,291 women) aged between 19 and 35 years in all judo weight categories competing in 128 international tournaments under the auspices of the European Judo Union (EJU), including European Judo Championships, in the period between 2005 and 2020. The participants were informed of the protocol and procedure of the EJU Injury registration form. Athletes signed the informed consent form. The EJU Injury registration form was approved by the Medical Commission of EJU. The study was approved by the Bioethics Committee at the Regional Medical Chamber (No. 287/KBL/OIL/2020).

2.2. Study Design

All relevant information was obtained using the questionnaire controlled and supervised by the European Judo Union (EJU) Medical Commissioner present at each competition. When judokas were injured, they were asked to complete this questionnaire and provide relevant information, with the help of the local medical staff and the EJU medical commissioner present. "Minor" injuries, such small nose bleeds or skin abrasions, which do not influence the athlete's performance in any way, were not counted. "Serious" injuries were defined as injuries so severe they needed transportation of the athlete to hospital. The Cronbach's alpha (=0.71, which is considered an acceptable value) was used to assess the validation of the EJU Injury registration form.

2.3. Data Acquisition

In the present study, an injury was defined as the physical condition which necessitated an intervention or medical advice by the medical team present at the judo tournament or a visit to the hospital. After each medical intervention, the injured athlete or the medical staff was asked to complete the medical form. The first part of the form asked the judokas to give general information, including their gender and weight category. In the second part, the medical staff was able to collect data on the anatomical location of the injury, type of injury, structure involved, side of the lesion, and whether the judoka was allowed to continue the fight. The diagnosis of the injury was always filled in on the medical form by the treating physician, either the team doctor or the physician of the local medical team. To ensure the privacy of the injured athlete, individual names were never mentioned. When the judoka had to be transferred to hospital, the injury was defined as "serious".

2.4. Statistical Analysis

The following variables were examined: gender, weight class, body regions, type of injury, and whether or not the athlete had to be transported to hospital, and the injury frequency of each body region was calculated. The Student's t-test and chi-square test were used to evaluate the differences in incidence rates of specific injuries regarding the sex and weight categories. Statistical significance was set at $p = 0.05$. Data were analyzed using Microsoft Windows SPSSWINN 21.0.

3. Results

Of the 699 injured judokas, 384 (54.9%) were men and 315 (45.1%) were women. Overall, 2.5% of all participating judokas needed medical assistance, with no significant difference between men and women ($p > 0.05$).

Table 1 presents the anatomical location of all injuries broken down into smaller units. A total of 696 Injury Registration Forms were filled in correctly in terms of anatomical location. The most frequently injured location was the knee (17.4%), closely followed by shoulder (15.7%) and elbow (14.2%). If we compare the three most frequently occurring anatomical locations in both genders, we find that there is no statistically significant difference in shoulder and knee injuries. However, women had statistically significant more elbow injuries when compared to men ($p < 0.01$).

Table 1. Distribution of injuries by anatomical location.

Anatomical Location	Number of Injuries	% of Total Injury	Men No/%	Women No/%	Δ%	p
Head and neck						
Head	26	3.7	22 (3.2)	4 (0.6)	2.6	<0.05
Neck	34	4.9	21 (3.0)	13 (1.9)	1.1	>0.25
Eye	63	9.1	35 (5.0)	28 (4.0)	1	>0.25
Nose	9	1.3	6 (0.7)	3 (0.4)	0.3	N/a
Mouth	10	1.4	7 (1.0)	3 (0.4)	0.6	N/a
Throat	8	1.1	3 (0.4)	5 (0.7)	0.3	N/a
	14	2	5 (0.7)	9 (1.3)	0.6	<0.05
Upper body						
Trunk	24	3.4	14 (2.0)	10 (1.4)	0.6	>0.20
Shoulder	109	15.7	63 (9.1)	46 (6.6)	2.5	>0.20
Back	11	1.6	6 (0.9)	5 (0.7)	0.2	N/a
Upper limb						
Elbow	99	14.2	44 (6.3)	55 (7.9)	1.6	<0.01
Hand	44	6.3	22 (3.2)	22 (3.2)	0	>0.25
Wrist	15	2.2	10 (1.4)	5 (0.7)	0.7	>0.10
Lower limb						
Knee	121	17.4	60 (8.6)	61 (8.8)	0.2	>0.15
Ankle	38	5.5	19 (2.7)	19 (2.7)	0	>0.25
Foot	20	2.9	14 (2.0)	6 (0.7)	1.3	<0.05
Femur	17	2.4	11 (1.6)	6 (0.7)	0.9	>0.10
Calf	13	1.9	9 (1.3)	4 (0.6)	0.7	N/a
Others	21	3	11	10		
Total	696		382	314		

N/a—not applicable.

Table 2 shows the type of injury which occurred during tournaments. On this subject, we received 695 correctly filled-in forms. The highest percentage rates were sprain (42.2%), occurring with equal frequency in men and women judokas. Soft tissue contusions were second, with an incidence of 23.1%, again occurring with equal frequency in men and women. Men experienced significantly more bleeding episodes than women. We caution that minor nose bleeds and superficial skin lesions were not counted, since they were not considered an injury and did not necessitate medical intervention. Sixty-one luxations occurred, 36 located at the shoulder and 10 at the elbow joint. Unconsciousness after strangling and choking techniques constituted a small percentage of the total number of injuries (6.8%).

Table 2. Characteristics of the injuries.

Injury	Number of Injury	%	Men No/%	Women No/%	Δ%	p
Sprain	293	42.2	151 (21,7)	142 (20.4)	1.3	>0.15
Contusion	160	23.1	89 (12.8)	71 (10.2)	2.6	>0.25
Luxation	61	8.8	34 (4.9)	27 (3.9)	1	>0.25
Unconsciousness	47	6.8	21 (3.0)	26 (3.7)	0.7	>0.25
Bleeding	50	7.1	36 (5.2)	14 (2.0)	3.2	<0.01
Fracture	30	4.3	17 (2.4)	13 (1.9)	0.5	>0.25
Rupture	28	4	18 (2.6)	10 (1.4)	0.8	>0.25
Commotio cerebri	19	2.7	11 (1.6)	8 (1.2)	0.4	>0.25
Others	7	1	4 (0.6)	3 (0.4)	0.2	N/a
Total	695		381	314		

N/a—not applicable.

Injuries were also classified according to their severity and the inability to continue fighting. A serious injury was defined as an injury which required transport to hospital. In the time span of our investigation, a total of 136 judokas suffered a serious injury, and 0.48% of all competitors needed transport to hospital. Of these 136 judokas, 72 were male and 64 were female ($p > 0.10$). The most common location of serious injuries was the shoulder: 36 judokas had to be transferred to hospital because of a shoulder injury. Hence, one-third of all judokas experienced serious shoulder injuries, and almost 26.5% of all serious injuries involved the shoulder. Thirty-two judokas experiencing elbow injuries were transferred to hospital. Of the elbow injuries, 32.3% were classified as serious, and 23.5% of all serious injuries were located at the elbow joint. There was a lower rate of severe knee injuries: 14.0% of knee injuries were serious, and 12.5% of all serious injuries were located at the knee joint. Thirty injuries were fractures, and of these, 26 (86.7%) were serious injuries. Sprains were the largest number of injuries (293), with 44 being serious. Of the 61 luxations, 35 (57.4%) were serious. Only 7.4% of all contusions were classified as serious. During the entire observation period, ten of the potentially very dangerous neck injuries had to be transferred to hospital. Four judokas had to be transferred to hospital after concussion/commotio cerebri. The short period of unconsciousness which occasionally occurs after strangling and choking techniques ("shime-waza") was never a reason for transfer to hospital (Table 3).

Table 3. Body areas and injuries classified as serious.

Anatomical Location	No of Injury	No of Serious Injury	% of Injuries in This Area Classified as Serious	% of All Serious Injuries
Shoulder	109	36	33	26.5
Elbow	99	32	32.3	23.5
Knee	121	17	14	12.5
Head	34	6	17.6	4.4
Ankle	38	6	15.8	4.4
Foot	20	6	30	4.4
Neck	63	10	15.9	7.4
Type of injury				
Sprain	293	44	15	32.3
Luxation	61	35	57.4	25.7
Fracture	30	26	86.7	19.1
Contusion	160	10	6.2	7.4

Table 3. Cont.

Anatomical Location	No of Injury	No of Serious Injury	% of Injuries in This Area Classified as Serious	% of All Serious Injuries
Rupture	28	9	32.1	6.6
Bleeding	50	5	10	3.7
Commotio cerebri	19	4	21	2.9
Unconsciousness	47	0	0	0

Figure 1 shows that in male judokas, the number of injuries per weight category was distributed as to be expected with the number of participants in each weight category. In women (Figure 2), there was a remarkably high incidence of injuries in the under 52 kg category, and a low incidence in the under 57 kg category.

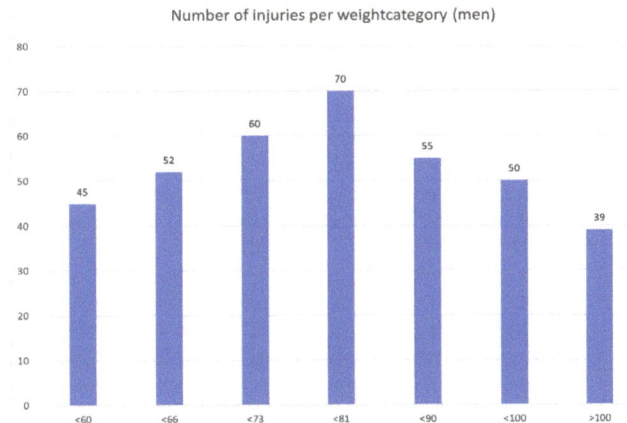

Figure 1. Distribution of injuries by weight category in men.

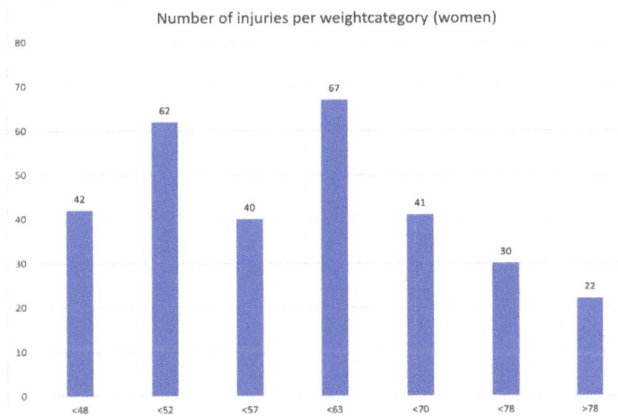

Figure 2. Distribution of injuries by weight category in women.

4. Discussion

The main findings of the present study is the higher frequency of injuries in female athletes, especially regarding injuries in the upper extremities in Europe's top-level judokas during competitions over a period of 15 years. We realise that many injuries also occur during training, but this study was designed only to determine injury incidence during top-level tournaments. The mechanism of injury in judo is linked to throwing and grappling techniques. According to some studies, most injuries affect the upper limbs, as the fight starts with both judokas standing [10,14,17–19].

Lower limbs are at a high risk of injury as well [13]. In two studies on the Korean Olympic team judokas, the knee was frequently injured [13], with 20% of the injuries occurring in the trunk, especially in the lumbar and thoracic spine. These injuries occurred during training, not during competition. We found that 30% of the injuries occurred in the lower limbs (most at the knee), and 20.7% of injuries in the trunk and shoulder combined. Comparing judo and wrestling, the most common injuries were in the lower (judo 61%; wrestling 41%, $p < 0.05$) and upper limbs (judo 30%; wrestling 32%) [2]. In the present study, the knee (17.4%), shoulder (15.7%), and elbow (14.2%) were the primary anatomical locations of an injury.

Regarding injury types, in most studies, contusions and abrasions were the most frequent injuries. In the present investigation, sprains were the most frequent injury type, followed by contusion. Overall, 42.2% of all injuries were sprains, and 23.1% of all injuries were contusions, with no statistically significant difference between the genders. In other studies, sprains mainly occurred in the knee, elbow, and ankle, and often the judokas suffered sprains of the acromioclavicular (AC) joint [18,20]. Frey et al., evaluating judo competition-related injuries during 21 seasons in France, showed that the six most frequently sprained joints accounted for over 75% of total sprains [18]. Additionally, the incidence for overall sprain injuries was significantly higher in female athletes (0.82% vs. 0.53%, respectively; $p < 0.001$). Our study did not provide evidence of any differences between sexes ($p > 0.05$). The high rate of sprains, mainly the acromioclavicular joint, elbow, and knee, can be explained by falls on the shoulder or the use of the arm as a stabilizer in abduction to defend from a throwing attack [18]. Sprains of the knee or ankle are likely related to the rotational maneuvers required to attack and defend. In the present study, 44 of 293 sprains were considered serious, and the judokas had to be hospitalized. On the other hand, only 10 contusions, mostly a consequence of a fall, were serious.

The third major injury among judokas in the present study was a fracture, with 30 cases, 26 of which were serious, requiring transport to hospital. In four cases, the treating physician decided not to transport the injured athlete to hospital. These were finger fractures, and these injuries were likely treated after travelling back to the athlete's home country. In the study of Frey et. al., clavicles were also the most commonly fractured bone [18], often from a direct fall onto the shoulder.

A major concern is cervical spine fracture, which can occur following hyperflexion or hyperextension of the cervical spine, or because of direct trauma or axial loading. Over the course of 15 years of injury recording, 10 neck injuries required transport to hospital.

In the present study, 47 of 695 medical interventions (6.8%) followed unconsciousness after a strangle/choke technique (shime-waza). In this case, judokas cannot stop the fight by themselves by tapping out, and the referee must immediately stop the fight. None of these were serious enough for the judoka to be transferred to hospital.

Concussions (commotio cerebri) were diagnosed only 19 times, and in four instances the judoka had to be transported to hospital [18,20–22].

There were no statistically significant differences in the occurrence of injury in the different weight categories, except a high injury rate in the women's under 52 kg weight class. Rapid weight loss can impair the psychological and physiological performance of judokas [23], but our data collection system did not allow us to collate data in this respect. Lightweight judokas are more prone to elbow injuries, and heavyweight judokas are more prone to knee injuries.

A new approach toward motor abilities development in judo, including agility, coordination, foot work, strength, and explosive power of both the lower and upper limbs may reduce the occurrence of injury. Improved motor skills may allow to better control the exposure to full-body contact, decreasing the risk of injuries and increasing performance.

4.1. Limitations

We collected data on a large cohort of elite judokas over a relatively long period of time. However, we acknowledge that we do not have data on the outcome of these injuries, on their treatment beyond what was collected at the time of injury, and on the outcome. For example, we do not know whether some of these injuries required surgery, whether the injured athletes had to stop training and competing for any length of time beyond what happened at a given tournament, and when a judoka returned to training and competition. All these issues, despite the logistic efforts necessary to collect such data, should be the subject of future endeavours.

4.2. Application

The quantitative and qualitative monitoring of injuries sustained by contestants in high-ranking judo competitions is conducted by the EJU, aiming to use the data to develop and constantly review the rules of judo competitions. Thanks to the information obtained from this type of reports, the EJU has already modified the relevant regulations on several occasions. For example, some throws or defense against throws which exposed players to an increased risk of injury have now been ruled illegal.

5. Conclusions

The overall incidence of injuries during Europe's high-level judo tournaments in the period 2005–2020 was 2.5%, with an incidence of serious injuries of 0.5%. Judo is therefore one of the Olympic sports with the lowest injury rate in competitions. The knee, shoulder, and elbow are the anatomical locations most prone to injury, with 20% of all injuries occurring in the upper limbs (including the shoulder) and 30% in the lower limbs. Sprains are the most frequent type of injury. There is no statistically significant difference between men and women in the overall injury rate, although women have significantly more elbow injuries. The women −52 kg weight category shows a remarkably higher injury incidence—this should be further investigated. It is remarkable that lightweights suffer more elbow injuries. Serious injuries are uncommon, and potentially very dangerous injuries, such as commotio cerebri and neck injuries, have a very low incidence rate. No judoka had to be transported to hospital after unconsciousness form strangulation/choking techniques.

What Are the New Findings?

- This study provides comprehensive data of injury rates and trends among male and female European elite judokas during international competitions.
- The women's under 52 kg weight class has a remarkably high injury incidence.
- Female judokas experience significantly more elbow injuries than men.
- Judo has an overall injury incidence of only 2.5% during top-level tournaments in Europe.
- Potentially very serious injuries, like commotio cerebri or neck trauma, are uncommon.
- Unconsciousness after choking techniques has, in this study, never led to hospitalisation.

Author Contributions: Conceptualization, W.B. and P.S.; methodology, W.B., P.S. and Ł.R.; software, G.B.; validation, N.M. (Nicola Maffulli), Ł.R. and N.M. (Nikos Malliaropoulos); formal analysis, W.B. and P.S.; investigation, W.J.; resources, Ł.R.; data curation, W.B. and K.M.; writing—original draft preparation, W.B., G.B. and Ł.R.; writing—review and editing, Ł.R.; visualization, P.S.; supervision, T.A.; project administration, P.S.; funding acquisition, W.B. and K.M. All authors have read and agreed to the published version of the manuscript.

Funding: This research received no external funding.

Institutional Review Board Statement: The study was conducted according to the guidelines of the Declaration of Helsinki and approved by the Ethics Committee of Regional Medical Board in Krakow (approval No. 287/KBL/OIL/2020).

Informed Consent Statement: Informed consent was obtained from all subjects involved in the study.

Data Availability Statement: The data presented in this study are available on request from the corresponding author.

Acknowledgments: A special thanks to all the members of the EJU Medical Commission, past and present, for all their efforts in collection all the data and Injury Registration Forms.

Conflicts of Interest: The authors declare no conflict of interest.

References

1. Kano, J. *Kodokan Judo*; Kodansha America: New York, NY, USA, 1986; pp. 42–44.
2. Witkowski, K.; Maslinski, J.; Szalek, M.; Cieslinski, W.; Migasiewicz, J. Risk related to passion–Comparative analysis of traumas on the example of judo and wrestling. *Arch. Budo Arch. Budo* **2015**, *11*, 411–415.
3. Frassinelli, S.; Zich, R. Identification of the Relationship between the Aspect Psychomotor and Effectiveness of Performance in Judo Athletes with a Fuzzy System. In Proceedings of XXXI URSI General Assembly Italy, 2014. Available online: http://old.ursi.org/proceedings/procGA14/papers/ursi_paper2598.pdf (accessed on 15 November 2020).
4. Amtmann, J.; Cotton, A. Strength and Conditioning for Judo. *Strength Cond. J.* **2005**, *27*, 26–31. [CrossRef]
5. Drapsin, M.; Drid, P.; Grujic, N.; Trivic, T. Fitness level of male competitive judo players. *J. Combat Sports Martial Arts* **2010**, *1*, 21–29.
6. Pocecco, E.; Gatterer, H.; Ruedl, G.; Burtscher, M. Specific exercise testing in judo athletes. *Arch. Budo* **2012**, *8*, 133–139. [CrossRef]
7. Frassinelli, S.; Niccolai, A.; Zich, R. An Approach to Physical Performance Analysis for Judo. *Int. J. Med. Health Biomed. Bioeng. Pharm. Eng.* **2017**, *11*, 413–419.
8. Mackala, K.; Stodolka, J.; Witkowski, K.; Vodicar, J.; Simenko, J. Acute effects of speed-jumping intervention training on selected motor ability determinants: Judo vs. soccer. *Arch. Budo* **2019**, *15*, 311–320.
9. Chen, S.-K.; Cheng, Y.-M.; Huang, P.-J.; Chou, P.-H.; Lin, Y.-C.; Hong, Y.-J. Investigation of Management Models in Elite Athlete Injuries. *Kaohsiung J. Med. Sci.* **2005**, *21*, 220–227. [CrossRef]
10. Green, C.M.; Petrou, M.J.; Fogarty-Hover, M.L.; Rolf, C.G. Injuries among judokas during competition. *Scand. J. Med. Sci. Sports* **2007**, *17*, 205–210. [CrossRef]
11. Koshida, S.; Deguchi, T.; Miyashita, K.; Iwai, K.; Urabe, Y. The common mechanisms of anterior cruciate ligament injuries in judo: A retrospective analysis. *Br. J. Sports Med.* **2008**, *44*, 856–861. [CrossRef]
12. Pocecco, E.; Ruedl, G.; Stankovic, N.; Sterkowicz, S.; Del Vecchio, F.B.; Gutiérrez-García, C.; Rousseau, R.; Wolf, M.; Kopp, M.; Miarka, B.; et al. Injuries in judo: A systematic literature review including suggestions for prevention. *Br. J. Sports Med.* **2013**, *47*, 1139–1143. [CrossRef]
13. Kim, K.-S.; Park, K.J.; Lee, J.; Kang, B.Y. Injuries in national Olympic level judo athletes: An epidemiological study. *Br. J. Sports Med.* **2015**, *49*, 1144–1150. [CrossRef]
14. Carvalho, M. Injury Profile and Risk Factors in a Young High Competitive Population of Judo Athletes. *Orthop. Sports Med.* **2018**, *1*. [CrossRef]
15. Jäggi, U.; Joray, C.P.; Brülhart, Y.; Luijckx, E.; Rogan, S. Injuries in the Martial Arts Judo, Taekwondo and Wrestling–A Systematic Review. *Sportverletz. Sportschaden.* **2015**, *29*, 219–225. [CrossRef] [PubMed]
16. Pierantozzi, E.; Muroni, R. Judo high level competitions injuries. *Medit. J. Musc. Surv.* **2009**, *7*, 26–29.
17. Engebretsen, L.; Soligard, T.; Steffen, K.; Alonso, J.M.; Aubry, M.; Budgett, R.; Dvorak, J.; Jegathesan, M.; Meeuwisse, W.H.; Mountjoy, M.; et al. Sports injuries and illnesses during the London Summer Olympic Games 2012. *Br. J. Sports Med.* **2013**, *47*, 407–414. [CrossRef]
18. Frey, A.; Lambert, C.; Vesselle, B.; Rousseau, R.; Dor, F.; Marquet, L.A.; Toussaint, J.F.; Crema, M.D. Epidemiology of Judo-Related Injuries in 21 Seasons of Competitions in France: A Prospective Study of Relevant Traumatic Injuries. *Orthop. J. Sports Med.* **2019**, *7*. [CrossRef] [PubMed]
19. Maciejewski, R.; Callanta, H. Injuries and training variables in Filipino judo athletes. *Biomed. Hum. Kinet.* **2016**, *8*, 165–172. [CrossRef]
20. Akoto, R.; Lambert, C.; Balke, M.; Bouillon, B.; Frosch, K.-H.; Höher, J. Epidemiology of injuries in judo: A cross-sectional survey of severe injuries based on time loss and reduction in sporting level. *Br. J. Sports Med.* **2017**, *52*, 1109–1115. [CrossRef]
21. Murayama, H.; Hitosugi, M.; Motozawa, Y.; Ogino, M.; Koyama, K. Rotational acceleration during head impact resulting from different judo throwing techniques. *Neurol. Med.-Chir.* **2014**, *54*, 374–378. [CrossRef] [PubMed]
22. Nambu, S.; Noji, M. Case of Fatal Head Trauma Experienced During Japanese Judo. *Curr. Sports Med. Rep.* **2014**, *13*, 11–15. [CrossRef]
23. Filaire, E.; Maso, F.; Degoutte, F.; Jouanel, P.; Lac, G. Food Restriction, Performance, Psychological State and Lipid Values in Judo Athletes. *Int. J. Sports Med.* **2001**, *22*, 454–459. [CrossRef]

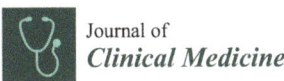

Article

Accuracy and Repeatability of Spatiotemporal Gait Parameters Measured with an Inertial Measurement Unit

Jorge Posada-Ordax [1], Julia Cosin-Matamoros [2,*], Marta Elena Losa-Iglesias [1], Ricardo Becerro-de-Bengoa-Vallejo [2], Laura Esteban-Gonzalo [2], Carlos Martin-Villa [2], César Calvo-Lobo [2] and David Rodriguez-Sanz [2]

[1] Facultad de Ciencias de la Salud, Universidad Rey Juan Carlos, 28933 Madrid, Spain; jorgesanidad@gmail.com (J.P.-O.); marta.losa@urjc.es (M.E.L.-I.)
[2] Facultad de Enfermería, Fisioterapia y Podología, Universidad Complutense de Madrid, 28040 Madrid, Spain; ribebeva@ucm.es (R.B.-d.-B.-V.); lesteb05@ucm.es (L.E.-G.); podologiamartinvilla@gmail.com (C.M.-V.); cescalvo@ucm.es (C.C.-L.); davidrodriguezsanz@ucm.es (D.R.-S.)
* Correspondence: juliacosin@hotmail.com

Abstract: In recent years, interest in finding alternatives for the evaluation of mobility has increased. Inertial measurement units (IMUs) stand out for their portability, size, and low price. The objective of this study was to examine the accuracy and repeatability of a commercially available IMU under controlled conditions in healthy subjects. A total of 36 subjects, including 17 males and 19 females were analyzed with a Wiva Science IMU in a corridor test while walking for 10 m and in a threadmill at 1.6 km/h, 2.4 km/h, 3.2 km/h, 4 km/h, and 4.8 km/h for one minute. We found no difference when we compared the variables at 4 km/h and 4.8 km/h. However, we found greater differences and errors at 1.6 km/h, 2.4 km/h and 3.2 km/h, and the latter one (1.6 km/h) generated more error. The main conclusion is that the Wiva Science IMU is reliable at high speeds but loses reliability at low speeds.

Keywords: accuracy; repeatability; inertial

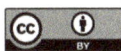

1. Introduction

In recent years, there has been increased interest in finding alternatives for the evaluation of mobility, among which inertial measurement units (IMUs) stand out because of their portability, size, and relatively low price [1]. Most publications that include a validation of an IMU compare its performance with optical motion-capture systems [2–6]. So far, the gold standards for gait analysis are optical motion capture systems, force platforms, and plantar pressure platforms, but these systems are expensive, space limited, and time consuming due to the placement of markers on the test subject. IMUs solve all of these problems.

Recent investigations on gait and posture assessment analysis show that an IMU could provide a new perspective for these functional tests as it allows for detailed space, time, and kinematic measurements of human motion on a continuous basis [7]. Mobile motion analysis systems are a promising element in aiding clinical decisions regarding the patient and could provide objective and quantifiable measures of gait, even for physicians with little experience in motion capture [8]. IMUs are increasingly being used for gait analysis because of their validity in healthy patients [9]. IMUs are also being used to study the spatial and temporal parameters of walking as predictors of falls [10] and as predictors of neurological diseases [11].

However, when used as a method of analysis, IMUs must comply with the principles of validity, objectivity, and repeatability [12]. Reliable repeatability is a prerequisite for the evolution of a patient over a period of time. Repeatability is necessary to differentiate between inaccurate measurements and actual changes in a patient's gait [12]. So far, research shows excellent repeatability for the analysis of gait [13,14], although there are some limitations, such as the calculation of parameters that depend on a spatial relationship of both feet, such as the width or length of the step [15]. Fariboz et al. provided information on the evaluation of the effects of medication in Parkinson's disease and demonstrated the applicability of inertial sensors to evaluate the disease [16]. The main purpose of this study was to evaluate the accuracy and repeatability of space-time parameters of walking with an IMU, called Wiva science, which is currently marketed, is simple to use and has a relatively low cost. Comparing it to other IMUs also marketed such as The Rehagate system, Physilog GaitUp and APDM Opal, our research team chose this device because it currently has few published studies and we believe that this study will be a novelty and will contribute to improving people's quality of life.

Therefore, we pose the following question: Are IMUs accurate for assessing gait in healthy patients without gait pathology?

2. Methods

In total, 36 healthy subjects participated in the present study. The exclusion criteria were recent and significant ligament damage, surgery, bone fractures, muscle damage in the lower extremities, abnormal gait patterns, contraindications to exercise, or other health conditions that could negatively affect the results of the study. A case-control study was done based on the guidelines of Strengthening the Reporting of Observational Research in Epidemiology (STROBE) [17]. The Declaration of Helsinki and human experimentation rules were followed [18]. This study was approved by the ethics committee of the Universidad Rey Juan Carlos de Madrid (internal registration number 2102201803818), and all participants signed an informed consent form before participating.

The accuracy and repeatability of a Wiva Science sensor (Wiva Science-LetSense Srl, Bologna, Italy; Figure 1) was tested by a subject walking on a treadmill and on normal ground. The treadmill was used to minimize the variability of walking among people between days [19]. For each condition, the IMU was placed in the sacral area of each subject, which was determined by palpation of the area by the investigator.

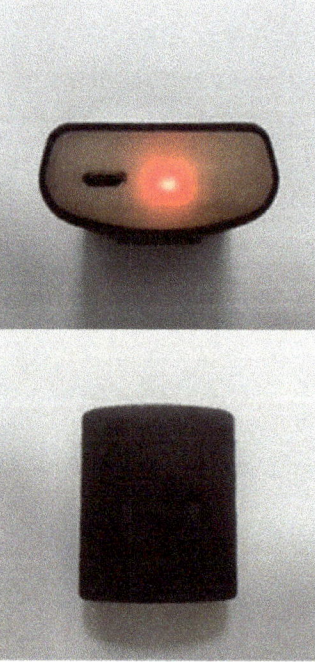

Figure 1. Wiva Science IMU. (Inertial Measurement Unit).

Intra-rater reliability (intraclass correlation coefficient (ICC) 0.91–0.98) and inter-rater reliability (ICC 0.80–0.87) have been established [20].

The subjects walked on the treadmill at 0.44 m/s (1.6 km/h), 0.67 m/s (2.4 km/h), 0.89 m/s (3.2 km/h), 1.11 m/s (4 km/h), and 1.33 m/s (4.8 km/s) for one minute at each speed. Subjects were given 15 s to adjust to each speed. In order to measure the repeatability of the IMU, the subjects returned for a second test. The protocol and the investigator were the same in both data-collection sessions. Subjects also performed several timed 10 m walking tests while wearing the IMU on normal ground. The subject walked for 10 m in a straight line, which included the subject's acceleration and deceleration distance. The subjects' normal speeds were estimated using the Wiva Science system and the 10 m distance. The subjects walked the 10 m three times at their normal speed, and the average was used in the statistical analysis.

The walking parameters of the IMU sensors were extracted using Biomech software (Version 1.6.1.14687, LetSense Group srl., Bologna, Italy, http://letsense.net (accessed on 11 December 2019)). The IMU measurements collected for the tests were validated with the speed data collected from the treadmill. The parameters studied were speed (m/min), step cadence (steps/min), stride length (m), stride length/height (%), average length (Emi) of step 1 (%), average length (Emi) of step 2 (%), average duration of step 1 (%), average duration of step 2 (%), position duration (% walking cycle), oscillation duration (% walking cycle), left foot bearing time (% gait cycle), right foot bearing time (% gait cycle), left foot swing time (% gait cycle), right foot swing time (% gait cycle), and surface speed (10 m). The measurements were taken as clinical standards. All participants did two tests separated by two days. All measurements were recorded by the same researcher.

2.1. Sample Size

A heterogeneous study sample was chosen since the measurement instrument is intended for different conditions. With an ICC of 0.90 and a confidence interval of ± 0.1, a sample of 35 participants was considered sufficient to perform the statistical calculations [21]. When testing reliability according to application in individual subjects and for use in clinical practice, a high ICC of 0.9 or 0.95 is recommended to increase the probability of measurement reliability [22,23].

We compared the sample size of this study with other research carried out to date. The RehaGait system was evaluated with 22 healthy subjects at different speeds on a treadmill [24], and Physilog GaitUp was evaluated with 14 individuals with stroke and 25 non-disabled elderly subjects using the "Up and Go" test [25]. The Valedo system was evaluated with 20 healthy subjects [26], the IMU Xsens MTx was evaluated with 10 subjects with Parkinson's disease in a walking test [27], and the InertiaCube3 was evaluated with 4 participants who had suffered strokes [28]. The IMU Shimmer3 sensor was evaluated with 4 subjects with Parkinson's disease and 11 healthy subjects [15], and the APDM Opal IMUs was evaluated on a treadmill with 19 healthy subjects and on regular ground with 14 healthy subjects [29].

2.2. Statistical Analysis

To interpret the ICC values, we used reference points proposed by Landis and Knoch [30] to indicate the following: 0.20 or less: mild; 0.21–0.40: fair; 0.41–0.60: moderate; 0.61–0.80: substantial; and 0.81 or greater: almost perfect. We followed Portney and Watkins' guidance that clinical measurements with reliability coefficients greater than 0.90 increase the probability of measurement reliability [23]. For each test within the session and between sessions, the ICC [31,32] was used to evaluate the reliability of each gait parameter.

All data analyses were performed in SPSS for Windows version 22 (SPSS Inc., Chicago, IL, USA). A Kolmogorov-Smirnov test was carried out to assess the normal distribution of the data. A descriptive statistical analysis was performed using the mean ± standard deviation (SD) and the 95% confidence interval. In addition, paired t-tests were performed to evaluate systematic differences in gait parameters between sessions. For the intersession evaluation, the mean value of the 14 measurements was analyzed.

The coefficients of variation (CVs) were calculated for absolute parameter comparison. The CV was calculated to measure the reliability of each session as the mean normalized to the SD. This value represents the variation between the tests normalized to the mean for each variable. A high CV value shows a greater heterogeneity of variable values. The statistical analysis was performed using the data from both feet.

Standard errors of the mean (SEMs) were calculated to measure the range of error for each gear parameter. The SEM was calculated between sessions from the ICC and SD as SEM = $s_x \cdot \sqrt{1 - r_{xx}}$, where s_x is the SD of the test data set, and r_{xx} is the confidence coefficient for these data, which is ICC in this case. Finally, the normality values (NVs) of the sample were defined for all the variables obtained with the Wiva Science system (NV = mean ± 1.96 * SD). From the result of each variable, NV was used to calculate the 95% confidence interval. A p-value < 0.05 with a 95% confidence interval was considered statistically significant for all tests.

Moreover, Bland and Altman plots were calculated to check agreement and heteroscedasticity [33].

3. Results

There were 36 subjects, including 17 males and 19 females with a mean age of 35.19 ± 11.79 years (19–64 years), mean weight of 74.83 ± 16.91 kg (47–107 kg), mean height of 171.69 ± 7.49 cm (157–192 cm), and mean body mass index (BMI) of 25.23 ± 4.34 (18.4–33.4). We found statistically significant differences in weight, height, and BMI (kg/cm^2) [34], as shown in Table 1.

Table 1. Demographic data of the sample.

Variable	Men (n = 17) Mean ± SD (Range)	Women (n = 19) Mean ± SD (Range)	Total (n = 36) Mean ± SD (Range)	p Value
AGE (years)	35.64 ± 13.19 (19–64)	34.78 ± 10.73 (22–62)	35.19 ± 11.79 (19–64)	0.8311
WEIGHT (kg)	86.29 ± 13.40 (60–107)	64.57 ± 12.70 (47–90)	74.83 ± 16.91 (47–107)	0.0000 *
SIZE (cm)	177.05 ± 5.58 (169–192)	166.89 ± 5.47 (157–177)	171.69 ± 7.49 (157–192)	0.0000 *
BMI	27.44 ± 3.55 (20.76–33.4)	23.25 ± 4.08 (18.4–31.14)	25.23 ± 4.34 (18.4–33.4)	0.0025 *

Abbreviations: cm: centimeters; kg: kilograms; BMI: body mass index; SD: standard deviation; 95% CI: 95% confidence interval; *: significant differences, p < 0.05.

High reliability was observed in all measurements in the first session (Table 2) with ICC > 0.81 except for the following variables: the average duration of step 1 at normal speed (ICC 0.41), 1.6, 2.4, 3.2 and 4 km/h (ICC: 0.28, ICC 0.73, ICC 0.39, and ICC 0.73, respectively); the average duration of step 2 at all speeds, which had low reliability (normal, 1.6, 2.4, 3.2 and 4 km/h had ICCs of 0.24, 0.22, 0.73, 0.37, and 0.75, respectively); the variable position duration at 1.6 km/h (ICC 0.72); the variable oscillation duration at 1.6 km/h (ICC 0.77); the variable left foot bearing time at 1.6 km/h and 3.2 km/h (ICC 0.38 and ICC 0.58 respectively); the variable right foot bearing time at normal speed (ICC 0.69) and 1.6 km/h (ICC 0.54); the variable left foot swing time at 1.6 km/h (ICC 0.49); and the variable right foot swing time at 1.6 km/h (ICC 0.48). The SEM was low except at normal speed, 1.6 and 2.4 km/h.

High reliability was observed in all measurements in the second session (Table 3) with ICC > 0.81 except for the following variables: the variable average duration of step 1 at all speeds (1.6 km/h, 2.4 km/h, 3.2 km/h, 4 km/h, 4.8 km/h: ICC 0.51, ICC 0.35, ICC 0.66, ICC 0.67, and ICC 0.31, respectively); the variable average duration of step 2 at all speeds (ICC 0.59, ICC 0.47, ICC 0.50, ICC 0.60, ICC 0.72, and ICC 0.34 respectively); the variable average duration of step 2 4.8 km/h (ICC 0.34); the variable oscillation duration at 1.6 km/h (ICC 0.78); the variable left foot bearing time at 1.6 km/h (ICC 0;63); the variable right foot bearing time at 1.6 km/h and 2.4 km/h (ICC 0.53 and ICC 0.80, respectively); the variable left foot swing time at 1.6 km/h (ICC 0.63); and the variable right foot swing time at 1.6 km/h (ICC 0.56). SEM was low except at normal speed, 1.6 km/h, and 2.4 km/h.

Table 2. Reliability analysis within the variables studied for the first session.

Variables	Mean (DS)	IC95%	CV (%)	ICC (2.1) (IC95%)	SEM	MDC	95% Normality Values
Normal speed	73.68 (12.63)	(69.56–77.81)	17.14	0.93	3.18	8.81	(48.93–98.44)
Speed 1.6 km/h	34.30 (7.16)	(31.96–36.64)	20.87	0.93	1.77	4.92	(20.27–48.33)
Speed 2.4 km/h	43.09 (6.63)	(40.93–45.26)	15.38	0.98	0.99	2.29	(30.10–56.09)
Speed 3.2 km/h	54.51 (8.20)	(51.83–57.19)	15.05	0.98	0.99	2.36	(38.42–70.59)
Speed 4 km/h	67.39 (9.29)	(64.36–70.43)	13.78	0.98	0.99	3.18	(49.18–85.61)
Speed 4.8 km/h	79.27 (10.47)	(75.85–82.69)	13.21	0.98	0.99	3.17	(58.74–99.79)
Step cadence normal speed	55.74 (4.29)	(54.34–57.14)	7.70	0.87	1.53	4.26	(47.32–64.16)
Step cadence 1.6 km/h	37.04 (7.94)	(34.44–39.64)	21.45	0.93	1.98	5.50	(21.46–52.62)
Step cadence 2.4 km/h	42.37 (4.83)	(40.80–43.95)	11.40	0.98	0.59	1.64	(32.90–51.84)
Step cadence 3.2 km/h	49.26 (3.99)	(47.96–50.57)	8.11	0.99	0.30	0.83	(41.43–57.10)
Step cadence 4 km/h	55.41 (3.41)	(54.30–56.53)	6.17	0.98	0.48	1.34	(48.71–62.12)
Step cadence 4.8 km/h	59.76 (3.14)	(58.7 –60.79)	5.26	0.98	0.37	1.02	(53.59–65.94)
Stride length normal speed	1.32 (0.25)	(1.25 –1.39)	15.50	0.96	0.04	0.11	(0.92–1.72)
Stride length 1.6 km/h	0.94 (0.17)	(0.89–1.00)	18.04	0.92	0.04	0.12	(0.61–1.28)
Stride length 2.4 km/h	1.02 (0.15)	(0.97–1.07)	14.95	0.98	0.01	0.05	(0.72–1.32)
Stride length 3.2 km/h	1.10 (0.15)	(1.05–1.15)	13.96	0.98	0.01	0.04	(0.80–1.41)
Stride length 4 km/h	1.21 (0.16)	(1.16–1.27)	13.48	0.98	0.01	0.05	(0.89–1.54)
Stride length 4.8 km/h	1.32 (0.18)	(1.26–1.38)	13.62	0.99	0.01	0.04	(0.97–1.68)
Stride length/height normal speed	79.16 (13.31)	(74.81–83.51)	16.81	0.96	2.33	6.46	(53.07–105.26)
Stride length/height 1.6 km/h	56.82 (13.30)	(52.48–61.17)	23.41	0.98	1.58	4.38	(30.75–82.90)
Stride length/height 2.4 km/h	61.50 (12.13)	(57.53–65.46)	19.72	0.99	1.04	2.90	(37.72–85.27)
Stride length/height 3.2 km/h	66.52 (11.91)	(62.63–70.42)	17.91	0.99	1.04	2.90	(43.16–89.89)
Stride length/height 4 km/h	73.07 (12.37)	(69.02–77.11)	16.93	0.99	1.09	3.02	(48.81–97.32)
Stride length/height 4.8 km/h	79.72 (13.76)	(75.22–84.22)	17.27	0.99	1.02	2.82	(52.73–106.71)
Average length of step 1—normal speed	0.66 (0.10)	(0.62–0.69)	15.98	0.95	0'02	0.06	(0.45–0.86)
Average length of step 1—1.6 km/h	0.47 (0.08)	(0.44–0.49)	17.64	0.95	0.01	0.04	(0.30–0.63)
Average length of step 1—2.4 km/h	0.51 (0.08)	(0.48–0.54)	16.07	0.98	0.01	0.03	(0.35–0.67)
Average length of step 1—3.2 km/h	0.55 (0.08)	(0.52–0.57)	15.16	0.98	0.01	0.03	(0.38–0.71)
Average length of step 1—4 km/h	0.60 (0.08)	(0.58–0.63)	13.95	0.97	0.01	0.03	(0.44–0.77)
Average length of step 1—4.8 km/h	0.66 (0.09)	(0.63–0.69)	14.20	0.98	0.01	0.03	(0.48–0.85)

Table 2. Cont.

Variables	Mean (DS)	IC95%	CV (%)	ICC (2.1) (IC95%)	SEM	MDC	95% Normality Values
Average length of step 2—normal speed	0.66 (0.10)	(0.62–0.69)	15.89	0.94	0.02	0.06	(0.45–0.86)
Average length of step 2—1.6 km/h	0.47 (0.08)	(0.44–0.49)	17.12	0.95	0.01	0.04	(0.31–0.62)
Average length of step 2—2.4 km/h	0.50 (0.07)	(0.48–0.53)	15.16	0.97	0.01	0.03	(0.35–0.65)
Average length of step 2—3.2 km/h	0.55 (0.07)	(0.53–0.58)	13.80	0.98	0.01	0.03	(0.40–0.70)
Average length of step 2—4 km/h	0.61 (0.08)	(0.58–0.63)	13.78	0.97	0.01	0.03	(0.44–0.77)
Average length of step 2—4.8 km/h	0.66 (0.09)	(0.63–0.69)	13.57	0.98	0.01	0.02	(0.48–0.83)
Average duration of step 1—normal speed	49.89 (2.18)	(49.17–50.60)	4.37	0.41	1.66	4.62	(45.61–54.17)
Average duration of step 1—1.6 km/h	49.42 (2.36)	(48.65–50.20)	4.77	0.28	2.00	5.55	(44.79–54.05)
Average duration of step 1—2.4 km/h	50.09 (1.58)	(49.57–50.69)	3.16	0.73	0.82	2.28	(46.98–53.20)
Average duration of step 1—3.2 km/h	49.82 (1.14)	(49.45–50.19)	2.29	0.39	0.89	2.46	(47.58–52.06)
Average duration of step 1—4 km/h	49.79 (1.17)	(49.40–50.17)	2.35	0.73	0.60	1.68	(47.49–52.08)
Average duration of step 1—4.8 km/h	49.97 (0.91)	(49.67–50.27)	1.83	0.88	0.31	0.87	(48.17–51.76)
Average duration of step 2—normal speed	50.29 (2.53)	(49.46–51.12)	5.04	0.24	2.20	6.12	(45.31–55.27)
Average duration of step 2—1.6 km/h	50.63 (2.28)	(49.88–51.38)	4.51	0.22	2.01	5.58	(46.15–55.11)
Average duration of step 2—2.4 km/h	49.92 (1.60)	(49.39–50.44)	3.21	0.73	0.82	2.27	(46.77–53.06)
Average duration of step 2—3.2 km/h	50.18 (1.14)	(49.80–50.55)	2.28	0.37	0.90	2.50	(47.93–52.42)
Average duration of step 2—4 km/h	50.21 (1.17)	(49.83–50.62)	2.33	0.75	0.58	1.62	(47.92–52.51)
Average duration of step 2—4.8 km/h	50.03 (0.91)	(49.73–50.33)	1.83	0.88	0.31	0.88	(48.23–51.83)
Position duration normal speed	63.67 (2.63)	(62.81–64.53)	4.14	0.91	0.75	2.10	(58.50–68.84)
Position duration 1.6 km/h	62.39 (2.56)	(61.55–63.22)	4.11	0.72	1.34	3.72	(57.35–67.42)
Position duration 2.4 km/h	62.92 (2.31)	(62.16–63.67)	3.67	0.88	0.77	2.13	(58.39–67.45)
Position duration 3.2 km/h	61.80 (1.99)	(61.14–62.45)	3.22	0.94	0.46	1.29	(57.88–65.71)
Position duration 4 km/h	60.98 (2.01)	(60.32–61.64)	3.30	0.98	0.28	0.78	(57.03–64.94)
Position duration 4.8 km/h	60.09 (1.83)	(59.48–60.69)	3.05	0.98	0.23	0.64	(56.48–63.69)

Table 2. *Cont.*

Variables	Mean (DS)	IC95%	CV (%)	ICC (2.1) (IC95%)	SEM	MDC	95% Normality Values
Oscillation duration normal speed	34.34 (2.72)	(33.45–35.23)	7.93	0.93	0.67	1.85	(29.00–39.68)
Oscillation duration 1.6 km/h	36.46 (2.41)	(35.67–37.25)	6.61	0.77	1.14	3.16	(31.74–41.19)
Oscillation duration 2.4 km/h	35.65 (2.33)	(34.89–36.41)	6.53	0.88	0.78	2.17	(31.08–40.22)
Oscillation duration 3.2 km/h	36.55 (2.03)	(35.89–37.21)	5.55	0.94	0.46	1.27	(32.57–40.53)
Oscillation duration 4 km/h	37.14 (2.02)	(36.48–37.80)	5.43	0.98	0.27	0.76	(33.18–41.10)
Oscillation duration 4.8 km/h	37.91 (1.80)	(37.32–38.50)	4.76	0.98	0.23	0.64	(34.37–41.45)
Left foot bearing time normal speed	63.62 (3.48)	(62.48–64.76)	5.47	0.91	0.99	2.74	(56.79–70.45)
Left foot bearing time 1.6 km/h	61.88 (3.68)	(60.67–63.08)	5.95	0.38	2.89	8.01	(54.65–69.10)
Left foot bearing time 2.4 km/h	62.93 (2.43)	(62.13–63.72)	3.82	0.89	0.80	2.23	(58.16–67.69)
Left foot bearing time 3.2 km/h	62.12 (3.62)	(60.94–63.30)	5.83	0.58	2.32	6.45	(55.02–69.22)
Left foot bearing time 4 km/h	60.85 (2.42)	(60.06–61.64)	3.97	0.94	0.57	1.59	(56.11–65.60)
Left foot bearing time 4.8 km/h	59.84 (2.23)	(59.11–60.57)	3.73	0.94	0.50	1.40	(55.46–64.22)
Right foot bearing time normal speed	63.72 (2.75)	(62.82–64.62)	4.32	0.69	1.53	4.24	(58.32–69.11)
Right foot bearing time 1.6 km/h	62.90 (3.43)	(61.78–64.03)	5.45	0.54	2.31	6.41	(56.18–69.63)
Right foot bearing time 2.4 km/h	62.91 (2.89)	(61.96–63.85)	4.59	0.83	1.17	3.24	(57.24–68.57)
Right foot bearing time 3.2 km/h	61.75 (2.10)	(61.06–62.44)	3.41	0.86	0.77	2.14	(57.62–65.88)
Right foot bearing time 4 km/h	61.12 (2.27)	(60.38–61.87)	3.71	0.92	0.62	1.74	(56.67–65.58)
Right foot bearing time 4.8 km/h	60.34 (2.02)	(59.67–61.00)	3.35	0.91	0.59	1.65	(56.36–64.31)
Left foot swing time normal speed	34.37 (3.54)	(33.21–35.53)	10.31	0.94	0.80	2.24	(27.42–41.32)
Left foot swing time 1.6 km/h	37.02 (3.33)	(35.93–38.11)	9.00	0.49	2.37	6.57	(30.48–43.56)
Left foot swing time 2.4 km/h	35.65 (2.43)	(34.85–36.45)	6.83	0.89	0.80	2.23	(30.87–40.43)
Left foot swing time 3.2 km/h	36.51 (2.40)	(35.72–37.29)	6.58	0.93	0.59	1.66	(31.80–41.22)
Left foot swing time 4 km/h	37.29 (2.42)	(36.49–38.08)	6.49	0.94	0.57	1.59	(32.54–42.03)
Left foot swing time 4.8 km/h	38.16 (2.20)	(37.44–38.87)	5.76	0.94	0.50	1.40	(33.84–42.47)

Table 2. Cont.

Variables	Mean (DS)	IC95%	CV (%)	ICC (2.1) (IC95%)	SEM	MDC	95% Normality Values
Right foot swing time normal speed	34.18 (2.71)	(33.30–35.07)	7.94	0.90	0.83	2.32	(28.86–39.51)
Right foot swing time 1.6 km/h	35.81 (3.60)	(34.64–36.99)	10.06	0.48	2.58	7.15	(28.75–42.88)
Right foot swing time 2.4 km/h	35.65 (2.92)	(34.69–36.60)	8.19	0.83	1.19	3.31	(29.92–41.37)
Right foot swing time 3.2 km/h	36.59 (2.14)	(35.89–37.29)	5.86	0.87	0.76	2.11	(32.39–40.80)
Right foot swing time 4 km/h	37.01 (2.27)	(36.27–37.75)	6.14	0.92	0.62	1.72	(32.56–41.47)
Right foot swing time 4.8 km/h	37.62 (2.01)	(37.01–38.33)	5.35	0.91	0.59	1.65	(33.71–41.62)

Abbreviations: km/h (kilometers per hour); IC (confidence interval); CV (coefficient of variation); ICC (coefficient of intraclass correlation); SEM (standard error of mean); MDC (minimum detectable change).

Table 3. Reliability analysis within the variables studied for the second session.

Variables	MEAN (DS)	IC95%	CV (%)	ICC (2,1) (IC95%)	SEM	MDC	95% NORMALITY VALUES
NORMAL SPEED	76.21 (11.86)	(72.34–80.08)	15.56	0.96	2.32	6.44	(52.96–99.45)
SPEED 1.6 km/h	34.77 (6.50)	(32.64–36.89)	18.70	0.93	1.71	4.75	(22.01–47.52)
SPEED 2.4 km/h	43.11 (6.52)	(40.98–45.24)	15.12	0.93	1.66	4.60	(30.33–55.89)
SPEED 3.2 km/h	55.03 (7.07)	(52.72–57.34)	12.85	0.98	0.74	2.06	(41.16–68.90)
SPEED 4 km/h	67.61 (9.14)	(64.62–70.59)	13.52	0.99	0.90	2.50	(49.68–85.53)
SPEED 4.8 km/h	79.79 (10.79)	(76.26–83.31)	13.52	0.98	1.15	3.18	(58.63–100.95)
STEP CADENCE NORMAL SPEED	56.90 (3.80)	(55.66–58.14)	6.68	0.96	0.67	1.86	(49.45–64.35)
STEP CADENCE 1.6 km/h	34.73 (6.15)	(32.72–36.74)	17.72	0.90	1.89	5.25	(22.66–46.80)
STEP CADENCE 2.4 km/h	40.74 (5.31)	(39.00–42.48)	13.04	0.88	1.82	5.06	(30.32–51.16)
STEP CADENCE 3.2 km/h	48.62 (3.63)	(47.43–49.81)	7.47	0.98	0.42	1.16	(41.50–55.74)
STEP CADENCE 4 km/h	55.13 (3.29)	(54.05–56.21)	5.97	0.99	0.25	0.70	(48.67–61.59)
STEP CADENCE 4.8 km/h	59.57 (3.07)	(58.57–60.58)	5.16	0.96	0.54	1.50	(53.55–65.60)
STRIDE LENGTH NORMAL SPEED	1.34 (0.19)	(1.27–1.40)	14.64	0.97	0.03	0.09	(0.95–1.72)
STRIDE LENGTH 1.6 km/h	1.01 (0.16)	(0.95–1.06)	16.42	0.98	0.02	0.05	(0.68–1.33)
STRIDE LENGTH 2.4 km/h	1.058 (0.13)	(1.01–1.10)	12.97	0.98	0.01	0.04	(0.78–1.32)
STRIDE LENGTH 3.2 km/h	1.13 (0.14)	(1.08–1.18)	12.55	0.99	0.01	0.03	(0.85–1.41)
STRIDE LENGTH 4 km/h	1.23 (0.17)	(1.17–0.28)	13.80	0.99	0.01	0.04	(0.89–1.56)
STRIDE LENGTH 4.8 km/h	1.34 (0.18)	(1.28–1.40)	14.02	0.99	0.01	0.04	(0.97–1.71)
STRIDE LENGTH/HEIGHT NORMAL SPEED	80.32 (12.34)	(76.29–84.35)	15.36	0.97	1.86	5.16	(56.13–104.51)
STRIDE LENGTH/HEIGHT 1.6 km/h	60.79 (12.73)	(56.64–64.95)	20.93	0.99	1.16	3.24	(35.84–85.75)
STRIDE LENGTH/HEIGHT 2.4 km/h	63.51 (11.29)	(59.82–67.20)	17.78	0.99	0.87	2.43	(41.37–85.65)

Table 3. Cont.

Variables	MEAN (DS)	IC95%	CV (%)	ICC (2,1) (IC95%)	SEM	MDC	95% NORMALITY VALUES
STRIDE LENGTH/HEIGHT 3.2 km/h	68.02 (10.93)	(64.45–71.59)	16.07	0.99	0.79	2.19	(46.59–89.45)
STRIDE LENGTH/HEIGHT 4 km/h	73.67 (12.37)	(69.63–77.71)	16.79	0.99	0.87	2.43	(49.43–97.92)
STRIDE LENGTH/HEIGHT 4.8 km/h	80.50 (13.92)	(75.95–85.04)	17.29	0.99	0.85	2.37	(53.20–107.79)
AVERAGE LENGTH OF STEP 1 NORMAL SPEED	0.67 (0.10)	(0.63–0.70)	15.00	0.96	0.02	0.05	(0.47–0.86)
AVERAGE LENGTH OF STEP 1 1.6 km/h	0.51 (0.08)	(0.48–0.53)	17.09	0.97	0.01	0.04	(0.33–0.68)
AVERAGE LENGTH OF STEP 1 2.4 km/h	0.53 (0.07)	(0.50–0.55)	13.73	0.96	0.01	0.04	(0.38–0.67)
AVERAGE LENGTH OF STEP 1 3.2 km/h	0.56 (0.07)	(0.53–0.58)	13.46	0.98	0.01	0.02	(0.41–0.71)
AVERAGE LENGTH OF STEP 1 4 km/h	0.61 (0.08)	(0.58–0.64)	14.08	0.98	0.01	0.02	(0.44–0.78)
AVERAGE LENGTH OF STEP 1 4.8 km/h	0.67 (0.09)	(0.64–0.70)	14.35	0.99	0.01	0.02	(0.48–0.86)
AVERAGE LENGTH OF STEP 2 NORMAL SPEED	0.67 (0.10)	(0.63–0.70)	15.12	0.96	0.02	0.05	(0.47–0.87)
AVERAGE LENGTH OF STEP 2 1.6 km/h	0.50 (0.08)	(0.47–0.52)	17.07	0.97	0.01	0.03	(0.33–0.66)
AVERAGE LENGTH OF STEP 2 2.4 km/h	0.52 (0.07)	(0.50–0.54)	13.68	0.96	0.01	0.03	(0.38–0.66)
AVERAGE LENGTH OF STEP 2 3.2 km/h	0.57 (0.07)	(0.54–0.59)	12.51	0.97	0.01	0.02	(0.43–0.70)
AVERAGE LENGTH OF STEP 2 4 km/h	0.61 (0.08)	(0.58–0.64)	14.39	0.98	0.01	0.02	(0.44–0.78)
AVERAGE LENGTH OF STEP 2 4.8 km/h	0.66 (0.09)	(0.63–0.70)	14.32	0.98	0.01	0.02	(0.48–0.85)
AVERAGE DURATION OF STEP 1 NORMAL SPEED	49.93 (2.36)	(49.16–50.71)	4.74	0.51	1.65	4.57	(45.29–54.58)
AVERAGE DURATION OF STEP 1 1.6 km/h	50.05 (2.98)	(49.08–51.03)	5.96	0.35	2.39	6.64	(44.20–55.91)
AVERAGE DURATION OF STEP 1 2.4 km/h	49.75 (1.67)	(49.20–50.30)	3.37	0.66	0.97	2.69	(46.47–53.04)
AVERAGE DURATION OF STEP 1 3.2 km/h	49.98 (1.31)	(49.55–50.41)	2.63	0.60	0.82	2.29	(47.39–52.56)
AVERAGE DURATION OF STEP 1 4 km/h	49.84 (1.07)	(49.48–50.19)	2.15	0.67	0.61	1.69	(47.73–51.94)
AVERAGE DURATION OF STEP 1 4.8 km/h	50.05 (1.12)	(49.68–50.41)	2.23	0.31	0.92	2.56	(47.85–52.24)
AVERAGE DURATION OF STEP 2 NORMAL SPEED	50.31 (2.09)	(49.62–50.99)	4.16	0.59	1.33	3.69	(46.20–54.42)
AVERAGE DURATION OF STEP 2 1.6 km/h	49.78 (3.14)	(48.75–50.80)	6.31	0.47	2.28	6.33	(43.61–55.94)

Table 3. Cont.

Variables	MEAN (DS)	IC95%	CV (%)	ICC (2,1) (IC95%)	SEM	MDC	95% NORMALITY VALUES
AVERAGE DURATION OF STEP 2 2.4 km/h	50.08 (2.01)	(49.43–50.74)	4.02	0.50	1.41	3.92	(46.13–54.03)
AVERAGE DURATION OF STEP 2 3.2 km/h	50.01 (1.30)	(49.58–50.44)	2.61	0.60	0.82	2.28	(47.44–52.57)
AVERAGE DURATION OF STEP 2 4 km/h	50.15 (1.07)	(49.80–50.50)	2.14	0.72	0.56	1.57	(48.04–52.25)
AVERAGE DURATION OF STEP 2 4.8 km/h	49.95 (1.11)	(49.59–50.31)	2.22	0.34	0.90	2.49	(47.77–52.13)
POSITION DURATION NORMAL SPEED	63.63 (2.86)	(62.69–64.56)	4.50	0.93	0.72	2.02	(58.00–69.25)
POSITION DURATION 1.6 km/h	63.25 (3.04)	(62.26–64.25)	4.81	0.82	1.28	3.56	(57.28–69.23)
POSITION DURATION 2.4 km/h	63.09 (2.78)	(62.19–64.00)	4.41	0.90	0.85	2.35	(57.64–68.55)
POSITION DURATION 3.2 km/h	61.77 (2.02)	(61.05–62.48)	3.56	0.98	0.30	0.84	(57.45–66.08)
POSITION DURATION 4 km/h	61.03 (2.28)	(60.29–61.78)	3.73	0.98	0.26	0.72	(56.56–65.50)
POSITION DURATION 4.8 km/h	60.13 (1.88)	(59.51–60.74)	3.13	0.98	0.24	0.68	(56.44–63.82)
OSCILLATION DURATION NORMAL SPEED	34.28 (2.72)	(33.39–35.17)	7.96	0.95	0.56	1.55	(28.93–39.63)
OSCILLATION DURATION 1.6 km/h	35.57 (3.12)	(34.55–36.59)	8.77	0.78	1.44	4.00	(29.45–41.69)
OSCILLATION DURATION 2.4 km/h	35.48 (2.72)	(34.59–36.37)	7.67	0.92	0.75	2.08	(30.14–40.82)
OSCILLATION DURATION 3.2 km/h	36.61 (2.24)	(35.88–37.34)	6.11	0.98	0.30	0.85	(32.22–41.00)
OSCILLATION DURATION 4 km/h	37.08 (2.29)	(36.33–37.83)	6.19	0.97	0.35	0.99	(32.58–41.58)
OSCILLATION DURATION 4.8 km/h	37.84 (1.89)	(37.22–38.46)	5.00	0.97	0.31	0.85	(34.13–41.56)
LEFT FOOT BEARING TIME NORMAL SPEED	63.45 (3.58)	(62.28–64.63)	5.65	0.92	0.99	2.75	(56.42–70.49)
LEFT FOOT BEARING TIME 1.6 km/h	63.53 (4.41)	(62.09–64.97)	6.94	0.63	2.65	7.35	(54.88–72.18)
LEFT FOOT BEARING TIME 2.4 km/h	63.06 (2.79)	(62.14–63.97)	4.42	0.87	0.98	2.73	(57.59–68.52)
LEFT FOOT BEARING TIME 3.2 km/h	61.99 (2.43)	(61.20–62.79)	3.92	0.96	0.45	1.24	(57.22–66.76)
LEFT FOOT BEARING TIME 4 km/h	60.87 (2.60)	(60.02–61.72)	4.27	0.95	0.52	1.46	(55.77–65.96)
LEFT FOOT BEARING TIME 4.8 km/h	59.98 (2.40)	(59.20–60.77)	4.00	0.91	0.69	1.92	(55.27–64.69)
RIGHT FOOT BEARING TIME NORMAL SPEED	63.80 (2.64)	(62.93–64.66)	4.15	0.83	1.06	2.95	(58.60–68.99)

Table 3. *Cont.*

Variables	MEAN (DS)	IC95%	CV (%)	ICC (2,1) (IC95%)	SEM	MDC	95% NORMALITY VALUES
RIGHT FOOT BEARING TIME 1.6 km/h	62.99 (4.50)	(61.51–64.43)	7.15	0.53	3.07	8.52	(54.15–71.82)
RIGHT FOOT BEARING TIME 2.4 km/h	63.08 (3.56)	(61.92–64.25)	5.65	0.80	1.58	4.39	(56.09–70.08)
RIGHT FOOT BEARING TIME 3.2 km/h	61.58 (2.65)	(60.71–62.44)	4.30	0.94	0.62	1.73	(56.38–66.77)
RIGHT FOOT BEARING TIME 4 km/h	61.20 (2.48)	(60.39–62.01)	4.06	0.97	0.40	1.12	(56.32–66.07)
RIGHT FOOT BEARING TIME 4.8 km/h	60.27 (1.96)	(59.63–60.91)	3.25	0.91	0.59	1.63	(56.42–64.12)
LEFT FOOT SWING TIME NORMAL SPEED	34.54 (3.42)	(33.33–35.57)	9.94	0.95	0.72	2.01	(27.73–41.16)
LEFT FOOT SWING TIME 1.6 km/h	35.29 (4.24)	(33.90–36.62)	12.02	0.63	2.57	7.14	(26.97–43.61)
LEFT FOOT SWING TIME 2.4 km/h	35.46 (2.91)	(34.51–36.41)	8.21	0.83	1.19	3.30	(29.75–41.16)
LEFT FOOT SWING TIME 3.2 km/h	36.38 (2.44)	(35.58–37.18)	6.72	0.96	0.45	1.27	(31.58–41.17)
LEFT FOOT SWING TIME 4 km/h	37.28 (2.59)	(36.43–38.12)	6.95	0.95	0.53	1.47	(32.19–42.36)
LEFT FOOT SWING TIME 4.8 km/h	38.03 (2.37)	(37.25–38.80)	6.25	0.91	0.69	1.91	(33.37–42.68)
RIGHT FOOT SWING TIME NORMAL SPEED	34.13 (2.60)	(33.28–34.98)	7.64	0.84	1.01	2.80	(29.02–39.24)
RIGHT FOOT SWING TIME 1.6 km/h	35.83 (4.70)	(34.30–37.37)	13.13	0.56	3.11	8.62	(26.61–45.06)
RIGHT FOOT SWING TIME 2.4 km/h	35.57 (3.38)	(34.46–36.68)	9.52	0.84	1.31	3.64	(28.93–42.21)
RIGHT FOOT SWING TIME 3.2 km/h	36.84 (2.63)	(35.98–37.70)	7.15	0.95	0.56	1.55	(31.67–42.00)
RIGHT FOOT SWING TIME 4 km/h	36.95 (2.48)	(36.13–37.76)	6.73	0.97	0.42	1.16	(32.07–41.82)
RIGHT FOOT SWING TIME 4.8 km/h	37.72 (1.94)	(37.09–38.36)	5.16	0.90	0.59	1.63	(33.90–41.54)

Abbreviations: km/h (kilometers per hour); IC (confidence interval); CV (coefficient of Variation); ICC (intraclass correlation coefficient); SEM (standard error of mean); MDC (minimum detectable change).

Comparing the differences between first and second session (Table 4), we observed a significant difference between the first and second sessions at normal speed ($p = 0.05$).

Table 4. Systematic differences between the first and second session.

Variables	Mean (DS) First Session	IC95%	Mean (DS) Second Session	IC95%	LoA	p VALUE
Normal speed	73.68 (12.63)	(69.56–77.81)	76.21 (11.86)	(72.34–80.08)	−2.52 (−12.48–7.43)	0.005 *
Speed 1.6 km/h	34.30 (7.16)	(31.96–36.64)	34.77 (6.50)	(32.64–36.89)	−0.47 (−10.39–9.46)	0.585
Speed 2.4 km/h	43.09 (6.63)	(40.93–45.26)	43.11 (6.52)	(40.98–45.24)	−0.02 (−5.15–5.12)	0.969
Speed 3.2 km/h	54.51 (8.20)	(51.83–57.19)	55.03 (7.07)	(52.72–57.34)	−0.52 (−6.19–5.15)	0.287
Speed 4 km/h	67.39 (9.29)	(64.36–70.43)	67.61 (9.14)	(64.62–70.59)	−0.21 (−4.43–4.01)	0.556
Speed 4.8 km/h	79.27 (10.47)	(75.85–82.69)	79.79 (10.79)	(76.26–83.31)	−0.52 (−4.72–3.68)	0.154
Step cadence normal speed	55.74 (4.29)	(54.34–57.14)	56.90 (3.80)	(55.66–58.14)	−1.16 (−4.49–2.17)	0.000 *
Step cadence 1.6 km/h	37.04 (7.94)	(34.44–39.64)	34.73 (6.15)	(32.72–36.74)	2.31 (−7.53–12.16)	0.009
Step cadence 2.4 km/h	42.37 (4.83)	(40.80–43.95)	40.74 (5.31)	(39.00–42.48)	1.63 (−3.01–6.27)	0.000 *
Step cadence 3.2 km/h	49.26 (3.99)	(47.96–50.57)	48.62 (3.63)	(47.43–49.81)	0.64 (−2.14–3.43)	0.010 *
Step cadence 4 km/h	55.41 (3.41)	(54.30–56.53)	55.13 (3.29)	(54.05–56.21)	0.28 (−1.69–2.26)	0.101
Step cadence 4.8 km/h	59.76 (3.14)	(58.73–60.79)	59.57 (3.07)	(58.57–60.58)	0.19 (−2.23–2.61)	0.368
Stride length normal speed	1.32 (0.25)	(1.25–1.39)	1.34 (0.19)	(1.27–1.40)	−0.02 (−0.14–0.10)	0.069
Stride length 1.6 km/h	0.94 (0.17)	(0.89–1.00)	1.01 (0.16)	(0.95–1.06)	−0.06 (−0.24–0.11)	0.000 *
Stride length 2.4 km/h	1.02 (0.15)	(0.97–1.07)	1.058 (0.13)	(1.01–1.10)	−0.03 (−0.16–0.09)	0.005 *
Stride length 3.2 km/h	1.10 (0.15)	(1.05–1.15)	1.13 (0.14)	(1.08–1.18)	−0.03 (−0.16–0.11)	0.032 *
Stride length 4 km/h	1.21 (0.16)	(1.16–1.27)	1.23 (0.17)	(1.17–1.28)	−0.01 (−0.09–0.07)	0.117
Stride length 4.8 km/h	1.32 (0.18)	(1.26–1.38)	1.34 (0.18)	(1.28–1.40)	−0.01 (−0.09–0.06)	0.056
Stride length/height normal speed	79.16 (13.31)	(74.81–83.51)	80.32 (12.34)	(76.29–84.35)	−1.16 (−8.69–6.37)	0.079
Stride length/height 1.6 km/h	56.82 (13.30)	(52.48–61.17)	60.79 (12.73)	(56.64–64.95)	−3.97 (−14.21–6.27)	0.000 *
Stride length/height 2.4 km/h	61.50 (12.13)	(57.53–65.46)	63.51 (11.29)	(59.82–67.20)	−2.01 (−9.86–5.84)	0.005 *
Stride length/height 3.2 km/h	66.52 (11.91)	(62.63–70.42)	68.02 (10.93)	(64.45–71.59)	−1.50 (−9.60–6.60)	0.036 *
Stride length/height 4 km/h	73.07 (12.37)	(69.02–77.11)	73.67 (12.37)	(69.63–77.71)	−0.61 (−5.37–4.15)	0.143
Stride length/height 4.8 km/h	79.72 (13.76)	(75.22–84.22)	80.50 (13.92)	(75.95–85.04)	−0.78 (−5.45–3.90)	0.060

Table 4. Cont.

Variables	Mean (DS) First Session	IC95%	Mean (DS) Second Session	IC95%	LoA	p VALUE
Average length step 1 normal speed	0.66 (0.10)	(0.62–0.69)	0.67 (0.10)	(0.63–0.70)	−0.01 (−0.07–0.05)	0.058
Average length step 1 1.6 km/h	0.47 (0.08)	(0.44–0.49)	0.51 (0.08)	(0.48–0.53)	−0.04 (−0.12–0.04)	0.000 *
Average length step 1 2.4 km/h	0.51 (0.08)	(0.48–0.54)	0.53 (0.07)	(0.50–0.55)	−0.02 (−0.08–0.04)	0.004 *
Average length step 1 3.2 km/h	0.55 (0.08)	(0.52–0.57)	0.56 (0.07)	(0.53–0.58)	−0.01 (−0.08–0.05)	0.026*
Average length step 1 4 km/h	0.60 (0.08)	(0.58–0.63)	0.61 (0.08)	(0.58–0.64)	−0.01 (−0.05–0.04)	0.140
Average length step 1 4.8 km/h	0.66 (0.09)	(0.63–0.69)	0.67 (0.09)	(0.64–0.70)	−0.01 (−0.05–0.04)	0.103
Average length step 2 normal speed	0.66 (0.10)	(0.62–0.69)	0.67 (0.10)	(0.63–0.70)	−0.01 (−0.08–0.06)	0.156
Average length step 2 1.6 km/h	0.47 (0.08)	(0.44–0.49)	0.50 (0.08)	(0.47–0.52)	−0.03 (−0.12–0.06)	0.001 *
Average length step 2 2.4 km/h	0.50 (0.07)	(0.48–0.53)	0.52 (0.07)	(0.50–0.54)	−0.02 (−0.09–0.06)	0.019 *
Average length step 2 3.2 km/h	0.55 (0.07)	(0.53–0.58)	0.57 (0.07)	(0.54–0.59)	−0.01 (−0.08–0.05)	0.061
Average length step 2 4 km/h	0.61 (0.08)	(0.58–0.63)	0.61 (0.08)	(0.58–0.64)	0.00 (−0.04–0.03)	0.202
Average length step 2 4.8 km/h	0.66 (0.09)	(0.63–0.69)	0.66 (0.09)	(0.63–0.70)	−0.01 (−0.05–0.03)	0.070
Average duration of step 1 normal speed	49.89 (2.18)	(49.17–50.60)	49.93 (2.36)	(49.16–50.71)	−0.05 (−2.44–2.34)	0.811
Average duration of step 1 1.6 km/h	49.42 (2.36)	(48.65–50.20)	50.05 (2.98)	(49.08–51.03)	−0.63 (−4.69–3.43)	0.078
Average duration of step 1 2.4 km/h	50.09 (1.58)	(49.57–50.69)	49.75 (1.67)	(49.20–50.30)	0.34 (−1.81–2.48)	0.075
Average duration of step 1 3.2 km/h	49.82 (1.14)	(49.45–50.19)	49.98 (1.31)	(49.55–50.41)	−0.16 (−1.61–1.29)	0.208
Average duration of step 1 4 km/h	49.79 (1.17)	(49.40–50.17)	49.84 (1.07)	(49.48–50.19)	−0.05 (−1.81–1.71)	0.739
Average duration of step 1 4.8 km/h	49.97 (0.91)	(49.67–50.27)	50.05 (1.12)	(49.68–50.41)	−0.08 (−1.41–1.25)	0.481
Average duration of step 2 normal speed	50.29 (2.53)	(49.46–51.12)	50.31 (2.09)	(49.62–50.99)	−0.02 (−2.45–2.42)	0.932
Average duration of step 2 1.6 km/h	50.63 (2.28)	(49.88–51.38)	49.78 (3.14)	(48.75–50.80)	0.85 (−3.69–5.39)	0.034 *
Average duration of step 2 2.4 km/h	49.92 (1.60)	(49.39–50.44)	50.08 (2.01)	(49.43–50.74)	−0.17 (−2.54–2.21)	0.415
Average duration of step 2 3.2 km/h	50.18 (1.14)	(49.80–50.55)	50.01 (1.30)	(49.58–50.44)	0.17 (−1.22–1.55)	0.165
Average duration of step 2 4 km/h	50.21 (1.17)	(49.83–50.62)	50.15 (1.07)	(49.80–50.50)	0.07 (−1.83–1.96)	0.680
Average duration of step 2 4.8 km/h	50.03 (0.91)	(49.73–50.33)	49.95 (1.11)	(49.59–50.31)	0.08 (−1.26–1.42)	0.507

Table 4. Cont.

Variables	Mean (DS) First Session	IC95%	Mean (DS) Second Session	IC95%	LoA	p VALUE
Position duration normal speed	63.67 (2.63)	(62.81–64.53)	63.63 (2.86)	(62.69–64.56)	0.04 (−1.79–1.88)	0.780
Position duration 1.6 km/h	62.39 (2.56)	(61.55–63.22)	63.25 (3.04)	(62.26–64.25)	−0.87 (−4.63–2.90)	0.010 *
Position duration 2.4 km/h	62.92 (2.31)	(62.16–63.67)	63.09 (2.78)	(62.19–64.00)	−0.18 (−3.03–2.67)	0.467
Position duration 3.2 km/h	61.80 (1.99)	(61.14–62.45)	61.77 (2.02)	(61.05–62.48)	0.03 (−1.82–1.88)	0.852
Position duration 4 km/h	60.98 (2.01)	(60.32–61.64)	61.03 (2.28)	(60.29–61.78)	−0.05 (−1.59–1.49)	0.695
Position duration 4.8 km/h	60.09 (1.83)	(59.48–60.69)	60.13 (1.88)	(59.51–60.74)	−0.04 (−1.39–1.30)	0.723
Oscillation duration normal speed	34.34 (2.72)	(33.45–35.23)	34.28 (2.72)	(33.39–35.17)	0.06 (−1.68–1.80)	0.684
Oscillation duration 1.6 km/h	36.46 (2.41)	(35.67–37.25)	35.57 (3.12)	(34.55–36.59)	0.89 (−2.29–4.08)	0.002 *
Oscillation duration 2.4 km/h	35.65 (2.33)	(34.89–36.41)	35.48 (2.72)	(34.59–36.37)	0.17 (−2.55–2.88)	0.478
Oscillation duration 3.2 km/h	36.55 (2.03)	(35.89–37.21)	36.61 (2.24)	(35.88–37.34)	−0.06 (−1.95–1.83)	0.721
Oscillation duration 4 km/h	37.14 (2.02)	(36.48–37.80)	37.08 (2.29)	(36.33–37.83)	0.06 (−1.53–1.66)	0.635
Oscillation duration 4.8 km/h	37.91 (1.80)	(37.32–38.50)	37.84 (1.89)	(37.22–38.46)	0.07 (−1.38–1.51)	0.585
Left foot bearing time normal speed	63.62 (3.48)	(62.48–64.76)	63.45 (3.58)	(62.28–64.63)	0.17 (−1.99–2.32)	0.367
Left foot bearing time 1.6 km/h	61.88 (3.68)	(60.67–63.08)	63.53 (4.41)	(62.09–64.97)	−1.65 (−7.56–4.25)	0.002 *
Left foot bearing time 2.4 km/h	62.93 (2.43)	(62.13–63.72)	63.06 (2.79)	(62.14–63.97)	−0.13 (−3.64–3.38)	0.667
Left foot bearing time 3.2 km/h	62.12 (3.62)	(60.94–63.30)	61.99 (2.43)	(61.20–62.79)	0.13 (−3.88–4.13)	0.715
Left foot bearing time 4 km/h	60.85 (2.42)	(60.06–61.64)	60.87 (2.60)	(60.02–61.72)	−0.02 (−2.06–2.02)	0.918
Left foot bearing time 4.8 km/h	59.84 (2.23)	(59.11–60.57)	59.98 (2.40)	(59.20–60.77)	−0.14 (−2.12–1.84)	0.403
Right foot bearing time normal speed	63.72 (2.75)	(62.82–64.62)	63.80 (2.64)	(62.93–64.66)	−0.08 (−2.82–2.66)	0.730
Right foot bearing time 1.6 km/h	62.90 (3.43)	(61.78–64.03)	62.99 (4.50)	(61.51–64.43)	−0.08 (−5.98–5.82)	0.873
Right foot bearing time 2.4 km/h	62.91 (2.89)	(61.96–63.85)	63.08 (3.56)	(61.92–64.25)	−0.18 (−3.64–3.28)	0.547
Right foot bearing time 3.2 km/h	61.75 (2.10)	(61.06–62.44)	61.58 (2.65)	(60.71–62.44)	0.17 (−2.46–2.81)	0.442
Right foot bearing time 4 km/h	61.12 (2.27)	(60.38–61.87)	61.20 (2.48)	(60.39–62.01)	−0.08 (−2.24–2.09)	0.686
Right foot bearing time 4.8 km/h	60.34 (2.02)	(59.67–61.00)	60.27 (1.96)	(59.63–60.91)	0.07 (−1.74–1.88)	0.670

Table 4. Cont.

Variables	Mean (DS) First Session	IC95%	Mean (DS) Second Session	IC95%	LoA	p VALUE
Left foot swing time normal speed	34.37 (3.54)	(33.21–35.53)	34.54 (3.42)	(33.33–35.57)	−0.08 (−2.33–2.18)	0.698
Left foot swing time 1.6 km/h	37.02 (3.33)	(35.93–38.11)	35.29 (4.24)	(33.90–36.62)	1.73 (−3.33–6.78)	0.000*
Left foot swing time 2.4 km/h	35.65 (2.43)	(34.85–36.45)	35.46 (2.91)	(34.51–36.41)	0.19 (−3.28–3.67)	0.516
Left foot swing time 3.2 km/h	36.51 (2.40)	(35.72–37.29)	36.38 (2.44)	(35.58–37.18)	0.13 (−1.87–2.14)	0.443
Left foot swing time 4 km/h	37.29 (2.42)	(36.49–38.08)	37.28 (2.59)	(36.43–38.12)	0.01 (−2.04–2.05)	0.961
Left foot swing time 4.8 km/h	38.16 (2.20)	(37.44–38.87)	38.03 (2.37)	(37.25–38.80)	0.13 (−1.89–2.14)	0.456
Right foot swing time normal speed	34.18 (2.71)	(33.30–35.07)	34.13 (2.60)	(33.28–34.98)	0.05 (−2.06–2.17)	0.771
Right foot swing time 1.6 km/h	35.81 (3.60)	(34.64–36.99)	35.83 (4.70)	(34.30–37.37)	−0.02 (−6.35–6.31)	0.971
Right foot swing time 2.4 km/h	35.65 (2.92)	(34.69–36.60)	35.57 (3.38)	(34.46–36.68)	0.08 (−3.01–3.16)	0.769
Right foot swing time 3.2 km/h	36.59 (2.14)	(35.89–37.29)	36.84 (2.63)	(35.98–37.70)	−0.25 (−2.83–2.34)	0.273
Right foot swing time 4 km/h	37.01 (2.27)	(36.27–37.75)	36.95 (2.48)	(36.13–37.76)	0.07 (−2.10–2.23)	0.724
Right foot swing time 4.8 km/h	37.62 (2.01)	(37.01–38.33)	37.72 (1.94)	(37.09–38.36)	−0.05 (−1.89–1.78)	0.733

Abbreviation: km/h (kilometers per hour); CI (confidence interval); SD (standard deviation); * (paired t-test significant differences, $p < 0.05$): LoA (limit of agreement).

4. Discussion

Assessing the reliability of any IMU or gait analysis system is essential to ensure the reliability of the measurements made by analyzing the gait parameters, a lack of errors in the operation of the devices, and a lack of human error. This study shows that the Wiva Science IMU has high reliability in its measurements, but we must mention that the reliability is reduced at lower speeds. At 4 km/h, no errors are observed in the measurements, and at 1.6 km/h, the results are most affected. This may be due to changes in the speed of the subject's walking and errors between both days of the test.

Furthermore, if we compare our study with others, we agree that ICCs are lower at slower speeds and higher ICCs at higher speeds or with normal gait velocity [24,35].

According to the validation research of the gait parameters studied with the IMU Free4Act [36] which could be classified as the predecessor of Wiva Science, they obtained lower ICC results the lower the study speeds were.

Comparing our investigation with the reliability and repeatability study of the IMU MTw sensors (MTw sensors, Xsens Technologies B.V., The Netherlands) [37] they performed the gait tests at a comfortable speed for the patient, 25 m for 1 min in 19 subjects. They obtained an ICC > 0.8 in all measurements including intrasession and intersession, being in agreement with our study by having good reliability and repeatability at a speed comfortable for the patient.

Furthermore, we believe that since the worst results were isolated and occurred at 1.6, 2.4 and 3.2 km/h speeds, they are not significant. Compared to other studies with high reliability results ICC > 0.81, it has the worst scores in stance time and swing time as our study [15]. With regard to the reproduction of the study, the subjects did not use footwear or clothing that could bias the measurements, such as socks or stockings, since they could alter the biomechanics of the participant.

The results of our research are similar to other researches where they have used inertial measurement units placed on the lower back [38,39] and having greater difficulty in measuring the parameters related to stance and swing times [40,41]. It is possible that this is due to the fact that they are more accurate in their measurements the more proximal their placement is to the foot [42]. However, the placement of the inertial measurement units in the sacral area, according to some authors, can reduce residual errors related to pelvic rotations and errors in gait measurements [43].

All of the research revealed positive results in terms of accuracy and repeatability, so we believe that using a sample of 36 healthy subjects for our research was sufficient. We must emphasize that we first placed the IMU in the subject's sacral area with an elastic belt supplied by the manufacturer, but it was not useful, and it even skewed the measurements during the repetition of the tests. Therefore, the device was held with hypoallergenic adhesive bandages. Another important limitation was the impossibility of limiting the tests from the Biomech software (Version 1.6.1.14687, LetSense Group srl., Bologna, Italy, http://letsense.net (accessed on 11 December 2019)), which was not able to eliminate the acceleration and deceleration times from the tests performed in a 10 m-long corridor at normal speed. A few studies have quantified events occurring at the initiation of gait using IMUs [44,45]. The total time spent between the two days of the test was approximately one and a half hours per subject, which was a source of fatigue for the participant.

5. Conclusions

We found no difference when we compared the variables between the first and second sessions at higher speeds (4 and 4.8 km/h). However, we found greater differences and errors at lower speeds of 3.2, 2.4 and 1.6 km/h, and the latter one generated more error. Based on the results of this study, we leave open future lines of investigation related to comparison between morphotypes of the foot and the behavior for walking evaluated with IMUs. In addition, we must test Wiva Science IMU at different walking speeds and find whether it is effectively unreliable at lower speeds. We must also evaluate its behavior at higher speeds.

Author Contributions: Conceptualization, J.P.-O. and C.M.-V.; methodology, M.E.L.-I., C.M.-V., C.C.-L., D.R.-S. and J.C.-M.; software, J.P.-O. and C.M.-V.; validation, R.B.-d.-B.-V., L.E.-G., C.C.-L. and J.C.-M.; formal analysis, L.E.-G. and C.C.-L.; investigation, J.P.-O., M.E.L.-I., R.B.-d.-B.-V., C.M.-V. and J.C.-M.; resources, L.E.-G. and C.C.-L.; data curation, J.P.-O.; writing—original draft preparation, D.R.-S.; writing—review and editing, D.R.-S.; visualization, D.R.-S.; supervision, M.E.L.-I. and R.B.-d.-B.-V.; project administration, R.B.-d.-B.-V.; funding acquisition, J.P.-O. All authors have read and agreed to the published version of the manuscript.

Funding: This research received no external funding.

Institutional Review Board Statement: The study was conducted according to the guidelines of the Declaration of Helsinki, and approved by the Institutional Review Board (or Ethics Committee) of Rey Juan Carlos University (protocol code 2102201803818 and approved the 18 April 2018).

Informed Consent Statement: Informed consent was obtained from all subjects involved in the study.

Conflicts of Interest: The authors declare no conflict of interest.

References

1. Cutti, A.; Ferrari, A.; Garofalo, P.; Raggi, M.; Cappello, A.; Ferrari, A. 'Outwalk': A protocol for clinical gait analysis based on inertial and magnetic sensors. *Med. Biol. Eng. Comput.* **2009**, *48*, 17–25. [CrossRef]
2. Taylor, L.; Miller, E.; Kaufman, K. Static and dynamic validation of inertial measurement units. *Gait Posture* **2017**, *57*, 80–84. [CrossRef]
3. Lee, M.; Youm, C.; Jeon, J.; Cheon, S.M.; Park, H. Validity of shoe-type inertial measurement units for Parkinson's disease patients during treadmill walking. *J. Neuroeng. Rehabil.* **2018**, *15*, 1–12. [CrossRef]

4. Lanovaz, J.L.; Oates, A.R.; Treen, T.T.; Unger, J.; Musselman, K.E. Gait & posture validation of a commercial inertial sensor system for spatiotemporal gait measurements in children. *Gait Posture* **2017**, *51*, 14–19. [CrossRef]
5. Adamowicz, L.; Gurchiek, R.D.; Ferri, J.; Ursiny, A.T.; Fiorentino, N.; Mcginnis, R.S. Validation of Novel Relative Orientation and Inertial Sensor-to-Segment Alignment Algorithms for Estimating 3D Hip Joint Angles. *Sensors* **2019**, *19*, 5143. [CrossRef] [PubMed]
6. Karatsidis, A.; Jung, M.; Schepers, H.M.; Bellusci, G.; de Zee, M.; Veltink, P.H. Musculoskeletal model-based inverse dynamic analysis under ambulatory conditions using inertial motion capture. *Med. Eng. Phys.* **2019**, *65*, 68–77. [CrossRef]
7. Fong, D.; Chan, Y. The Use of Wearable Inertial Motion Sensors in Human Lower Limb Biomechanics Research: A Systematic Review. *Sensors* **2010**, *10*, 11556–11565. [CrossRef]
8. Chen, S.; Lach, J.; Lo, B.; Yang, G.Z. Toward Pervasive Gait Analysis With Wearable Sensors: A Systematic Review. *IEEE J. Biomed. Health Inform.* **2016**, *20*, 1521–1537. [CrossRef]
9. Orlowski, K.; Eckardt, F.; Herold, F.; Aye, N.; Edelmann-Nusser, J.; Witte, K. Examination of the reliability of an inertial sensor-based gait analysis system. *Biomed. Tech.* **2017**, *62*, 615–622. [CrossRef]
10. Barak, Y.; Wagenaar, R.C.; Holt, K.G. Gait characteristics of elderly people with a history of falls: A dynamic approach. *Phys. Ther.* **2006**, *86*, 1501–1510. [CrossRef] [PubMed]
11. IJmker, T.; Lamoth, C.J.C. Gait and cognition: The relationship between gait stability and variability with executive function in persons with and without dementia. *Gait Posture* **2012**, *35*, 126–130. [CrossRef]
12. Larrinaga, F.; Carrasco, R.A. Virtual connection tree concept application over CDMA based cellular systems. *IEE Colloq.* **1997**, *26*, 217–238.
13. Kavanagh, J.J.; Morrison, S.; James, D.A.; Barrett, R. Reliability of segmental accelerations measured using a new wireless gait analysis system. *J. Biomech.* **2006**, *39*, 2863–2872. [CrossRef]
14. Schwesig, R.; Kauert, R.; Wust, S.; Becker, S.; Leuchte, S. Reliability of the novel gait analysis system RehaWatch. *Biomed. Tech.* **2010**, *55*, 109–115. [CrossRef]
15. Kluge, F.; Gaßner, H.; Hannink, J.; Pasluosta, C.; Klucken, J.; Eskofier, B.M. Towards mobile gait analysis: Concurrent validity and test-retest reliability of an inertial measurement system for the assessment of spatio-temporal gait parameters. *Sensors* **2017**, *17*, 1522. [CrossRef]
16. Rahimi, F.; Bee, C.; Duval, C.; Boissy, P.; Edwards, R.; Jog, M. Using ecological whole body kinematics to evaluate effects of medication adjustment in Parkinson disease. *J. Parkinsons Dis.* **2014**, *4*, 617–627. [CrossRef]
17. Vandenbroucke, J.P.; von Elm, E.; Altman, D.G.; Gtzsche, P.C.; Mulrow, C.D.; Pocock, S.J.; Poole, C.; Schlesselman, J.J.; Egger, M.; Initiative, S. Strengthening the Reporting of Observational Research in Epidemiology (STROBE): Explanation and elaboration. *Int. J. Surg.* **2014**, *12*, 1500–1524. [CrossRef]
18. World Medical Association. World Medical Association Declaration of Helsinki. JAMA [Internet] 2013 Nov 27 [cited 2018 Jan 14]; 310, 2191. Available online: http://www.ncbi.nlm.nih.gov/pubmed/24141714 (accessed on 15 March 2021).
19. Hollman, J.H.; Watkins, M.K.; Imhoff, A.C.; Braun, C.E.; Akervik, K.A.; Ness, D.K. A comparison of variability in spatiotemporal gait parameters between treadmill and overground walking conditions. *Gait Posture* **2016**, *43*, 204–209. [CrossRef]
20. Gijon-nogueron, G.; Sanchez-rodriguez, R.; Lopezosa-reca, E.; Cervera-marin, J.A.; Martinez-quintana, R.; Martinez-nova, A. Normal Values of the Foot Posture Index in a Young Adult Spanish Population. *J. Am. Pod. Med. Assoc.* **2015**, *105*, 42–46. [CrossRef]
21. Giraudeau, B.; Mary, J.Y. Planning a reproducibility study: How many subjects and how many replicates per subject for an expected width of the 95 per cent confidence interval of the intraclass correlation coefficient. *Stat. Med.* **2001**, *20*, 3205–3214. [CrossRef] [PubMed]
22. De Vet, H.C.W.; Terwee, C.B.; Mokkink, L.B.; Knol, D.L. *Measurement in Medicine: A Practical Guide (Practical Guides to Biostatistics and Epidemiology)*; Cambridge University (England) Press: Cambridge, UK, 2011; Volume 96, Available online: https://www.cambridge.org/ (accessed on 21 June 2020).
23. Portney, L.G.; Watkins., M.P. *Foundations of Clinical Research: Applications to Practice*, 3rd ed.; F.A. Davis Company (Pennsylvania): Philadelphia, PA, USA, 2009.
24. Donath, L.; Faude, O.; Lichtenstein, E.; Nuesch, C.; Mündermann, A. Validity and reliability of a portable gait analysis system for measuring spatiotemporal gait characteristics: Comparison to an instrumented treadmill. *J. Neuroeng. Rehabil.* **2016**, *13*, 1–9. [CrossRef]
25. Wüest, S.; Massé, F.; Aminian, K.; Gonzenbach, R.; De Bruin, E.D. Reliability and validity of the inertial sensor-based Timed "Up and Go" test in individuals affected by stroke. *J. Rehabil. Res. Dev.* **2016**, *53*, 599–610. [CrossRef]
26. Bauer, C.M.; Rast, F.M.; Ernst, M.J.; Kool, J.; Oetiker, S.; Rissanen, S.M.; Kankaanpää, M. Concurrent validity and reliability of a novel wireless inertial measurement system to assess trunk movement. *J. Electromyogr. Kinesiol.* **2015**, *25*, 782–790. [CrossRef] [PubMed]
27. Esser, P.; Dawes, H.; Collett, J.; Feltham, M.G.; Howells, K. Validity and inter-rater reliability of inertial gait measurements in Parkinson's disease: A pilot study. *J. Neurosci. Methods* **2012**, *205*, 177–181. [CrossRef] [PubMed]
28. Perez-Cruzado, D.; Gonzalez-Sanchez, M.; Cuesta-Vargas, A.I. Parameterization and reliability of single-leg balance test assessed with inertial sensors in stroke survivors: A cross-sectional study. *Biomed. Eng. Online* **2014**, *13*, 1–12. [CrossRef]

29. Washabaugh, E.P.; Kalyanaraman, T.; Adamczyk, P.G.; Claflin, E.S.; Krishnan, C. Validity and repeatability of inertial measurement units for measuring gait parameters. *Gait Posture* **2017**, *55*, 87–93. [CrossRef]
30. Landis, J.R.; Koch, G.G. The measurement of observer agreement for categorical data. *Biometrics* **1977**, *33*, 159–174. [CrossRef]
31. Dobbs, R.J.; Charlett, A.; Bowes, S.G.; O'Neill, C.J.A.; Weller, C.; Hughes, J.; Dobbs, S.M. Is this walk normal? *Age Ageing* **1993**, *22*, 27–30. [CrossRef]
32. Lord, S.R.; Lloyd, D.G.; Nirui, M.; Raymond, J.; Williams, P.; Stewart, R.A. The effect of exercise on gait patterns in older women: A randomized controlled trial. *J. Gerontol.* **1996**, *51*, M64–M70. [CrossRef]
33. Bland, J.M.; Altman, D.G. Statistical methods for assessing agreement between two methods of clinical measurement. *Lancet* **1986**, *1*, 307–310. [CrossRef]
34. Garrow, J.S. *Quetelet Index as Indicator of Obesity*; Lancet: London, UK, 1986; Volume 1, p. 1219.
35. Papi, E.; Osei-Kuffour, D.; Chen, Y.A.; McGregor, A.H. Use of wearable technology for performance assessment: A validation study. *Med. Eng. Phys.* **2015**, *37*, 698–704. [CrossRef]
36. Buganè, F.; Benedetti, M.G.; Casadio, G.; Attala, S.; Biagi, F.; Manca, M.; Leardini, A. Estimation of spatial-temporal gait parameters in level walking based on a single accelerometer: Validation on normal subjects by standard gait analysis. *Comput. Methods Programs Biomed.* **2012**, *108*, 129–137. [CrossRef]
37. Hamacher, D.; Taylor, W.R.; Singh, N.B.; Schega, L. Towards clinical application: Repetitive sensor position re-calibration for improved reliability of gait parameters. *Gait Posture* **2014**, *39*, 1146–1148. [CrossRef]
38. Zijlstra, W.; Hof, A.L. Assessment of spatio-temporal gait parameters from trunk accelerations during human walking. *Gait Posture* **2003**, *18*, 1–10. [CrossRef]
39. Moon, Y.; Mcginnis, R.S.; Seagers, K.; Motl, R.W.; Sheth, N.; Wright, A.; Ghaffari, R.; Sosnoff, J.J. Monitoring gait in multiple sclerosis with novel wearable motion sensors. *PLoS ONE* **2017**, *12*, e0171346. [CrossRef]
40. Aminian, K.; Najafi, B.; Büla, C.; Leyvraz, P.; Robert, P. Spatio-temporal parameters of gait measured by an ambulatory system using miniature gyroscopes. *J. Biomech.* **2002**, *35*, 689–699. [CrossRef]
41. Pappas, I.P.I.; Popovic, M.R.; Keller, T.; Dietz, V.; Morari, M. A Reliable Gait Phase Detection System. IEEE Trans. *Neural Syst. Rehabil. Eng.* **2001**, *9*, 113–125. [CrossRef]
42. Iosa, M.; Picerno, P.; Paolucci, S.; Morone, G. Wearable Inertial Sensors for Human Movement Analysis Wearable Inertial Sensors for Human Movement Analysis. *Expert Rev. Med. Devices* **2016**, *13*, 641–659. [CrossRef]
43. Shin, S.H.; Park, C.G. Adaptive step length estimation algorithm using optimal parameters and movement status awareness. *Med. Eng. Phys.* **2011**, *33*, 1064–10671. [CrossRef]
44. Martinez-mendez, R.; Sekine, M.; Tamura, T. Detection of anticipatory postural adjustments prior to gait initiation using inertial wearable sensors. *J. Neuroeng. Rehabil.* **2011**, 1–10. [CrossRef]
45. Bonora, G.; Carpinella, I.; Cattaneo, D.; Chiari, L.; Ferrarin, M. A new instrumented method for the evaluation of gait initiation and step climbing based on inertial sensors: A pilot application in Parkinson's disease. *J. Neuroeng. Rehabil.* **2015**, 1–12. [CrossRef]

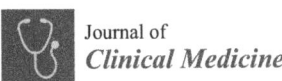

Journal of Clinical Medicine

Article

Effects of Whole-Body Vibration and Balance Training on Female Athletes with Chronic Ankle Instability

Wen-Dien Chang [1], Shuya Chen [2] and Yung-An Tsou [3,4,*]

1. Department of Sport Performance, National Taiwan University of Sport, Taichung 404401, Taiwan; changwendien@ntus.edu.tw
2. Department of Physical Therapy and Graduate Institute of Rehabilitation Science, China Medical University, Taichung 40402, Taiwan; sychen@mail.cmu.edu.tw
3. Department of Otolaryngology-Head and Neck Surgery, China Medical University Hospital, Taichung 40402, Taiwan
4. Department of Audiology and Speech-Language Pathology, Asia University, Taichung 41354, Taiwan
* Correspondence: d22052121@gmail.com; Tel.: +886-4-2205-3366

Abstract: We explored the effects of 6-week whole-body vibration (WBV) and balance training programs on female athletes with chronic ankle instability (CAI). This randomized controlled study involved female athletes with dominant-leg CAI. The participants were randomly divided into three groups: WBV training (Group A), balance training (Group B), and nontraining (control group; Group C). Groups A and B performed three exercise movements (double-leg stance, one-legged stance, and tandem stance) in 6-week training programs by using a vibration platform and balance ball, respectively. The Star Excursion Balance Test (SEBT), a joint position sense test, and an isokinetic strength test were conducted. In total, 63 female athletes with dominant-leg CAI were divided into three study groups (all $n = 21$). All of them completed the study. We observed time-by-group interactions in the SEBT ($p = 0.001$) and isokinetic strength test at 30°/s of concentric contraction (CON) of ankle inversion ($p = 0.04$). Compared with the control group, participants of the two exercise training programs improved in dynamic balance, active repositioning, and 30°/s of CON and eccentric contraction of the ankle invertor in the SEBT, joint position sense test, and isokinetic strength test, respectively. Furthermore, the effect sizes for the assessed outcomes in Groups A and B ranged from very small to small. Female athletes who participated in 6-week training programs incorporating a vibration platform or balance ball exhibited very small or small effect sizes for CAI in the SEBT, joint position sense test, and isokinetic strength test. No differences were observed in the variables between the two exercise training programs.

Keywords: chronic ankle instability; whole-body vibration; balance training

Citation: Chang, W.-D.; Chen, S.; Tsou, Y.-A. Effects of Whole-Body Vibration and Balance Training on Female Athletes with Chronic Ankle Instability. *J. Clin. Med.* **2021**, *10*, 2380. https://doi.org/10.3390/jcm10112380

Academic Editors: David Rodríguez-Sanz and Yasuhito Tanaka

Received: 9 March 2021
Accepted: 24 May 2021
Published: 28 May 2021

Publisher's Note: MDPI stays neutral with regard to jurisdictional claims in published maps and institutional affiliations.

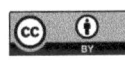

Copyright: © 2021 by the authors. Licensee MDPI, Basel, Switzerland. This article is an open access article distributed under the terms and conditions of the Creative Commons Attribution (CC BY) license (https://creativecommons.org/licenses/by/4.0/).

1. Introduction

Lateral ankle sprain is one of the most common sports injuries and often causes a decrease in neuromuscular control and loss of proprioception [1]. Neuromuscular control helps maintain the functional stability of the ankle, whereas proprioception influences ankle joint position and sense of movement. Impairments in these functions cause reduced dynamic balance and reaction time of the ankle joint during exercise [2]. An ankle sprain resulting in damage to the lateral ankle capsuloligamentous complex can cause sequelae, such as recurring ankle sprains. It decreases ankle function as well as causing a loose feeling, and this postinjury symptom is classified as chronic ankle instability (CAI) [3]. Athletes with CAI may experience limited functionality of their lower extremities, which may affect their sports performance [4]. Therefore, specific balance exercises for athletes with CAI are critical in rehabilitation and training programs and could effectively reduce the risk of ankle sprain during sports activities.

Balance training is a progressive type of exercise performed on an unstable surface, and the resultant efferent output causes changes in α motor neuron excitability [5]. Balance training was used to improve muscle excitability in the ankle joint and increase motor control for CAI [6]. Whole-body vibration (WBV) training is another popular method used in CAI rehabilitation [7]. WBV training was performed on an oscillating vibration platform, which activates muscle spindles to facilitate tonic vibration reflex [8]. This training also enhances α motor neuron excitability and the synchronization of motor units to increase motor control in the ankle [9]. To the best of our knowledge, there have only been a few studies comparing the effects between WBC and traditional balance training on CAI. Therefore, WBV and balance training programs were designed and used for athletes with CAI in the current study.

For basketball and volleyball players, ankle stability and motor control are crucial for ground impact during jumping and landing. The dominant leg is a commonly discussed factor in these types of actions by injured athletes because it plays a critical role in object manipulation and lead-out movements [10]. However, the nondominant leg performs a stabilizing and supporting role in sports activities [10]. Therefore, the dominant leg is highly susceptible to sports injuries such as ankle sprain and may suddenly become injured during jumping and landing on an unstable surface. A study by van Melick et al. revealed that female athletes were more likely to jump using the dominant leg than male athletes [11]. A systematic review revealed that female athletes sustained ankle sprains more often than male athletes [12]. Sex-related differences in the epidemiology of ankle injuries were noted in sports injury protection [12]. Ristolainen et al. indicated female athletes tend to have a higher risk of sport-related ankle injury than male athletes [13]. Therefore, importance needs to be placed on an effective strategy of rehabilitation for female athletes. Previous studies have also reported a high incidence of ankle injuries in basketball and volleyball players [14,15]. Therefore, investigating the effects of specific interventions for CAI in female basketball and volleyball athletes is essential. Our study aim was to compare the effects of 6-week WBV and balance training on dominant-leg CAI in female athletes.

2. Methods

This study was a randomized controlled trial approved by the Institutional Review Board of China Medical University Hospital (CRREC-106-063). Participants with CAI were recruited from women's basketball and volleyball teams at neighboring colleges. For inclusion criteria, female athletes had to have a history of at least one ankle sprain, lateral ankle instability of the dominant leg with a severity score ≤24 measured using the Cumberland Ankle Instability Tool, and a continual feeling of the ankle "giving way" after one year [16]. The dominant leg was used for lead-out movements and was determined as the foot used to kick a ball [10]. Exclusion criteria were acute ankle sprain, a history of surgery in both legs, and any musculoskeletal diseases of the lower extremities. The sample size calculation using G*Power software reported by Sefton et al. [17] was used, which resulted in a total of 21 participants. We also tried to use the statistical power of 80%, α level of 0.05, and effect size (f = 0.25) to calculate via G*Power software (version 3.1.9.2; Heinrich-Heine-Universität, Düsseldorf, Germany). A total sample size of 46 was calculated and required. In the current study, the estimated sample size was set to at least 48 participants (16 participants per group), which was a statistically adequate sample size.

2.1. Study Procedures

This experimental trial was conducted at the end of the semester, and there was no practice or competition during this study period. The participants were randomly divided into three groups: Group A, who completed a 6-week WVB training program; Group B, who completed a 6-week balance training program; and Group C, who did not participate in a training program (Figure 1). All participants continued their normal daily activity and were instructed not to receive any treatments or therapy for CAI. The participants were assessed before and after the study. The participants underwent three assessments, the Star Excursion Balance Test (SEBT), a joint position sense test, and an isokinetic strength test, consecutively, and their performance was evaluated by the same physiotherapist. The participants and researchers were not blinded to the study process.

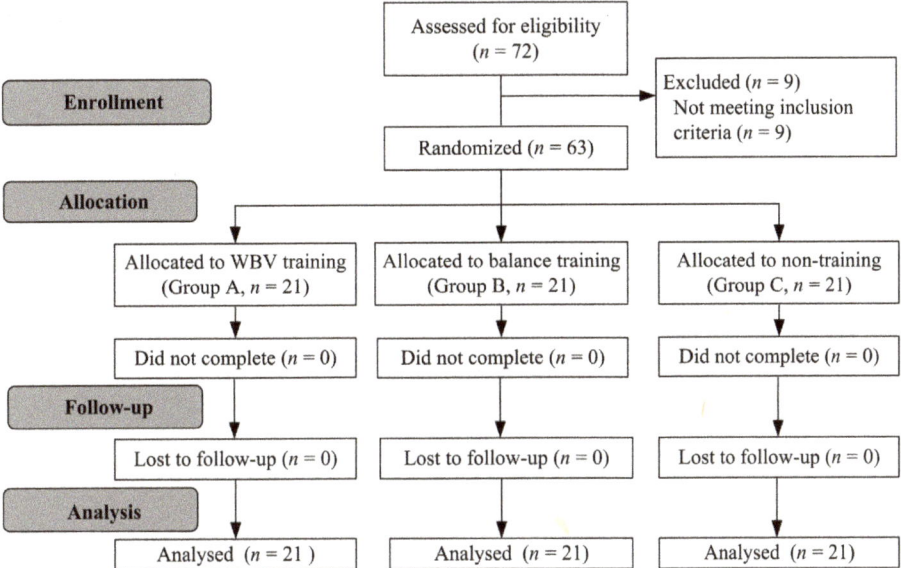

Figure 1. Flowchart of the current study. WBV: whole-body vibration.

2.2. Exercise Training Program

Groups A and B performed the same exercises during the 6-week training programs, but Group A used a vibration platform (AIBI Power Shaper, AIBI Fitness, Singapore), and Group B used a balance ball (BOSU Balance Trainer, Fitness Quest, Ashland, OH, USA). Group A performed the exercises while standing on the vibration platform, which operated at a frequency and amplitude of 5 Hz and 3 mm, respectively. Group B participants performed the exercises on the balance ball. Participants in both groups were asked to maintain balance on either leg or an affected leg while having eyes closed. Both training programs were conducted respectively three times per week for 6 weeks and consisted of a 5-min warm-up exercise, a 20-min main exercise, and a 5-min cool-down exercise. They were designed with standard exercise prescription and clinical experience by one physical therapist. The main exercise comprised three exercise movements: a double-leg stance, a one-legged stance, and a tandem stance (Figure 2). Weeks 1–3 consisted of four sets of 45-s exercises with a 40-s rest interval between exercises, and weeks 4–6 consisted of five sets of 45-s exercises with a 30-s rest interval between exercises. The training programs in Group A and B were identical in the current study, except standing on different training devices. Group C participants were encouraged to continue their normal daily activity and avoid additional training programs or therapeutic exercise.

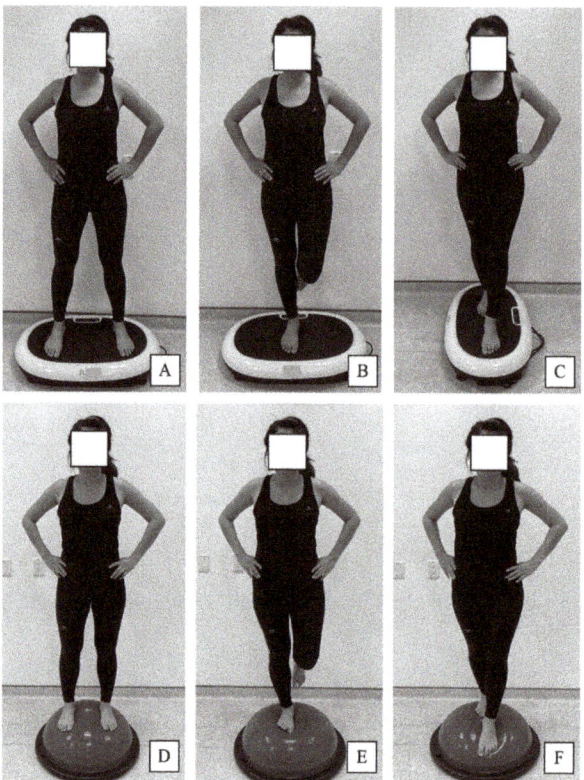

Figure 2. Demonstration of exercises on the vibration platform (**A–C**) and balance ball (**D–F**). (**A,D**): double-leg stance; (**B,E**): one-legged stance; (**C,F**): tandem stance.

2.3. Assessments

2.3.1. Star Excursion Balance Test

The SEBT was used to measure dynamic balance. The SEBT exhibited moderate-to-favorable interrater reliability (intraclass correlation coefficients [ICC] = 0.67–0.97) in an assessment of ankle instability [18]. An asterisk comprising eight tape segments joined at the center was placed on the floor. The tape segments were extended in eight directions (i.e., anterior, anterolateral, anteromedial, posteromedial, posterior, posterolateral, medial, and lateral) from the center at 45° angles [19]. The participants were asked to stand at the center of the asterisk using the leg with the involved ankle and then lightly touch the asterisk with the contralateral leg as far as possible in a direction chosen by the physiotherapist. The participants were instructed to maintain their balance in the one-legged stance by using the leg with the involved ankle and then return the contralateral leg to its initial position. Reach distances in the eight directions were recorded following three consecutive tests. The length of the involved leg was measured from the anterior superior iliac spine to the medial malleolus. The average reach distances in each direction were normalized according to the length of the involved leg and represented as a percentage.

2.3.2. Joint Position Sense Test

The SYSTEM 3 PRO dynamometer (Biodex Medical Systems, Shirley, NY, USA) was used to conduct a joint position sense test measuring active and passive repositioning. The dynamometer exhibited medium-to-high reliability in an assessment of joint kinesthesia ability (r = 0.6–0.8) [20]. The participants laid in a supine position while blindfolded, and the involved ankle was placed on the ankle inversion-eversion footplate of the dynamometer with a plantar flexion of 15°. Three reference angles were established for ankle inversion, neutral ankle position, and ankle eversion (15°, 0°, and 10°, respectively), and the participants were asked to actively and passively reproduce the angle. The absolute value of the joint angle error represents the actual difference between the reference angle and the matching angle [21].

In active repositioning, the involved ankle was first placed in a neutral position and then moved to the inversion or eversion reference angle for 10 s. The participants were asked to actively reproduce the angle three times; the corresponding angles produced by the participants were then recorded. In passive repositioning, the involved ankle was also first placed in a neutral position and then moved to the inversion or eversion reference angle for 10 s. The involved ankle was then passively inverted and everted through a full range of motion by using 5°/s of angular velocity and stopped at the original reference angle by using a hand-held switch. Three passive repositioning trials were completed to reproduce the reference angle, and the corresponding angles were recorded. The average absolute values of the joint angle errors were subsequently analyzed.

2.3.3. Isokinetic Strength Test

The SYSTEM 3 PRO dynamometer was also used to conduct the isokinetic strength test. The dynamometer exhibited high reliability (ICC coefficients = 0.87–0.96) and was effective in measuring the isokinetic strength of ankle joints [22]. Ankle invertor and evertor muscle strength was measured in terms of concentric contraction (CON) and eccentric contraction (ECC) at velocities of 30°/s and 120°/s, respectively [23]. Prior to testing, the participants warmed up for 10 min using general range-of-motion exercises for ankle joints. The participants sat in a chair with the backrest at a seatback tilt of 70°, and their trunks and pelvises were fixed with straps. The involved leg was fixed with a strap, and the involved foot was secured to ankle attachments with two straps. The tested ankle was positioned with 20° of plantar flexion, and the rotational axis of the dynamometer was leveled at the subtalar joint. Three repetitions were performed at velocities of 30°/s and 120°/s with 1-min rest intervals between each repetition [24]. The CON and ECC of the ankle inversion and eversion were calculated as peak torque normalized according to body weight. The respective ratios of inversion and eversion for ECC or CON at 30°/s and 120°/s were also calculated.

2.4. Statistical Analysis

Statistical analysis was performed using SPSS version 25.0 (SPSS, Chicago, IL, USA). The Shapiro–Wilk test was used to verify the normality of the data to ensure the normal distribution of all assessed variables ($p > 0.05$). Descriptive statistics were used, and all data are presented as the mean ± standard deviation. An analysis of variance (ANOVA) and chi-squared test were used for continuous and categorical variables, respectively, to compare the differences within groups. The results of the SEBT, joint position sense test, and isokinetic strength test were analyzed using a two-way repeated-measures ANOVA (three groups × two times) followed by a Bonferroni post hoc test. Effect size (d) was classified according to the scale of Cohen [25] into very small (<0.2), small (0.2–0.5), medium (0.5–0.8), and large (>0.8), and the effects of Groups A and B were determined to respectively compare Group C. Multivariable linear regression analysis was used to evaluate the association of main outcome measurements between the two training groups and the non-training group. Multivariable modelling was performed with R^2 and β coefficients and specified as the change values of assessment variables for the prediction. The α level for all statistical analyses was set at 0.05.

3. Results

Sixty-three female athletes (50 basketball players and 13 volleyball players) with dominant-leg CAI participated following the inclusion criteria in our study. The participants were randomly divided using a random number generator into Groups A, B, and C (all n = 21, Figure 1). After the study process, no participants dropped out, and no participants reported adverse reactions. All of the participants completed the study. The demographics are presented in Table 1, and no significant differences were observed within the three groups (all $p > 0.05$).

Table 1. Demographics of the participants.

	Group A (n = 21)	Group B (n = 21)	Group C (n = 21)	p
Age (y)	20.31 ± 1.28	20.43 ± 1.25	21.23 ± 1.47	0.08
Height (cm)	168.34 ± 5.78	166.8 ± 6.84	169.53 ± 4.78	0.32
Weight (kg)	61.01 ± 22.39	58.83 ± 13.14	58.67 ± 16.54	0.89
Dominant leg (Lt/Rt)	5/16	4/17	5/16	0.91
Composite score of CAIT	19.21 ± 1.89	19.14 ± 2.01	19.25 ± 1.91	0.89

Left, Lt; Right. Rt; Cumberland Ankle Instability Tool, CAIT.

The ANOVA outcomes are summarized in Table 2. In the results of multivariable linear regression (Table 3), the R^2 values were 0.80 and 0.93 in Group A and B, respectively. Significant relationships between the change in values in active repositioning and 30°/s of ECC ankle inversion were noted ($p < 0.05$). Results of the SEBT among the three groups are presented in Table 4. To calculate the composite score of SEBT, the main effects of group ($F_{(2, 60)} = 5.30$, $p = 0.03$), time ($F_{(2, 60)} = 67.78$, $p = 0.001$), and time × group ($F_{(2, 60)} = 17.84$, $p = 0.001$) were observed. Post hoc tests indicated no significant differences in the SEBT within the groups before assessment in terms of composite score and individual directions ($p > 0.05$). Between Groups A and C, the anteromedial ($p = 0.01$, effect size: d = 1.25, 95% CI = 0.59–1.91), posterolateral ($p = 0.03$, effect size: d = 1.05, 95% CI = 0.41–1.70), and lateral ($p = 0.03$, effect size: d = 1.09, 95% CI = 0.44–1.74) directions in the SEBT were significantly different. However, no significant difference was observed in composite scores on the SEBT within the two groups ($p > 0.05$). Moreover, the results indicated that the SEBT composite score and individual directions were higher in Group B than in Group C (all $p < 0.05$). Within the two groups, a small effect size in composite score on the SEBT was observed (d = 2.34, 95% CI = 1.55–3.12), and very small to small effect sizes were observed for all individual directions (anterior, d = 1.70, 95% CI = 1.00–2.41; anterolateral, d = 1.53, 95% CI = 0.84–2.22; anteromedial, d = 1.88, 95% CI = 1.15–2.60; posteromedial, d = 1.21, 95% CI = 0.55–1.86; posterior, d = 1.74, 95% CI = 1.03–2.45; posterolateral, d = 2.13, 95% CI = 1.38–2.89; medial, d = 1.32, 95% CI = 0.65–1.99; and lateral, d = 2.18, 95% CI = 1.41–2.94).

Table 2. Outcome of ANOVA with the factors for the assessed variables.

Assessed Variables	Group			Time			Time × Group		
	F	p	ηp²	F	p	ηp²	F	p	ηp²
Composite of star excursion balance test	5.30	0.03	0.54	67.78	0.001	0.87	17.84	0.001	0.79
Active repositioning									
15° of ankle inversion	3.35	0.08	0.42	12.37	0.006	0.55	0.48	0.63	0.09
0° in ankle neutral position	6.59	0.01	0.59	12.26	0.006	0.54	1.58	0.25	0.26
10° of ankle eversion	0.51	0.61	0.10	8.27	0.01	0.45	1.60	0.25	0,27
Passive repositioning									
15° of ankle inversion	1.27	0.32	0.22	1.15	0.32	0.10	0.34	0.71	0.07
0° in ankle neutral position	0.16	0.84	0.03	0.67	0.42	0.06	0.18	0.83	0.03
10° of ankle eversion	0.56	0.58	0.11	0.70	0.41	0.06	0.87	0.44	0.16
Ankle inversion									
30°/s COM (N-m/kg)	3.01	0.10	0.40	0.04	0.82	0.01	4.49	0.04	0.50
30°/s ECC (N-m/kg)	14.02	0.002	0.75	5.56	0.04	0.35	0.71	0.51	0.13
120°/s COM (N-m/kg)	1.42	0.28	0.24	2.44	0.14	0.19	0.97	0.41	0.17
120°/s ECC (N-m/kg)	1.83	021	029	001	056	001	022	045	0.04
Ankle eversion									
30°/s COM (N-m/kg)	1.53	0.26	0.25	2.76	0.12	0.21	0.53	0.60	0.10
30°/s ECC (N-m/kg)	0.16	0.85	0.03	0.49	0.48	0.04	0.22	0.80	0.04
120°/s COM (N-m/kg)	2.73	0.11	0.37	4.12	0.07	0.45	4.07	0.06	0.47
120°/s ECC (N-m/kg)	0.34	0.71	0.07	4.72	0.06	0.32	3.22	0.09	0.41

COM: concentric contraction; ECC: eccentric contraction.

Table 3. The main outcome measurements in two training groups using linear regression analysis.

	Group A			Group B		
	B	95% CI	p	B	95% CI	p
Composite of star excursion balance test	2.52	−8.29–13.34	0.58	−2.92	−6.68–0.84	0.10
Active repositioning						
15° of ankle inversion	−0.05	−0.19−−0.09	0.03	0.01	−0.08–0.12	0.71
0° in ankle neutral position	0.30	0.04–0.56	0.02	−0.02	−0.13−−0.001	0.04
10° of ankle eversion	−0.05	−0.25–0.15	0.55	0.02	−0.04–0.10	0.38
Passive repositioning						
15° of ankle inversion	−0.15	−0.32–0.01	0.05	−0.02	−0.09–0.03	0.34
0° in ankle neutral position	−0.02	−0.15–0.11	0.69	0.02	−0.03–0.07	0.36
10° of ankle eversion	0.05	−0.09–0.21	0.41	−0.009	−0.07–0.05	0.73
Ankle inversion						
30°/s COM (N-m/kg)	−0.07	−0.15−−0.01	0.04	−0.01	−0.03–0.008	0.17
30°/s ECC (N-m/kg)	0.04	−0.14–0.23	0.56	−0.005	−0.05–0.04	0.80
120°/s COM (N-m/kg)	−0.03	−0.11–0.04	0.31	−0.006	−0.03–0.02	0.64
120°/s ECC (N-m/kg)	0.03	−0.09–0.16	0.53	0.002	−0.02–0.03	0.88
Ankle eversion						
30°/s COM (N-m/kg)	−0.02	−0.09–0.04	0.36	−0.02	−0.04–0.005	0.09
30°/s ECC (N-m/kg)	0.02	−0.07–0.12	0.60	−0.01	−0.04–0.02	0.48
120°/s COM (N-m/kg)	0.06	−0.06–0.18	0.26	−0.005	−0.03–0.02	0.69
120°/s ECC (N-m/kg)	−0.07	−0.25–0.10	0.34	−0.01	−0.04–0.008	0.13

COM: concentric contraction; ECC: eccentric contraction.

Table 4. Results of star excursion balance test in three group.

	Group A		Group B		Group C	
	Pre-	Post-	Pre-	Post-	Pre-	Post-
Anterior	80.63 ± 9.78	88.27 ± 10.83	76.16 ± 7.56	91.30 ± 4.94 +	78.31 ± 12.40	81.45 ± 6.48
Anterolateral	72.35 ± 8.26	79.61 ± 15.14	71.74 ± 7.73	82.71 ± 8.54 +	75.65 ± 5.36	72.93 ± 2.88
Anteromedial	87.01 ± 15.30	93.69 ± 9.58 *	85.18 ± 6.14	98.25 ± 7.07 +	87.99 ± 11.85	80.63 ± 11.20
Posteromedial	81.27 ± 13.50	91.08 ± 13.51	85.59 ± 10.64	98.59 ± 11.04 +	85.20 ± 9.91	84.71 ± 11.86
Posterior	71.62 ± 13.16	85.42 ± 16.69	70.49 ± 13.95	97.33 ± 12.54 +	73.53 ± 10.34	79.50 ± 7.21
Posterolateral	68.10 ± 10.76	80.14 ± 12.39 *	63.37 ± 13.12	91.65 ± 13.01 +	68.17 ± 13.02	69.68 ± 6.47
Medial	87.27 ± 16.96	93.62 ± 8.91	84.64 ± 6.90	97.73 ± 4.82 +	86.84 ± 8.54	91.15 ± 5.10
Lateral	64.73 ± 13.36	70.33 ± 13.39 *	65.85 ± 13.26	85.58 ± 16.49 +	67.41 ± 8.20	59.69 ± 3.06
Composite	76.62 ± 9.80	85.27 ± 11.76	75.38 ± 5.83	92.89 ± 7.80 +	77.89 ± 4.60	77.47 ± 5.07

* $p < 0.05$, Group A vs. Group C, between-group using Bonferroni test; + $p < 0.05$, Group B vs. Group C, between-group using Bonferroni test.

The changes in active and passive repositioning data before and after assessment for the three groups are presented in Table 5. During active repositioning, for an ankle inversion of 15°, the main effects of group ($F_{(2, 60)} = 3.35$, $p = 0.08$), time ($F_{(2, 60)} = 12.37$, $p = 0.006$), and time × group ($F_{(2, 60)} = 0.48$, $p = 0.63$) were observed. For the neutral ankle position, the main effects of group ($F_{(2, 60)} = 6.59$, $p = 0.01$), time ($F_{(2, 60)} = 12.26$, $p = 0.006$), and time × group ($F_{(2, 60)} = 1.58$, $p = 0.25$) were observed. For an ankle eversion of 10°, the main effects of group ($F_{(2, 60)} = 0.51$, $p = 0.61$), time ($F_{(2, 60)} = 8.27$, $p = 0.01$), and time × group ($F_{(2, 60)} = 1.60$, $p = 0.25$) were observed. During passive repositioning, for an ankle inversion of 15°, neutral ankle position, and an ankle eversion of 10°, no statistical significance was observed in the main effects of group, time, and time × group ($p > 0.05$).

Table 5. Results of joint position sense measurements in three group.

	Group A		Group B		Group C	
	Pre-	Post-	Pre-	Post-	Pre-	Post-
Active repositioning						
15° of ankle inversion	7.78 ± 5.60	4.67 ± 2.49 *	7.32 ± 3.67	5.14 ± 1.84 +	8.33 ± 1.40	6.73 ± 1.66
0° in ankle neutral position	6.94 ± 3.83	4.55 ± 2.87 *	9.52 ± 2.71	6.55 ± 1.40 +	9.06 ± 2.94	9.25 ± 1.02
10° of ankle eversion	7.22 ± 4.94	4.35 ± 2.24 *	7.65 ± 3.31	4.55 ± 2.16 +	7.00 ± 4.10	6.84 ± 2.92
Passive repositioning						
15° of ankle inversion	6.17 ± 4.72	5.55 ± 3.45	6.45 ± 3.56	4.23 ± 1.07	7.67 ± 4.43	4.79 ± 2.51
0° in ankle neutral position	6.78 ± 3.32	5.21 ± 3.47	5.40 ± 3.03	5.16 ± 3.86	5.86 ± 4.31	5.16 ± 3.12
10° of ankle eversion	6.41 ± 3.42	4.50 ± 2.74	6.75 ± 2.69	6.25 ± 3.62	6.45 ± 4.36	6.70 ± 3.78

* $p < 0.05$, Group A vs. Group C, between-group using Bonferroni test; + $p < 0.05$, Group B vs. Group C, between-group using Bonferroni test.

For active repositioning data, the within-group analysis of Group A revealed a significant decrease in neutral ankle position ($p = 0.04$) but no significant decreases for an ankle inversion of 15° ($p = 0.16$) and an ankle eversion of 10° ($p = 0.13$). In Group B, significant decreases for an ankle inversion of 15° ($p = 0.01$), neutral ankle position ($p = 0.02$), and an ankle eversion of 10° ($p = 0.01$) were observed. Post hoc tests indicated no significant differences within the three groups before assessment. Compared with Group C, Groups A and B exhibited significant decreases for an ankle inversion of 15°, neutral ankle position, and an ankle eversion of 10° ($p < 0.05$). Very small to small effect sizes were observed for an ankle inversion of 15° (d = −0.97, 95% CI = −1.61 to −0.33), neutral ankle position (d = −2.18, 95% CI = −2.94 to −1.41), and an ankle eversion of 10° (d = −0.95, 95% CI = −1.59 to −0.31) after assessment between Groups A and C. Between Groups A and C, small to medium effect sizes were also observed for an ankle inversion of 15° (d = −0.90, 95% CI = −1.54 to −0.27), neutral ankle position (d = −2.20, 95% CI = −2.97 to −1.43), and an ankle eversion of 10° (d = −0.89, 95% CI = −1.52 to −0.25) after assessment.

The CON and ECC data before and after assessment for the three groups are presented in Table 6. For 30°/s of CON ankle inversion, the main effects of group ($F_{(2, 60)}$ = 3.01, p = 0.10), time ($F_{(2, 60)}$ = 0.04, p = 0.82), and time × group ($F_{(2, 60)}$ = 4.49, p = 0.04) were observed. For 30°/s of ECC ankle inversion, the main effects of group ($F_{(2, 60)}$ = 14.02, p = 0.002), time ($F_{(2, 60)}$ = 5.56, p = 0.04), and time × group ($F_{(2, 60)}$ = 0.71, p = 0.51) were observed. Post hoc tests indicated no significant differences within the three groups for 30°/s of CON and ECC ankle inversion before assessment, but the number of ankle invertor muscle contractions in Group C was significantly lower than those in Groups A and B for 30°/s of CON (p = 0.01 and p = 0.02, respectively) and 30°/s of ECC (p = 0.01 and p = 0.001, respectively). Very small effect sizes were observed in 30°/s of CON ankle inversion after assessment in Group A (d = 1.24, 95% CI = 0.58–1.90) and Group B (d = 1.13, 95% CI = 0.47–1.78) compared with Group C. Small effect sizes were also observed in 30°/s of ECC ankle inversion after assessment in Group A (d = 1.15, 95% CI = 0.49–1.80) and Group B (d = 1.37, 95% CI = 0.69–2.04) compared with Group C. However, no significant main effects of group, time, and time × group (p > 0.05) were observed in 30°/s of ECC and CON ankle eversion. In addition, for 120°/s of CON and ECC ankle inversion or eversion, no statistical significance was observed in the main effects of group, time, and time × group (p > 0.05). Regarding the analysis of the ratios of inversion and eversion for ECC or CON at 30°/s and 120°/s, no isokinetic parameters were statistically significant after using two-way repeated-measures ANOVA (p > 0.05).

Table 6. Results of isokinetic strength test in three groups.

	Group A		Group B		Group C	
	Pre-	Post-	Pre-	Post-	Pre-	Post-
Ankle inversion						
30°/s COM (N-m/kg)	28.47 ± 9.79	32.27 ± 9.25 *	27.52 ± 9.26	29.91 ± 6.80 +	26.89 ± 11.14	21.90 ± 7.35
30°/s ECC (N-m/kg)	30.23 ± 6.53	33.15 ± 9.75 *	29.73 ± 5.61	32.45 ± 6.17 +	23.06 ± 9.06	23.31 ± 7.13
120°/s COM (N-m/kg)	26.81 ± 7.14	32.00 ± 10.89	23.11 ± 11.33	26.44 ± 7.35	24.45 ± 12.83	24.35 ± 10.40
120°/s ECC (N-m/kg)	29.61 ± 11.18	31.75 ± 9.42	26.05 ± 8.83	23.96 ± 8.17	26.63 ± 11.22	27.27 ± 10.77
Ankle eversion						
30°/s COM (N-m/kg)	22.87 ± 5.36	26.74 ± 6.79	20.40 ± 8.85	21.39 ± 8.61	20.12 ± 4.00	21.61 ± 8.83
30°/s ECC (N-m/kg)	28.18 ± 6.09	30.83 ± 7.15	28.20 ± 8.24	29.73 ± 7.24	28.59 ± 7.99	27.74 ± 8.80
120°/s COM (N-m/kg)	24.84 ± 8.86	29.22 ± 8.18	21.00 ± 12.16	32.08 ± 3.48	21.08 ± 4.30	22.39 ± 4.91
120°/s ECC (N-m/kg)	29.65 ± 7.10	32.90 ± 8.28	26.72 ± 10.23	35.64 ± 5.74	29.87 ± 8.91	28.35 ± 7.10
Angular velocity (30°/s)						
COMeverton/COMinverton	0.85 ± 0.25	0.90 ± 0.36	0.76 ± 0.23	0.81 ± 0.45	0.84 ± 0.31	0.90 ± 0.43
ECCeverton/ECCinverton	0.97 ± 0.29	1.02 ± 0.43	0.96 ± 0.25	0.98 ± 0.35	0.95 ± 0.32	0.98 ± 0.48
ECCeverton/COMinverton	1.05 ± 0.30	1.07 ± 0.46	1.21 ± 0.47	1.06 ± 0.44	1.09 ± 0.64	1.23 ± 0.52
Angular velocity (120°/s)						
COMeverton/COMinverton	1.05 ± 0.46	1.05 ± 0.52	1.08 ± 0.49	1.01 ± 0.34	1.27 ± 0.29	1.04 ± 0.38
ECCeverton/ECCinverton	1.20 ± 0.72	1.13 ± 0.51	1.14 ± 0.55	1.21 ± 0.46	1.16 ± 0.33	1.11 ± 0.46
ECCevertor/COMinvertor	1.18 ± 0.43	1.15 ± 0.49	1.31 ± 0.67	1.22 ± 0.38	1.25 ± 0.39	1.20 ± 0.49

* p < 0.05, Group A vs. Group C, between-group using Bonferroni test; + p < 0.05, Group B vs. Group C, between-group using Bonferroni test; concentric contraction, CON; eccentric contraction, ECC.

4. Discussion

Compared with the control group, the female athletes with dominant-leg CAI improved in the SEBT, the active repositioning portion of the joint position sense test, and 30°/s of CON and ECC of the ankle invertor in the isokinetic strength test after completing a 6-week WVB or balance training program. However, very small to small effect sizes for the assessed outcomes were observed between the exercise programs and control groups.

Sixty-three female athletes (50 basketball players and 13 volleyball players) with CAI participated in the study. Some prospective studies have reported that 19%–20% of ankle sprain rates occur in female basketball players [26,27]. Compared with male athletes, female athletes often experience greater laxity in the ankle joint and its ligaments.

These sex-specific differences are caused by variations in hormone levels [28]. In addition, because the dominant leg is preferentially used for jumping and landing in basketball and volleyball, 80% of CAI in the dominant ankle is due to participation in sports [26]. Balance exercise programs have been designed specifically for female athletes, and the resulting improvements in balance and stability after completing such programs could reduce the risk of contact ankle sprains [29]. To our knowledge, the current study is the first to compare two exercise training programs with a control group. After 6 weeks, the WVB training group performed better than the balance training group did, and both groups exhibited improvements in dynamic balance, joint position sense, and isokinetic muscle strength after assessment. However, compared with the control group, both groups contributed to very small or small effect sizes of the assessed variables.

Balance deficit is the main cause of increased risk of recurring ankle sprain [30]. The exercise training programs, i.e., WBV and balance training, also play a decisive role in the rehabilitation process after an ankle sprain [31,32]. Some studies have suggested that balance training, especially by using the BOSU Balance Trainer, effectively reduces the balance deficit in patients with CAI [33,34]. WBV training is a popular method used for CAI rehabilitation and mitigating ankle instability. WBV training can increase α and γ neuron excitability and improve muscle spindle sensitivity, resulting in decreased muscular reaction time [8,9]. Therefore, the effects of WBV training on CAI could enhance ankle posture control during the SEBT, a dynamic balance measurement tool. Compared with the control group, female athletes with CAI experienced enhanced dynamic balance through WBV training and by using the BOSU Balance Trainer, both of which resulted in similar effects. However, both training programs contributed to very small or small effect sizes for CAI. Rendos et al. observed that WBV training does not cause acute dynamic balance improvements in patients with CAI [35]. Sierra-Guzmán et al. observed that compared with a control group, athletes with CAI exhibited moderate effect sizes (d = 0.54) in a composite score of SEBT after 6-week programs combining WBV training and the BOSU Balance Trainer [36]. Cloak et al. also observed a significant increase in the SEBT and revealed that 6-week programs combining WBV and a wobble board were effective for athletes with CAI [7]. Established programs combined with WBV may be a potential rehabilitation strategy for athletes with CAI, and should be studied in the future.

The joint position sense test measures joint kinesthesia and is used to measure the sensorimotor deficit of CAI [37]. Compared with the control group, athletes who underwent 6-week programs incorporating WBV training and the BOSU Balance Trainer showed improvement in the active repositioning of joint position sense at an ankle inversion of 15°, neutral ankle position, and an ankle eversion of 10°, but no significant improvement in passive repositioning ($p > 0.05$). Sousa et al. indicated that CAI could cause a decrease in joint position sense during ankle inversion, consequently affecting functional ankle movement [38]. In the current study, the reduced joint position error in ankle inversion and eversion is the contraction that was improved by both balance training programs. During active repositioning, the detection of movement sensation is markedly enhanced by ankle muscle contraction. We observed that the enhancement in active repositioning was better than that in passive repositioning because of the increase in spindle afferent activity and muscle strength [39]. Otzel et al. applied WBV at 35 Hz for CAI rehabilitation and reported no improvement in joint position accuracy or proprioception [40]. In the current study, the WBV training with a frequency of 5 Hz could improve the joint kinesthesia ability of ankle inversion and eversion in active repositioning for CAI, and the effects were the same as the balance training program. Baumbach et al. indicated that the frequency of WBV may be a key factor in CAI rehabilitation [41]. A frequency of <10 Hz is used for relaxing muscles; a frequency between 10 Hz and 20 Hz is used for coordination exercises, and a frequency >20 Hz is used for enhancing muscle contractions in WBV training [42]. However, the effects of various WBV frequencies on joint position sense in CAI are unknown, and additional research on this issue is warranted.

Regarding ankle strength, Wilkerson et al. reported significantly greater deficits in inversion strength than in eversion strength by using an isokinetic dynamometer [43]. Concentric invertor strength deficits are commonly found in patients with CAI, resulting in deep peroneal nerve dysfunction or selective neuromuscular inhibition after ankle sprain [44]. Ko et al. analyzed isokinetic ankle invertor and evertor muscle strength at angular velocities of 30°/s and 120°/s in patients with CAI and observed a severe invertor strength deficit at an angular velocity of 30°/s [45]. In our findings, the ECC and CON invertor strengths at 30°/s of angular velocity in the WBV and balance training group were significantly higher than those in the control group ($p < 0.05$). However, no significant differences in ECC and CON at angular velocities of 30°/s and 120°/s were observed in both groups before and after assessment ($p > 0.05$). Three exercise movements (double-leg stance, one-legged stance, and tandem stance) were applied in our training program, which consisted of 6-week programs incorporating static balance training exercises on a vibration platform or balance ball. During the exercises, the athletes (who had CAI) were instructed to maintain their balance on an unstable surface. The low frequency of 5 Hz of WBV in addition to static posture control exercises improved the ankle invertor strengths in ECC and CON at an angular velocity of 30°/s. This strategy can be used as ankle invertor strength training for mitigating strength deficits in patients with CAI. The resultant increase in invertor isokinetic strength at a low angular velocity could be applied to reduce the capacity of control lateral postural sway during weight-bearing activities and to alleviate CAI symptoms [46].

Some studies have suggested that patients with CAI possess limited evertor isokinetic strength in injured ankles [47,48] and that an increase in evertor strength could assist the lateral ligaments in supporting a sudden ankle inversion movement [49]. The ECC of eversion/CON of inversion strength ratio, which is a functional agonist/antagonist strength ratio, is focused on outcome measurements for patients with CAI. Because normal movement patterns of lower extremities and gait patterns involve the interaction of agonist and antagonist strength, the strength ratio was used as an indicator of rehabilitation training for patients with CAI [50]. Brent et al. used the ankle eversion/inversion strength ratio to assess the outcomes of a 6-week strength training program for CAI and indicated that the balance of ankle eversion and inversion strength can support injured ligaments and improve ankle stability [49]. In the current study, the ankle eversion isokinetic strength and eversion/inversion isokinetic strength ratio at 30°/s and 120°/s angular velocities and the ECC of eversion/COM of inversion strength ratio did not exhibit significant differences within and between the groups ($p > 0.05$). Brent et al. reported that ankle invertor and evertor strength was significantly increased in college students with CAI after a 6-week strength training program [49]. Mohd Salim et al. also observed that the ankle eversion/inversion strength ratio improved in the ankles of patients with CAI after a 1-week standard physiotherapy program [51]. These studies suggest that ankle eversion or inversion strength in the ankles of patients with CAI could be increased compared with those with healthy ankles after specific exercise training for mitigating CAI [49,51]. However, we are the first to further examine the ECC and CON of eversion and inversion strengths at various angular velocities and compare training and nontraining groups in the context of the ankles of patients with CAI. Research on this topic is rare, and comparing the effects of ankle eversion or inversion on isokinetic strength after a balance training program specific to patients with CAI remains challenging.

This study had several limitations. First, the participants with CAI self-reported their symptoms and ankle sprain history, which could be misleading when determining CAI status. Second, dorsiflexion and plantar flexion movements were not involved in the measurement of joint position sense and isokinetic strength. The anterior and posterior kinetic chain involving ankle stability was not discussed after the training programs. Third, lack of long-term follow-up could not confirm the cure of CAI or long-term effects. Four, our exercise training programs may be of insufficient duration and exercise implementation as normal fitness training. Our results revealed that there were very small or small effect sizes for CAI in dynamic balance, joint kinesthesia ability, and muscle strength of the ankle invertor and evertor after 6-week WBV or balance training. We researched the effects of the 20-min exercise comprised of three exercise movements performed on a balance ball or vibration platform. The variability of movement design may be inadequate, and the progress of training intensity maybe also insufficient, resulting in a very small or small effects on improvement of muscle strength, proprioception and balance ability. Investigation on the effects on different program designs of WBV or balance training in future studies is recommended.

5. Conclusions

Compared with the control group, female athletes who participated in 6-week exercise training programs incorporating a vibration platform and balance ball exhibited very small or small effect sizes for CAI in the SEBT, the joint position sense test, and the isokinetic strength test; in addition, COM and ECC at an ankle inversion of 30°/s were enhanced. We observed no differences among the variables within the two exercise training programs. A balance training program combining WBV training with a balance ball may be a potentially effective strategy for mitigating CAI, but further research is required to confirm these results.

Author Contributions: W.-D.C. and Y.-A.T. contributed to designing the method, and wrote the first draft of the report, with input from the other authors. S.C. conducted the data analyses. All authors have read and agreed to the published version of the manuscript.

Funding: This research received no funding.

Institutional Review Board Statement: The study was conducted according to the guidelines of the Declaration of Helsinki, and approved by the Internal Review Board of China Medical University Hospital (CRREC-106-063).

Informed Consent Statement: Informed consent was obtained from all subjects involved in the study.

Data Availability Statement: Data is contained within the article.

Conflicts of Interest: The authors declare no conflict of interests regarding the publication of this paper.

Abbreviations

WBV	whole-body vibration
CAI	chronic ankle instability
SEBT	Star Excursion Balance Test
CON	concentric contraction
ECC	eccentric contraction

References

1. Sierra-Guzmán, R.; Jiménez, F.; Abián-Vicén, J. Predictors of chronic ankle instability: Analysis of peroneal reaction time, dynamic balance and isokinetic strength. *Clin. Biomech.* **2018**, *54*, 28–33. [CrossRef]
2. Eechaute, C.; Vaes, P.; Duquet, W. The dynamic postural control is impaired in patients with chronic ankle instability: Reliability and validity of the multiple hop test. *Clin. J. Sport Med.* **2009**, *19*, 107–114. [CrossRef]
3. Delahunt, E.; Coughlan, G.F.; Caulfield, B.; Nightingale, E.J.; Lin, C.W.; Hiller, C.E. Inclusion criteria when investigating insufficiencies in chronic ankle instability. *Med. Sci. Sports Exerc.* **2010**, *42*, 2106–2121. [CrossRef]
4. Schiftan, G.S.; Ross, L.A.; Hahne, A.J. The effectiveness of proprioceptive training in preventing ankle sprains in sporting populations: A systematic review and meta-analysis. *J. Sci. Med. Sport.* **2015**, *18*, 238–244. [CrossRef] [PubMed]
5. De Ridder, R.; Willems, T.; Vanrenterghem, J.; Roosen, P. Influence of balance surface on ankle stabilizing muscle activity in subjects with chronic ankle instability. *J. Rehabil. Med.* **2015**, *47*, 632–638. [CrossRef]
6. Levin, O.; Vanwanseele, B.; Thijsen, J.R.; Helsen, W.F.; Staes, F.F.; Duysens, J. Proactive and reactive neuromuscular control in subjects with chronic ankle instability: Evidence from a pilot study on landing. *Gait Posture* **2015**, *41*, 106–111. [CrossRef] [PubMed]

7. Cloak, R.; Nevill, A.; Day, S.; Wyon, M. Six-week combined vibration and wobble board training on balance and stability in footballers with functional ankle instability. *Clin. J. Sport Med.* **2013**, *23*, 384–391. [CrossRef] [PubMed]
8. Cardinale, M.; Bosco, C. The use of vibration as an exercise intervention. *Exerc. Sport Sci. Rev.* **2003**, *31*, 3–7. [CrossRef] [PubMed]
9. Pollock, R.D.; Woledge, R.C.; Martin, F.C.; Newham, D.J. Effects of whole body vibration on motor unit recruitment and threshold. *J. Appl. Physiol.* **2012**, *112*, 388–395. [CrossRef]
10. Peters, M. Footedness: Asymmetries in foot preference and skill and neuropsychological assessment of foot movement. *Psychol. Bull.* **1988**, *103*, 179–192. [CrossRef] [PubMed]
11. van Melick, N.; Meddeler, B.M.; Hoogeboom, T.J.; Nijhuis-van der Sanden, M.W.G.; van Cingel, R.E.H. How to determine leg dominance: The agreement between self-reported and observed performance in healthy adults. *PLoS ONE* **2017**, *12*, e0189876. [CrossRef] [PubMed]
12. Caldemeyer, L.E.; Brown, S.M.; Mulcahey, M.K. Neuromuscular training for the prevention of ankle sprains in female athletes: A systematic review. *Phys. Sportsmed.* **2020**, *48*, 363–369. [CrossRef] [PubMed]
13. Ristolainen, L.; Heinonen, A.; Waller, B.; Kujala, U.M.; Kettunen, J.A. Gender differences in sport injury risk and types of inju-ries: A retrospective twelve-month study on cross-country skiers, swimmers, long-distance runners and soccer players. *J. Sports Sci. Med.* **2009**, *8*, 443–451. [PubMed]
14. Hosea, T.M.; Carey, C.C.; Harrer, M.F. The gender issue: Epidemiology of ankle injuries in athletes who participate in basketball. *Clin. Orthop. Relat. Res.* **2000**, *372*, 45–49. [CrossRef] [PubMed]
15. Brumitt, J.; Mattocks, A.; Loew, J.; Lentz, P. Preseason functional performance test measures are associated with injury in female college volleyball players. *J. Sport Rehabil.* **2020**, *29*, 320–325. [CrossRef] [PubMed]
16. Gribble, P.A.; Delahunt, E.; Bleakley, C.M.; Caulfield, B.; Docherty, C.L.; Fong, D.T.; Fourchet, F.; Hertel, J.; Hiller, C.E.; Kaminski, T.W.; et al. Selection criteria for patients with chronic ankle instability in controlled research: A position statement of the International Ankle Consortium. *J. Athl. Train.* **2014**, *49*, 121–127. [CrossRef] [PubMed]
17. Sefton, J.M.; Yarar, C.; Hicks-Little, C.A.; Berry, J.W.; Cordova, M.L. Six weeks of balance training improves sensorimotor function in individuals with chronic ankle instability. *J. Orthop. Sports Phys. Ther.* **2011**, *41*, 81–89. [CrossRef]
18. Hertel, J.; Miller, S.; Denegar, C. Intratester and intertester reliability during the Star Excursion Balance Tests. *J. Sport Rehab.* **2000**, *9*, 104–116. [CrossRef]
19. Hertel, J.; Braham, R.A.; Hale, S.A.; Olmsted-Kramer, L.C. Simplifying the star excursion balance test: Analyses of subjects with and without chronic ankle instability. *J. Orthop. Sports Phys. Ther.* **2006**, *36*, 131–137. [CrossRef]
20. Sekir, U.; Yildiz, Y.; Hazneci, B.; Ors, F.; Saka, T.; Aydin, T. Reliability of a functional test battery evaluating functionality, proprioception, and strength in recreational athletes with functional ankle instability. *Eur. J. Phys. Rehabil. Med.* **2008**, *44*, 407–415.
21. Brown, C.; Ross, S.; Mynark, R.; Guskiewics, K. Assessing functional ankle instability with joint position sense, time to stabilization, and electromyography. *J. Sport Rehabil.* **2004**, *13*, 122–134. [CrossRef]
22. Tankevicius, G.; Lankaite, D.; Krisciunas, A. Test-retest reliability of biodex system 4 pro for isometric ankle-eversion and -inversion measurement. *J. Sport Rehabil.* **2013**, *22*, 212–215. [CrossRef] [PubMed]
23. Fish, M.; Milligan, J.; Killey, J. Is it possible to establish reference values for ankle muscle isokinetic strength? A meta-analytical study. *Isokinet. Exerc. Sci.* **2014**, *22*, 85–97. [CrossRef]
24. Kaminski, T.W.; Buckley, B.D.; Powers, M.E.; Hubbard, T.J.; Ortiz, C. Effect of strength and proprioception training on eversion to inversion strength ratios in subjects with unilateral functional ankle instability. *Br. J. Sports Med.* **2003**, *37*, 410–415. [CrossRef] [PubMed]
25. Cohen, J. *Statistical Power Analysis for the Behavioral Sciences*, 2nd ed.; Lawrence Erlbaum Associates: Hillsdale, NJ, USA, 1988.
26. Willems, T.M.; Witvrouw, E.; Delbaere, K.; Philippaerts, R.; De Bourdeaudhuij, I.; De Clercq, D. Intrinsic risk factors for inversion ankle sprains in females—A prospective study. *Scand. J. Med. Sci. Sports* **2005**, *15*, 336–345. [CrossRef] [PubMed]
27. Beynnon, B.D.; Renström, P.A.; Alosa, D.M.; Baumhauer, J.F.; Vacek, P.M. Ankle ligament injury risk factors: A prospective study of college athletes. *J. Orthop. Res.* **2001**, *19*, 213–220. [CrossRef]
28. Quatman, C.E.; Ford, K.R.; Myer, G.D.; Paterno, M.V.; Hewett, T.E. The effects of gender and pubertal status on generalized joint laxity in young athletes. *J. Sci. Med. Sport* **2008**, *11*, 257–263. [CrossRef]
29. Frank, R.M.; Romeo, A.A.; Bush-Joseph, C.A.; Bach, B.R., Jr. Injuries to the female athlete in 2017: Part II: Upper and lower-extremity injuries. *JBJS Rev.* **2017**, *5*, e5. [CrossRef]
30. Pierobon, A.; Raguzzi, I.; Soliño, S.; Salzberg, D.; Vuoto, T.; Gilgado, D.; Perez Calvo, E. Minimal detectable change and reliability of the star excursion balance test in patients with lateral ankle sprain. *Physiother. Res. Int.* **2020**, *25*, 1850. [CrossRef]
31. Halabchi, F.; Hassabi, M. Acute ankle sprain in athletes: Clinical aspects and algorithmic approach. *World J. Orthop.* **2020**, *11*, 534–558. [CrossRef] [PubMed]
32. D'Hooghe, P.; Cruz, F.; Alkhelaifi, K. Return to play after a lateral ligament ankle sprain. *Curr. Rev. Musculoskelet. Med.* **2020**, *13*, 281–288. [CrossRef] [PubMed]
33. Laudner, K.G.; Koschnitzky, M.M. Ankle muscle activation when using the Both Sides Utilized (BOSU) balance trainer. *J. Strength Cond. Res.* **2010**, *24*, 218–222. [CrossRef] [PubMed]
34. Strøm, M.; Thorborg, K.; Bandholm, T.; Tang, L.; Zebis, M.; Nielsen, K.; Bencke, J. Ankle joint control during single-legged balance using common balance training devices–implications for rehabilitation strategies. *Int. J. Sports Phys. Ther.* **2016**, *11*, 388–399. [PubMed]

35. Rendos, N.K.; Jun, H.P.; Pickett, N.M.; Lew Feirman, K.; Harriell, K.; Lee, S.Y.; Signorile, J.F. Acute effects of whole body vibration on balance in persons with and without chronic ankle instability. *Res. Sports Med.* **2017**, *25*, 391–407. [CrossRef] [PubMed]
36. Sierra-Guzmán, R.; Jiménez-Diaz, F.; Ramírez, C.; Esteban, P.; Abián-Vicén, J. Whole-body-vibration training and balance in recreational athletes with chronic ankle instability. *J. Athl. Train.* **2018**, *53*, 355–363. [CrossRef] [PubMed]
37. Xue, X.; Ma, T.; Li, Q.; Song, Y.; Hua, Y. Chronic ankle instability is associated with proprioception deficits: A systematic review with meta-analysis. *J. Sport Health Sci.* **2020**, *2020*, 1–10. [CrossRef]
38. Sousa, A.S.P.; Leite, J.; Costa, B.; Santos, R. Bilateral proprioceptive evaluation in individuals with unilateral chronic ankle instability. *J. Athl. Train.* **2017**, *52*, 360–367. [CrossRef]
39. Lönn, J.; Crenshaw, A.G.; Djupsjöbacka, M.; Pedersen, J.; Johansson, H. Position sense testing: Influence of starting position and type of displacement. *Arch. Phys. Med. Rehabil.* **2000**, *81*, 592–597. [CrossRef]
40. Otzel, D.M.; Hass, C.J.; Wikstrom, E.A.; Bishop, M.D.; Borsa, P.A.; Tillman, M.D. Motoneuron function does not change following whole-body vibration in individuals with chronic ankle instability. *J. Sport Rehabil.* **2019**, *28*, 614–622. [CrossRef]
41. Baumbach, S.F.; Fasser, M.; Polzer, H.; Sieb, M.; Regauer, M.; Mutschler, W.; Schieker, M.; Blauth, M. Study protocol: The effect of whole body vibration on acute unilateral unstable lateral ankle sprain—A biphasic randomized controlled trial. *BMC Musculoskelet. Disord.* **2013**, *14*, 22. [CrossRef]
42. Rittweger, J.; Just, K.; Kautzsch, K.; Reeg, P.; Felsenberg, D. Treatment of chronic lower back pain with lumbar extension and whole-body vibration exercise: A randomized controlled trial. *Spine* **2002**, *27*, 1829–1834. [CrossRef] [PubMed]
43. Wilkerson, G.B.; Pinerola, J.J.; Caturano, R.W. Invertor vs. evertor peak torque and power deficiencies associated with lateral ankle ligament injury. *J. Orthop. Sports Phys. Ther.* **1997**, *26*, 78–86. [CrossRef]
44. Hertel, J. Functional snatomy, pathomechanics, and pathophysiology of lateral ankle instability. *J. Athl. Train.* **2002**, *37*, 364–375. [PubMed]
45. Ko, K.R.; Lee, H.; Lee, W.Y.; Sung, K.S. Ankle strength is not strongly associated with postural stability in patients awaiting surgery for chronic lateral ankle instability. *Knee Surg. Sports Traumatol. Arthrosc.* **2020**, *28*, 326–333. [CrossRef]
46. Munn, J.; Beard, D.J.; Refshauge, K.M.; Lee, R.Y. Eccentric muscle strength in functional ankle instability. *Med. Sci. Sports Exerc.* **2003**, *35*, 245–250. [CrossRef]
47. Willems, T.; Witvrouw, E.; Verstuyft, J.; Vaes, P.; De Clercq, D. Proprioception and muscle strength in subjects with a history of ankle sprains and chronic instability. *J. Athl. Train.* **2002**, *37*, 487–493.
48. Bosien, W.R.; Staples, S.; Russell, S.W. Residual disability following acute ankle sprains. *J. Bone Jt. Surg. Am.* **1955**, *37*, 1237–1243. [CrossRef] [PubMed]
49. Brent, I.S.; Carrie, L.D.; Janet, S.; Joanne, K.; John, S. Ankle strength and force sense after a progressive, 6-week strength training programme in people with functional ankle instability. *J. Athl. Train.* **2012**, *47*, 282–288.
50. Yildiz, Y.; Aydin, T.; Sekir, U.; Hazneci, B.; Komurcu, M.; Kalyon, T.A. Peak and end range eccentric evertor/concentric invertor muscle strength ratios in chronically unstable ankles: Comparison with healthy individuals. *J. Sports Sci. Med.* **2003**, *2*, 70–76.
51. Mohd Salim, N.S.; Umar, M.A.; Shaharudin, S. Effects of the standard physiotherapy programme on pain and isokinetic ankle strength in individuals with grade I ankle sprain. *J. Taibah. Univ. Med. Sci.* **2018**, *13*, 576–581. [CrossRef] [PubMed]

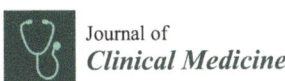

Article

Risk Factors for Non-Contact Lower-Limb Injury: A Retrospective Survey in Pediatric-Age Athletes

Yanfei Guan [1], Shannon S. D. Bredin [1], Jack Taunton [2], Qinxian Jiang [3], Nana Wu [1], Yongfeng Li [4] and Darren E. R. Warburton [1,5,*]

[1] Physical Activity Promotion and Chronic Disease Prevention Unit, School of Kinesiology, Faculty of Education, University of British Columbia, Vancouver, BC V6T 1Z4, Canada; yanfei.guan@ubc.ca (Y.G.); shannon.bredin@ubc.ca (S.S.D.B.); nana.wu@ubc.ca (N.W.)
[2] Allan McGavin Sport Medicine Centre, Faculty of Medicine, University of British Columbia, Vancouver, BC V6T 1Z3, Canada; jack.taunton@ubc.ca
[3] Department of Physical Education, Weifang Medical University, Weifang 261053, China; qinxian.jiang@wfmc.edu.cn
[4] College of Sports and Health, Shandong Sport University, Ji'nan 250102, China; liyongfeng@sdpei.edu.cn
[5] Experimental Medicine Program, Faculty of Medicine, University of British Columbia, Vancouver, BC V6T 1Z4, Canada
* Correspondence: darren.warburton@ubc.ca; Tel.: +1-604-822-4603

Abstract: Background: Risk factors for non-contact lower-limb injury in pediatric-age athletes and the effects of lateral dominance in sport (laterally vs. non-laterally dominant sports) on injury have not been investigated. Purpose: To identify risk factors for non-contact lower-limb injury in pediatric-age athletes. Methods: Parents and/or legal guardians of 2269 athletes aged between 6–17 years were recruited. Each participant completed an online questionnaire that contained 10 questions about the athlete's training and non-contact lower-limb injury in the preceding 12 months. Results: The multivariate logistic regression model determined that lateral dominance in sport (adjusted OR (laterally vs. non-laterally dominant sports), 1.38; 95% CI, 1.10–1.75; $p = 0.006$), leg preference (adjusted OR (right vs. left-leg preference), 0.71; 95% CI, 0.53–0.95; $p = 0.023$), increased age (adjusted OR, 1.21; 95% CI, 1.16–1.26; $p = 0.000$), training intensity (adjusted OR, 1.77; 95% CI, 1.43–2.19; $p = 0.000$), and training frequency (adjusted OR, 1.36; 95% CI, 1.25–1.48; $p = 0.000$) were significantly associated with non-contact lower-limb injury in pediatric-age athletes. Length of training ($p = 0.396$) and sex ($p = 0.310$) were not associated with a non-contact lower-limb injury. Conclusions: Specializing in laterally dominant sports, left-leg preference, increase in age, training intensity, and training frequency indicated an increased risk of non-contact lower-limb injury in pediatric-age athletes. Future research should take into account exposure time and previous injury.

Keywords: injury risk; pediatric sport; lateral dominance; injury prediction

1. Introduction

The injury rate is high in children and adolescents participating in sports activities [1–4]. Radelet et al. [4] reported that the injury rate ranged from 1.0 to 2.3 per 100 athlete exposures in 7 to 13-year-old children in community sports. In 12 to 15-year-old students, the injury rate in sports activities was 60.85 injuries/100 students/year [1]. Compared to adults, children and adolescents are more vulnerable to sports injuries due to the stage of maturation in growth cartilage and the musculoskeletal system [4,5]. Both acute and overuse injuries in growth cartilage may result in the permanent alteration of bone and muscle growth, which may have a long-term impact such as disability in later life if the injury is not properly treated [6,7].

A number of survey studies have investigated sports injury and related risk factors in children and adolescents [1–4,8,9], demonstrating that the most common sport injuries occur to the lower limbs, with the ankle and knee the most frequently injured locations [1,2,8].

Although contact injuries account for the majority of sport injuries [8,10], some non-contact injuries (e.g., ankle sprains and muscle strains) are found to be the most common injuries across sports [2,10]. Further, non-contact injuries are often associated with modifiable risk factors such as neuromuscular disorders, overtraining, and being unfit [11]. However, there is a lack of survey-based research investigating the risk factors for non-contact lower-limb injury in pediatric-age athletes. This is an important cohort to focus research on, especially considering that children as young as 6 years of age (or even younger) engage in competitive sport training [12].

Regardless of the mechanism (contact vs. non-contact) of injury, studies have reported a range of risk factors for sports injury in children and adolescents, including training duration [8], impact [4,8], age [13], sex [13], previous injury [2,13], amount of physical activity [3], and stage of maturity [3]. To date, there is a lack of research examining the potential effects of lateral dominance in sport (laterally dominant vs. non-laterally dominant sport) on the risk of injury in the lower limbs. Laterally dominant sports (or asymmetric sports, e.g., fencing, badminton, and soccer) are characterized by the two sides of the lower limbs frequently performing in different patterns [14] or performing movements that are directed towards one side [15]. For example, in the lunge movement, which is frequently performed in fencing, tennis, and badminton, the dominant leg performs as the leading leg while the non-dominant leg performs as the supporting leg [14]. This asymmetric movement may cause lateral dominance and relative adaptions of the dominant leg in the long-term [14]. In contrast, non-laterally dominant sports (or symmetric sports, e.g., running, swimming) are characterized by both sides of the lower limbs equally involved in the movements, requiring equal mastery of techniques with the dominant and non-dominant leg [15]. Compared with non-laterally dominant sports, long-term training in laterally dominant sports may cause greater inter-limb asymmetry which has been associated with an increased risk of lower-limb injury [16,17]. To date, there is no evidence available in the literature reporting the injury rate between athletes specialized in laterally dominant vs. non-laterally dominant sports. Therefore, it is unknown empirically whether the laterally dominant moving pattern in laterally dominant sports will increase the risk of lower-limb injury.

The purpose of this study was to examine the effects of lateral dominance in sports (laterally dominant vs. non-laterally dominant sports) on non-contact lower-limb injury, and to identify risk factors of non-contact lower-limb injury in pediatric-age athletes. It was hypothesized that pediatric-age athletes specialized in laterally dominant sports would sustain a greater risk of non-contact lower-limb injury compared to those specialized in non-laterally dominant sports.

2. Method

2.1. Participants

Parents and/or legal guardians of pediatric-age athletes training in sports clubs and/or school teams were eligible to participate in the online survey, if the athletes met the following criteria: (1) were between the ages of 6 and 17 years, (2) specialized in only one sport, and (3) maintained regular training in the preceding 12 months. The levels of competition of the athletes were not limited. Informed consent was received upon completion and submission of the survey. The investigation received approval from, and was executed in exact accordance with, the ethical guidelines set forth by the University of British Columbia's Clinical Research Ethics Board and the Shandong Sport University's Human Ethics Committee for research involving human participants according to the standards established by the Declaration of Helsinki.

2.2. Questionnaire

The content of the questionnaire (Supplementary File) was developed based on previous surveys [4,5]. The parents and/or legal guardians were asked to answer 10 questions, reporting their child's age (y), sex, sport, dominant leg (right, left leg), length of training (y), training frequency (1, 2, 3, 4, 5 or more sessions/wk), training intensity (low, moderate, high), whether their children suffered any non-contact lower-limb injury (during training or competition) causing time loss for at least one day from participation in sports activities during the preceding 12 months, and the location and type of the injury. The question types included fill-in-the-blank questions (age, sex, sport, length of training), single-choice questions (dominant leg, training frequency, training intensity, presence or absence of injury), and multiple-choice questions (location and type of injury). A day lost due to injury was any day (including the day in which the participant was injured) where the participant was not permitted to or not able to participate in sporting activities in an unrestricted manner [18]. Participants were not asked about lower-limb injuries that occurred at a time other than during training or competition, or were caused by contact with equipment or another player. If the athlete sustained more than one injury during the preceding 12 months, participants were asked to report all the injuries [19]. Survey development included examination of the validity of the content. The questionnaire was reviewed by a sports medicine researcher, an athletic trainer, a physical education teacher, a sport psychologist, and three professors in the area of kinesiology. A pilot test was conducted in a taekwondo club before the actual large-scale survey was disseminated.

2.3. Procedures

Participant information and the link to an online questionnaire were sent to coaches. The coaches were contacted and identified by the members of the research team. The coaches were asked to send the questionnaire to the parents and/or legal guardians of the athletes who met the inclusion criteria of this study by email. The parents and/or legal guardians of the athletes completed and submitted the questionnaire online. All responses were anonymous. The survey was available online from June 2019 to June 2020.

2.4. Data Analyses

The criterion variable, non-contact lower-limb injury, was analyzed as a categorical variable (presence or absence of injury). The presence of injury was defined as a positive response to the question: "During the preceding 12 months, did you suffer any non-contact lower-limb injury causing time loss for at least one day from participation in sport activities?" The predictor variables were age (y), sex (female vs. male), leg preference (left vs. right leg), sport category (laterally dominant vs. non-laterally dominant sport), length of training (y), training frequency (sessions/wk), and training intensity (low, moderate, high). The continuous measurements (age and length of training) were described as mean ± standard deviation. The other measurements were described with frequencies and percentages.

2.5. Statistical Analyses

Normality and homoscedasticity assumption of the continuous data (age and length of training) were examined using the Kolmogorov-Smirnov and Levene's test, respectively. The Mann–Whitney U test was conducted to compare age and length of training between the injured and non-injured athletes as data were not normally distributed. Chi-square tests were employed to compare the proportion of injured athletes based on sex (males, females), training intensity (low, moderate, high intensity), training frequency (1, 2, 3, 4, 5 or more times/wk), leg preference (right, left leg), and sport category (non-laterally, laterally dominant sports).

A multivariate logistic regression model was used to calculate the adjusted odds ratio (OR) and 95% confidence interval (CI) for each predictor variable. Participants with missing data were excluded from related analyses. All statistical analyses were conducted using SPSS 23 with the alpha level set a priori at 0.05.

3. Results

A total of 2294 questionnaires were submitted. Any response was excluded if there was no response for the question of presence or absence of injury. Data from 2269 questionnaires were included in the final analyses. From these responses, 750 athletes (33.1%) specialized in laterally dominant sports (tennis, table tennis, soccer, badminton, fencing, long jump, shot put, high jump, baseball, and softball), and 1519 athletes (66.9%) specialized in non-laterally dominant sports (swimming, running, cycling, skating, basketball, taekwondo, rope skipping, dance, hockey, volleyball, traditional martial art, judo, kickboxing, karate, roller skating, gymnastics, and boxing). A total of 576 (25.4%) athletes sustained non-contact lower-limb injury causing time loss ($\geq$1 day) from participation in sport activities during the preceding 12 months. The ankle (12.1%), thigh (10.8%), and knee (10.6%) were most commonly reported as the location of injury (Figure 1). Ligament sprain (15.7%) and muscle strain (8.5%) were the most commonly reported non-contact lower-limb injuries (Figure 2).

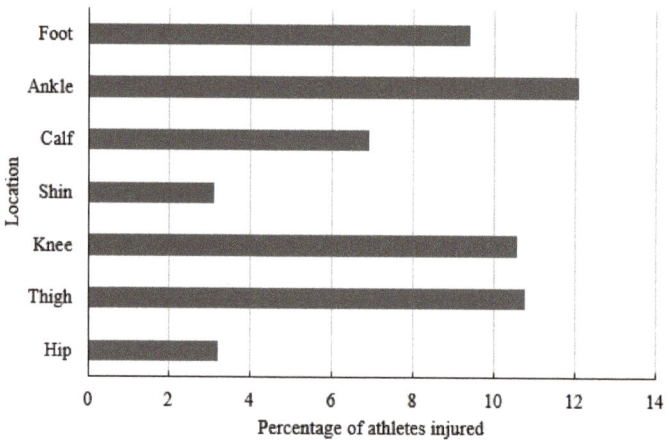

Figure 1. Injury breakdown by location.

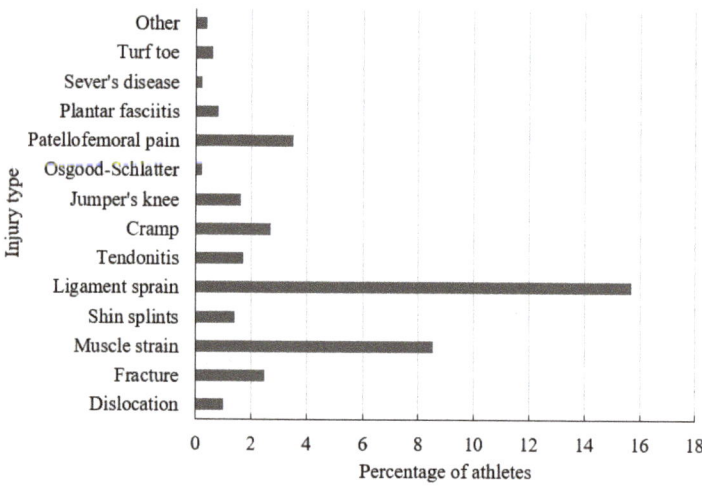

Figure 2. Injury breakdown by type.

The injured group showed significantly greater age (mean rank: 1417.58 vs. 1009.82, $n = 2227$, $p = 0.000$) and length of training (mean rank: 1192.72 vs. 971.22, $n = 2059$, $p = 0.000$) compared to the non-injured participants (Table 1). Results of the Chi-square tests (Table 2) showed that the injury rate increased with increasing training intensity (χ^2 (2, 2265) = 151.794, $p = 0.000$, Cramér's V = 0.259) and training frequency

(χ^2 (4, 2267) = 183.817, p = 0.000, Cramér's V = 0.285); the injury rate in laterally dominant sports was significantly greater compared to the non-laterally dominant sports (χ^2 (1, 2269) = 15.673, p = 0.000, Cramér's V = 0.083).

Table 1. Mann–Whitney U tests for the comparison of age and length of training between non-injured and injured pediatric-age athletes.

Variable	Non-Injured (Mean Rank)	Injured (Mean Rank)	p
Age (n = 2227)	1009.82	1417.58	0.000
Length of training (n = 2059)	971.22	1192.71	0.000

Table 2. Chi-square tests comparing the proportion of non-injured vs. injured pediatric-age athletes for each predictor variable.

Variable	Non-Injured		Injured		χ^2	p	Cramér's V
	n	Percentage	n	Percentage			
Sex					0.003	0.957	0.001
Female	527	74.5%	180	25.5%			
Male	1166	74.6%	396	25.4%			
Leg preference					1.131	0.288	0.022
Right	1438	75.1%	477	24.9%			
Left	249	72.4%	95	27.6%			
Training intensity					151.794	0.000	0.259
Low	523	83.5%	103	16.5%			
Moderate	1090	75.4%	355	24.6%			
High	77	39.7%	117	60.3%			
Training frequency					183.817	0.000	0.285
1 time/wk	678	84.4%	125	15.6%			
2 times/wk	620	80.5%	150	19.5%			
3 times/wk	191	63.2%	111	36.8%			
4 times/wk	78	53.1%	69	46.9%			
≥5 times/wk	125	51%	120	49%			
Sport category					15.673	0.000	0.083
LD sport	521	69.5%	229	30.5%			
NLD sport	1172	77.2%	347	22.8%			

LD, laterally dominant sport; NLD, non-laterally dominant sport.

In the multivariate logistic regression model (Table 3), risk of non-contact lower-limb injury increased with increasing age (adjusted OR, 1.21 for an increase of 1 year; 95% CI, 1.16–1.26; p = 0.000), training intensity (adjusted OR, 1.77 for an increase of 1 level; 95% CI, 1.43–2.19; p = 0.000), and training frequency (adjusted OR, 1.36 for an increase of 1 training day per week; 95% CI, 1.25–1.48; p = 0.000). Athletes specialized in laterally dominant sports showed a greater risk of non-contact lower-limb injury compared to those specialized in non-laterally dominant sports (adjusted OR, 1.38; 95% CI, 1.10–1.75; p = 0.006). Right-leg preference indicated lower risk of non-contact lower-limb injury compared to left-leg preference (adjusted OR, 0.71; 95% CI, 0.53–0.95; p = 0.023).

Table 3. Multivariate logistic regression analysis for predicting non-contact lower-limb injury in pediatric-age athletes.

Variable	Adjusted OR (95% CI)	p
Age (y)	1.21 (1.16–1.26)	0.000
Length of training (y)	1.03 (0.96–1.11)	0.396
Training intensity	1.77 (1.43–2.19)	0.000
Training frequency (sessions/wk)	1.36 (1.25–1.48)	0.000
Sex		
Female vs. Male	0.88 (0.70–1.12)	0.310
Sport category		
LD vs. NLD sport	1.38 (1.10–1.75)	0.006
Limb preference		
Right vs. Left leg	0.71 (0.53–0.95)	0.023

LD, laterally dominant; NLD, non-laterally dominant; OR, odds ratio; CI, confidence interval.

4. Discussion

4.1. Injury Analyses

This is the first survey study to our knowledge focusing on non-contact lower-limb injury in pediatric-age athletes. Our results showed that 25.4% of the athletes in our respondent sample sustained a non-contact lower-limb injury ($\geq$1-day time loss from sport activities) in a 12-month period. It is difficult to make age-matched comparisons between our results and previous findings because of the lack of research focusing on non-contact lower-limb injury in children and adolescents. Brumitt et al. [20] reported the same injury rate (25.4%) when examining non-contact lower-back and lower-limb injury ($\geq$1-day time loss from sport activities) in 169 male collegiate basketball players in one season. However, the rate of non-contact lower-limb injury varies greatly in other studies: Stiffler et al. [21] reported that 19.4% of 147 collegiate athletes sustained non-contact injuries in the knee or ankle in one academic year; while, Izovska et al. [22] reported that 33.6% of 227 professional soccer athletes sustained non-contact lower-limb injuries in one season. This range in injury rate may be influenced by the definition of injury used in the research and differences in participant characteristics across studies.

Our results showed that ligament sprain (15.7%) and muscle strain (8.5%) were the most frequently occurring injuries. This result is consistent with previous findings generated from 9th to 12th grade students [5] and 12 to 15-year-old students [2] in sport activities. Further, our results showed that ankle (12.1%), thigh (10.8%), and knee (10.6%) were the most frequently injured locations. Similarly, ankle and knee were also reported as the most frequently injured locations in adolescent (aged 14.67 $\pm$ 2.08 y) soccer players during training and competition [8], 5 to 17-year-old children and adolescents in sports activities [9], and 12 to 15-year-old students in sports activities [2]. The high rate of injury in these locations may be related to the anatomy of the knee and ankle [23], and the imbalance in force absorption of the quadriceps and hamstrings in sports activities [24]. The preponderance of injuries to the ankle and knee implies particular emphasis in injury prevention and sport training education in this area.

4.2. Effects of Lateral Dominance in Sport on Non-Contact Lower-Limb Injury

This is the first study to compare the rate of sport injury in athletes specialized in laterally dominant vs. non-laterally dominant sports. Results of the Chi-square test showed that the rate of non-contact lower-limb injury was significantly greater in athletes specialized in laterally dominant sports (30.5%) vs. non-laterally dominant sports (22.8%). The multivariate logistic regression model showed supportive results, wherein athletes specialized in laterally dominant sports were 1.38 times more likely to sustain a non-contact lower-limb injury compared to athletes specialized in non-laterally dominant sports after controlling for the effects of other factors. Cumulatively, these results suggest that pediatric-age athletes specialized in laterally dominant sports may need close monitoring for non-contact lower-limb injury by the coaches, athletic trainers, medical staff, and parents. We speculate that the long-term use of a laterally dominant moving pattern may result in greater inter-limb asymmetry in athletes specialized in laterally dominant sports, leading to greater odds of non-contact lower-limb injury. Future research is warranted to examine this postulation further.

To date, there is a lack of research in terms of classifying laterally dominant and non-laterally dominant sports in the literature. The present study suggests a way to classify laterally and non-laterally dominant sports on the basis of the pattern of movement in lower extremities in a sport. Sport that requires a large amount of movement characterized by the two sides performing/functioning differently was classified as a laterally dominant (or asymmetric) sport in the present study. For example, in the lunge, which is frequently performed in fencing, tennis, and badminton, the dominant leg performs as the leading leg and the non-dominant leg performs as the supporting leg [14]. In contrast, a non-laterally dominant (or symmetric) sport was classified as a sport where both legs are expected to be equally involved, such as running, swimming, and cycling [15]. In addition, a sport that requires a large amount of single-leg jumps (e.g., basketball and volleyball) or single-leg support/drive (e.g., kickboxing, taekwondo) on both sides was also classified as a non-laterally dominant (or symmetric) sport in the present study, despite the fact that the dominant leg is usually more involved than the non-dominant leg in practical action [15]. The method suggested in the present study could be used by future research with a need to classify laterally dominant and non-laterally dominant sports.

4.3. Other Risk Factors for Non-Contact Lower-Limb Injury

Our results indicated that the risk of non-contact lower-limb injury increased with age in pediatric-age athletes. A number of studies have demonstrated similar findings. Cuff, Loud, and O'Riordan [5] reported that the risk of overuse injuries increased with age in 9th to 12th grade students. Bijur, Trumble, Harel, Overpeck, Jones, and Scheidt [9] reported that the rate of sports injury increased with age in 5 to 17-year-old children. In addition, Michaud, Renaud, and Narring [3] reported that the rate of sports injury increased with age in 9 to 16-year-old students. The heightened risk of sports injury with increasing age may stem from the increased level of competition and time participating in sport as a function of age [13]. Taken together, these findings suggest that pediatric-age athletes may need close monitoring for injury, especially as they get older. However, findings in the literature were not always consistent. Some studies demonstrated that age was not associated with the risk of sport injury in junior high school students aged between 12 and 15 years [1], or in adolescent male soccer athletes aged 14.7 ± 2.1 years [8]. The inconsistency of findings may be attributed to differences in age stages and definition of injury across studies. We suggest future studies include participants with a wide range of ages (e.g., from 6 to 17 years) when evaluating the relationship between age and sport injury in pediatric-age athletes.

Currently, there is a lack of research concerning the effects of training frequency and intensity on sports injury. Our results indicate that the risk of non-contact lower-limb injury increased with increasing training frequency (1, 2, 3, 4, 5 or more sessions/week) in pediatric-age athletes. An increase of one training session per week increased the risk of non-contact lower-limb injury by 1.36 times. This finding suggests that coaches in youth sports training may need to reduce training frequency to prevent injury in pediatric-age athletes when required, although the effects of training duration in one training session have not been considered in the present study. Another consideration is that the training frequency of athletes who play on multiple teams (for the same sport) may not be scheduled by one coach. It is recommended that pediatric-age athletes play on only one team at a time to help decrease training frequency and the risk of injury. Our results also indicate that an increase of one level (low, moderate, high) in training intensity increases the odds of non-contact lower-limb injury by 1.77 times when controlling for the effects of other factors. It should be noted that there was no clear boundary of each intensity level (low, moderate, high) in the present study, and the training intensity was self-evaluated by the participants, which may have led to the underreporting of injury cases. Nevertheless, the present study provides preliminary evidence on the effects of training frequency and intensity on non-contact lower-limb injury in pediatric-age athletes.

With respect to the effects of length of training on sports injury, results are inconclusive in the present study. Although the injured group showed a greater length of training than the non-injured group, results of the multivariate logistic regression model showed no association between length of training and non-contact lower-limb injury after controlling for the effects of other factors. Available evidence on the influence of length of training on sports injury is scarce. Bastos, Vanderlei, Vanderlei, Júnior, and Pastre [8] reported that male soccer athletes (14.7 ± 2.1 years) with a training duration greater than 5 years sustained sports injury more frequently compared to those with a shorter training duration. The greater length of training demonstrates greater exposure time to training and competition, which may contribute to a greater risk of injury [25]. Further, with the increase in length of training, games may become more competitive, which may also increase the risk of injury [26].

Regarding the effects of sex (male vs. female) on the risk of sport injury, a systematic review focusing on children and adolescents has reported that boys are generally at greater risk of sports injury compared to girls because of their larger body mass, which may cause increased forces in jumping, sprinting, and pivoting in boys [13]. However, girls showed a greater risk of sports injury compared with boys in specific sports including soccer, basketball, and baseball, which may be related to the physiological and anatomical characteristics of girls [13]. Focusing on non-contact lower-limb injury, our results showed that there was no difference in the risk of injury between boys and girls. This might be attributed to the variance in the sporting backgrounds of the participants in the present study. Overall, practitioners should pay attention to the differences between sports and consider the potential effects of sex (male vs. female) on the risk of injury in pediatric-age athletes.

Another finding is that left-leg preference indicates a greater risk of non-contact lower-limb injury compared to right-leg preference, suggesting that pediatric-age athletes with left-leg preference may need close monitoring for non-contact lower-limb injury. This finding is consistent with previous research examining risk factors for injury in 12 to 18-year-old [27] and 7 to 12-year-old soccer athletes [28]. The reasons for these findings are unclear. It has been suggested that these findings may be associated with the environmental biases in a right-handed world and differences in function related to neurologic development [29]. This is an area for further research.

4.4. Limitations

We acknowledge the limitations of the present study. Non-contact lower-limb injuries were self-reported by parents/guardians in the present study, which may lead to underreporting of injury cases. It may also cause recall bias as the parents need to remember events up to 12 months before, as well as classify injuries by themselves instead of medically trained staff. Further, it has been suggested that the effects of previous injury [1,2] and exposure time to sports [3,30] should be considered when evaluating injury risk; however, these two factors were not included in the present study. Therefore, our findings did not take into account the effects of exposure time and previous injury.

5. Conclusions

Pediatric-age athletes who specialize in laterally dominant sports may demonstrate a greater risk of non-contact lower-limb injury compared to those specialized in non-laterally dominant sports. Left-leg preference, increase in age, training intensity, and training frequency were also associated with a greater risk of non-contact lower-limb injury in pediatric-age athletes. These findings should be utilized with caution as exposure time and previous injuries were not included. However, this study provides useful findings in evaluating the risk of non-contact lower-limb injury in pediatric-age athletes, and the effects of lateral dominance in sport (laterally vs. non-laterally dominant sport) on injury. Future research should include more comprehensive predictor variables to further examine risk factors of non-contact lower-limb injury in pediatric-age athletes. Future research should also explore whether the greater odds of non-contact lower-limb injury in pediatric-age athletes specialized in laterally dominant vs. non-laterally dominant sports is a result of greater inter-limb asymmetry.

Supplementary Materials: The following are available online at https://www.mdpi.com/article/10.3390/jcm10143171/s1, Supplementary File: Questionnaire for Training Information and Non-Contact Lower-Limb In-jury in Pediatric-age Athletes.

Author Contributions: Conceptualization, Y.G. and D.E.R.W.; Methodology, Y.G., S.S.D.B., J.T., Q.J. and D.E.R.W.; Validation, S.S.D.B., J.T., Q.J., Y.L. and D.E.R.W.; Formal analysis, Y.G. and N.W.; Investigation, Y.G., Y.L. and N.W.; Resources, Y.G., Y.L. and D.E.R.W.; Data curation, Y.G. and D.E.R.W.; Writing—original draft preparation, Y.G.; Writing—review and editing, Y.G., S.S.D.B., J.T., Q.J., N.W. and D.E.R.W.; supervision, S.S.D.B. and D.E.R.W. All authors have read and agreed to the published version of the manuscript.

Funding: This research received no external funding.

Institutional Review Board Statement: The study was conducted according to the guidelines of the Declaration of Helsinki, and approved by the University of British Columbia's Clinical Research Ethics Board (H18-02252) and the Shandong Sport University's Human Ethics Committee for research involving human participants according to the standards established by the Declaration of Helsinki.

Informed Consent Statement: Informed consent was received upon completion and submission of the survey.

Data Availability Statement: The data presented in this study are available on request from the corresponding author.

Conflicts of Interest: The authors declare no conflict of interest.

References

1. Emery, C.; Tyreman, H. Sport participation, sport injury, risk factors and sport safety practices in Calgary and area junior high schools. *Paediatr. Child Health* **2009**, *14*, 439–444. [CrossRef]
2. Emery, C.A.; Meeuwisse, W.H.; Mcallister, J.R. Survey of sport participation and sport injury in Calgary and area high schools. *Clin. J. Sport Med.* **2006**, *16*, 20–26. [CrossRef]
3. Michaud, P.; Renaud, A.; Narring, F. Sports activities related to injuries? A survey among 9–19 year olds in Switzerland. *Inj. Prev.* **2001**, *7*, 41–45. [CrossRef]
4. Radelet, M.A.; Lephart, S.M.; Rubinstein, E.N.; Myers, J.B. Survey of the injury rate for children in community sports. *Pediatrics* **2002**, *110*, e28. [CrossRef]
5. Cuff, S.; Loud, K.; O'Riordan, M.A. Overuse injuries in high school athletes. *Clin. Pediatr.* **2010**, *49*, 731–736. [CrossRef]
6. Micheli, L.J.; Klein, J. Sports injuries in children and adolescents. *Br. J. Sports Med.* **1991**, *25*, 6. [CrossRef] [PubMed]
7. Patel, D.R.; Nelson, T.L. Sports injuries in adolescents. *Med. Clin. N. Am.* **2000**, *84*, 983–1007. [CrossRef]
8. Bastos, F.N.; Vanderlei, F.M.; Vanderlei, L.C.M.; Júnior, J.N.; Pastre, C.M. Investigation of characteristics and risk factors of sports injuries in young soccer players: A retrospective study. *Int. Arch. Med.* **2013**, *6*, 14. [CrossRef]
9. Bijur, P.E.; Trumble, A.; Harel, Y.; Overpeck, M.D.; Jones, D.; Scheidt, P.C. Sports and recreation injuries in US children and adolescents. *Arch. Pediatr. Adolesc. Med.* **1995**, *149*, 1009–1016. [CrossRef] [PubMed]
10. Hootman, J.M.; Dick, R.; Agel, J. Epidemiology of collegiate injuries for 15 sports: Summary and recommendations for injury prevention initiatives. *J. Athl. Train.* **2007**, *42*, 311–319.
11. Gonell, A.C.; Romero, J.P.; Soler, L.M. Relationship between the Y balance test scores and soft tissue injury incidence in a soccer team. *Int. J. Sports Phys. Ther.* **2015**, *10*, 955–966. [PubMed]
12. Malina, R.M. Early sport specialization: Roots, effectiveness, risks. *Curr. Sports Med. Rep.* **2010**, *9*, 364–371. [CrossRef]
13. Emery, C.A. Risk factors for injury in child and adolescent sport: A systematic review of the literature. *Clin. J. Sport Med.* **2003**, *13*, 256–268. [CrossRef]
14. Guan, Y.; Guo, L.; Wu, N.; Zhang, L.; Warburton, D.E. Biomechanical insights into the determinants of speed in the fencing lunge. *Eur. J. Sport Sci.* **2018**, *18*, 201–208. [CrossRef]
15. Upper Body Anthropometrical Differences Amongst Participants of Asymmetrical (Fast Bowlers in Cricket) and Symmetrical (Crawl Stroke Swimmers) Sport and Sedentary Individuals in South Africa. Available online: http://hdl.handle.net/10394/228 (accessed on 9 May 2021).

16. Knapik, J.J.; Bauman, C.L.; Jones, B.H.; Harris, J.M.; Vaughan, L. Preseason strength and flexibility imbalances associated with athletic injuries in female collegiate athletes. *Am. J. Sports Med.* **1991**, *19*, 76–81. [CrossRef]
17. Ford, K.R.; Myer, G.D.; Hewett, T.E. Valgus knee motion during landing in high school female and male basketball players. *Med. Sci. Sports Exerc.* **2003**, *35*, 1745–1750. [CrossRef] [PubMed]
18. Rauh, M.J.; Margherita, A.J.; Rice, S.G.; Koepsell, T.D.; Rivara, F.P. High school cross country running injuries: A longitudinal study. *Clin. J. Sport Med.* **2000**, *10*, 110–116. [CrossRef] [PubMed]
19. Read, P.J.; Oliver, J.L.; Croix, M.; Myer, G.D.; Lloyd, R.S. A prospective investigation to evaluate risk factors for lower extremity injury risk in male youth soccer players. *Scand. J. Med. Sci. Sports* **2018**, *28*, 1244–1251. [CrossRef] [PubMed]
20. Brumitt, J.; Nelson, K.; Duey, D.; Jeppson, M.; Hammer, L. Preseason Y Balance Test Scores are not associated with noncontact time-loss lower quadrant injury in male collegiate basketball players. *Sports* **2019**, *7*, 4. [CrossRef] [PubMed]
21. Stiffler, M.R.; Bell, D.R.; Sanfilippo, J.L.; Hetzel, S.J.; Pickett, K.A.; Heiderscheit, B.C. Star excursion balance test anterior asymmetry is associated with injury status in division I collegiate athletes. *J. Orthop. Sports Phys. Ther.* **2017**, *47*, 339–346. [CrossRef] [PubMed]
22. Izovska, J.; Mikic, M.; Dragijsky, M.; Zahalka, F.; Bujnovsky, D.; Hank, M. Pre-season bilateral strength asymmetries of professional soccer players and relationship with non-contact injury of lower limb in the season. *Sport Mont* **2019**, *17*, 107–110.
23. Tham, S.C.; Tsou, I.Y.; Chee, T.S. Knee and ankle ligaments: Magnetic resonance imaging findings of normal anatomy and at injury. *Ann. Acad. Med. Singap.* **2008**, *37*, 324.
24. Read, P.J.; Oliver, J.L.; Croix, M.B.D.S.; Myer, G.D.; Lloyd, R.S. Neuromuscular risk factors for knee and ankle ligament injuries in male youth soccer players. *Sports Med.* **2016**, *46*, 1059–1066. [CrossRef] [PubMed]
25. Stege, J.; Stubbe, J.; Verhagen, E.; Van Mechelen, W. Risk factors for injuries in male professional soccer: A systematic review. *Br. J. Sports Med.* **2011**, *45*, 375–376. [CrossRef]
26. Brito, J.; Rebelo, A.; Soares, J.M.; Seabra, A.; Krustrup, P.; Malina, R.M. Injuries in youth soccer during the preseason. *Clin. J. Sport Med.* **2011**, *21*, 259–260. [CrossRef] [PubMed]
27. Emery, C.A.; Meeuwisse, W.H.; Hartmann, S.E. Evaluation of risk factors for injury in adolescent soccer: Implementation and validation of an injury surveillance system. *Am. J. Sports Med.* **2005**, *33*, 1882–1891. [CrossRef]
28. Rössler, R.; Junge, A.; Chomiak, J.; Němec, K.; Dvorak, J.; Lichtenstein, E.; Faude, O. Risk factors for football injuries in young players aged 7 to 12 years. *Scand. J. Med. Sci. Sports* **2018**, *28*, 1176–1182. [CrossRef]
29. Graham, C.J.; Cleveland, E. Left-handedness as an injury risk factor in adolescents. *J. Adolesc. Health* **1995**, *16*, 50–52. [CrossRef]
30. Taunton, J.; Ryan, M.; Clement, D.; Mckenzie, D.; Lloyd-Smith, D.; Zumbo, B. A prospective study of running injuries: The Vancouver Sun Run "In Training" clinics. *Br. J. Sports Med.* **2003**, *37*, 239–244. [CrossRef]

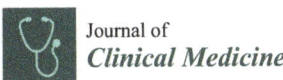

Article

Impact of a Breathing Intervention on Engagement of Abdominal, Thoracic, and Subclavian Musculature during Exercise, a Randomized Trial

Petr Bahenský [1,*], Václav Bunc [2], Renata Malátová [1], David Marko [1], Gregory J. Grosicki [3] and Jan Schuster [1]

1. Department of Sports Studies, Faculty of Education, University of South Bohemia, 371 15 České Budějovice, Czech Republic; malatova@pf.jcu.cz (R.M.); David.Marko@seznam.cz (D.M.); jan.schuster@seznam.cz (J.S.)
2. Sports Motor Skills Laboratory, Faculty of Sports, Physical Training and Education, Charles University, 165 52 Prague, Czech Republic; Bunc@ftvs.cuni.cz
3. Department of Health Sciences and Kinesiology, Biodynamics and Human Performance Center, Armstrong Campus, Georgia Southern University, Savannah, GA 31419, USA; ggrosicki@georgiasouthern.edu
* Correspondence: pbahensky@pf.jcu.cz; Tel.: +42-038-777-3171

Abstract: Background: Breathing technique may influence endurance exercise performance by reducing overall breathing work and delaying respiratory muscle fatigue. We investigated whether a two-month yoga-based breathing intervention could affect breathing characteristics during exercise. Methods: Forty-six endurance runners (age = 16.6 ± 1.2 years) were randomized to either a breathing intervention or control group. The contribution of abdominal, thoracic, and subclavian musculature to respiration and ventilation parameters during three different intensities on a cycle ergometer was assessed pre- and post-intervention. Results: Post-intervention, abdominal, thoracic, and subclavian ventilatory contributions were altered at 2 W·kg^{-1} (27:23:50 to 31:28:41), 3 W·kg^{-1} (26:22:52 to 28:31:41), and 4 W·kg^{-1} (24:24:52 to 27:30:43), whereas minimal changes were observed in the control group. More specifically, a significant ($p < 0.05$) increase in abdominal contribution was observed at rest and during low intensity work (i.e., 2 and 3 W·kg^{-1}), and a decrease in respiratory rate and increase of tidal volume were observed in the experimental group. Conclusions: These data highlight an increased reliance on more efficient abdominal and thoracic musculature, and less recruitment of subclavian musculature, in young endurance athletes during exercise following a two-month yoga-based breathing intervention. More efficient ventilatory muscular recruitment may benefit endurance performance by reducing energy demand and thus optimize energy requirements for mechanical work.

Keywords: breathing pattern; breathing exercise; load; diaphragm; adolescents

1. Introduction

The physiological implications of reductions in physical activity due to an environment that is oversaturated with technological innovation are only beginning to be realized [1,2]. Adverse changes in respiratory patterns are just one of these deleterious adaptations, and dysfunctional breathing has become increasingly common with an expected prevalence of between 60–80% in otherwise healthy adults [3].

Gas exchange during normal activity is coordinated by inspiratory and expiratory processes involving synchronized movement of the upper and lower chest, abdomen, and diaphragm [4–7]. In the resting state, breathing is regulated by an expansion of the lower chest and anteroposterior movement of the sternal bones that is facilitated by the diaphragm and intercostal muscles that account for ~2–5% of whole-body oxygen consumption at rest. During intensive muscle work, respiratory energy demand can increase several times. In the case of trained athletes, it reaches up to 10% of the total energy consumption during moderately demanding activity [8–10]. Meanwhile, excess

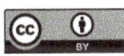

involvement of areas of the upper chest distinctly characterizes respiratory inefficiency and potential breathing disorders [4,11], which may become increasingly relevant during high intensity work where ventilatory oxygen demand may comprise 15% (or more) of whole-body oxygen consumption [8–10].

Though inter-individual variability characterized by differential involvement of abdominal, thoracic, and subclavian body sectors in breathing patterns have been observed [12], systematic analysis of the effect of breathing technique on athletic performance is vastly understudied [13]. However, the influence of breathing patterns on performance has recently come to the forefront of physical activity research [14], and the role of the diaphragm during high-intensity work has received significant attention [13,15]. In individuals with dysfunctional respiration, the pain threshold is lowered, and control of motor functions and movement dysfunctions are impaired, all of which may adversely affect the individual's physical performance [16]. Pertinently, increasing diaphragmatic respiratory involvement reduces breathing effort, improves ventilation efficiency, reduces dyspnea, improves exercise tolerance, and can be trained [17–20]. Thus, there is great incentive to elucidate techniques to improve respiratory efficiency as a potential means to improve athletic performance [21–23].

Specific respiratory (inspiratory) muscle training (IMT) improves the function of the inspiratory muscles. According to literature and clinical experience, there are three established methods: (1) resistive load, (2) threshold load, and (3) normocapnic hyperpnea. Each training method and the associated devices have specific characteristics [24]. Setting up an IMT should start with specific diagnostics of respiratory muscle function and be followed by detailed individual introduction to training. Changing respiratory muscular activity through strengthening of inspiratory muscles may attenuate disease risk. Weakness or fatigue of the diaphragm and the accessory muscles of inspiration is widely recognized as a cause of failure to wean from mechanical ventilation [25]. The influence of IMT on exercise performance has also been surveyed. Faghy and Brown [22] provided evidence for the ability of IMT training to improve exercise performance (time trial) with thoracic load carriage.

Many methods can be used to evaluate the respiratory pattern [26], the most common of which are palpation, chest circumference, plethysmography of the whole body, chest skiagram, spirometry or various instruments recording changes in height of individual torso segments, or through a three-dimensional system [27–29]. Estimation of chest wall motion by surface measurements allows one-dimensional measurements of the chest wall by assessment with an optical reflectance system [30] or by three-dimensional tracking [31,32]. Chest wall volume changes can be assessed by optoelectronic plethysmography [33] or by optoelectronic plethysmography [34]. Building upon these techniques, our group used a respiratory muscle dynamometer to measure instantaneous values of involvement of the ventilatory musculature (MD03 muscle dynamometer) [11,35,36]. Using this dynamometer, the present study evaluated whether two-months of a yoga breathing exercise program may influence breathing characteristics during various intensities of exercise in young healthy athletes.

Based on previous work by our group [37], we hypothesized that the breathing exercise program would modulate respiratory musculature contribution. We anticipated greater involvement of the musculature of the lower torso (i.e., abdomen and thoracic sectors) and less upper-body contribution (i.e., subclavian) during exercise following the yoga-based breathing intervention.

2. Materials and Methods

2.1. Subjects

Forty-six adolescent distance runners (14–18 years) participated in our study: 23 males (age = 16.4 ± 1.1, height = 177.1 ± 5.8 cm, weight = 62.4 ± 5.8 kg) and 23 females (age = 16.8 ± 1.1, height = 168.5 ± 4.4 cm, weight = 55.9 ± 4.0 kg). All participants reported a history of endurance running of at least six times a week for the past year. They are all members of the same training group, and thus training volume and intensity were comparable throughout the duration of the study. Participants were randomly allocated to an experimental group (n = 23), which took part in an eight-week breathing intervention, or a control group (n = 23), which continued training but did not carry out the yoga-based breathing intervention. One participant did not complete the intervention for medical reasons unrelated to the intervention and was excluded from the study. The two groups, both experimental and control, followed the same training program, the only difference being that the experimental group performed the yoga-based breathing intervention. A randomization sequence has been generated using Randomization.org. An independent person not involved in this study made the computer-generated randomization sequence. The study protocol was reviewed and approved by the local ethics committee on 19 October 2018 (002/2018) and followed the guidelines of the World Medical Assembly Declaration of Helsinki. This research is a clinical trial (NCT04950387). Written informed consent to participate was provided by guardians and verbal assessment was provided by the participants.

2.2. Study Design

2.2.1. Measurement of Sectors Engagement

The testing took place in the Laboratory of Load Diagnostics at Department of Sports Studies, Faculty of Education, University of South Bohemia. We evaluated ventilatory musculature involvement in three basic areas (Figure 1; abdominal = red sensor, thoracic = green sensor, and subclavian = blue sensor) using a muscle dynamometer MD03 as previously described [35,36].

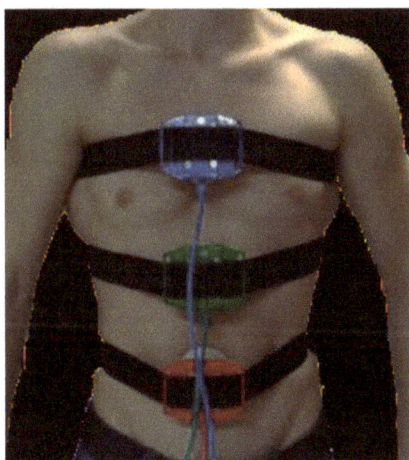

Figure 1. The positions of the location of probes on the body.

The device is a four-channel digital muscle dynamometer that, by design, allows instantaneous values of muscle force to be measured in relation to time (i.e., both the force size and its dynamics can be evaluated). In general, different muscles and muscle groups on the human body can be measured. MD03 is made up of four muscle probes (we used three probes) that attach themselves to the human body with belts. Greater muscle involvement in the segment of interest at a higher tidal volume results in higher dynamometer pressure values. The probes contain a strain transducer to a digital signal that is transmitted to a microprocessor evaluation unit that adjusts digital signals from the probes into a compatible form with a USB input to a notebook. Probe attachment sites were selected based on the kinematics of the aforementioned thoracic sectors.

The first probe was placed in the lower respiratory sector on the ventral side of the level L4–5. The second probe was placed on the ventral side just below the sternum (between ribs 8 and 9). The third probe was characterized by upper respiratory musculature involvement and was placed between ribs 3 and 4 on the ventral side on the sternum. Chest compression and expansion during respiration change the force applied to the individual sensors in the attached belt.

2.2.2. Measurement of Ventilatory Parameters

Inspiratory and expiratory forces exerted on individual probes located in the given breathing sectors were recorded for 60 s and minute averages were determined for each probe. After 60 s of resting data acquisition using both spontaneous and deep breathing, participants underwent an incremental test on a cycle ergometer (Lode, Groningen, The Netherlands) and oxygen consumption, tidal volume, respiratory rate, and minute ventilation were continuously monitored (Metalyzer B3, Cortex, Leipzig, Germany). The exercise protocol consisted of a graded exercise test that was made relative to participant body weight (i.e., $W \cdot kg^{-1}$) and began with a 4-minute stage at $1\ W \cdot kg^{-1}$ followed by three, two-minute stages (for partial stabilization of ventilation parameters) at progressive intensities (2, 3, 4 $W \cdot kg^{-1}$) as we have described previously [38,39] and cadence was standardized to 95–100 $rev \cdot min^{-1}$. Ventilatory muscular involvement of the abdominal, thoracic, and subclavian body sectors was monitored during the last minute of each of the three submaximal intensities.

2.2.3. Breathing Exercise Program

The training program lasted eight weeks. The experimental group performed yoga-based breathing exercises daily. In the first week of the breathing intervention, training took place in the form of three supervised group sessions [37]. In the following weeks, there were always two group training sessions, each lasted ~30 min. On unsupervised days, participants were asked to perform exercises individually at home for at least 10 min. Information about the length of each individual's training session was recorded in a diary by the participant.

The design of the breathing exercise program was based on yoga, and the aim was to activate the diaphragm and become aware of individual breathing sectors. As such, breath training included a variety of exercises, such as breathing wave training, full breathing (breathing into all sectors), and paced breathing (breathing in a specified rhythm). The exercises were performed in various positions, including lying down, sitting in the kneeling position, sitting, kneeling, and standing (see Supplementary Material). All breathing was performed through the nose. At the beginning of the intervention, the participants breathed spontaneously, later switching to prolonging the inspiratory and expiratory phases. They started with a 1:1 ratio of inhale to exhale length. Gradually, the pre-exhalation and pre-exhalation phases of breath holding were included: inspiration-6 periods, holding breath-3 periods, exhaling-6 periods, holding breath-3 periods. Each of the participants adapted the exercise to their individual respiratory rate. Each of the exercises was repeated six times. The exercises were slow, with a deep focus on breathing, in line with the movement. Very important was the perception of the direction of movement and expansion of the chest, the behavior of the axis of the body (head, spine, pelvis), which they learned during the introductory meetings [37]. The control group did not participate in any form of breathing training and were told to go about their lives as usual.

The follow-up testing, which was the same as the aforementioned described graded maximal test on the cycle ergometer, was performed after eight weeks of intervention.

2.3. Statistical Analysis

Data are presented as mean ± SD. The normality of data was confirmed using the Shapiro–Wilk test. A two-way repeated-measures ANOVA (group × intensity) was used to compare changes in the involvement of individual breathing sectors and respiratory rate in the intervention and control groups. Significant interactions were examined using Bonferroni adjusted simple main effect post hoc comparisons. An alpha-level of 0.05 was used to assess statistical significance for all comparisons. Subsequently, effect size was determined using Cohen's d. The Pearson correlation coefficient was used to examine relationships between changes in tidal volume and pressure values on the dynamometer. The alpha-level was set to 0.05. The data processing was done in Excel 2016 (Microsoft, Oregon, WA, USA) and Statistica 12 (StatSoft, Tulsa, OK, USA).

3. Results

Participants carried out the yoga-based breathing program for an average of 13.3 ± 2.8 min per day during the two-month period. In the experimental group, there was a significant increase in the involvement of the abdominal segment during deep breathing and at 2 and 3 W·kg^{-1} ($p < 0.05$; see Figure 2 and Table 1). The only significant change in thoracic involvement was seen at 3 W·kg^{-1} ($p < 0.01$). In subclavian respiration, there was no significant change in involvement at any of the intensities, even at rest or at rest during deep resting breathing. In the control group, there was no significant change in the involvement of individual breathing sectors at rest or at any load level ($p > 0.05$; Table 1).

Table 1. Average values measured by probes and standard deviations of pressure on individual breathing sectors at rest and at different load intensities in the experimental group (EG) and control group (CG).

Breathing Sector	Time [n·cm^{-2}]	Rest [n·cm^{-2}]	Deep–Rest [n·cm^{-2}]	2 W·kg^{-1} [n·cm^{-2}]	3 W·kg^{-1} [n·cm^{-2}]	4 W·kg^{-1} [n·cm^{-2}]
abdominal EG	pre	0.54 ± 0.33	0.93 ± 0.36	1.38 ± 0.74	1.43 ± 0.66	1.54 ± 0.62
	post	0.94 ± 0.37 [l]	1.79 ± 0.76 [l,**]	2.01 ± 0.90 [m,*]	2.04 ± 1.01 [m,*]	1.91 ± 0.75 [m]
chest EG	pre	0.46 ± 0.35	0.82 ± 0.56	1.32 ± 0.88	1.31 ± 0.75	1.59 ± 0.89
	post	0.65 ± 0.38 [m]	1.34 ± 0.91 [m]	1.79 ± 0.75 [m]	2.19 ± 1.31 [m,**]	2.16 ± 1.24 [m]
subclavian EG	pre	0.65 ± 0.49	1.43 ± 0.79	2.92 ± 1.99	3.00 ± 1.39	3.59 ± 1.94
	post	0.83 ± 0.42 [s]	1.66 ± 0.97 [s]	2.70 ± 0.99	2.83 ± 0.88 [*]	3.08 ± 1.26 [s]
abdominal CG	pre	0.56 ± 0.36	0.91 ± 0.40	1.33 ± 0.67	1.39 ± 0.55	1.55 ± 0.60
	post	0.57 ± 0.39	0.89 ± 0.42	1.35 ± 0.70	1.42 ± 0.52	1.54 ± 0.62
chest CG	pre	0.48 ± 0.34	0.85 ± 0.57	1.35 ± 0.90	1.36 ± 0.69	1.58 ± 0.90
	post	0.46 ± 0.37	0.88 ± 0.59	1.35 ± 0.85	1.37 ± 0.72	1.56 ± 0.88
subclavian CG	pre	0.60 ± 0.45	1.45 ± 0.82	2.95 ± 2.01	3.03 ± 1.43	3.49 ± 1.45
	post	0.63 ± 0.42	1.49 ± 0.88	2.91 ± 1.95	2.98 ± 1.35	3.40 ± 1.42

Note: * $p < 0.05$, ** $p < 0.01$, Cohen's d: [s] small effect size, [m] medium effect size, [l] large effect size.

As a result of the breathing exercise intervention, the experimental group experienced a significant reduction ($p < 0.05$) of respiratory rate under load 3 and 4 W·kg^{-1}, with medium (4 W·kg^{-1}) or small (rest, deep rest, 2 and 3 W·kg^{-1}) effect sizes. We noted a significant increase of tidal volume at 2 W·kg^{-1}, there are changes with small effect size, during all intensities of load. Minute ventilation and oxygen consumption were not significantly altered (see Table 2). The overall effect of breathing exercise intervention in all phases on changes of respiratory rate and tidal volume was confirmed at level $p < 0.01$.

Table 2. Percent change in respiratory rate (RR), tidal volume (V$_T$), minute ventilatory volume (V$_E$) and oxygen consumption (VO$_2$) after breathing exercises intervention versus exercise prior to breathing exercises intervention at different intensities in the experimental group (EG) and control group (CG).

		Rest	Deep-Rest	2 W·kg^{-1}	3 W·kg^{-1}	4 W·kg^{-1}
EG	RR	−3.12 [s]	−3.97 [s]	−5.85 [s]	−7.18 [s,*]	−8.36 [m,**]
	V$_T$	-	-	10.60 [s,*]	7.33 [s]	6.00 [s]
	V$_E$	-	-	2.48	−0.60	−2.89
	VO$_2$	-	-	−0.27	−0.15	−0.10
CG	RR	−1.32	−1.40	0.05	−0.07	0.45
	V$_T$	-	-	−0.60	−0.15	0.07
	V$_E$	-	-	1.72	−0.65	−0.31
	VO$_2$	-	-	0.39	0.55	0.30

Note: ANOVA: * $p < 0.05$, ** $p < 0.01$, Cohen's d: [s] small effect size, [m] medium effect size.

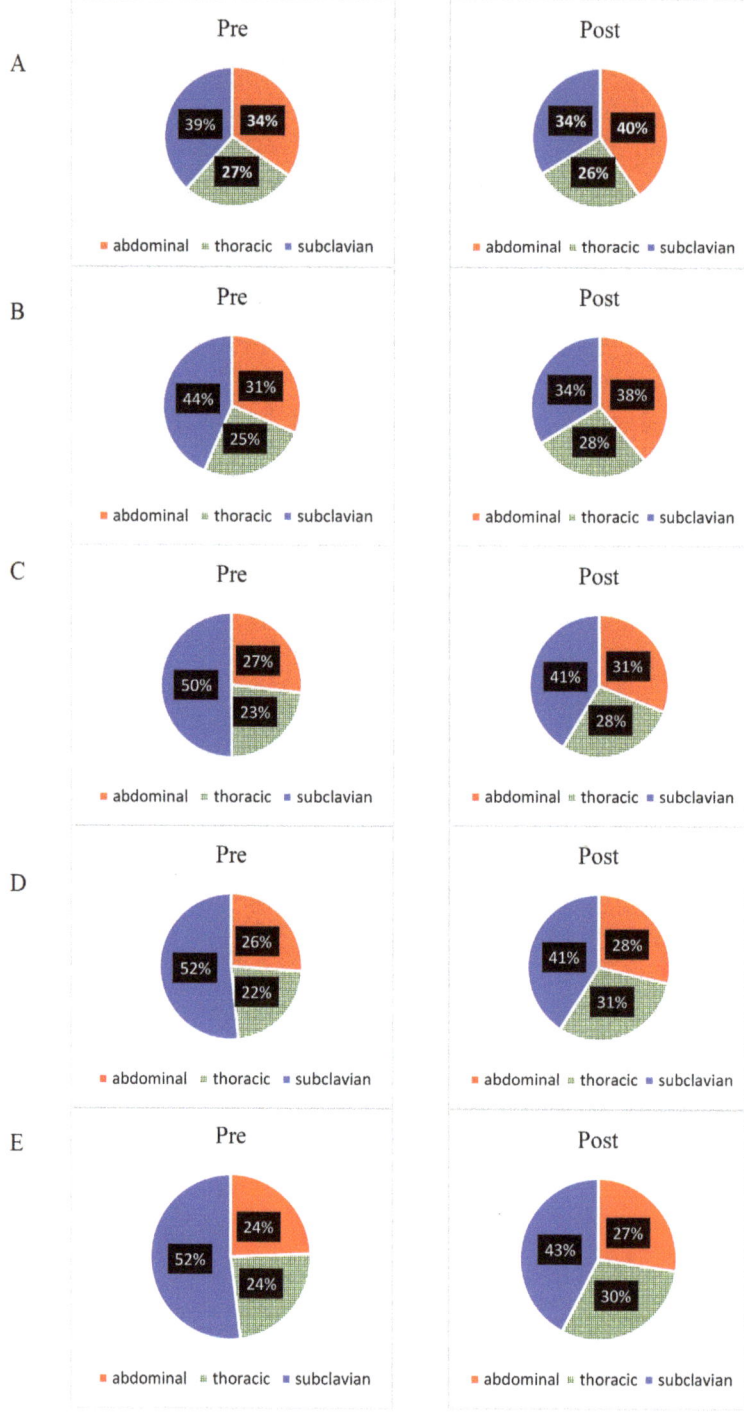

Figure 2. Engagement of breathing sectors at rest (**A**), during deep breathing (**B**), under load 2 W·kg^{-1} (**C**), under load 3 W·kg^{-1} (**D**), under load 4 W·kg^{-1} (**E**) pre and post intervention.

Changes in tidal volume were significantly related to abdominal probe pressure at all intensities (see Table 3).

Table 3. Pearson correlation coefficient of change in tidal volume and abdominal probe pressure.

Correlation	2 W·kg^{-1}	3 W·kg^{-1}	4 W·kg^{-1}
V_T and abdominal sector engagement	0.452 *	0.584 *	0.531 *

Note: * $p < 0.05$.

In all intensities, greater abdominal and less subclavian percentage contribution was noted (see Figure 2).

4. Discussion

The primary finding of the present study was an alternation in breathing patterns at rest, and during cycling exercise at various intensities, in young healthy individuals following an eight-week breathing intervention. This finding corroborates previous research by our group in showing greater and more efficient abdominal contribution to respiration following a breathing intervention [37]. Moreover, it is worthy to note that the respiratory musculature involvement following the intervention was close to what may be recommended [4].

Physical exertion often increases the perception of respiratory effort in healthy people and leads to a feeling of dyspnea. Sports activities, be it intensive, short duration ($\geq$85% of the maximum oxygen uptake) or less intense, longer-lasting duration ("ultramarathon" etc.) can lead to fatigue of the inspiratory and/or expiratory muscles [24]. Moreover, tired respiratory muscles impair athletic performance. During physical activity and sport, work of the respiratory muscles is compounded by greater demand for postural stabilization and movement efficiency [40]. Body stability is impaired when the respiratory muscles are tired, which can increase the risk of tripping or falling [24].

Respiratory therapy is an integral part of treatment for many patients with various diseases. Respiratory contributions have been shown to limit exercise in patients with heart failure. The manner in which the respiratory system limits exercise is due to abnormalities in ventilation, perfusion, or both ventilation and perfusion inspiratory muscle weakness may induce several impairments in both healthy and athletic individuals [22]. Similarly, studies have demonstrated that inspiratory muscle strength also has an important role in the pathophysiology of exercise limitation in several clinical conditions. Indeed, IMT is becoming an effective complementary treatment with positive effects on muscle strength and exercise capacity. More recently, studies have found that maximal inspiratory pressure (MIP) is strongly correlated with VO_2 peak in patients after acute myocardial infarction and heart failure, reinforcing the influence of the inspiratory muscles on functional capacity [41]. The exercises primarily reduced end-expiratory lung volume rather than end-inspiratory lung volume, which is constrained by the presence of a thoracic load. Consequently, the training stimuli may be targeting and strengthening the inspiratory muscles throughout an operational range, which may not be utilised during exercise with load carriage. Importantly, previous work has identified that fatigue of the expiratory muscles is not an influencing factor in determining operational lung volumes, despite reduced end-expiratory time and increased peak gastric and esophageal pressures, and it may be more appropriate to assess influences that inhibit flow [42]. In general, the IMT performed at an intensity of 30% MIP resulted in decreased cardiac sympathetic modulation (LF) and increased parasympathetic (HF) at rest in patients with hypertension, heart failure, and diabetes mellitus [43]. Nevertheless, this measure has been questioned as interventions can elicit either complex non-linear reciprocal or parallel changes in either division of ANS, and these complex interactions can influence the calculation and interpretation of LF/HF [44]. However, applying IMT to different diseases, associated with a variety of training protocols, as well as few studies found in the literature, makes the effects of IMT on cardiovascular autonomic control inconclusive. Inspiratory muscle training promotes changes in cardiovascular autonomic responses in humans [43]. Though inspiratory muscle training seems to improve maximal inspiratory pressure, it remains unclear whether these benefits translate to weaning success and a shorter duration of mechanical ventilation [25].

It is important to note that all participants were encouraged to breathe spontaneously during the testing period to ensure that any observed changes were in fact attributable to the intervention. Interestingly, the observed significant increase in abdominal contribution to breathing was noted at rest and during light/moderate intensities (2 and 3 W·kg^{-1}), but not at the greatest load (i.e., 4 W·kg^{-1}). Greater involvement of the thoracic musculature was also observed at lower (i.e., 3 W·kg^{-1}) but not the greatest workload. This may be ascribed to greater anaerobic energy contribution at the greatest workload and thus the need for excess ventilation to remove rapidly accumulating CO_2 [13,45]. However, of relevance was the observation of a trend towards a reduction in subclavian involvement at the higher workload in the experimental group. At the same time, there was a decrease in respiratory rate, an increase in tidal volume while maintaining the minute ventilation volume and oxygen consumption. Reduced subclavian involvement together with decreased respiratory rate and increased tidal volume at the same minute ventilation volume and same VO_2 denotes greater respiratory efficiency and thus greater oxygen availability for mechanical musculature. At the same time, a decrease in respiratory rate also signals a decrease in respiratory work as one of the possible effects of a targeted breathing exercise program. A link has been shown between an increase of pressure on the abdominal probes and an increase of tidal volume. Furthermore, the increased contribution of the abdominal sector to respiration, together with the decreased respiratory rate, and increased tidal volume with the similar minute ventilation, indicates an improved breathing economy [38,46]. This is important as respiratory muscle efficiency is one of the conditions for good performance in endurance.

At rest, and during deep breathing, greater recruitment of abdominal muscles helps to optimize respiratory efficiency and delay the onset of respiratory muscle fatigue. However, during submaximal exercise, a significant alteration in respiratory musculature characterized by a reduction in abdominal and increased subclavian contribution is observed. Our results suggest that while it is possible to manipulate spontaneous breathing patterns during exercise, these benefits may be limited to lighter loads that are likely below the ventilatory threshold. However, reduced respiratory rate following breath training at both low and high workloads may be of benefit across a range of exercise performance disciplines.

The present findings should be interpreted in the context of the population; a greater training effect may be anticipated in adolescents in whom respiratory patterns during exercise are not as well engrained [47]. Like previous research in the field, we strategically selected an eight-week training intervention [48–51]. Future studies to determine the possible benefits of shorter breath training interventions, as well as the persistence of these adaptations if breath training is stopped, are warranted. Other limitations of the present work include our relatively modest sample size as well as that much of the training was performed at-home without direct supervision. Verification of these findings in non-athletic populations and potentially less healthy individuals, such as those with breathing illnesses, would also be of interest.

5. Conclusions

These data highlight an increased reliance on more efficient abdominal and thoracic musculature, and less recruitment of subclavian musculature, in young endurance athletes following a two-month breathing intervention. More efficient ventilatory muscular recruit at both lower and higher intensities during exercise may benefit endurance performance by reducing oxygen demand of the ventilator musculature and thus increasing oxygen availability for mechanical work.

Supplementary Materials: The following are available online at https://www.mdpi.com/article/10.3390/jcm10163514/s1.

Author Contributions: Conceptualization, P.B., R.M., and D.M.; methodology, P.B., V.B., R.M., D.M., G.J.G., and J.S.; software, P.B. and D.M.; validation, P.B., V.B., R.M., and D.M.; formal analysis, P.B., D.M., and J.S.; investigation, P.B., R.M. and D.M.; resources, P.B., R.M., D.M., and J.S.; data curation, P.B., V.B., and G.J.G.; writing—original draft preparation, P.B., V.B. and G.J.G.; writing—review and editing, P.B., V.B., R.M., D.M., G.J.G., and J.S.; visualization, P.B.; supervision, P.B., V.B., and G.J.G.; project administration, P.B., R.M., D.M., and J.S.; funding acquisition, P.B. and R.M. All authors have read and agreed to the published version of the manuscript.

Funding: This research was funded by the Grant Agency of University of South Bohemia within the framework of Team grant project No. 021/2019/S.

Institutional Review Board Statement: The study was conducted according to the guidelines of the Declaration of Helsinki, and approved by the Ethics Committee of Faculty of Education, University of South Bohemia, Ref. No.: 001/2018, from 19 October 2018.

Informed Consent Statement: Informed consent was obtained from all subjects involved in the study.

Data Availability Statement: Data sharing not applicable.

Conflicts of Interest: The authors declare no conflict of interest. The funders had no role in the design of the study; in the collection, analyses, or interpretation of data; in the writing of the manuscript, or in the decision to publish the results.

References

1. Bravo-Sánchez, A.; Morán-García, J.; Abián, P.; Abián-Vicén, J. Association of the Use of the Mobile Phone with Physical Fitness and Academic Performance: A Cross-Sectional Study. *Int. J. Environ. Res. Public Health* **2021**, *18*, 1042. [CrossRef] [PubMed]
2. Eitivipart, A.C.; Viriyarojanakul, S.; Redhead, L. Musculoskeletal disorder and pain associated with smartphone use: A systematic review of biomechanical evidence. *Hong Kong Physiother. J.* **2018**, *38*, 77–90. [CrossRef] [PubMed]
3. Depiazzi, J.; Everard, M.L. Dysfunctional breathing and reaching one's physiological limit as causes of exercise-induced dyspnoea. *Breathe* **2016**, *12*, 120–129. [CrossRef]
4. Chaitow, L.; Bradley, D.; Gilbert, C. *Multidisciplinary Approaches to Breathing Pattern Disorders*; Churchill Livingstone: London, UK, 2002.
5. Kaminoff, L. What yoga therapists should know about the anatomy of breathing. *Int. J. Yoga Therap.* **2006**, *16*, 67–77. [CrossRef]
6. Pryor, J.A.; Prasad, S.A. *Physiotherapy for Respiratory and Cardiac Problems*; Churchill Livingstone: Edinburgh, UK, 2002.
7. Yuan, G.; Drost, N.A.; McIvor, R.A. Respiratory Rate and Breathing Pattern. *McMaster Univ. Med J.* **2013**, *10*, 23–25.
8. Aaron, E.A.; Johnson, B.D.; Seow, C.K.; Dempsey, J.A. Oxygen cost of exercise hyperpnea: Measurement. *J. Appl. Physiol.* **1992**, *72*, 1810–1817. [CrossRef] [PubMed]
9. Guenette, J.A.; Sheel, A.W. Physiological consequences of a high work of breathing during heavy exercise in humans. *J. Sci. Med. Sport* **2007**, *10*, 341–350. [CrossRef]
10. McArdle, W.D.; Katch, F.I.; Katch, V.L. *Essentials of Exercise Physiology*; Lippincott Williams and Wilkins: Baltimore, MD, USA, 2016.
11. Malátová, R.; Bahenský, P.; Mareš, M.; Rost, M. Breathing pattern of restful and deep breathing. In *Proceedings of the 11th International Conference on Kinanthropology, Brno, Czech Republic, 29 Novermber–1 December 2017*; Zvonař, M., Sajdlová, Z., Eds.; Masarykova Univerzita: Brno, Czech Republic, 2017.
12. Benchetrit, G. Breathing pattern in humans: Diversity and individuality. *Respir. Physiol.* **2000**, *122*, 123–129. [CrossRef]
13. Clifton-Smith, T. Breathing pattern disorders and the athlete. In *Recognizing and Treating Breathing Disorders E-Book: A Multidisciplinary Approach*; Churchill Livingstone: London, UK, 2014. [CrossRef]
14. Chaitow, L.; Bradley, D.; Gilbert, C. *Recognizing and Treating Breathing Disorders. A Multidisciplinary Approach*, 2nd ed.; Churchill Livingston: London, UK, 2014.
15. Hodges, P.W.; Heijnen, I.; Gandevia, S.C. Postural activity of the diaphragm is reduced in humans when respiratory demand increases. *J. Physiol.* **2001**, *537*, 999–1008. [CrossRef]
16. Weavil, J.C.; Amann, M. Neuromuscular fatigue during whole body exercise. *Curr. Opin. Physiol.* **2019**, *10*, 128–136. [CrossRef]
17. Hruzevych, I.; Boguslavska, V.; Kropta, R.; Galan, Y.; Nakonechnyi, I.; Pityn, M. The effectiveness of the endogenous-hypoxic breathing in the physical training of skilled swimmers. *J. Phys. Educ. Sport* **2017**, *17*, 1009–1016. [CrossRef]
18. Kisner, C.; Colby, L.A. Management of pulmonary conditions. In *Therapeutic Exercise: Foundations and Techniques*, 5th ed.; FA Davis Company: Philadelphia, PA, USA, 2007; pp. 851–882.
19. Szczepan, S.; Danek, N.; Michalik, K.; Wróblewska, Z.; Zatoń, K. Influence of a Six-Week Swimming Training with Added Respiratory Dead Space on Respiratory Muscle Strength and Pulmonary Function in Recreational Swimmers. *Int. J. Environ. Res. Public Health* **2020**, *17*, 5743. [CrossRef] [PubMed]
20. Verges, S.; Lenherr, O.; Haner, A.C.; Schulz, C.; Spengler, C.M. Increased fatigue resistance of respiratory muscles during exercise after respiratory muscle endurance training. *Am. J. Physiol. Regul. Integr. Comp. Physiol.* **2006**, *292*, R1246–R1253. [CrossRef] [PubMed]

21. Aliverti, A. The respiratory muscles during exercise. *Breathe* **2016**, *12*, 165–168. [CrossRef] [PubMed]
22. Faghy, M.A.; Brown, P.I. Functional training of the inspiratory muscles improves load carriage performance. *Ergonomics* **2019**, *62*, 1439–1449. [CrossRef] [PubMed]
23. Hinde, K.L.; Low, C.; Lloyd, R.; Cooke, C.B. Inspiratory muscle training at sea level improves the strength of inspiratory muscles during load carriage in cold-hypoxia. *Ergonomics* **2020**, *63*, 1584–1598. [CrossRef]
24. Göhl, O.; Walker, D.J.; Walterspacher, S.; Langer, D.; Spengler, C.M.; Wanke, T.; Petrovic, M.; Zwick, R.H.; Stieglitz, S.; Glöckl, R.; et al. Atemmuskeltraining: State-of-the-Art [Respiratory Muscle Training: State of the Art]. *Pneumologie* **2016**, *70*, 37–48. [CrossRef]
25. Moodie, L.; Reeve, J.; Elkins, M. Inspiratory muscle training in mechanically ventilated patients. *J. Physiother.* **2011**, *57*, 213–221. [CrossRef]
26. Sclauser Pessoa, I.M.; Franco Parreira, V.; Fregonezi, G.A.; Sheel, A.W.; Chung, F.; Reid, W.D. Reference values for maximal inspiratory pressure: A systematic review. *Can. Respir. J.* **2014**, *21*, 43–50. [CrossRef]
27. Bockenhauer, S.E.; Chen, H.; Julliard, K.N.; Weedon, J. Measuring thoracic excursion: Reliability of the cloth tape measure technique. *J. Am. Osteopath. Assoc.* **2007**, *107*, 191–196.
28. Cahalin, L.P. Pulmonary evaluation. In *Cardiovaskular and Pulmonary Physical Therapy*; DeTurkW, E., Cahalin, L.P., Eds.; McGraw-Hill: New York, NY, USA, 2004.
29. Kaneko, H.; Horie, J. Breathing movements of the chest and abdominal wall in healthy subjects. *Respir. Care* **2012**, *57*, 1442–1451. [CrossRef] [PubMed]
30. Cala, S.J.; Kenyon, C.M.; Ferrigno, G.; Carnevali, P.; Aliverti, A.; Pedotti, A.; Macklem, P.T.; Rochester, D.F. Chest wall and lung volume estimation by optical reflectance motion analysis. *J. Appl. Physiol.* **1996**, *81*, 2680–2689. [CrossRef]
31. Aliverti, A.; Cala, S.J.; Duranti, R.; Ferrigno, G.; Kenyon, C.M.; Pedotti, A.; Scano, G.; Sliwinski, P.; Macklem, P.T.; Yan, S. Human respiratory muscle actions and control during exercise. *J. Appl. Physiol.* **1997**, *83*, 1256–1269. [CrossRef]
32. Ferrigno, G.; Carnevali, P.; Aliverti, A.; Molteni, F.; Beulcke, G.; Pedotti, A. Three-dimensional optical analysis of chest wall motion. *J. Appl. Physiol.* **1994**, *77*, 1224–1231. [CrossRef]
33. Hostettler, S.; Illi, S.K.; Mohler, E.; Aliverti, A.; Spengler, C.M. Chest wall volume changes during inspiratory loaded breathing. *Respir. Physiol. Neurobiol.* **2011**, *175*, 130–139. [CrossRef]
34. Romagnoli, I.; Gorini, M.; Gigliotti, F.; Bianchi, R.; Lanini, B.; Grazzini, M.; Stendardi, L.; Scano, G. Chest wall kinematics, respiratory muscle action and dyspnoea during arm vs. leg exercise in humans. *Acta Physiol.* **2006**, *188*, 63–73. [CrossRef] [PubMed]
35. Malátová, R.; Pučelík, J.; Rokytová, J.; Kolář, P. The objectification of therapeutical methods used for improvement of the deep stabilizing spinal system. *Neuroendocrinol. Lett.* **2007**, *28*, 315–320.
36. Malátová, R.; Pučelík, J.; Rokytová, J.; Kolář, P. Technical means for objectification of medical treatments in the area of the deep stabilisation spinal system. *Neuroendocrinol. Lett.* **2008**, *29*, 125–130.
37. Malátová, R. The Importance of Breathing Stereotype and Intervention Possibilities. Post Doctoral Thesis, Brno, Czech Republic, 2021.
38. Bahenský, P.; Bunc, V.; Marko, D.; Malátová, R. Dynamics of ventilation parameters at different load intensities and the options to influence it by a breathing exercise. *J. Sports Med. Phys. Fit.* **2020**, *60*, 1101–1109. [CrossRef] [PubMed]
39. Bahenský, P.; Marko, D.; Grosicki, G.J.; Malátová, R. Warm-up breathing exercises accelerate VO_2 kinetics and reduce subjective strain during incremental cycling exercise in adolescents. *J. Phys. Educ. Sport* **2020**, *20*, 3361–3367. [CrossRef]
40. Gandevia, S.C.; Butler, J.E.; Hodges, P.W.; Taylor, J.L. Balancing acts: Respiratory sensations, motor control and human posture. *Clin. Exp. Pharmacol. Phys.* **2002**, *29*, 118–121. [CrossRef]
41. Cipriano, G.F.; Cipriano, G., Jr.; Santos, F.V.; Güntzel Chiappa, A.M.; Pires, L.; Cahalin, L.P.; Chiappa, G.R. Current insights of inspiratory muscle training on the cardiovascular system: A systematic review with meta-analysis. *Integr. Blood Press. Control* **2019**, *12*, 1–11. [CrossRef]
42. Taylor, B.J.; How, S.C.; Romer, L.M. Expiratory Muscle Fatigue Does Not Regulate Operating Lung Volumes during High-Intensity Exercise in Healthy Humans. *J. Appl. Physiol.* **2013**, *114*, 1569–1576. [CrossRef]
43. de Abreu, R.M.; Rehder-Santos, P.; Minatel, V.; Dos Santos, G.L.; Catai, A.M. Effects of inspiratory muscle training on cardiovascular autonomic control: A systematic review. *Auton. Neurosci.* **2017**, *208*, 29–35. [CrossRef]
44. Billman, G.E. The LF/HF ratio does not accurately measure cardiac sympathovagal balance. *Front. Physiol.* **2013**, *4*, 26. [CrossRef] [PubMed]
45. Hodges, P.W.; Gandevia, S.C. Activation of the human diaphragm during a repetitive postural task. *J. Physiol.* **2000**, *522*, 165–175. [CrossRef]
46. Bahenský, P.; Malátová, R.; Bunc, V. Changed dynamic ventilation parameters as a result of a breathing exercise intervention programme. *J. Sports Med. Phys. Fit.* **2019**, *59*, 1369–1375. [CrossRef]
47. Kenney, W.L.; Wilmore, J.H.; Costill, D.L. *Physiology of Sport and Exercise*; Human Kinetics: Champaign, IL, USA, 2015.
48. Hamdouni, H.; Kliszczewski, B.; Zouhal, H.; Rhibi, F.; Ben Salah, F.Z.; Ben Abderrahmann, A. Effect of three fitness programs on strength, speed, flexibility and muscle power on sedentary subjects. *J. Sports Med. Phys. Fit.* **2021**. [CrossRef]
49. Karthik, P.S.; Chandrasekhar, M.; Ambareesha, K.; Nikhil, C. Effect of pranayama and suryanamaskar on pulmonary functions in medical students. *J. Clin. Diagn. Res.* **2014**, *8*, 4–6. [CrossRef]

50. Langer, D.; Ciavaglia, C.; Faisal, A.; Webb, K.A.; Neder, J.A.; Gosselink, R.; Dacha, S.; Topalovic, M.; Ivanova, A.; O'Donnel, D.E.; et al. Inspiratory muscle training reduces diaphragm activation and dyspnea during exercise in COPD. *J. Appl. Physiol.* **2018**, *125*, 381–392. [CrossRef]
51. Radhakrishnan, K.; Sharma, V.K.; Subramanian, S.K. Does treadmill running performance, heart rate and breathing rate response during maximal graded exercise improve after volitional respiratory muscle training? *Br. J. Sports Med.* **2017**. [CrossRef] [PubMed]

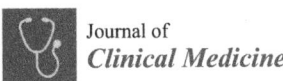

Article

Composite Score of Readiness (CSR) as Holistic Profiling of Functional Deficits in Footballers Following ACL Reconstruction

Łukasz Oleksy [1,2,3,*], Anna Mika [4], Aleksandra Królikowska [5], Maciej Kuchciak [6], Magda Stolarczyk [7], Renata Kielnar [8], Henryk Racheniuk [9], Jan Szczegielniak [9], Edyta Łuszczki [8] and Artur Stolarczyk [1]

1. Orthopaedic and Rehabilitation Department, Medical University of Warsaw, 02-091 Warsaw, Poland; drstolarczyk@gmail.com
2. Oleksy Medical & Sports Sciences, 37-100 Łańcut, Poland
3. Polish Strength and Conditioning Association, 44-141 Gliwice, Poland
4. Institute of Clinical Rehabilitation, University of Physical Education in Krakow, 31-571 Kraków, Poland; anna.mika@awf.krakow.pl
5. Department of Sports Medicine, Faculty of Health Sciences, Wroclaw Medical University, 50-367 Wroclaw, Poland; aleksandra.krolikowska@umed.wroc.pl
6. Department of Physical Education, University of Rzeszow, 35-959 Rzeszow, Poland; mkuchciak@ur.edu.pl
7. Third Clinic of Internal Medicine and Cardiology, Medical University of Warsaw, 02-091 Warsaw, Poland; magda.stolarczyk@wum.edu.pl
8. Institute of Health Sciences, Medical College of Rzeszow University, 35-959 Rzeszow, Poland; kielnarrenata@o2.pl (R.K.); eluszczki@ur.edu.pl (E.Ł.)
9. Institute of Physiotherapy, Faculty of Physical Education and Physiotherapy, Opole University of Technology, 46-020 Opole, Poland; h.racheniuk@po.edu.pl (H.R.); j.szczegielniak@po.edu.pl (J.S.)
* Correspondence: loleksy@oleksy-fizjoterapia.pl

Abstract: Background: The decision to return to sport (RTS) after anterior cruciate ligament (ACL) reconstruction is difficult; thus, coaching staff require a readable, easy-to-use, and holistic indication of an athlete's readiness to play. Purpose: To present the Composite Score of Readiness (CSR) as a method providing a single score for RTS tests after ACL reconstruction. Methods: The study comprised 65 male football players (age 18–25 years), divided into three groups: ACL group—subjects after ACL rupture and reconstruction, Mild Injury (MI) group—subjects after mild lower limb injuries, and Control (C) group—subjects without injuries. The CSR was calculated based on three performed tests (Y-balance test, Functional Movement Screen, and Tuck Jump Assessment) and expressed as the sum of z-scores. The CSR index allows highlighting an athlete's functional deficits across tests relative to the evaluated group. Results: The CSR indicated that relative to the group of athletes under the study, similar functional deficits were present. Comparing athletes following ACL reconstruction to both the MI and C groups, in the majority of subjects, the CSR index was below zero. The correlation between CSR and raw tests results indicated that the CSR is most strongly determined by YBT. Conclusion: The CSR is a simple way to differentiate people after serious injuries (with large functional deficits) from people without injuries or with only small deficits. Because the CSR is a single number, it allows us to more easily interpret the value of functional deficits in athletes, compared to rating those deficits based on raw tests results.

Keywords: anterior cruciate ligament (ACL); composite score of readiness (CSR); injury prevention; rehabilitation; football; soccer

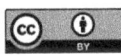

1. Introduction

Anterior cruciate ligament (ACL) injuries are very common in sports [1]. The most important goal for athletes after ACL reconstruction is a successful return to play [1,2]. It has been reported that from 78% to 98% of professional athletes, and 65% of amateurs, return to pre-injury level [3]. However, 74% of ACL re-injuries occur within the first

2 years [3]. After ACL reconstruction, the deficits were observed in postural stability as well as in alterations in knee and hip function. It was suggested that they might be associated with pathological movement patterns leading to further tissue overloads, and often, to ACL re-injury [4–6]. It has been suggested that return-to-sport (RTS) testing after ACL reconstruction should include several tests, such as isokinetic strength, hop test, and a jump landing task assessed with the Landing Error Scoring System or Tuck Jump Assessment (TJA) [6–9]. Additionally, movement patterns, mobility, and stability evaluation with the Functional Movement Screen (FMS) and dynamic balance via the Y-balance test (YBT) or the star excursion balance test were also recommended [9].

The decision to RTS after ACL reconstruction is difficult for clinicians to make. Moreover, the coaching staff require a readable, easy-to-use, and holistic indication of an athlete's readiness to play [10]. This has raised a need to provide a single score to assess athletes' RTS, rather than separately discussing each individual test result [10,11]. As we know, the athletes are regularly put through many tests whose individual results collected together produce an overwhelming amount of data [10–12]. Some authors propose identifying fewer but more predictive tests [8,13]. Others provide us with strategies that aim to reduce the data without decreasing the number of performed tests, such as Total Score of Athleticism (TSA), a single score of an athlete's holistic athleticism introduced by Turner [10]. This way of assessment, by creating a single index, is already known in the literature. Such indices were used in gait evaluation [14–17]. The Gait Deviation Index (GDI), Gillette Gait Index (GGI), or Normalcy Index (NI) were derived to calculate the amount by which a subject's gait deviates from an average normal profile and to represent this deviation as a single number [14–17]. The other index, called "Total Score of Athleticism (TSA)", was described by Thurner et al. [10,11], and allowed coaches to examine the athleticism level of individual athletes relative to their teammates. This approach provided coaches with quick and easy-to-read data indicating how well each athlete performed in the tests relative to their teammates, and which areas are strengths, and which are weaknesses [10,11].

It is known that for coaches, most important is that the evaluation and interpretation of test results for a given athlete are clear and easy to interpret and that they are read in the same way by others. Direct reference to the baseline value (indicating a correct result) may allow for a precise assessment of the size of an athlete's deficits. Following the TSA model, we would like to propose the injury risk index called "Composite Score of Readiness (CSR)". This study is the first in which a single score index for RTS evaluation is described, which may differentiate athletes following a serious injury such as ACL reconstruction from athletes after mild musculoskeletal injuries and healthy controls. This index may allow assessing the level of functional deficits in these athletes. Therefore, the purpose of this study was to present the Composite Score of Readiness (CSR) as a method providing a single score for RTS tests after ACL reconstruction.

2. Methods

2.1. Participants

The studied participants involved 65 male football players belonging to regional teams participated in this study. Basing on a medical interview and gathered medical documentation, the players were divided into three groups, named consecutively "Group 1 (ACL)", "Group 2 (MI)", and "Group 3 (C)". The three groups were similar in age, body weight, and body height, as presented in Table 1. Based on medical interviews and gathered medical documentation, they were free of the following diagnosed medical problems: currently experiencing pain and movement restriction, respiratory and circulatory system diseases, bilateral injuries in the lower limbs in the history, injuries of the trunk in the past, injuries of upper limbs in the past, and they gave consent to participate in research. The inclusion criteria in Group I were: clearance to play by an orthopedic specialist after primary unilateral ACL rupture and following arthroscopic reconstruction underwent during the 3 years before the research; bone–patellar, tendon–bone, or hamstring tendon autografts used during ACL reconstruction; no abnormalities and no history of injury in the contralateral knee; no to all of the following procedures: medial and/or lateral meniscectomy, medial and/or lateral meniscal transplant, posterior cruciate ligament repair, and medial or/and lateral collateral ligament repair/reconstruction osteoarthritis surgery in the ACL-reconstructed knee other than shaving; the lack of any upper limbs and trunk injuries in the past. The inclusion criteria in Group 2: clearance to play by an orthopedic specialist after grade I or "mild" lower limb muscle injury according to Grassi et al. [18] and following conservative treatment undergone during the 3 years before the research; no history of any other injuries in lower limbs, the lack of any upper limbs and trunk injuries in the past. The inclusion criteria in Group 3, a control group, was the lack of any lower and upper limbs and trunk injuries in the past.

Table 1. Subjects characteristics.

	Group 1	Group 2	Group 3
Number of subjects (n)	24	21	20
Height (cm)	175 ± 4	177 ± 6	178 ± 6
Weight (kg)	77.3 ± 7.6	74.3 ± 9.1	75.8 ± 8.8
Age	22.7 ± 3.6	20.5 ± 3.7	23.1 ± 2.8

No significant difference was found for any variable.

Group 1 (ACL) (n = 24)—subjects after ACL rupture and reconstruction in previous 2–3 years who passed RTS including orthopedic and manual tests performed by a physiotherapist, muscle strength evaluation and hop tests, and were cleared to play (involved leg—after ACL reconstruction, uninvolved leg—contralateral limb without ACL injury);

Group 2 (MI) (n = 21)—subjects after mild lower limb injury in previous 2–3 years (involved leg—after mild injury, uninvolved leg—contralateral limb without injury);

Group 3 (C) (n = 20)—control group without injuries (the left limb was the equivalent of the involved limb and the right limb was the equivalent of the uninvolved limb).

The study participants were informed in detail about the research protocol and gave their written informed consent to participate in the study. Informed consent was acquired from the parent for participants under the age of 18. Approval of the Ethical Committee of Regional Medical Chamber in Kraków was obtained for this study (16/KBL/OIL/2016). All procedures were performed in accordance with the 1964 Declaration of Helsinki and its later amendments.

2.2. Procedures

A 5 min warm-up included general, non-specific exercises, which prepared the entire body for the performed tests. Then, each subject performed testing trials for each test to become fully familiar with the nature of the measurements. The protocol included the FMS test, the YBT, and TJA with 15 min intervals between the tests. An experienced researcher blinded to the subject group allocation performed all tests.

2.3. Functional Movement Screen

The FMS test (Functional Movement Systems Inc., Chatham, VA, USA), which includes assessment of body asymmetries and recognition of poor quality movement patterns, was performed according to the original methodology reported by Cook et al. [19–21]. FMS test inter-rater reliability was ICC = 0.87–0.89, and intra-rater was ICC = 0.81–0.91 [22,23].

2.4. Y-Balance Test

The YBT test (Move2Perform, Evansville, IN, USA) was conducted according to the criteria described by Plisky et al. [24,25]. Three reach trials were performed in each direction, first standing on the uninvolved leg and then on the involved (on the right leg and then on the left in the control group) [25]. The intra-rater reliability of the YBT was ICC = 0.85–0.91 and inter-rater reliability was ICC = 0.85–0.93 [25,26].

3. Tuck Jump Assessment

TJA was carried out according to previously described protocols [27,28]. Jumping efforts were recorded with the resolution 736 × 352 and 125 fps frame rate using the NiNOX 125 camcorder (NiNOX 125, Noraxon USA, Scottsdale, AZ, USA) from the sagittal and frontal plane view. Technique flaws were scored according to previously published form [28]. The reported TJA intra-tester mean percentage of exact agreement ranged between 87.2% and 100%, with kappa values of k = 0.86–1.0 [29].

3.1. Composite Score of Readiness (CSR)

The CSR was calculated from the 3 performed tests (FMS, YBT, and TJA) [10,11]. The CSR was the sum of z-scores, which represented the number of standard deviations by which the value of a raw score was above or below the mean of the measured variables. Raw scores above the mean have positive z-scores, while for those below the mean, the z-scores are negative. The z-scores were then summed to form a single score. Because z-scores and SD are unitless, the results can be summed across all tests. The CSR allows highlighting an athlete's functional deficits across tests relative to the evaluated group. The interpretation of the CSR is based on the methodology described by Thurner et al. [10,11]. If zero represents the group average, any value above zero means that the athlete is better than average, while values below 0 indicate worse performance.

- The mean ± 1 SD contains ~68% of all test scores;
- The mean ± 2 SD ~95%;
- The mean ± 3 SD ~99%.

Two types of CSR were calculated. One type is the CSR, in which the z-score for individual athletes was calculated relative to their own group.

CSR_A—calculated for athletes after ACL reconstruction relative to the group of athletes also after ACL reconstruction;

CSR_M—calculated for athletes after mild lower limb injuries relative to the group of athletes with similar mild lower limb injuries;

CSR_H—calculated for athletes without injuries relative to the group of similar athletes without injuries.

Then, the value of the CSR index for each athlete was converted relative to the remaining 2 groups. In this way, the relative CSR index was created, showing the size of the functional deficits of a given athlete in relation to different reference groups.

CSR_{A-M}—calculated for athletes after ACL reconstruction relative to the group of athletes with mild lower limb injuries;

CSR_{A-H}—calculated for athletes after ACL reconstruction relative to the group of athletes without injuries;

CSR_{M-H}—calculated for athletes after mild lower limb injuries relative to the group of athletes without injuries.

3.2. Statistical Analysis

Statistical analysis was performed using STATISTICA 12.0 Pl software. All evaluated variables were reported as the arithmetic mean (x) and standard deviation (SD). The data were evaluated for normality with Shapiro–Wilk test. The t-test was used to determine the differences between groups. Additionally, Pearson's linear correlation coefficient (r) was calculated (below 0.50—poor; between 0.50 and 0.75—moderate; between 0.75 and 0.90—good; above 0.90—excellent). Statistical significance was set at the level of ($p < 0.05$).

4. Results

All CSR indices were normally distributed ($p > 0.05$). They are graphically presented in Figure 1, highlighting particular athletes' performance relative to their group. Zero represents the team average in terms of CSR (sum of performed tests). Bars above the zero line represent athletes better than average, while bars below the line indicate worse than average athletes.

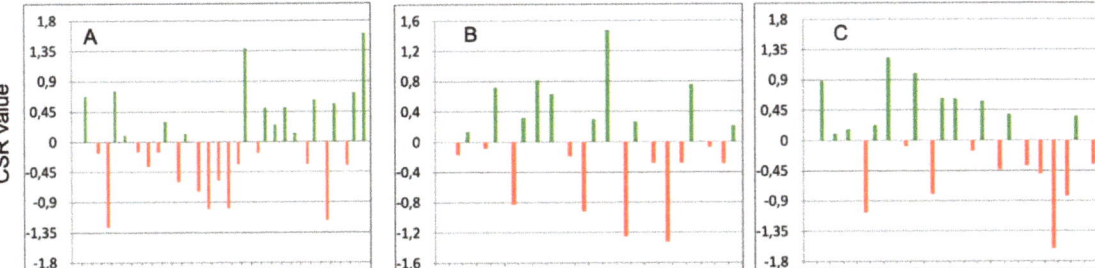

Figure 1. The values of CSR_A (**A**), CSR_M (**B**), and CSR_H (**C**) in athletes relative to the own group. Zero represents the group average CSR value; green bars indicate positive value (it means that the particular athlete is better than average); red bars indicate negative value (it means that the particular athlete is worse than average).

It has been shown that the CSR_A in 15 athletes was below zero (Figure 1A). The CSR_M was below zero in 11 athletes (Figure 1B), while the CSR_H in 10 athletes did not exceed zero (Figure 1C). This means that relative to the own group, athletes represented similar functional deficits. The CSR_A, CSR_M, and CSR_H indices allow demonstrating who, within the group, exhibits better and who exhibits worse performance.

Comparing athletes after ACL reconstruction to both the MI and C groups, it can be seen that in the majority of subjects, the CSR_{A-M} (Figure 2A) and CSR_{A-H} indices (Figure 2B) were below zero. It has been demonstrated that athletes with severe injury, similar to ACL reconstruction, despite passing the RTS, are in a functionally worse state compared to athletes with mild injuries or healthy ones. On the other hand, when comparing athletes with mild injuries to those healthy, they did not differ significantly from each other because the number of positive and negative CSR_{M-H} indices was similar (Figure 2C).

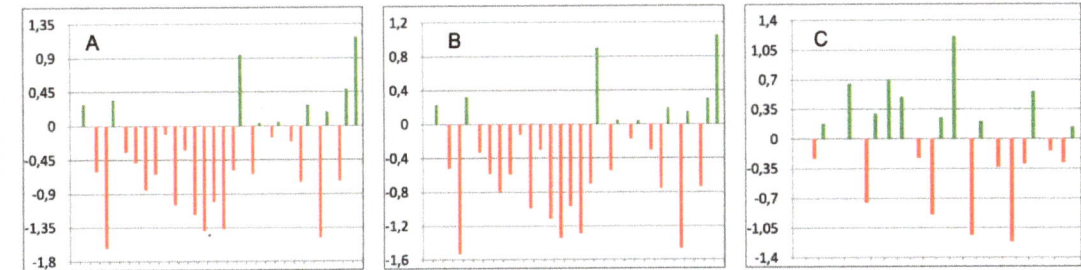

Figure 2. The values of CSR_{A-M} (**A**), CSR_{A-H} (**B**), and CSR_{M-H} (**C**) when comparing athletes after ACL reconstruction to both the MI and C groups. Zero represents the group average CSR value; green bars indicate positive value (it means that the particular athlete is better than average); red bars indicate negative value (it means that the particular athlete is worse than average).

The analysis of differences between the presented CSR indices showed similar results. The values of the CSR_{M-H} were significantly higher than CSR_{A-M} (Figure 3A). This difference was more visible when the CSR_{A-H} was compared to CSR_{M-H} and it was significant (Figure 3B). However, when CSR_{A-M} and CSR_{A-H} were compared, the values were similar, while the difference was non-significant ($p > 0.05$) (Figure 3C).

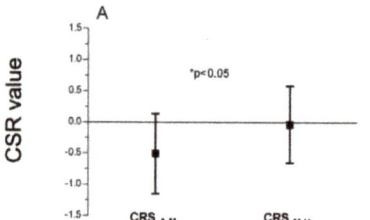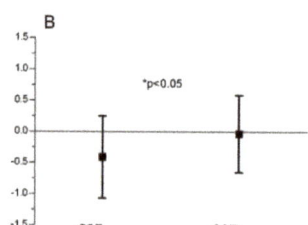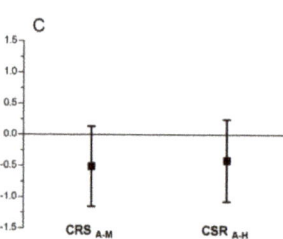

Figure 3. The difference between (**A**) CSR_{A-M} and CSR_{M-H}; (**B**) between CSR_{A-H} and CSR_{M-H}; (**C**) between CSR_{A-M} and CSR_{A-H}.

The correlation between CSR indices and raw test results indicated that the CSR is determined most strongly by YBT (Table 2). There was a strong and significant relationship between the composite score of the YBT test and each of the three CSR indices (r = 0.9–0.93) (Table 2). Interestingly, analyzing the correlation between the value of each CSR and the YBT components, it was noted that the relationship was good and significant for all reaching directions of both limbs but was stronger in the posterolateral and posteromedial directions (r = 0.79–0.85). The anterior direction demonstrated a moderate relationship (r = 0.57–0.64). Both the FMS and TJA tests presented a much weaker relationship with the CSR indices. The relationship between the FMS composite score and CSR was poor (r = 0.35–0.38). Between the TJA composite score and the CSR, the correlation was also poor and non-significant (r = 0.30–0.35) (Table 2).

Table 2. The relationship between CSR and raw tests results.

Outcome Measure	Side	CSR_A	CSR_{A-M}	CSR_{A-H}
FMS Composite Score (points)		0.38 *	0.35	0.38 *
TJA Composite Score (points)		0.36	0.30	0.35
YBT Composite Score (%)	I	0.92 *	0.93 *	0.92 *
	U	0.90 *	0.92 *	0.90 *
YBT Anterior Reach (%)	I	0.56 *	0.60 *	0.57 *
	U	0.59 *	0.64 *	0.59 *
YBT Posterolateral Reach (%)	I	0.85 *	0.83 *	0.85 *
	U	0.83 *	0.83 *	0.84 *
YBT Posteromedial Reach (%)	I	0.82 *	0.82 *	0.81 *
	U	0.80 *	0.79 *	0.79 *

(I) Involved side; (U) uninvolved side. CSR_A—index calculated for athletes after ACL reconstruction relative to the group of athletes also after ACL reconstruction. CSR_{A-M}—index calculated for athletes after ACL reconstruction relative to the group of athletes with mild lower limbs injuries. CSR_{A-H}—index calculated for athletes after ACL reconstruction relative to the group of athletes without injuries. (TJA) Tuck Jump Assessment; (FMS) Functional Movement Screen; (YBT) Y-balance test. Values are expressed as Pearson correlation coefficient (r). * $p < 0.05$.

5. Discussion

The most important information from this study is that the CSR is a simple way to differentiate athletes with severe functional deficits following serious injuries such as ACL rupture and reconstruction from those without injuries or with only small functional deficits. This difference may be expressed as one index, which is easy to interpret. We have also noted that athletes after ACL reconstruction are in a functionally worse state than athletes following mild injuries or those who are healthy.

Unfortunately, as indicated by some authors, passing the RTS criteria did not result in a decreased risk of ACL re-injury, suggesting that some functional deficits are still present and may not be diagnosed during evaluation [30,31]. The RTS may include many tests, and there is no consensus as to which are the most sensitive and valid. Moreover, many of them may be difficult to rate unambiguously, especially when a number of tests are performed by the athlete and provide non-homogenous results. Very often, coaches and athletes are not interested in the raw score of the test, which may be difficult for interpretation, but they require a simple indication of an athlete's readiness-to-play after ACL reconstruction.

This manner of assessment, through a one-number index, has been discussed in the literature on the subject of gait pattern disorder assessment [14–17] or in the evaluation of athletes' sports level [10,11]. The single number reflects the value by which a subject's gait deviates from the average for normal gait [14–17]. Additionally, the TSA is a method providing a single score of holistic athleticism, from fitness tests and informing how well someone performed relative to the others taking part in the test [10,11]. Therefore, we suggest that the CSR may be a good tool for properly discriminating athletes with high functional deficits after serious injuries such as ACL rupture and reconstruction from athletes with mild injuries or from healthy ones. The CSR may allow to easily rate the severity of post-injury functional deficits in relation to the reference value (the value close to zero). According to the methodology described by Thurner et al. [10,11], a score of one indicates that an athlete has obtained a better score than 84% of his/her group, while a score of two indicates a score better than 97%.

In the present study, the CSR_A, CSR_M, and CSR_H indices allowed to show who, within the group, demonstrates better and who demonstrates worse performance. As was presented, when compared athletes with similar functional deficiencies, those with greater and those with smaller deficits can be distinguished. However, based on this type of CSR, we do not know the size of these deficits in relation to the normal values, e.g., in healthy controls without injuries. Only by comparing athletes after ACL reconstruction to other reference groups (healthy or mildly injured) can the size of these deficits be observed. In our study, by comparing athletes post-ACL reconstruction to both the MI and C groups, it could be seen that the majority exhibited CSR indices below zero. It was shown that athletes with severe injuries, such as ACL reconstruction, despite passing the RTS, were in a functionally worse state compared to those with mild injuries or healthy individuals. On the other hand, comparing athletes with mild injuries to healthy subjects, they did not differ significantly from each other because the amount of positive and negative indices was similar.

It has been recommended that RTS testing after ACL reconstruction should incorporate several tests, but it is unclear which are most associated with a successful RTS [8,9]. The TJA was reported to identify players at risk of ACL injuries by identifying side-to-side asymmetries, neuromuscular imbalances, as well as jumping and landing technique flaws [7]. The FMS has been suggested as an effective tool during RTS evaluation [24], while its limited usage has been underlined by others [32,33]. Chorba et al. [34] have reported that the FMS was unable to differentiate between subjects who had not experienced any ACL rupture and those who had. Moreover, it was shown that ACL injuries alter movement patterns, but the FMS test is unable to detect them, and these deficits may increase the risk of re-injury [35]. Additionally, the application of YBT in RTS screening provides equivocal results. Some researchers have indicated the usefulness of YBT [36–38], while others have not found any differences in YBT scores among athletes following ACL reconstruction who were or were not cleared for return to unrestricted activity [39]. In the current study, it has been reported that CRS calculated from FMS, YBT, and TJA tests indicated that athletes after ACL reconstruction are in a functionally worse state than those following mild injuries or without injuries.

A crucial issue, which was also underlined by Thurner et al. [10,11], is that the diagnostic value of such an index may be influenced by the kind of applied test as well as by the amount (number) of the tests from which z-scores are summed. They have reported that the validity of the TSA index was largely determined by the relevance of the implemented fitness tests [10,11]. This problem may also be a weakness of the CSR index. Therefore, we have analyzed which test influenced the final index the most; thus, in other words, which test is most indicative of functional deficits related to ACL reconstruction. Our results allowed us to suggest that CSR is determined most strongly by YBT. Interestingly, analyzing the correlation between the value of each CSR and the YBT components (not only a composite score), it was noted that the relationship was good and significant for all reaching directions of both limbs but was stronger in the posterolateral and posteromedial directions. The anterior direction (considered by many authors to be the most deficient in people after ACL) showed a moderate relationship. On the other hand, both the FMS and TJA tests presented a much weaker association with the CSR indices. This means that these tests are less indicative for assessing the size of functional deficits in athletes after ACL reconstruction. However, this issue requires further research to see which tests are the most sensitive in detecting specific deficiencies post-ACL reconstruction. Another critical aspect that requires further research is the analysis of individual test components because, as has been shown in our research, the composite score of a given test does not always provide the same information as its individual elements. Perhaps, most optimal would be an index created from parts of the tests and not only from their composite results.

This study also has some limitations which should be addressed. We calculated the CSR only from three tests (FMS, YBT, TJA). Perhaps, if more tests would be included in CSR calculations, its diagnostic value would be more substantial, and the CSR itself would be more comprehensive. Additionally, because psychological factors have emerged as important in the RTS process, it seems required to include psychological tests as a component of CSR. Therefore, there is a need for future research, including a broader selection of tests. Moreover, the utility of CSR should be assessed in future studies concerning its reliability, sensitivity to rehabilitation interventions, and predictability of RTS outcomes.

6. Conclusions

The CSR is a simple way to differentiate individuals following serious injuries (with large functional deficits) from those without injuries or with only small deficits. Because the CSR is a single number, it allows easier interpretation of the functional deficit size in athletes than if rating those deficits from raw tests results.

Author Contributions: Ł.O.: conceptualization, methodology, investigation, resources, data curation, formal analysis, writing—original draft, supervision, and funding acquisition. A.M.: methodology, investigation, resources, data curation, formal analysis, and writing—original draft. A.K.: methodology, resources, and writing—review and editing. M.K.: methodology, investigation, resources, data curation, and writing—review and editing. M.S.: methodology and writing—review and editing. R.K.: methodology and writing—review and editing. H.R.: methodology and writing—review and editing. J.S.: methodology and writing—review and editing. E.Ł.: methodology and writing—review and editing. A.S.: methodology, writing review and editing, and funding acquisition. All authors have read and agreed to the published version of the manuscript.

Funding: This research received no external funding.

Institutional Review Board Statement: Approval of the Ethical Committee of Regional Medical Chamber in Kraków was obtained for this study (protocol number 16/KBL/OIL/2016; date of approval 10/02/2016). All procedures were performed in accordance with the 1964 Declaration of Helsinki and its later amendments.

Informed Consent Statement: Informed consent was obtained from all subjects involved in the study.

Data Availability Statement: All data generated or analyzed during this study are included in this published article.

Conflicts of Interest: The authors declare no conflict of interest.

References

1. Ross, B.J.; Savage-Elliott, I.; Brown, S.M.; Mulcahey, M.K. Return to Play and Performance After Primary ACL Reconstruction in American Football Players: A Systematic Review. *Orthop. J Sports Med.* **2020**, *8*, 2325967120959654. [CrossRef]
2. Welling, W.; Benjaminse, A.; Seil, R.; Lemmink, K.; Zaffagnini, S.; Gokeler, A. Low rates of patients meeting return to sport criteria 9 months after anterior cruciate ligament reconstruction: A prospective longitudinal study. *Knee Surg. Sports Traumatol. Arthrosc.* **2018**, *26*, 3636–3644. [CrossRef]

3. Welling, W.; Benjaminse, A.; Lemmink, K.; Gokeler, A. Passing return to sports tests after ACL reconstruction is associated with greater likelihood for return to sport but fail to identify second injury risk. *Knee* **2020**, *27*, 949–957. [CrossRef] [PubMed]
4. Hoog, P.; Warren, M.; Smith, C.A.; Chimera, N.J. Functional hop tests and Tuck Jump Assessment scores between female division I collegiate athletes participating in high versus low ACL injury prone sports: A cross sectional analysis. *Int. J. Sports Phys. Ther.* **2016**, *11*, 945–953. [PubMed]
5. Myer, G.D.; Ford, K.R.; Hewett, T.E. Rationale and clinical techniques for anterior cruciate ligament injury prevention among female athletes. *J. Athl. Train.* **2004**, *39*, 352–364. [PubMed]
6. Lai, C.C.H.; Ardern, C.L.; Feller, J.A.; Webster, K.E. Eighty-three per cent of elite athletes return to preinjury sport after anterior cruciate ligament reconstruction: A systematic review with meta-analysis of return to sport rates, graft rupture rates and performance outcomes. *Br. J. Sports Med.* **2018**, *52*, 128–138. [CrossRef]
7. Arundale, A.J.H.; Kvist, J.; Hägglund, M.; Fältström, A. Tuck Jump score is not related to hopping performance or patient-reported outcome measures in female soccer players. *Int. J. Sports Phys. Ther.* **2020**, *15*, 395–406. [CrossRef]
8. Webster, K.E.; Feller, J.A. Who Passes Return-to-Sport Tests, and Which Tests Are Most Strongly Associated with Return to Play After Anterior Cruciate Ligament Reconstruction? *Orthop. J. Sports Med.* **2020**, *8*, 2325967120969425.
9. Bishop, C. Assessing movement using a variety of screening tests. *Prof. Strength Cond.* **2015**, *37*, 17–26.
10. Turner, A.N.; Jones, B.; Stewart, P.; Bishop, C.; Parmar, N.; Chavda, S.; Read, P. Total score of athleticism: Holistic athlete profiling to enhance decision-making. *Strength Cond. J.* **2019**, *41*, 91–101. [CrossRef]
11. Turner, A. Total Score of Athleticism: A strategy for assessing an athlete's athleticism. *Prof. Strength Cond.* **2014**, *33*, 13–17.
12. Madsen, L.P.; Booth, R.L.; Volz, J.D.; Docherty, C.L. Using Normative Data and Unilateral Hopping Tests to Reduce Ambiguity in Return-to-Play Decisions. *J. Athl. Train.* **2020**, *55*, 699–706. [CrossRef] [PubMed]
13. Hewett, T.E.; Webster, K.E.; Hurd, W.J. Systematic Selection of Key Logistic Regression Variables for Risk Prediction Analyses: A Five-Factor Maximum Model. *Clin. J. Sport Med.* **2019**, *29*, 78–85. [CrossRef] [PubMed]
14. Cretual, A.; Bervet, K.; Ballaz, L. Gillette Gait Index in adults. *Gait Posture* **2010**, *32*, 307–310. [CrossRef] [PubMed]
15. Schwartz, M.H.; Rozumalski, A. The Gait Deviation Index: A new comprehensive index of gait pathology. *Gait Posture* **2008**, *28*, 351–357. [CrossRef]
16. McMulkin, M.L.; MacWilliams, B.A. Application of the Gillette Gait Index, Gait Deviation Index and Gait Profile Score to multiple clinical pediatric populations. *Gait Posture* **2015**, *41*, 608–612. [CrossRef]
17. Romei, M.; Galli, M.; Motta, F.; Schwartz, M.; Crivellini, M. Use of the normalcy index for the evaluation of gait pathology. *Gait Posture* **2004**, *19*, 85–90. [CrossRef]
18. Grassi, A.; Quaglia, A.; Canata, G.L.; Zaffagnini, S. An update on the grading of muscle injuries: A narrative review from clinical to comprehensive systems. *Joints* **2016**, *4*, 39–46. [CrossRef]
19. Cook, G.; Burton, L.; Kiesel, K.; Rose, G.; Bryant, M.F. *Functional Movement Systems: Screening, Assessment, Corrective Strategies*; On Target Publications: Aptos, CA, USA, 2010.
20. Cook, G.; Burton, L.; Hoogenboom, B.J.; Voight, M. Functional movement screening: The use of fundamental movements as an assessment of function—Part 2. *Int. J. Sports Phys. Ther.* **2014**, *9*, 549–563.
21. Cook, G.; Burton, L.; Hoogenboom, B.J.; Voight, M. Functional movement screening: The use of fundamental movements as an assessment of function—Part 1. *Int. J. Sports Phys. Ther.* **2014**, *9*, 396–409.
22. Gribble, P.A.; Brigle, J.; Pietrosimone, B.G.; Pfile, K.R.; Webster, K.A. Intrarater reliability of the functional movement screen. *J. Strength Cond. Res.* **2013**, *27*, 978–981. [CrossRef]
23. Smith, C.A.; Chimera, N.J.; Wright, N.J.; Warren, M. Interrater and intrarater reliability of the functional movement screen. *J. Strength Cond. Res.* **2013**, *27*, 982–987. [CrossRef] [PubMed]
24. Chimera, N.J.; Smith, C.A.; Warren, M. Injury history, sex, and performance on the functional movement screen and Y balance test. *J. Athl. Train.* **2015**, *50*, 475–485. [CrossRef] [PubMed]
25. Brumitt, J.; Nelson, K.; Duey, D.; Jeppson, M.; Hammer, L. Preseason Y Balance Test Scores are not Associated with Noncontact Time-Loss Lower Quadrant Injury in Male Collegiate Basketball Players. *Sports* **2018**, *7*, 4. [CrossRef] [PubMed]
26. Shaffer, S.W. Y-balance test: A reliability study involving multiple raters. *Mil. Med.* **2013**, *178*, 1264–1270. [CrossRef]
27. Frost, D.M.; Beach, T.A.; Campbell, T.L.; Callaghan, J.P.; McGill, S.M. An appraisal of the Functional Movement Screen™ grading criteria—Is the composite score sensitive to risky movement behavior? *Phys. Ther. Sport.* **2015**, *16*, 324–330. [CrossRef]
28. Lininger, M.R.; Smith, C.A.; Chimera, N.J.; Hoog, P.; Warren, M. Tuck Jump Assessment: An Exploratory Factor Analysis in a College Age Population. *J. Strength Cond. Res.* **2017**, *31*, 653–659. [CrossRef]
29. Herrington, L.; Myer, G.D.; Munro, A. Intra and inter-tester reliability of the tuck jump assessment. *Phys. Ther. Sport.* **2013**, *14*, 152–155. [CrossRef]
30. Losciale, J.M.; Zdeb, R.M.; Ledbetter, L.; Reiman, M.P.; Sell, T.C. The association between passing return-to-sport criteria and second anterior cruciate ligament injury risk: A systematic review with meta-analysis. *J. Orthop. Sports Phys. Ther.* **2019**, *49*, 43–54. [CrossRef] [PubMed]
31. Webster, K.E.; Hewett, T.E. What is the evidence for and validity of return-to-sport testing after anterior cruciate ligament reconstruction surgery? A systematic review and meta-analysis. *Sports Med.* **2019**, *49*, 917–929. [CrossRef]
32. Hoover, D. Predictive validity of the Functional Movement Screen in a population of recreational runners training for a half marathon. In Proceedings of the American College of Sports Medicine Annual Meeting, Indianapolis, IN, USA, 28–31 May 2008.

33. Munce, T.A. Using functional movement tests to assess injury risk and predict performance in Collegiate basketball players. In Proceedings of the American College of Sports Medicine Annual Meeting, San Francisco, CA, USA, 29 May–2 June 2012.
34. Chorba, R.S.; Chorba, D.J.; Bouillon, L.E.; Overmyer, C.A.; Landis, J.A. Use of a functional movement screening tool to determine injury risk in female collegiate athletes. *N. Am. J. Sports Phys. Ther.* **2010**, *5*, 47–54.
35. Stergiou, N.; Ristanis, S.; Moraiti, C.; Georgoulis, A.D. Tibial rotation in anterior cruciate ligament (ACL)-deficient and ACL-reconstructed knees: A theoretical proposition for the development of osteoarthritis. *Sports Med.* **2007**, *37*, 601–613. [CrossRef]
36. Butler, R.J.; Lehr, M.E.; Fink, M.L.; Kiesel, K.B.; Plisky, P.J. Dynamic balance performance and noncontact lower extremity injury in college football players: An initial study. *Sports Health* **2013**, *5*, 417–422. [CrossRef] [PubMed]
37. Miller, M.M.; Trapp, J.L.; Post, E.G.; Trigsted, S.M.; McGuine, T.A.; Brooks, M.A.; Bell, D.R. The Effects of Specialization and Sex on Anterior Y-Balance Performance in High School Athletes. *Sports Health* **2017**, *9*, 375–382. [CrossRef] [PubMed]
38. Gonell, A.C.; Romero, J.A.P.; Soler, L.M. Relationship between the Y balance test scores and soft tissue injury incidence in a soccer team. *Int. J. Sports Phys. Ther.* **2015**, *10*, 955–966.
39. Mayer, S.W.; Queen, R.M.; Taylor, D.; Moorman, C.T., 3rd; Toth, A.P.; Garrett, W.E., Jr.; Butler, R.J. Functional Testing Differences in Anterior Cruciate Ligament Reconstruction Patients Released Versus Not Released to Return to Sport. *Am. J. Sports Med.* **2015**, *43*, 1648–1655. [CrossRef] [PubMed]

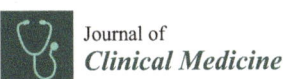

Review

Criterion-Related Validity of Field-Based Fitness Tests in Adults: A Systematic Review

Jose Castro-Piñero [1,2], Nuria Marin-Jimenez [1,2,*], Jorge R. Fernandez-Santos [1,2], Fatima Martin-Acosta [1,2], Victor Segura-Jimenez [1,2], Rocio Izquierdo-Gomez [1,2], Jonatan R. Ruiz [3] and Magdalena Cuenca-Garcia [1,2]

[1] GALENO Research Group, Department of Physical Education, Faculty of Education Sciences, University of Cádiz, Avenida República Saharaui s/n, Puerto Real, 11519 Cádiz, Spain; jose.castro@uca.es (J.C.-P.); jorgedelrosario.fernandez@uca.es (J.R.F.-S.); fatima.martin@uca.es (F.M.-A.); victor.segura@uca.es (V.S.-J.); rocio.izquierdo@uca.es (R.I.-G.); magdalena.cuenca@uca.es (M.C.-G.)
[2] Instituto de Investigación e Innovación Biomédica de Cádiz (INiBICA), 11009 Cádiz, Spain
[3] PROmoting FITness and Health through Physical Activity Research Group (PROFITH), Sport and Health University Research Institute (iMUDS), Department of Physical and Sports Education, School of Sports Science, University of Granada, 18007 Granada, Spain; ruizj@ugr.es
* Correspondence: nuria.marin@uca.es; Tel.: +34-956-016-253

Citation: Castro-Piñero, J.; Marin-Jimenez, N.; Fernandez-Santos, J.R.; Martin-Acosta, F.; Segura-Jimenez, V.; Izquierdo-Gomez, R.; Ruiz, J.R.; Cuenca-Garcia, M. Criterion-Related Validity of Field-Based Fitness Tests in Adults: A Systematic Review. *J. Clin. Med.* **2021**, *10*, 3743. https://doi.org/10.3390/jcm10163743

Academic Editors: David Rodríguez-Sanz and Naama W. Constantini

Received: 8 June 2021
Accepted: 15 August 2021
Published: 23 August 2021

Publisher's Note: MDPI stays neutral with regard to jurisdictional claims in published maps and institutional affiliations.

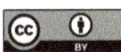

Copyright: © 2021 by the authors. Licensee MDPI, Basel, Switzerland. This article is an open access article distributed under the terms and conditions of the Creative Commons Attribution (CC BY) license (https://creativecommons.org/licenses/by/4.0/).

Abstract: We comprehensively assessed the criterion-related validity of existing field-based fitness tests used to indicate adult health (19–64 years, with no known pathologies). The medical electronic databases MEDLINE (via PubMed) and Web of Science (all databases) were screened for studies published up to July 2020. Each original study's methodological quality was classified as high, low and very low, according to the number of participants, the description of the study population, statistical analysis and systematic reviews which were appraised via the AMSTAR rating scale. Three evidence levels were constructed (strong, moderate and limited evidence) according to the number of studies and the consistency of the findings. We identified 101 original studies (50 of high quality) and five systematic reviews examining the criterion-related validity of field-based fitness tests in adults. Strong evidence indicated that the 20 m shuttle run, 1.5-mile, 12 min run/walk, YMCA step, 2 km walk and 6 min walk test are valid for estimating cardiorespiratory fitness; the handgrip strength test is valid for assessing hand maximal isometric strength; and the Biering–Sørensen test to evaluate the endurance strength of hip and back muscles; however, the sit-and reach test, and its different versions, and the toe-to-touch test are not valid for assessing hamstring and lower back flexibility. We found moderate evidence supporting that the 20 m square shuttle run test is a valid test for estimating cardiorespiratory fitness. Other field-based fitness tests presented limited evidence, mainly due to few studies. We developed an evidence-based proposal of the most valid field-based fitness tests in healthy adults aged 19–64 years old.

Keywords: cardiorespiratory fitness; muscular strength; motor fitness and flexibility; validation; fitness testing; adulthood

1. Introduction

Physical fitness is an integrated measure of all the functions and structures involved in performing physical activity [1]. Nowadays, physical fitness is one surrogate marker of overall adult health (19–64 years), especially cardiorespiratory fitness and muscular strength. Cardiorespiratory fitness is inversely associated with cardiovascular diseases [2], obesity [3], osteoporosis [4] diabetes [5], different cancer types [6,7], and is a predictor of all-cause of mortality [8–12] and cardiovascular disease [10,12–15]. Likewise, in the psychological sphere, high levels of cardiorespiratory fitness are associated with well-being [16,17], improved cognitive function [18] and a reduced risk of Alzheimer's disease [19] and other mental conditions such as anxiety, panic and depression [20]. Muscular strength demonstrates a protective effect against all-cause mortality [21,22]; and is inversely associated with weight gain and adiposity-related hypertension occurrence and the prevalence and incidence of the metabolic syndrome, [22] and mental health clinical presentations [23,24]. Consequently, physical fitness assessment is a vital tool of prevention and health diagnoses.

Laboratory testing is an objective and accurate method of assessing physical fitness. However, due to the cost of sophisticated instruments, time constraints and the need for qualified technicians, laboratory testing is limited to sport clubs, schools, population-based studies, and offices or clinical settings. However, field-based fitness testing can offer useful and practical alternatives as screening tools, since they are relatively safe and time-efficient, involve minimal equipment and low cost, and can be easily administered to multiple people simultaneously.

The validity of field-based fitness tests needs to be considered when deciding which test to use [25]. Criterion-related validity refers to the extent to which a field-based test of a physical fitness component correlates with the criterion measure (i.e., the gold standard) [26]. Since the early interest in physical fitness testing in the 1950–1960s, many field-based fitness tests have been proposed [27]. It would be desirable to summarise the criterion-related validity of the existing field-based fitness tests in adults. There have been attempts to summarize the criterion-related validity of a certain test [28,29] or several tests with a common characteristic [30–32]; however, no attempts have been made to summarise the criterion-related validity of all the existing field-based fitness tests in adults.

Therefore, the aim of the present systematic review was to comprehensively study the criterion-related validity of the existing field-based fitness tests used in adults. The findings of this review will provide an evidence-based proposal for most valid field-based fitness tests for healthy adults, aged 19–64 years old.

2. Materials and Methods

The review was registered in PROSPERO (registration number: CRD42019118482) and the applied methodology followed the guidelines drawn in the Preferred Reporting Items for Systematic Reviews and Meta-Analysis (PRISMA) statement [33].

2.1. Literature Search

The search was performed in the MEDLINE (via Pubmed) and Web of Science electronic databases from inception until July 2020. We screened studies conducted for criterion-related validity in adults, where one or more field-based fitness tests were carried out. Thus, the keywords selected were based on terms related to "criterion-related validity", "adults" and "field-based fitness test". The search syntax was adapted to the indexing terms of each database (see Supplementary Material 1). Searching was restricted to articles published in humans and the English or Spanish languages.

2.2. Eligibility Criteria

The inclusion criteria for this systematic review were the (1) age criterion: adults (19–64 years old). During this review, we faced the problem that some studies sampled adults and older adults, or adults or adolescents together. In these cases, we observed whether these studies performed stratified analyses by age groups, isolating the adult population from the rest; if so, the study was included and information concerning the adult population reported. In contrast, when the authors analysed the whole sample together, we only included the study if the age of the sample was predominantly within our study age range; (2) participants: the study population was based on a generally healthy population, who did not present any injury, physical and/or mental disabilities, irrespective of body mass index (BMI), diabetes or other cardiovascular risks (i.e., hypertension, hypercholesterolemia, lipid profiles, glucose levels, insulin sensitivity); and (3) study design: original studies or systematic reviews/meta-analysis. The original studies that were selected for the analysis of their criterion-related validity but which were also included in the selected systematic reviews were excluded; (4) language criterion: articles were only published in English or Spanish; (5) topic criterion: studies examining the criterion-related validity of the field-based fitness test. Studies examining the relationship between field-based fitness tests were excluded. Likewise, studies that analysed the criterion-related validity of tests designed for exclusive use in sports or clinical settings were not included.

Two authors (J.C.P. and J.R.F.S.) independently assessed the titles and abstracts of the articles retrieved by the search strategy for eligibility. Then, the full texts of the selected articles were acquired, and the same two researchers independently screened them to determine whether to include the article based on the inclusion criteria. When no consensus was reached between both researchers, a third research (N.M.J.) made the final decision with regard to inclusion. Reasons for the exclusion of identified articles were recorded.

2.3. Data Extraction

Two researchers (N.M.J. and F.M.A.) independently extracted the following information from each eligible original study according to the standardized form: (1) the author's name; (2) participants (sex and number); (3) age of participants; (4) filed-based test; (5) criterion measure (gold standard); (6) statistical methods; (7) main outcome; and (8) conclusions.

The same researchers independently extracted the following information from the systematic reviews: (1) author's name, date and years covered by the review; (2) type of review and number of included studies; (3) age of participants; (4) filed-based test; (5) criterion measure (gold standard); (6) main outcome; and (7) conclusions.

Disagreements in the extracted data were discussed between studies until a consensus was reached.

2.4. Criteria for Risk of Bias Assessment

Due to the heterogeneity of statistical methods employed by the original studies selected, the high number of tests included, and the limited number of studies per test, a meta-analysis was not conducted. An assessment of risk of bias in selected original studies and systematic reviews was made for each eligible study by two studies (N.M.J. and F.M.A.) independently. Discrepancies were solved in a consensus meeting. Inter-rater agreement for the risk of bias between researchers was calculated by the percentage agreement (96% (Kappa = 0.962) before consensus, and 100% agreement after consensus meeting).

The assessing risk of bias criteria in original studies were determined according to quality assessment list employed by Castro-Piñero et al. [27], which include the three following criteria: (1) the adequate number of participants; (2) an adequate description of the study population; and (3) adequate statistical analysis (see Supplementary Table S1). Each criterion was rated from 0 to 2, being 2 the best score. For all studies, a total score was calculated by counting up the number of positive items (a total score between 0 and 6). Studies were categorized as very low quality (0–2), low quality (3–4) and high quality (5–6).

The methodological quality of each systematic review was appraised using the 'Assessment of Multiple Systematic Reviews' (AMSTAR) rating scale [34]. AMSTAR contains 11-items to assess the methodological aspects of reviews with items scored as 1 if the answer was "Yes", and 0 if the answer was "No", "Cannot Answer" or "Not Applicable" (see Supplementary Table S2). The total score ranged from 0 to 11. The item on conflict of interest requires that the systematic review and all primary studies be assessed. We modified this item to only assess the review itself as Biddle et al. [35] proposed, given that PRISMA does not require a conflict-of-interest assessment for each primary study. The final quality rates were computed by tertiles, where the first tertile ranged from 0 to 3 points (low quality); the second tertile from 4 to 7 points (medium quality); and the third tertile from 8 to 11 points (high quality).

2.5. Levels of Evidence

Three evidence levels [27] were constructed: (1) strong evidence: consistent findings in three or more high-quality studies; (2) moderate evidence: consistent findings in two high-quality studies; and (3) limited evidence: consistent findings in multiple low-quality studies, inconsistent results found in multiple high-quality studies, or results based on one single study. The degree of criterion-related validity of the field-based fitness test will be discussed for those tests on which we found strong or moderate evidence that the test is (or not) valid. The results of low- or very low-quality studies can be seen in the Supplementary Material 2.

3. Results

The literature search yielded 9202 and 27 additional records were identified through other sources (see the PRISMA flowchart in Figure 1). After the removal of duplicate references (1805 studies), and the screening of titles and abstracts (7233 studies), we excluded 9038 studies. A total of 191 full-text studies were assessed for eligibility, and 85 studies (six systematic reviews) were excluded due to reasons indicated in Figure 1.

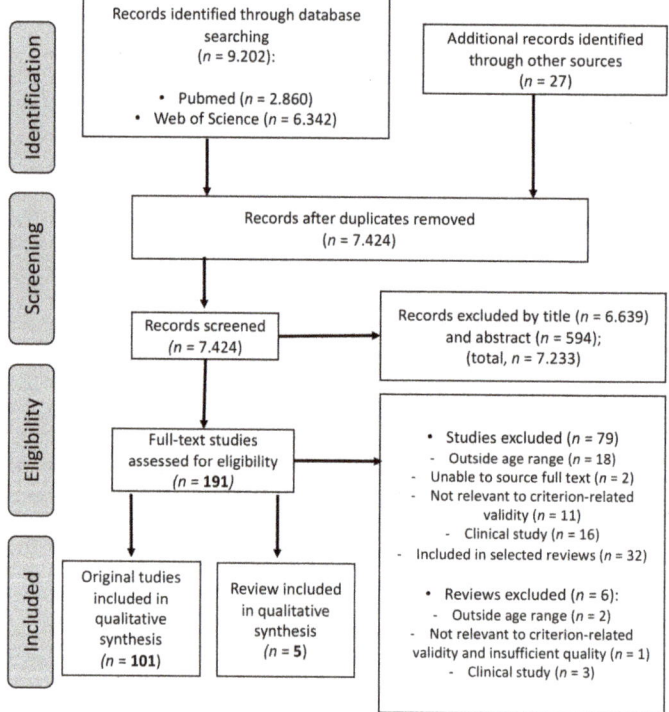

Figure 1. Flow chart of retrieved and selected articles.

Finally, a total of 101 original studies (see Supplementary Table S3) addressed the criterion-related validity of field-based fitness tests in adults aged 19–64 years. The sample size involved 10,632 participants (see Supplementary Table S4). Eighty-six and seventy-eight original studies reported female (n = 5539) and male (n = 4722) sample proportions, respectively; however, in 7 seven studies, sex was not specified.

A total of four meta-analyses [28–31] and one systematic review [32] were included in the present systematic review (see Supplementary Table S2). The sample size involved 9985 participants with ages ranging from 19 to 64 years (see Supplementary Table S5).

3.1. Quality Assessment

Of the 101 original studies included in the present systematic review, 11 and 40 studies were classified as very low (a total score less than 2) and low quality (a total score of 3 and 4), respectively (see Supplementary Table S3). A total of 50 original studies were classified as high-quality (a total score higher than 4). Of these 40, nine and one analysed the criterion-related validity of cardiorespiratory fitness, muscular strength and flexibility field-based fitness tests in adults, respectively. No study of those classified as high quality analysed the criterion-related validity of motor fitness (i.e., speed, agility, balance and coordination).

Two meta-analyses [28,30] and one systematic review [32] were ranked as high quality (all eight points), and two meta-analyses [29,31] were ranked as medium quality (both seven points) (see Supplementary Table S2). Three of them assessed the criterion-related validity of field-based cardiorespiratory fitness tests: the 20 m shuttle run test [28]; distance and time-based run/walk tests [30]; and the step tests [32]—whilst and two of them studied the criterion-related validity of the sit-and-reach [31] and toe-to-touch tests [29].

* References of high-quality studies are presented in Supplementary Material 3.

3.2. Criterion-Related Validity

Table 1 shows a summary of the different levels of evidence found for the criterion-related validity of cardiorespiratory fitness tests.

Table 1. Levels of evidence of cardiorespiratory fitness tests.

Field-Based Fitness Test	Strong	Moderate	Limited
Shuttle run tests			
20 m shuttle run	●		
20 m square shuttle		●	
Incremental shuttle walk			■
Distance and time-based run/walk test			
1.5-mile run/walk	●		
12 min run/walk	●		
5000 m run/walk	◐		
3 miles run/walk	◐		
2 miles run/walk	◐		
3.000 m run/walk	◐		
1000 m run/walk	◐		
600 m run/walk	◐		
600 yd run/walk	◐		
½-mile run/walk	◐		
¼-mile run/walk	◐		
9 min run/walk			●
2 km walk	●		
6 min walk	●		
1-mile walk			■
¼-mile walk			●
3 min walk			●
Treadmill jogging			■
Mankato submaximal exercise			●
Modified Astrand–Ryhming			●
University Montreal			●
Ruffier			○

Table 1. *Cont.*

Field-Based Fitness Test	Strong	Moderate	Limited
Step tests			
YMCA step		●	
Chester step			▨
Modified Harvard step			●
6 min single 15 cm-step			●
Modified Canadian aerobic fitness step			●
Tecumseh step			●
Astrand–Ryhming step			●
Danish step			○
Queen's College step			▨
2 min step			○

● Indicates high validity; ○ moderate validity; ◐ low/null validity; ▨ inconclusive validity.

3.2.1. Cardiorespiratory Fitness

Distance and Time-Based Run/Walk Tests

Seventeen high-quality studies examined the criterion-related validity of the distance run/walk or walk tests (see Supplementary Table S4). Four and two studies showed that the 2 km walk [36–39] and 1.5-mile run/walk [40,41] tests, respectively, were valid for assessing cardiorespiratory fitness (r = 0.80–0.93, all $p < 0.05$). Four studies [42–45] observed that the 1-mile walk test was an accurate test for estimating VO_{2max} (r = 0.81–0.88, all $p < 0.05$), while another two studies [46,47] showed that it was not a valid test (r = 0.69, 13.3% E, $p < 0.05$; mean differences range from 2.360 to 9.131 mL/kg/min, all $p < 0.001$, respectively). The treadmill jogging test reported contradictory results: one study [48] found it to have high validity for assessing cardiorespiratory fitness (r = 0.84, both $p < 0.001$); whereas another study [41] revealed that it was not a valid test (r = 0.50, $p < 0.05$).

Five high-quality studies investigated the criterion-related validity of the time-based run/walk or walk tests (see Supplementary Table S4). These studies showed that the 3 min walk, [49] 6 min walk, [50–52] and the 12 min run/walk [41] tests were valid for assessing cardiorespiratory fitness (r = 0.70–0.95, all $p < 0.05$). Additionally, one original high-quality study reported that the University Montreal test [53] was valid for estimating cardiorespiratory fitness (r = 0.71, $p < 0.001$; mean difference = 0.025 ± 7.445 mL/kg/min., $p > 0.05$).

A meta-analysis [30] consisting of 102 studies on adults determined that the criterion-related validity of the distance run/walk field tests for estimating cardiorespiratory fitness ranged from low to high, with the 1.5-mile (r_p = 0.80; 95% CI: 0.72–0.80) and 12 min run/walk tests (r_p = 0.79; 95% CI: 0.71–0.87) being the best predictors (see Supplementary Table S5).

Twenty-Metre Shuttle Run Test

Nine high-quality studies analysed the criterion-related validity of the 20 m shuttle run test [41,54–58] or modifications of it [55,57,59–61] (see Supplementary Table S4). Four studies [41,55–57] reported that the 20 m shuttle run was a valid test for assessing cardiorespiratory fitness (r = 0.82–0.94, all $p < 0.05$). However, one study [58] concluded that this test was not valid for assessing cardiorespiratory fitness (mean differences range from −0.54 ± 6.23 to −2.94 ± 6.55 mL/kg/min, all $p < 0.01$). Two studies [59,60] proved that the incremental shuttle walk test was not valid (r = 0.72, 19% E, both $p < 0.001$), while one study [61] found that this test was valid for assessing cardiorespiratory fitness (mean difference = 0.14 ± 9.27 mL/kg/min, $p > 0.05$). Moreover, two studies [55,57] reported that the 20 m square shuttle run test was valid (r = 0.95, both $p < 0.001$).

A meta-analysis [28] which included 24 studies in adults found that the 20 m shuttle run test had a moderate-to-high criterion-related validity for estimating VO_{2max} (r_p = 0.79–0.94; 95% CI: 0.56–1.00) (see Supplementary Table S5).

Step Tests

Eleven high-quality studies analysed the criterion-related validity of the step tests (see Supplementary Table S4). Four studies observed that the Danish step [62], the Queen's College step [63], and the 2 min step [64] tests were not valid for estimating VO_{2max} (r = 0.034–0.72, all $p < 0.05$). However, another eight studies proved the validity of the modified Canadian aerobic fitness [65], 6 min single 15 cm step [66], YMCA step [67–71], Tecumseh step [70] and modified Harvard step [72] tests (r = 0.80–0.91, all $p < 0.05$).

A systematic review [32] comprised of 11 studies on adults investigated the criterion-related validity of the step tests (see Supplementary Table S5). Validity measures were varied, and a broad range of correlation coefficients were reported across the 11 studies (r = 0.469–0.95; all $p < 0.005$) with conflicting results in most of the step test protocols. The study concluded that the Chester step test was the best predictor for assessing cardiorespiratory fitness.

3.2.2. Muscular Strength

Table 2 shows a summary of the different levels of evidence found for the criterion-related validity of muscular strength, flexibility and motor fitness tests.

Table 2. Levels of evidence of muscular strength, flexibility and motor fitness tests.

Field-Based Fitness Test	Strong	Moderate	Limited
Maximal isometric strength			
Handgrip strength (TKK)	●		
Handgrip strength (Jamar)		◐	
Handgrip strength (DynEx)			▪
Hip and back endurance strength			
Biering–Sørensen	●		
Abdominal endurance strength			
Prone bridging			●
Original/modifications curl-up			○
Lower body endurance strength			
Sit-to-stand			▪
Lower body explosive strength			
Sargent jump			●
Upper body endurance strength			
Original/modification flexed-arm hang			▪
Baumgartner modified pull-up			▪
Standard push-up			▪
Hand-release push-up			▪
Bent-knee push-up			▪
Revised push-up			▪
Lower back flexibility			
Original/modifications sit-and-reach	○		
Hamstring flexibility			
Original/modifications sit-and-reach	◐		
Toe-touch	◐		
Agility			
Ten-step			◐
Balance			
Romberg test			▪

● Indicates high validity; ○ moderate validity; ◐ low/null validity; ▪ inconclusive validity.

Maximal Isometric Strength

Four high-quality studies assessed the criterion-related validity of hand maximal isometric strength, using the handgrip strength tests (see Supplementary Table S4). Three high-quality studies reported that the TKK dynamometer [73–75] was valid (mean difference range −0.20, $p > 0.05$ to 2.02 kg $p < 0.001$) ($r = 0.98$, $p < 0.001$). However, three studies showed inconclusive results about the validity of the DynEx dynamometer [73,75,76], and two studies observed that the Jamar dynamometer [73,76] was less accurate than the TKK and DynEx dynamometer for estimating hand maximal isometric strength.

Endurance Strength

Four high-quality studies assessed the criterion-related validity of trunk endurance strength (see Supplementary Table S4). Two studies [77,78] suggested that the Biering–Sørensen ($r = 0.84$–98, $p < 0.01$) test was valid, whereas another study [79] reported acceptable validity ($r = 0.60$–0.71, $p < 0.05$). One study showed that the prone bridging test [80] was valid for assessing trunk endurance strength (no mean difference, $p > 0.05$).

Explosive Strength

Only one high-quality study assessed the criterion-related validity of explosive strength (see Supplementary Table S4). This study concluded that the Sargent test [81] was not valid (mean difference: 4.4 ± 5.1, $p < 0.001$) for estimating lower body explosive strength.

3.2.3. Flexibility

Only one study [82] that examined the criterion-related validity of flexibility tests was classified as high quality (see Supplementary Table S4). They found that the sit-and-reach was not a valid test ($r = 0.44$–0.48, $p < 0.05$).

A meta-analysis [31] which included 28 studies on adults (see Supplementary Table S5) found that the sit-and-reach test and its different versions, had moderate validity for estimating hamstring extensibility (r_p ranged from 0.49; 95% CI: 0.29–0.68 to 0.68; 95% CI: 0.55–0.80), but a low validity for estimating lumbar extensibility (r_p ranged from 0.16; 95% CI: −0.10–0.41 to 0.35; 95% CI: 0.15–0.54). Moreover, another meta-analysis [29] carried out on adults (of six studies) reported that the toe-touch test had moderate validity for assessing hamstring extensibility ($r_p = 0.66$; 95% CI: 0.56–1.00).

3.2.4. Motor Fitness

No study investigating the criterion-related validity of motor fitness tests was classified as high quality (see Supplementary Table S3).

4. Discussion

The present systematic review comprehensively studied the criterion-related validity of the existing field-based fitness tests used in adults. The findings of this review provide an evidence-based proposal for most valid field-based fitness tests for adult population.

4.1. Cardiorespiratory Fitness

The gold standard to assess VO_{2max} is the Douglas bag method, although there is agreement that the respiratory gas analyser is a valid method of assessing oxygen uptake [83]. All high-quality studies measured VO_{2max} or peak oxygen consumption when performing a submaximal/maximal treadmill or cycle test, except Manttari et al. [52], who directly measured VO_{2max} when performing the 6 min walk test.

4.1.1. Distance and Time-Based Run/Walk Tests

The run/walk field tests are probably the most widely used tests [27,84], however, until recently, there was no consensus regarding the most appropriate distance or time to use for these tests [85]. Mayorga et al. [30] performed a meta-analysis which examined the criterion-related validity of the 5000 m, 3 mile, 2 mile, 3000 m, 1.5-mile, 1-mile,

1000 m, $\frac{1}{2}$-mile, 600 m, 600 yd, $\frac{1}{4}$-mile, 15 min, 12 min, 9 min, and 6 min run/walk tests. They found that the criterion-related validity of the run/walk tests, only considering the performance score, ranged from low to high, with the 1.5-mile and the 12 min run/walk tests being the most appropriate tests for estimating cardiorespiratory fitness in adults aged 19–64 years. Sex, age or VO_{2max} level did not affect criterion-related validity, whereas when multiple predictors (i.e., performance score, sex, age or body mass) were considered, the criterion-related validity values were higher. In this sense, two high-quality original studies reinforced these results, and showed that the 12 min [41] and the 1.5-mile [40,41] run/walk tests were fairly accurate for estimating cardiorespiratory fitness in adults aged 18–26 years (r = 0.87–0.93, $p < 0.05$).

Overall, the run/walk tests are not user-friendly tests, due to the difficulty of developing an appropriate pace, which may affect the test outcome (some participants start too fast, so they are unable to maintain their speed throughout the test; others start too slow, so when they wish to increase their speed the test is already finished). These problems are more likely to occur in longer distance tests. Other factors affecting the test outcome include the individual's willingness to endure the discomfort of strenuous exercise, a short attention span, poor motivation, and limited interest in a monotonous task [86–88].

The 2 km and 6 min walk tests are probably the most widely used walk tests in adults [39,51]. Both tests require submaximal effort, thus avoiding the problem of enduring the discomfort of strenuous exercise. In addition, it allows to evaluate those people with a low level of physical fitness or is unable to run. Three high-quality studies [36,37,39] observed that Oja's equation derived from the 2 km walk test has high validity (r = 0.80–0.87, all $p < 0.05$) in untrained and/or overweight/obese adults aged 20–64 years. One high-quality study reported that the 2 km walk test [38] is a reasonably valid field test for estimating the cardiorespiratory fitness of moderately active adults aged 35–45 years, but not in adults with very high maximal aerobic power.

Many studies developed prediction equations for the 6 min test based on spirometry [89]. However, only three high-quality studies [50–52] analysed the criterion-related validity of the 6 min test based on VO_{2max} in adults. They showed a moderate-to-high validity (r = 0.70–0.93, all $p < 0.001$) in obese and healthy adults aged 18–64 years. Burr et al. [90] suggested that, on its own, the 6 min walk test can be useful to discriminate between broad categories of high, moderate and low fitness, but that this approach may be associated with a degree of error, especially in the high fitness group.

According to these findings, the 2 km and 6 min walk tests are valid for use in adults aged 19–64 years with low or moderate fitness levels, but not in adults with a high fitness level.

Regarding the 1 mile walk test, conflicting results were found, especially when examining the accuracy of the Kline's [42] and Dolgener's [46] equations in adults aged 19–64 years.

4.1.2. Twenty-Metre Shuttle Run Test

The 20 m shuttle run test was developed by Leger at al. [91] to solve the pace issue of the run/walk tests. The test consists of 1 min stages of continuous running at an increasing speed. Recently, a meta-analysis [28] showed that the performance score of the 20 m shuttle run test had a moderate-to-high criterion-related validity for estimating VO_{2max} (r_p = 0.66–0.84) in youth and adults aged 18–64 years, higher than when other variables (i.e., sex, age or body mass) were accounted for (r_p = 0.78–0.95). This study also reported that Leger's protocol had a greater average criterion-related validity coefficient (r_p = 0.84; 95% CI: 0.80–0.89) than Eurofit, QUB and Dong-HO protocols; and Leger's protocol was statistically higher for adults (r_p = 0.94, 0.87–1.00) than for children (r_p = 0.78; 95% CI: 0.72–0.85). These values are higher than those reported for the 1500 m and 12 min run/walk tests [30]. Moreover, the meta-analysis showed that sex did not seem to affect the criterion-related validity values.

On the other hand, Cooper et al. [54] showed that Brewer's protocol and equation were not valid for assessing active young people aged 18–26 years (mean difference = 1.8 ± 6.3 mL/kg/min; p = 0.004). In line with these findings, Kim et al. [58] observed that Leger's protocol and equation were more accurate than Brewer's protocol and equation (mean difference −0.54 mL/kg/min; %CV: 1.39 vs. mean difference −2.944 mL/kg/min; %CV: 8.87) in Korean adults, especially in women. Nonetheless, the authors suggested the need to develop new equations for Korean adults.

It is important to note that the 20 m square shuttle run test [55,57] was proposed as an alternative to the 20 m shuttle run test to reduce the test's turning angle from 180 to 90. This test was the best predictor of VO_{2max} than the 20 m shuttle run test in young male adults aged 18–25 years.

4.1.3. Step Tests

Step tests are a safe, simple, inexpensive and practical method of assessing cardiorespiratory fitness under submaximal conditions, which require minimum space [32]; they are also a great alternative to laboratory tests in clinical settings. There are a wide variety of step test protocols which differ in terms of stepping frequency, test duration and number of test stages. Bennett et al. [32] analysed the criterion-related validity of different step tests (the Chester step test, a personalised step test, the STEP tool step test, the Queen's College step test, the Skubic and Hodgkins step test, a height-adjusted, rate-specific, single-state step test, the Astrand–Ryhming step test, and a modified YMCA 3 min step test) in adults aged 18–64 years. The validity of these tests ranged from moderate to high, and they suggested that the Chester step test was the most valid step test to evaluate cardiorespiratory fitness in adults. However, this systematic review only included two studies with contradictory results, similarly to the Queen's College step test.

Analysing the 12 high-quality studies that examined the criterion-related validity of the step tests in adults aged 19–64 years, we can conclude that the YMCA step test [67,71] seemed to be the most appropriate step test to estimate VO_{2max} in adults aged 19–64 years. However, it is important to note that there is no single equation, since the result of the equation depends on the sample used. Santo and Golding [92] even altered the protocol by adjusting the step height to the individual participant's height in order to increase the accuracy of this test.

4.1.4. Levels of Evidence

Strong evidence indicated that (a) the 20 m shuttle run test using Leger's equation, the 2 km walk using Oja's equation, the 6 min and the YMCA step tests are valid for estimating cardiorespiratory fitness; and (b) the criterion-related validity of the distance and time-based run/walk tests range from low to high, with the 1.5-mile and 12 min run/walk tests being the best predictors. Moderate evidence indicated that the 20 m square shuttle run test is valid for estimating cardiorespiratory fitness. Due to the inconsistent results found in high-quality studies, limited evidence was found for the validity of the 1-mile walk, treadmill jogging, incremental shuttle walking, Chester, and Queen's College step tests. Due to the low number of high-quality studies, limited evidence indicated that (a) the 3 min walk, the $\frac{1}{4}$-mile walk, Mankato submaximal, modified Astrand–Ryhming, University Montreal, modified Canadian aerobic fitness step, 6 min single 15 cm step, Tecumseh step, modified Harvard step and Astrand–Ryhming Step tests are valid for estimating cardiorespiratory fitness; and (b) the YMCA cycle, Ruffier, Danish step, and 2 min step tests are not valid for estimating cardiorespiratory fitness. Due to the consistent results found in multiple low-quality studies, limited evidence supported using the 6 min step test for estimating cardiorespiratory fitness.

4.2. Muscular Strength

The specificity of the type of muscular work performed and the use of different energy systems are both major challenges for establishing a gold standard method for maximal, endurance and explosive muscular strength tests [93]. One repetition maximum (1RM) and repetitions to a certain percentage of 1RM (i.e., 50% of 1RM or 70% of 1RM) [27], isokinetic dynamometer strength [94–96], and electromyography [78,80] were used as gold standards.

4.2.1. Maximal Isometric Strength

The TKK dynamometer [73–75] seemed the most appropriate test to assess maximal isometric strength in adults. All the studies used the "known weights" as the criterion reference.

Several studies examined whether the elbow position (extended or flexed at 90 degrees) affected the hand maximal isometric strength score in children [75], adolescents [97] and young adults [98]. They observed that performing the handgrip strength test with the elbow extended seems the most appropriate protocol to evaluate hand maximal isometric strength in these populations—which is in accordance with the protocol recommended by the American Center for Disease Control and Prevention [99].

Ruiz et al. [100] also investigated whether the position (grip span) on the standard grip dynamometer determined the hand maximal isometric strength in adults. They found that when measuring hand maximal isometric strength in women, hand size must be taken into consideration, providing the mathematical equation ($y = x/5 + 1.5$ cm) to adapt optimal grip span (y) to hand size (x). In adult men, optimal grip span could be set at a fixed value (5.5 cm) and is not influenced by hand size.

Importantly, just like the step test, the handgrip strength test can be very useful in clinical settings because it requires minimal equipment and space, is time-efficient and easy to administer.

4.2.2. Endurance Strength

The Biering–Sørensen test, a trunk holding test in an antigravity prone position, is commonly used to measure the back and hip muscle endurance strength, which is associated with lower back pain [101]. Mannion et al. [77] and Coorevits et al. [78] showed that the test endurance time was highly associated with isometric/endurance hip and back musculature strength (r = 0.84–98, $p < 0.01$). On the other hand, Kankaanpää et al. [79], found that this association was moderate (r = 0.60–0.71, $p < 0.05$). However, when BMI (r= −0.49–0.51, $p < 0.001$) in women and age (r = 0.25–0.29, $p < 0.05$) in men were accounted for in the prediction model, the explained variance increased considerably. Thus, the Biering–Sørensen test might be considered as valid for measuring back muscle endurance strength.

Assessing abdominal muscle functionality is clinically relevant since it is considered to be related to lower back pain [102,103]. The curl-up test, or its different versions, was the field test originally used to assess this capacity. In the present review, no original studies evaluating the criterion-related validity of this test were classified as high quality. An alternative of the curl-up test could be the prone bridging test, an isometric holding test in prone position which is currently being used to supposedly measure abdominal endurance strength. The prone bridging test time is inversely associated with lower back pain [104,105]. In relation to the validity of this test, De Blaiser et al. [80] found a higher activation of the abdominal core musculature during the test than for the back and hip musculature, showing a high association between test time and abdominal endurance strength. Future high-quality studies are necessary to clarify the validity of this test.

It should be noted that no study that analysed the criterion-related validity of lower and upper body endurance strength tests were classified as high quality.

4.2.3. Explosive Strength

The standing long jump is proposed in health-related fitness test batteries in preschool children [106], as well as children and adolescents [107] to assess lower body explosive strength, given its criterion-related and predictive validity. However, to our knowledge, the criterion-related validity of this test has not been studied. Bui et al. observed that the Sargent jump test [81] is not appropriate to evaluate lower body explosive strength, because its overestimates the height of a vertical jump and its accuracy is reduced as the jump height increases (mean difference: 4.4 ± 5.1, $p < 0.001$). Due to the close relationship that lower body maximal/explosive strength has on adult health [22,23], more high-quality studies are required to analyse the criterion-related validity of these tests in future research.

4.2.4. Levels of Evidence

Strong evidence indicated that (a) the handgrip strength test with the elbow extended and with the grip span adapted to the hand size and sex (using the TKK dynamometer) is a valid test for assessing hand maximal isometric strength; and (b) the Biering–Sørensen test offers a valid test for assessing endurance strength of hip and back muscles. Moderate evidence indicated that handgrip strength (Jamar) has acceptable validity for assessing hand maximal isometric strength. Due to (a) the low number of high-quality studies, limited evidence (only one study) was found supporting the use of prone bridging for assessing abdominal endurance strength and the Sargent jump test for assessing lower body explosive strength; (b) the inconsistent results found in multiple high-quality studies, limited evidence was found for the validity of using handgrip strength (DynEx) for assessing hand maximal isometric strength; and (c) the consistent results found in multiple low or very low-quality studies, the curl-up test, or its different versions, are not valid for assessing abdominal endurance strength.

4.3. Flexibility

Radiography seems to be the best criterion measurement of flexibility, but goniometry is also used as a criterion measure [108,109].

Goniometers are relatively easy to obtain; nevertheless, their use requires a certain technical qualification since it is a sensitive method, and thus it is not feasible for use in all settings [110]. Traditionally, the sit-and-reach test, originally designed by Wells and Dillon [111], and its different versions, are included in the fitness test batteries for measuring hamstring and lower back flexibility, which are probably the most widely used measures of flexibility [27].

Mayorga et al. [31] performed a meta-analysis to analyse the criterion-related validity of the sit-and-reach and its different versions (modified sit-and-reach, back-saver sit-and-reach, modified back-saver sit-and-reach, V sit-and-reach, modification V sit-and-reach, unilateral sit-and-reach and chair sit-and-reach). These tests showed moderate validity for estimating hamstring extensibility, but low validity for estimating lumbar extensibility. They also found that the classic sit-and-reach test had the highest criterion-related validity coefficient in both hamstring and lumbar extensibility, compared to the other test, which does not seem to justify the use of the classic protocol modifications in order to solve the problems attributed to itself (i.e., the length proportion between the upper and lower limbs or the position of the head and ankles).

The toe-touch test is another field-based test for measuring hamstring flexibility, in which the individuals were assessed standing instead of sitting on the floor [112]. Although this test is easy to administer and can be an alternative to the sit-and-reach test, when the participant has problems being measured sitting, it is not proposed for any filed-based fitness test battery. A meta-analysis [29] analysed the criterion-related validity of the toe-touch test for measuring hamstring flexibility, reporting similar validity coefficients to those of the classic sit-and-reach.

It is interesting to highlight that Nuzzo [113] has recently suggested that flexibility should be invalidated as a major component of fitness, due to its lack of predictive and concurrent validity in terms of meaningful health and performance outcomes.

Levels of Evidence

Strong evidence indicated that (a) the sit-and-reach test and its modified versions have moderate validity for estimating hamstring extensibility, but low validity for estimating lumbar extensibility; and (b) the toe-to-touch test has moderate validity for estimating hamstring extensibility.

4.4. Motor Fitness

The validity of motor fitness tests is the least studied in adults. None of the three studies that analysed the criterion-related validity in motor fitness tests were classified as high quality. Given that the motor fitness tests (i.e., gait/walking speed, balance, timed up and go) are associated with all-cause mortality [114–116], falls and fractures [117], disability in activities of daily living [118] and depression [119], it would be useful to know their criterion-related validity.

Levels of Evidence

Due to the consistent results found in multiple low-quality studies, we found limited evidence that the ten-step test had moderate validity in assessing agility.

5. Conclusions

The systematic review emphasized important major points regarding the criterion-related validity of adult field-based fitness tests (Figure 2):

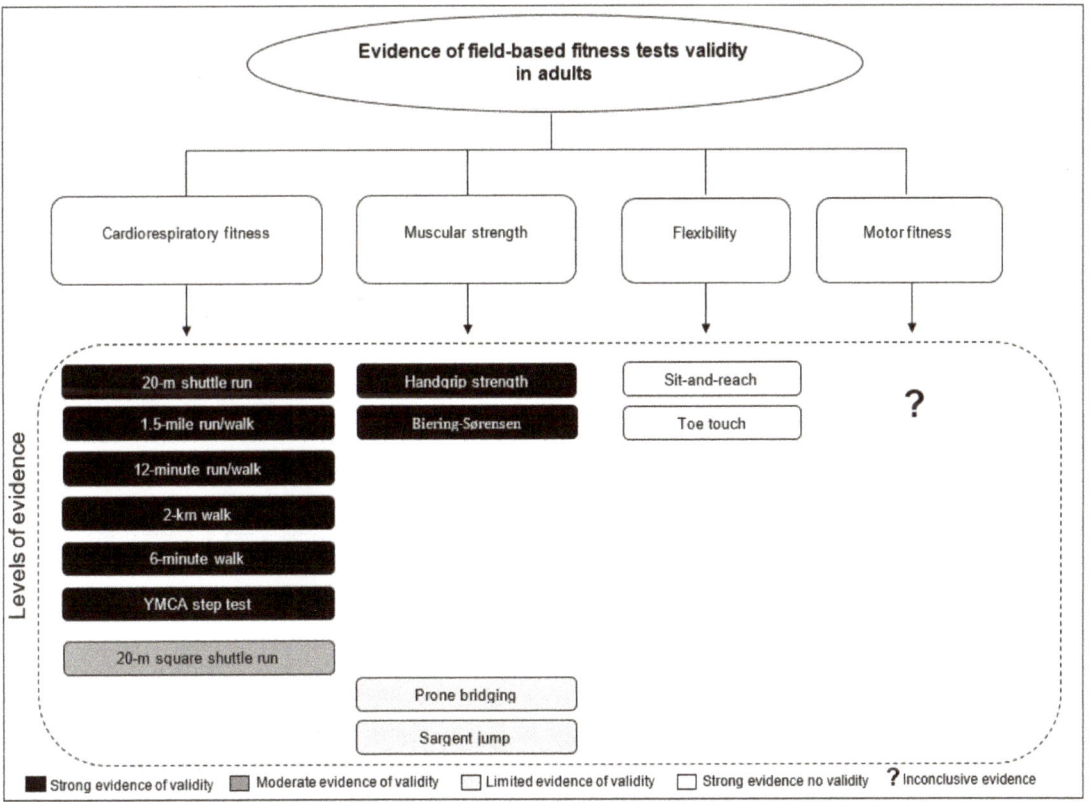

Figure 2. Major points regarding criterion-related validity of adult field-based fitness tests.

Cardiorespiratory fitness: the 20 m shuttle run tests best assessed cardiorespiratory fitness using Leger's equation. Alternatively, the 1.5-mile, 12 min run/walk and YMCA step tests were other cardiorespiratory testing options. When low-level cardiorespiratory fitness existed, or if running was possible, the 2 km, then Oja's equation or 6 min walk tests were appropriate alternatives.

Muscular strength: strong evidence indicated that (a) the handgrip strength test, with the elbow extended and with the grip span adapted to the individual's hand size (using the TKK dynamometer), offers a valid means to assess hand maximal isometric strength; and (b) the Biering–Sørensen test estimated the endurance strength of hip and back muscles. Limited evidence (only one study) supported the prone bridging and Sargent jump tests as abdominal endurance strength and lower body explosive strength surrogate markers, respectively.

Flexibility: strong evidence supported the sit-and-reach test and its different versions, and that the toe-to-touch tests is not valid for assessing hamstring and lower back flexibility.

Motor fitness: limited evidence about the criterion-related validity of motor fitness existed.

When there are problems of space and time, as in clinical settings, the YMCA step and the handgrip strength tests are good alternatives for assessing cardiorespiratory fitness and isometric muscular strength, respectively.

Supplementary Materials: The following are available online at https://www.mdpi.com/article/10.3390/jcm10163743/s1: Supplementary Tables and Supplementary Material.

Author Contributions: J.C.-P. and M.C.-G. conceived the study idea. J.C.-P. led the writing of the review and carried out methodological aspects with N.M.-J., F.M.-A. and J.R.F.-S., F.M.-A., V.S.-J., R.I.-G. and J.R.R. contributed writing—review and editing the final manuscript. All authors discussed the results and contributed to the final manuscript, and agreed with the order of presentation of the authors. All authors have read and agreed to the published version of the manuscript.

Funding: This project was supported by Ministry of Economy, Industry and Competitiveness in the 2017 call for R&D Projects of the State Program for Research, Development and Innovation Oriented to the Challenges of the Company; National Plan for Scientific and Technical Research and of Innovation 2017-2020 (DEP2017-88043-R); and the Regional Government of Andalusia and University of Cadiz: Research and Knowledge Transfer Fund (PPIT-FPI19).

Institutional Review Board Statement: Not applicable.

Informed Consent Statement: Not applicable.

Conflicts of Interest: The authors declare no conflict of interest.

References

1. Castillo Garzon, M.J.; Ortega Porcel, F.B.; Ruiz Ruiz, J. Improvement of physical fitness as anti-aging intervention. *Med. Clin.* **2005**, *124*, 146–155.
2. LaMonte, M.J.; Barlow, C.E.; Jurca, R.; Kampert, J.B.; Church, T.S.; Blair, S.N. Cardiorespiratory fitness is inversely associated with the incidence of metabolic syndrome: A prospective study of men and women. *Circulation* **2005**, *112*, 505–512. [CrossRef]
3. Fung, M.D.; Canning, K.L.; Mirdamadi, P.; Ardern, C.I.; Kuk, J.L. Lifestyle and weight predictors of a healthy overweight profile over a 20-year follow-up. *Obesity* **2015**, *23*, 1320–1325. [CrossRef] [PubMed]
4. Howe, T.E.; Rochester, L.; Neil, F.; Skelton, D.A.; Ballinger, C. Exercise for improving balance in older people. *Cochrane Database Syst. Rev.* **2011**, *11*, Cd004963. [CrossRef] [PubMed]
5. Balducci, S.; Cardelli, P.; Pugliese, L.; D'Errico, V.; Haxhi, J.; Alessi, E.; Iacobini, C.; Menini, S.; Bollanti, L.; Conti, F.G.; et al. Volume-dependent effect of supervised exercise training on fatty liver and visceral adiposity index in subjects with type 2 diabetes The Italian Diabetes Exercise Study (IDES). *Diabetes Res. Clin. Pract.* **2015**, *109*, 355–363. [CrossRef] [PubMed]
6. Pletnikoff, P.P.; Laukkanen, J.A.; Tuomainen, T.P.; Kauhanen, J.; Rauramaa, R.; Ronkainen, K.; Kurl, S. Cardiorespiratory fitness, C-reactive protein and lung cancer risk: A prospective population-based cohort study. *Eur. J. Cancer* **2015**, *51*, 1365–1370. [CrossRef] [PubMed]
7. Sui, X.; Lee, D.C.; Matthews, C.E.; Adams, S.A.; Hebert, J.R.; Church, T.S.; Lee, C.D.; Blair, S.N. Influence of cardiorespiratory fitness on lung cancer mortality. *Med. Sci. Sports Exerc.* **2010**, *42*, 872–878. [CrossRef]
8. Blair, S.N.; Kohl, H.W., 3rd; Paffenbarger, R.S., Jr.; Clark, D.G.; Cooper, K.H.; Gibbons, L.W. Physical fitness and all-cause mortality. A prospective study of healthy men and women. *JAMA* **1989**, *262*, 2395–2401. [CrossRef]
9. Farrell, S.W.; Fitzgerald, S.J.; McAuley, P.A.; Barlow, C.E. Cardiorespiratory fitness, adiposity, and all-cause mortality in women. *Med. Sci. Sports Exerc.* **2010**, *42*, 2006–2012. [CrossRef]

10. Barry, V.W.; Baruth, M.; Beets, M.W.; Durstine, J.L.; Liu, J.; Blair, S.N. Fitness vs. fatness on all-cause mortality: A meta-analysis. *Prog. Cardiovasc. Dis.* **2014**, *56*, 382–390. [CrossRef]
11. Ortega, F.B.; Lavie, C.J.; Blair, S.N. Obesity and Cardiovascular Disease. *Circ. Res.* **2016**, *118*, 1752–1770. [CrossRef]
12. McAuley, P.A.; Beavers, K.M. Contribution of cardiorespiratory fitness to the obesity paradox. *Prog. Cardiovasc. Dis.* **2014**, *56*, 434–440. [CrossRef]
13. Lavie, C.J.; McAuley, P.A.; Church, T.S.; Milani, R.V.; Blair, S.N. Obesity and cardiovascular diseases: Implications regarding fitness, fatness, and severity in the obesity paradox. *J. Am. Coll. Cardiol.* **2014**, *63*, 1345–1354. [CrossRef]
14. Lavie, C.J.; Ozemek, C.; Carbone, S.; Katzmarzyk, P.T.; Blair, S.N. Sedentary Behavior, Exercise, and Cardiovascular Health. *Circ. Res.* **2019**, *124*, 799–815. [CrossRef]
15. Barry, V.W.; Caputo, J.L.; Kang, M. The Joint Association of Fitness and Fatness on Cardiovascular Disease Mortality: A Meta-Analysis. *Prog. Cardiovasc. Dis.* **2018**, *61*, 136–141. [CrossRef]
16. Oktay, A.A.; Lavie, C.J.; Kokkinos, P.F.; Parto, P.; Pandey, A.; Ventura, H.O. The Interaction of Cardiorespiratory Fitness With Obesity and the Obesity Paradox in Cardiovascular Disease. *Prog. Cardiovasc. Dis.* **2017**, *60*, 30–44. [CrossRef] [PubMed]
17. Delextrat, A.A.; Warner, S.; Graham, S.; Neupert, E. An 8-Week Exercise Intervention Based on Zumba Improves Aerobic Fitness and Psychological Well-Being in Healthy Women. *J. Phys. Act. Health* **2016**, *13*, 131–139. [CrossRef] [PubMed]
18. Ortega, F.B.; Lee, D.C.; Sui, X.; Kubzansky, L.D.; Ruiz, J.R.; Baruth, M.; Castillo, M.J.; Blair, S.N. Psychological well-being, cardiorespiratory fitness, and long-term survival. *Am. J. Prev. Med.* **2010**, *39*, 440–448. [CrossRef] [PubMed]
19. Boots, E.A.; Schultz, S.A.; Oh, J.M.; Larson, J.; Edwards, D.; Cook, D.; Koscik, R.L.; Dowling, M.N.; Gallagher, C.L.; Carlsson, C.M.; et al. Cardiorespiratory fitness is associated with brain structure, cognition, and mood in a middle-aged cohort at risk for Alzheimer's disease. *Brain Imaging Behav.* **2015**, *9*, 639–649. [CrossRef] [PubMed]
20. Willis, B.L.; Gao, A.; Leonard, D.; Defina, L.F.; Berry, J.D. Midlife fitness and the development of chronic conditions in later life. *Arch. Intern. Med.* **2012**, *172*, 1333–1340. [CrossRef] [PubMed]
21. Zhu, N.; Jacobs, D.R., Jr.; Schreiner, P.J.; Launer, L.J.; Whitmer, R.A.; Sidney, S.; Demerath, E.; Thomas, W.; Bouchard, C.; He, K.; et al. Cardiorespiratory fitness and brain volume and white matter integrity: The CARDIA Study. *Neurology* **2015**, *84*, 2347–2353. [CrossRef] [PubMed]
22. Garcia-Hermoso, A.; Cavero-Redondo, I.; Ramirez-Velez, R.; Ruiz, J.R.; Ortega, F.B.; Lee, D.C.; Martinez-Vizcaino, V. Muscular Strength as a Predictor of All-Cause Mortality in an Apparently Healthy Population: A Systematic Review and Meta-Analysis of Data From Approximately 2 Million Men and Women. *Arch. Phys. Med. Rehabil.* **2018**, *99*, 2100–2113.e5. [CrossRef]
23. Garcia-Hermoso, A.; Ramirez-Velez, R.; Peterson, M.D.; Lobelo, F.; Cavero-Redondo, I.; Correa-Bautista, J.E.; Martinez-Vizcaino, V. Handgrip and knee extension strength as predictors of cancer mortality: A systematic review and meta-analysis. *Scand. J. Med. Sci. Sports* **2018**, *28*, 1852–1858. [CrossRef] [PubMed]
24. Kettunen, O.; Kyrolainen, H.; Santtila, M.; Vasankari, T. Physical fitness and volume of leisure time physical activity relate with low stress and high mental resources in young men. *J. Sports Med. Phys. Fit.* **2014**, *54*, 545–551.
25. Currell, K.; Jeukendrup, A.E. Validity, reliability and sensitivity of measures of sporting performance. *Sports Med.* **2008**, *38*, 297–316. [CrossRef] [PubMed]
26. Docherty, D. Field tests and test batteries. In *Measurement in Pediatric Exercise Science*; Docherty, D., Ed.; Human Kinetics: Champaign, IL, USA, 1996; pp. 285–334.
27. Castro-Pinero, J.; Artero, E.G.; Espana-Romero, V.; Ortega, F.B.; Sjostrom, M.; Suni, J.; Ruiz, J.R. Criterion-related validity of field-based fitness tests in youth: A systematic review. *Br. J. Sports Med.* **2009**, *44*, 934–943. [CrossRef]
28. Mayorga-Vega, D.; Aguilar-Soto, P.; Viciana, J. Criterion-related validity of the 20-m shuttle run test for estimating cardiorespiratory fitness: A meta-analysis. *J. Sports Sci. Med.* **2015**, *14*, 536–547.
29. Mayorga-Vega, D.; Viciana, J.; Cocca, A.; Merino-Marban, R. Criterion-related validity of toe-touch test for estimating hamstring extensibility: A metaanalysis. *J. Hum. Sport Exerc.* **2014**, *9*, 188–200. [CrossRef]
30. Mayorga-Vega, D.; Bocanegra-Parrilla, R.; Ornelas, M.; Viciana, J. Criterion-related validity of the distance- and time-based walk/run field tests for estimating cardiorespiratory fitness: A systematic review and Meta-analysis. *PLoS ONE* **2016**, *11*, e0151671. [CrossRef]
31. Mayorga-Vega, D.; Merino-Marban, R.; Viciana, J. Criterion-related validity of sit-and-reach tests for estimating hamstring and lumbar extensibility: A meta-analysis. *J. Sports Sci. Med.* **2014**, *13*, 1–14. [PubMed]
32. Bennett, H.; Parfitt, G.; Davison, K.; Eston, R. Validity of submaximal step tests to estimate maximal oxygen uptake in healthy adults. *Sports Med.* **2016**, *46*, 737–750. [CrossRef]
33. Moher, D.; Liberati, A.; Tetzlaff, J.; Altman, D.G. Preferred reporting items for systematic reviews and meta-analyses: The PRISMA statement. *PLoS Med.* **2009**, *6*, e1000097. [CrossRef]
34. Shea, B.J.; Hamel, C.; Wells, G.A.; Bouter, L.M.; Kristjansson, E.; Grimshaw, J.; Henry, D.A.; Boers, M. AMSTAR is a reliable and valid measurement tool to assess the methodological quality of systematic reviews. *J. Clin. Epidemiol.* **2009**, *62*, 1013–1020. [CrossRef] [PubMed]
35. Biddle, S.J.; García Bengoechea, E.; Wiesner, G. Sedentary behaviour and adiposity in youth: A systematic review of reviews and analysis of causality. *Int. J. Behav. Nutr. Phys. Act.* **2017**, *14*, 43. [CrossRef] [PubMed]
36. Oja, P.; Laukkanen, R.; Pasanen, M.; Tyry, T.; Vuori, I. A 2-km walking test for assessing the cardiorespiratory fitness of healthy adults. *Int. J. Sports Med.* **1991**, *12*, 356–362. [CrossRef]

37. Laukkanen, R.; Oja, P.; Pasanen, M.; Vuori, I. Validity of a two kilometre walking test for estimating maximal aerobic power in overweight adults. *Int. J. Obes. Relat. Metab. Disord.* **1992**, *16*, 263–268.
38. Laukkanen, R.M.T.; Oja, P.; Pasanen, M.E.; Vuori, I.M. Criterion validity of a two-kilometer walking test for predicting the maximal oxygen uptake of moderately to highly active middle-aged adults. *Scand. J. Med. Sci. Sports* **1993**, *3*, 267–272. [CrossRef]
39. Laukkanen, R.M.T.; Kukkonen-Harjula, T.K.; Oja, P.; Pasanen, M.E.; Vuori, I.M. Prediction of change in maximal aerobic power by the 2-km walk test after walking training in middle-aged adults. *Int. J. Sports Med.* **2000**, *21*, 113–116. [CrossRef]
40. Larsen, G.E.; George, J.D.; Alexander, J.L.; Fellingham, G.W.; Aldana, S.G.; Parcell, A.C. Prediction of maximum oxygen consumption from walking, jogging, or running. *Res. Q. Exerc. Sport* **2002**, *73*, 66–72. [CrossRef]
41. McNaughton, L.; Hall, P.; Cooley, D. Validation of several methods of estimating maximal oxygen uptake in young men. *Percept. Mot. Ski.* **1998**, *87*, 575–584. [CrossRef]
42. Kline, C.; Porcari, J.P.; Hintermeister, R.; Freedson, P.S.; Ward, A.; McCarron, R.F.; Ross, J.; Rippe, J. Estimation of from a one-mile track walk, gender, age and body weight. *Med. Sports Exerc.* **1987**, *19*, 253–259.
43. George, J.D.; Fellingham, G.W.; Fisher, A.G. A modified version of the Rockport Fitness Walking Test for college men and women. *Res. Q. Exerc. Sport* **1998**, *69*, 205–209. [CrossRef]
44. Lunt, H.; Roiz De Sa, D.; Roiz De Sa, J.; Allsopp, A. Validation of one-mile walk equations for the estimation of aerobic fitness in British military personnel under the age of 40 years. *Mil. Med.* **2013**, *178*, 753–759. [CrossRef]
45. Greenhalgh, H.A.; George, J.D.; Hager, R.L. Cross-validation of a quarter-mile walk test using two VO2 max regression models. *Meas. Phys. Educ. Exerc. Sci.* **2001**, *5*, 139–151. [CrossRef]
46. Dolgener, F.A.; Hensley, L.D.; Marsh, J.J.; Fjelstul, J.K. Validation of the Rockport Fitness Walking Test in college males and females. *Res. Q. Exerc. Sport* **1994**, *65*, 152–158. [CrossRef]
47. Seneli, R.M.; Ebersole, K.T.; O'Connor, K.M.; Snyder, A.C. Estimated VO2max from the Rockport Walk Test on a Nonmotorized Curved Treadmill. *J. Strength Cond. Res.* **2013**, *27*, 3495–3505. [CrossRef] [PubMed]
48. George, J.D.; Vehrs, P.R.; Allsen, P.E.; Fellingham, G.W.; Fisher, A.G. Development of a submaximal treadmill jogging test for fit college-aged individuals. *Med. Sci. Sports Exerc.* **1993**, *25*, 643–647. [CrossRef]
49. Cao, Z.-B.; Miyatake, N.; Aoyama, T.; Higuchi, M.; Tabata, I. Prediction of maximal oxygen uptake from a 3-minute walk based on gender, age, and body composition. *J. Phys. Act. Health* **2013**, *10*, 280–287. [CrossRef]
50. Di Thommazo-Luporini, L.; Pinheiro Carvalho, L.; Luporini, R.; Trimer, R.; Falasco Pantoni, C.B.; Catai, A.M.; Arena, R.; Borghi-Silva, A. The six-minute step test as a predictor of cardiorespiratory fitness in obese women. *Eur. J. Phys. Rehabil. Med.* **2015**, *51*, 793–802. [PubMed]
51. Di Thommazo-Luporini, L.; Carvalho, L.P.; Luporini, R.L.; Trimer, R.; Falasco Pantoni, C.B.; Martinez, A.F.; Catai, A.M.; Arena, R.; Borghi-Silva, A. Are cardiovascular and metabolic responses to field walking tests interchangeable and obesity-dependent? *Disabil. Rehabil.* **2016**, *38*, 1820–1829. [CrossRef]
52. Manttari, A.; Suni, J.; Sievanen, H.; Husu, P.; Vaha-Ypya, H.; Valkeinen, H.; Tokola, K.; Vasankari, T. Six-minute walk test: A tool for predicting maximal aerobic power (VO2 max) in healthy adults. *Clin. Physiol. Funct. Imaging* **2018**. [CrossRef] [PubMed]
53. Bonet, J.B.; Magalhaes, J.; Viscor, G.; Pages, T.; Javierre, C.F.; Torrella, J.R. A field tool for the aerobic power evaluation of middle-aged female recreational runners. *Women Health* **2020**, *60*, 839–848. [CrossRef] [PubMed]
54. Cooper, S.M.; Baker, J.S.; Tong, R.J.; Roberts, E.; Hanford, M. The repeatability and criterion related validity of the 20 m multistage fitness test as a predictor of maximal oxygen uptake in active young men. *Br. J. Sports Med.* **2005**, *39*, e19. [CrossRef] [PubMed]
55. Flouris, A.D.; Koutedakis, Y.; Nevill, A.; Metsios, G.S.; Tsiotra, G.; Parasiris, Y. Enhancing specificity in proxy-design for the assessment of bioenergetics. *J. Sci. Med. Sport* **2004**, *7*, 197–204. [CrossRef]
56. Metsios, G.S.; Flouris, A.D.; Koutedakis, Y.; Nevill, A. Criterion-related validity and test-retest reliability of the 20m square shuttle test. *J. Sci. Med. Sport* **2008**, *11*, 214–217. [CrossRef]
57. Flouris, A.D.; Metsios, G.S.; Koutedakis, Y. Enhancing the efficacy of the 20 m multistage shuttle run test. *Br. J. Sports Med.* **2005**, *39*, 166–170. [CrossRef]
58. Kim, J.; Jung, S.H.; Cho, H.C. Validity and Reliability of Shuttle-Run Test in Korean Adults. *Int. J. Sports Med.* **2011**, *32*, 580–585. [CrossRef]
59. Jurio-Iriarte, B.; Gorostegi-Anduaga, I.; Rodrigo Aispuru, G.; Perez-Asenjo, J.; Brubaker, P.H.; Maldonado-Martin, S. Association between Modified Shuttle Walk Test and cardiorespiratory fitness in overweight/obese adults with primary hypertension: EXERDIET-HTA study. *J. Am. Soc. Hypertens.* **2017**, *11*, 186–195. [CrossRef] [PubMed]
60. Jurio-Iriarte, B.; Brubaker, P.H.; Gorostegi-Anduaga, I.; Corres, P.; Martinez Aguirre-Betolaza, A.; Maldonado-Martin, S. Validity of the modified shuttle walk test to assess cardiorespiratory fitness after exercise intervention in overweight/obese adults with primary hypertension. *Clin. Exp. Hypertens.* **2018**, *41*, 336–341. [CrossRef] [PubMed]
61. Lima, L.P.; Leite, H.R.; Matos, M.A.; Neves, C.D.C.; Lage, V.; Silva, G.P.D.; Lopes, G.S.; Chaves, M.G.A.; Santos, J.N.V.; Camargos, A.C.R.; et al. Cardiorespiratory fitness assessment and prediction of peak oxygen consumption by Incremental Shuttle Walking Test in healthy women. *PLoS ONE* **2019**, *14*, e0211357. [CrossRef]
62. Aadahl, M.; Zacho, M.; Linneberg, A.; Thuesen, B.H.; Jorgensen, T. Comparison of the Danish step test and the watt-max test for estimation of maximal oxygen uptake: The Health2008 study. *Eur. J. Prev. Cardiol.* **2013**, *20*, 1088–1094. [CrossRef]
63. Kumar, S.K.; Khare, P.; Jaryal, A.K.; Talwar, A. Validity of heart rate based nomogram fors estimation of maximum oxygen uptake in Indian population. *Indian J. Physiol. Pharmacol.* **2012**, *56*, 279–283. [PubMed]

64. Ricci, P.A.; Cabiddu, R.; Jürgensen, S.P.; André, L.D.; Oliveira, C.R.; Di Thommazo-Luporini, L.; Ortega, F.P.; Borghi-Silva, A. Validation of the two-minute step test in obese with comorbibities and morbidly obese patients. *Braz. J. Med Biol. Res.* **2019**, *52*, e8402. [CrossRef] [PubMed]
65. Weller, I.M.; Thomas, S.G.; Cox, M.H.; Corey, P.N. A study to validate the Canadian Aerobic Fitness Test. *Can. J. Public Health* **1992**, *83*, 120–124. [CrossRef]
66. Carvalho, L.P.; Di Thommazo-Luporini, L.; Aubertin-Leheudre, M.; Bonjorno Junior, J.C.; de Oliveira, C.R.; Luporini, R.L.; Mendes, R.G.; Lopes Zangrando, K.T.; Trimer, R.; Arena, R.; et al. Prediction of cardiorespiratory fitness by the six-minute step test and its association with muscle strength and power in sedentary obese and lean young women: A cross-sectional study. *PLoS ONE* **2015**, *10*, e0145960. [CrossRef] [PubMed]
67. Teren, A.; Zachariae, S.; Beutner, F.; Ubrich, R.; Sandri, M.; Engel, C.; Loeffler, M.; Gielen, S. Incremental value of veterans specific activity questionnaire and the ymca-step test for the assessment of cardiorespiratory fitness in population-based studies. *Eur. J. Prev. Cardiol.* **2016**, *23*, 1221–1227. [CrossRef] [PubMed]
68. Beutner, F.; Ubrich, R.; Zachariae, S.; Engel, C.; Sandri, M.; Teren, A.; Gielen, S. Validation of a brief step-test protocol for estimation of peak oxygen uptake. *Eur. J. Prev. Cardiol.* **2015**, *22*, 503–512. [CrossRef] [PubMed]
69. Lee, O.; Lee, S.; Kang, M.; Mun, J.; Chung, J. Prediction of maximal oxygen consumption using the Young Men's Christian Association-step test in Korean adults. *Eur. J. Appl. Physiol.* **2019**, *119*, 1245–1252. [CrossRef] [PubMed]
70. Kieu, N.T.V.; Jung, S.J.; Shin, S.W.; Jung, H.W.; Jung, E.S.; Won, Y.H.; Kim, Y.G.; Chae, S.W. The validity of the YMCA 3-minute step test for estimating maximal oxygen uptake in healthy Korean and Vietnamese adults. *J. Lifestyle Med.* **2020**, *10*, 21–29. [CrossRef]
71. Hong, S.H.; Yang, H.I.; Kim, D.I.; Gonzales, T.I.; Brage, S.; Jeon, J.Y. Validation of submaximal step tests and the 6-min walk test for predicting maximal oxygen consumption in young and healthy participants. *Int. J. Environ. Res. Public Health* **2019**, *16*, 4858. [CrossRef]
72. Hansen, D.; Jacobs, N.; Thijs, H.; Dendale, P.; Claes, N. Validation of a single-stage fixed-rate step test for the prediction of maximal oxygen uptake in healthy adults. *Clin. Physiol. Funct. Imaging* **2016**, *36*, 401–406. [CrossRef] [PubMed]
73. Espana-Romero, V.; Artero, E.G.; Santaliestra-Pasias, A.M.; Gutierrez, A.; Castillo, M.J.; Ruiz, J.R. Hand span influences optimal grip span in boys and girls aged 6 to 12 years. *J. Hand Surg.* **2008**, *33*, 378–384. [CrossRef] [PubMed]
74. Cadenas-Sanchez, C.; Sanchez-Delgado, G.; Martinez-Tellez, B.; Mora-Gonzalez, J.; Löf, M.; España-Romero, V.; Ruiz, J.R.; Ortega, F.B. Reliability and validity of different models of TKK hand dynamometers. *Am. J. Occup. Ther.* **2016**, *70*, 7004300010. [CrossRef] [PubMed]
75. Kolimechkov, S.; Castro-Piñero, J.; Petrov, A.; Alexandrova, A. The effect of elbow position on the handgrip strength test in children: Validity and reliability of TKK 5101 and DynX dynamometers. *Pedagog. Phys Cult Sports* **2020**, *24*, 240–247. [CrossRef]
76. Shechtman, O.; Gestewitz, L.; Kimble, C. Reliability and validity of the DynEx dynamometer. *J. Hand Ther.* **2005**, *18*, 339–347. [CrossRef] [PubMed]
77. Mannion, A.F.; Dolan, P. Electromyographic median frequency changes during isometric contraction of the back extensors to fatigue. *Spine* **1994**, *19*, 1223–1229. [CrossRef]
78. Coorevits, P.; Danneels, L.; Cambier, D.; Ramon, H.; Vanderstraeten, G. Assessment of the validity of the Biering-Sørensen test for measuring back muscle fatigue based on EMG median frequency characteristics of back and hip muscles. *J. Electromyogr. Kinesiol.* **2008**, *18*, 997–1005. [CrossRef]
79. Kankaanpää, M.; Laaksonen, D.; Taimela, S.; Kokko, S.M.; Airaksinen, O.; Hänninen, O. Age, sex, and body mass index as determinants of back and hip extensor fatigue in the isometric Sørensen back endurance test. *Arch. Phys. Med. Rehabil.* **1998**, *79*, 1069–1075. [CrossRef]
80. De Blaiser, C.; De Ridder, R.; Willems, T.; Danneels, L.; Roosen, P. Reliability and validity of trunk flexor and trunk extensor strength measurements using handheld dynamometry in a healthy athletic population. *Phys. Ther. Sport* **2018**, *34*, 180–186. [CrossRef]
81. Bui, H.T.; Farinas, M.-I.; Fortin, A.-M.; Comtois, A.-S.; Leone, M. Comparison and analysis of three different methods to evaluate vertical jump height. *Clin. Physiol. Funct. Imaging* **2015**, *35*, 203–209. [CrossRef]
82. Kawano, M.M.; Ambar, G.; Oliveira, B.I.R.; Boer, M.C.; Cardoso, A.P.R.G.; Cardoso, J.R. Influence of the gastrocnemius muscle on the sit-and-reach test assessed by angular kinematic analysis. *Braz. J. Phys. Ther.* **2010**, *14*, 10–15. [CrossRef] [PubMed]
83. Bassett, D.R., Jr.; Howley, E.T.; Thompson, D.L.; King, G.A.; Strath, S.J.; McLaughlin, J.E.; Parr, B.B. Validity of inspiratory and expiratory methods of measuring gas exchange with a computerized system. *J. Appl. Physiol.* **2001**, *91*, 218–224. [CrossRef] [PubMed]
84. Meredith, M.D.; Welk, G.J. *Fitnessgram & Activitygram Test Administration Manual*, 4th ed.; Human Kinetics: Champaign, IL, USA, 2010.
85. Ruiz, J.R.; Ortega, F.B.; Castro-Piñero, J. Validity and reliability of the 1/4 mile run-walk test in physically active children and adolescents. *Nutr. Hosp.* **2014**, *31*, 875–882.
86. Krahenbuhl, G.S.; Pangrazi, R.P.; Burkett, L.N.; Schneider, M.J.; Petersen, G. Field estimation of VO2 max in children eight years of age. *Med. Sci. Sports* **1977**, *9*, 37–40. [CrossRef] [PubMed]
87. McCormack, W.P.; Cureton, K.J.; Bullock, T.A.; Weyand, P.G. Metabolic determinants of 1-mile run/walk performance in children. *Med. Sci. Sports Exerc.* **1991**, *23*, 611–617. [CrossRef]
88. Shephard, R.J. Tests of maximum oxygen intake. A critical review. *Sports Med.* **1984**, *1*, 99–124. [CrossRef]

89. Duncan, M.J.; Mota, J.; Carvalho, J.; Nevill, A.M. An Evaluation of Prediction Equations for the 6 Minute Walk Test in Healthy European Adults Aged 50–85 Years. *PLoS ONE* **2015**, *10*, e0139629.
90. Burr, J.F.; Bredin, S.S.; Faktor, M.D.; Warburton, D.E. The 6-minute walk test as a predictor of objectively measured aerobic fitness in healthy working-aged adults. *Physician Sportsmed.* **2011**, *39*, 133–139. [CrossRef]
91. Leger, L.A.; Mercier, D.; Gadoury, C.; Lambert, J. The multistage 20 m shuttle run test for aerobic fitness. *J. Sports Sci.* **1988**, *6*, 93–101. [CrossRef]
92. Santo, A.; Golding, L.A. Predicting maximum oxygen uptake from a modified 3-minute step test. *Res. Q. Exer. Sport* **2003**, *74*, 110–115. [CrossRef]
93. Mayhew, J.L.; Ball, T.E.; Ward, T.E.; Hart, C.L.; Arnold, M.D. Relationships of structural dimensions to bench press strength in college males. *J. Sports Med. Phys. Fit.* **1991**, *31*, 135–141.
94. Stark, T.; Walker, B.; Phillips, J.K.; Fejer, R.; Beck, R. Hand-held dynamometry correlation with the gold standard isokinetic dynamometry: A systematic review. *PM R.* **2011**, *3*, 472–479. [CrossRef] [PubMed]
95. Paul, D.J.; Nassis, G.P. Testing strength and power in soccer players: The application of conventional and traditional methods of assessment. *J. Strength Cond. Res.* **2015**, *29*, 1748–1758. [CrossRef] [PubMed]
96. De Ste Croix, M.; Deighan, M.; Armstrong, N. Assessment and interpretation of isokinetic muscle strength during growth and maturation. *Sports Med.* **2003**, *33*, 727–743. [CrossRef] [PubMed]
97. España-Romero, V.; Ortega, F.B.; Vicente-Rodríguez, G.; Artero, E.G.; Rey, J.P.; Ruiz, J.R. Elbow position affects handgrip strength in adolescents: Validity and reliability of Jamar, DynEx, and TKK dynamometers. *J. Strength Cond. Res.* **2010**, *24*, 272–277. [CrossRef] [PubMed]
98. Balogun, J.A.; Akomolafe, C.T.; Amusa, L.O. Grip strength: Effects of testing posture and elbow position. *Arch. Phys. Med. Rehabil.* **1991**, *72*, 280–283. [PubMed]
99. *NHANES, Muscle Strength Procedures Manual*; National Health and Nutrition Examination Survey (NHANES); CDC: Druid Hills, GA, USA, 2013.
100. Ruiz-Ruiz, J.; Mesa, J.L.; Gutiérrez, A.; Castillo, M.J. Hand size influences optimal grip span in women but not in men. *J. Hand Surg.* **2002**, *27*, 897–901. [CrossRef] [PubMed]
101. Kim, W.J.; Kim, K.J.; Song, D.G.; Lee, J.S.; Park, K.Y.; Lee, J.W.; Chang, S.H.; Choy, W.S. Sarcopenia and Back Muscle Degeneration as Risk Factors for Back Pain: A Comparative Study. *Asian Spine J.* **2020**, *14*, 364–372. [CrossRef]
102. Abdelraouf, O.R.; Abdel-Aziem, A.A. The relationship between core endurance and back dysfunction in collegiate male athletes with and without nonspecific low back pain. *Int. J. Sports Phys. Ther.* **2016**, *11*, 337–344.
103. Ozcan Kahraman, B.; Salik Sengul, Y.; Kahraman, T.; Kalemci, O. Developing a Reliable Core Stability Assessment Battery for Patients with Nonspecific Low Back Pain. *Spine* **2016**, *41*, E844–E850. [CrossRef]
104. Arab, A.M.; Salavati, M.; Ebrahimi, I.; Ebrahim Mousavi, M. Sensitivity, specificity and predictive value of the clinical trunk muscle endurance tests in low back pain. *Clin. Rehabil.* **2007**, *21*, 640–647. [CrossRef]
105. del Pozo-Cruz, B.; Mocholi, M.H.; del Pozo-Cruz, J.; Parraca, J.A.; Adsuar, J.C.; Gusi, N. Reliability and validity of lumbar and abdominal trunk muscle endurance tests in office workers with nonspecific subacute low back pain. *J. Back Musculoskelet. Rehabil.* **2014**, *27*, 399–408. [CrossRef] [PubMed]
106. Ortega, F.B.; Cadenas-Sanchez, C.; Sanchez-Delgado, G.; Mora-Gonzalez, J.; Martinez-Tellez, B.; Artero, E.G.; Castro-Pinero, J.; Labayen, I.; Chillon, P.; Lof, M.; et al. Systematic review and proposal of a field-based physical fitness-test battery in preschool children: The PREFIT battery. *Sports Med.* **2015**, *45*, 533–555. [CrossRef]
107. Ruiz, J.R.; Castro-Piñero, J.; Espana-Romero, V.; Artero, E.G.; Ortega, F.B.; Cuenca, M.M.; Jimenez-Pavon, D.; Chillon, P.; Girela-Rejon, M.J.; Mora, J.; et al. Field-based fitness assessment in young people: The ALPHA health-related fitness test battery for children and adolescents. *Br. J. Sports Med.* **2011**, *45*, 518–524. [CrossRef]
108. Leighton, J.R. An instrument and technic for the measurement of range of joint motion. *Arch. Phys. Med. Rehabil.* **1955**, *36*, 571–578.
109. Kanbur, N.O.; Duzgun, I.; Derman, O.; Baltaci, G. Do sexual maturation stages affect flexibility in adolescent boys aged 14 years? *J. Sports Med. Phys. Fit.* **2005**, *45*, 53–57.
110. Castro-Pinero, J.; Chillon, P.; Ortega, F.B.; Montesinos, J.L.; Sjostrom, M.; Ruiz, J.R. Criterion-related validity of sit-and-reach and modified sit-and-reach test for estimating hamstring flexibility in children and adolescents aged 6-17 years. *Int. J. Sports Med.* **2009**, *30*, 658–662. [CrossRef] [PubMed]
111. Wells, K.F.; Dillon, E.K. The sit-and-reach. A test of back and leg flexibility. *Res. Q. Exerc. Sport* **1952**, *23*, 115–118. [CrossRef]
112. Kraus, H.; Hirschland, R. Minimum muscular fitness of the school children. *Res. Q.* **1954**, *25*, 178–188. [CrossRef]
113. Nuzzo, J.L. The Case for Retiring Flexibility as a Major Component of Physical Fitness. *Sports Med.* **2020**, *50*, 853–870. [CrossRef] [PubMed]
114. Elbaz, A.; Sabia, S.; Brunner, E.; Shipley, M.; Marmot, M.; Kivimaki, M.; Singh-Manoux, A. Association of walking speed in late midlife with mortality: Results from the Whitehall II cohort study. *Age* **2013**, *35*, 943–952. [CrossRef] [PubMed]
115. Niiranen, T.J.; Enserro, D.M.; Larson, M.G.; Vasan, R.S. Multisystem Trajectories Over the Adult Life Course and Relations to Cardiovascular Disease and Death. *J. Gerontol. Ser. A Biol. Sci. Med. Sci.* **2019**, *74*, 1778–1785. [CrossRef] [PubMed]
116. Cooper, R.; Strand, B.H.; Hardy, R.; Patel, K.V.; Kuh, D. Physical capability in mid-life and survival over 13 years of follow-up: British birth cohort study. *BMJ* **2014**, *348*, g2219. [CrossRef]

117. Nitz, J.C.; Stock, L.; Khan, A. Health-related predictors of falls and fractures in women over 40. *Osteoporos. Int.* **2013**, *24*, 613–621. [CrossRef] [PubMed]
118. Wang, D.X.M.; Yao, J.; Zirek, Y.; Reijnierse, E.M.; Maier, A.B. Muscle mass, strength, and physical performance predicting activities of daily living: A meta-analysis. *J. Cachexia Sarcopenia Muscle* **2020**, *11*, 3–25. [CrossRef] [PubMed]
119. Briggs, R.; Carey, D.; Claffey, P.; McNicholas, T.; Donoghue, O.; Kennelly, S.P.; Kenny, R.A. Do Differences in Spatiotemporal Gait Parameters Predict the Risk of Developing Depression in Later Life? *J. Am. Geriatr. Soc.* **2019**, *67*, 1050–1056. [CrossRef] [PubMed]

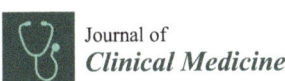

Article

The Effect of Submaximal Exercise Followed by Short-Term Cold-Water Immersion on the Inflammatory State in Healthy Recreational Athletes: A Cross-Over Study

Marta Pawłowska [1,*], Celestyna Mila-Kierzenkowska [1], Tomasz Boraczyński [2], Michał Boraczyński [3], Karolina Szewczyk-Golec [1,*], Paweł Sutkowy [1], Roland Wesołowski [1], Małgorzata Smoguła [1] and Alina Woźniak [1]

1. Department of Medical Biology and Biochemistry, Ludwik Rydygier Collegium Medicum in Bydgoszcz, Nicolaus Copernicus University in Toruń, 85-092 Bydgoszcz, Poland; celestyna_mila@cm.umk.pl (C.M.-K.); p.sutkowy@cm.umk.pl (P.S.); roland@cm.umk.pl (R.W.); malgorzata.smogula@gmail.com (M.S.); al1103@cm.umk.pl (A.W.)
2. Department of Health Sciences, Olsztyn University, 10-283 Olsztyn, Poland; boraczynski@osw.edu.pl
3. Department of Health Sciences, Collegium Medicum, University of Warmia and Mazury, 10-561 Olsztyn, Poland; michal.boraczynski@gmail.com
* Correspondence: marta.pawlowska@cm.umk.pl (M.P.); karosz@cm.umk.pl (K.S.-G.); Tel.: +48-52-585-38-22 (M.P.)

Abstract: Cold-water immersion (CWI) after exercise is a method used by sportsmen to improve recovery. The aim of the study was to assess the effect of a 3 min CWI on the inflammatory state by measuring levels of interleukin 6 (IL-6), interleukin 10 (IL-10), tumor necrosis factor α (TNF-α), and transforming growth factor β1 (TGF-β1), and activities of α1-antitrypsin (AAT) and lysosomal enzymes, including arylsulfatase (ASA), acid phosphatase (AcP), and cathepsin D (CTS D), in the blood of healthy recreational athletes. Male volunteers (n = 22, age 25 ± 4.8 yr) performed a 30 min submaximal aerobic exercise, followed by a 20 min rest at room temperature (RT-REST) or a 20 min rest at room temperature with an initial 3 min 8 °C water bath (CWI-REST). Blood samples were taken at baseline, immediately after exercise, and after 20 min of recovery. The IL-6, IL-10, and TNF-α levels and the AAT activity increased significantly immediately after exercise. The IL-6 level was significantly higher after CWI-REST than after RT-REST. No changes in the activities of the lysosomal enzymes were observed. The effect of a 3 min CWI on the level of inflammatory markers during post-exercise recovery was limited. Thus, it might be considered as a widely available method of regeneration for recreational athletes.

Keywords: cold-water immersion; cytokines; exercise; inflammation; lysosomal enzymes; regeneration method; recovery

Citation: Pawłowska, M.; Mila-Kierzenkowska, C.; Boraczyński, T.; Boraczyński, M.; Szewczyk-Golec, K.; Sutkowy, P.; Wesołowski, R.; Smoguła, M.; Woźniak, A. The Effect of Submaximal Exercise Followed by Short-Term Cold-Water Immersion on the Inflammatory State in Healthy Recreational Athletes: A Cross-Over Study. *J. Clin. Med.* **2021**, *10*, 4239. https://doi.org/10.3390/jcm10184239

Academic Editor: David Rodríguez-Sanz

Received: 27 July 2021
Accepted: 16 September 2021
Published: 18 September 2021

Publisher's Note: MDPI stays neutral with regard to jurisdictional claims in published maps and institutional affiliations.

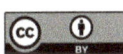

Copyright: © 2021 by the authors. Licensee MDPI, Basel, Switzerland. This article is an open access article distributed under the terms and conditions of the Creative Commons Attribution (CC BY) license (https://creativecommons.org/licenses/by/4.0/).

1. Introduction

Physical exercise is known to enhance and maintain overall health and wellness [1]. However, regular exercise and its effects may induce physical stress. After training, increases in inflammatory marker levels, including interleukin-6 (IL-6), interleukin-10 (IL-10), C-reactive protein (CRP), α1-antitrypsin (AAT), and others, can be observed [2,3]. Moreover, muscular exercise results in an acute increase in the production of reactive oxygen species (ROS), as evidenced by elevated biomarkers of oxidative damage in both the blood and skeletal muscles [4,5]. High levels of ROS lead to membrane lipid peroxidation, protein modifications, and DNA damage [6]. Proinflammatory cytokines, such as tumor necrosis factor α (TNF-α), activate neutrophils and initiate a local inflammatory response. Neutrophils migrate from the blood to damaged myocytes, which is accompanied by the production of ROS [7]. Structural changes in muscle fibers are also accompanied by an increased release of some intracellular enzymes, including lysosomal enzymes participating in intracellular macromolecule digestion [8]. Lysosomal enzymes may be released from cells after physical exercise, affecting the inflammatory response [9]. Taking these processes into consideration, regeneration between training sessions is the key to obtaining high training effectiveness and proper body adaptation to long-term physical effort [6].

Many athletes are interested in regeneration methods based on the exposure of the body to low ambient temperatures, i.e., during a bath in cold water. A rapid increase of body temperature after the end of the low temperature exposure causes increases in the blood flow, leading to better removal of waste metabolites and inflammatory mediators released by damaged tissue [10]. In addition, CWI may reduce muscle tension and fatigue, reduce joint pain, and improve general well-being, thus ensuring better sports performance [11]. Other popular methods of cold therapy include ice packs and whole-body cryotherapy (WBC) sessions [12]. WBC involves exposing the body to extreme low temperature (-100 °C to -160 °C) for 1–3 min. WBC also has a positive effect on the oxidant-antioxidant balance of the athlete's organism, soothing oxidative stress associated with intense physical effort [8]. However, WBC systems are quite expensive. As CWI is easier to administer for athletes and is a more cost-effective method of recovery with the use of cold than WBC (while providing the same or even greater benefits), it remains the more common method among individuals and teams [13]. There exists a long-standing belief that CWI reduces inflammation in tissues within and around the injured sites in skeletal muscle. Nevertheless, not much is yet known about the effects of cold exposure on pro- and anti-inflammatory cytokines. Moreover, previous research has mainly focused on the effects of CWI on the performance in the professional athlete population, and there is no research on CWI outcomes in the general population and recreational athletes [14]. It is noteworthy that the use of different cooling methods and a wide variety of exercise protocols during experiments resulted in a general dispute as to what types of exercise might benefit from CWI and which method of CWI is the most appropriate [15]. In addition, only a few studies have investigated the effect of post-exercise CWI on inflammatory markers over periods of less than two hours. Thus, establishing the minimum duration of CWI necessary to obtain a beneficial effect on the inflammatory state seems to be an issue of great interest.

Taking into account the unexplained issues of the impact of short CWI on inflammation, the aim of the present study was to determine if a 3 min CWI applied post-exercise is long enough to diminish the level of inflammatory markers in the blood of recreational athletes. For this purpose, concentrations of selected cytokines, including IL-6, IL-10, TNF-α, and transforming growth factor $\beta 1$ (TGF-$\beta 1$), as well as activities of AAT and selected lysosomal enzymes, including arylsulfatase (ASA), acid phosphatase (AcP), and cathepsin D (CTS D), were measured in the blood of young healthy recreational athletes who performed a 30 min submaximal aerobic exercise followed by a 20 min rest at room temperature with or without an initial 3 min cold-water bath.

2. Materials and Methods

2.1. Participants

Twenty-two young healthy recreationally trained male athletes who participated in the summer camp voluntarily agreed to participate in the study. The research included men who had never used cold-water immersion before the study period. The inclusion and exclusion criteria are described in Table 1.

The International Physical Activity Questionnaire (IPAQ) was used to assess the level of physical activity of the subjects during the last 7 days before the study. The IPAQ is expressed in MET $\times$ min/week. One MET is equal to 3.5 mL O_2/min/kg and represents the baseline oxygen consumption [16]. The included participants had a weekly physical activity level ranging between moderate and high. The range of practiced sports or physical workouts included running, strength or cardio workouts in the gym, gymnastics, swimming, tennis, cycling, and football. The category "moderate" means that the participants met at least one of the following criteria: (I) 3 or more days of vigorous activity of at least 20 min per day, (II) 5 or more days of moderate-intensity activity or walking of at least 30 min per day, and

(III) 5 or more days of any combination of walking, moderate-intensity, or high-intensity activities, achieving a minimum of at least 600 MET × min per week. The category "high" means that the participants met at least one of the following criteria: (I) vigorous-intensity activity of at least 3 days and accumulating at least 1500 MET × min/week, (II) 7 or more days of any combination of walking, moderate-intensity, or vigorous-intensity activities achieving a minimum of at least 3000 MET × min/week [16]. In the period just before or during the study, the subjects did not change their eating habits as well as the type and intensity of physical activity. People treated for any comorbidities, smoking cigarettes and under therapies that could affect the inflammatory state were excluded from the study. All the participants were informed about the purpose of the research and the potential risks, and they provided informed consent. The subjects were required to complete the baseline examination and two experimental sessions separated by 7 days. The research had the approval of the Bioethics Committee at Collegium Medicum in Bydgoszcz of the Nicolaus Copernicus University in Toruń (KB 278/2016).

Table 1. Eligibility criteria.

Inclusion Criteria
• Age 18–30 years • Weekly physical activity level ranging between moderate and high • Willingness to volunteer to participate in the trial and sign the informed consent form
Exclusion Criteria
• Cold-water immersion use before the study period • Active smoking or illicit drug use • Obesity • Cardiovascular diseases • Pulmonary diseases • Energy-restricted diet

2.2. Baseline Examination

The anthropometric evaluation and body composition of the participants, including body height (BH, cm), body weight (BM, kg), body mass index (BMI, kg/m^2), body fat (BF, %), and total body water mass (TBW, kg), were determined using a Tanita bioelectric impedance analyzer—BC 418 MA (Tanita Corporation, Tokyo, Japan). A physical working capacity-170 (PWC170) test was performed to determine the aerobic fitness of the participants [17]. The PWC170 test consisted of two 5 min standard exercise sessions on a bicycle ergometer (Monark Ergomedic 828 E, Vansbro, Sweden). The load for the second exercise test was increased to obtain but not exceed a heart rate (HR) of 170 beats per minute (bpm). The PWC170 index was calculated based on the mean of the HR values recorded at the end of each 5-min exercise period. The HR was measured using a cardiofrequency meter (Polar Electro Oy, Espoo, Finland). The load (power expressed in watts, W) was calculated during exercise at a HR of 170 bpm. The test result was calculated using the following formula: PWC170 = P1 + (P2 − P1)/(170 − HR1) (HR2 − HR1), where P1 means power of the first exercise test, P2—power of the second exercise test, HR1—HR during the first exercise test, HR2—HR during the second exercise test. The value of the PWC170 correlates well with the maximum oxygen consumption (VO$_2$ max), which is the primary oxygen function index [18]. The VO$_2$ max variables of all participants were calculated according to the Astrand–Ryhming normogram, using the values of PWC170 test [19]. For rating perceived exertion (RPE), the Borg Category Ratio-10 (CR10) scale was used (with a range of values from "0" to "10"). The first rate means "no exertion at all", whereas the last rate means "extremely strong" effort. There is also an exertion rate over 10, marked as "*". It is an exertion that makes the subject "unable to continue" the exercise bout. The RPE scale was used in both study sessions after a 30 min exercise period [20]. All measurements were performed by the same experienced investigator.

2.3. Study Design

The research project was divided into two sessions. The participants were assigned to either control condition (Session 1) or cold-water immersion (Session 2) in a counterbalanced crossover order. During Session 1, the volunteers were subjected to a 30 min exercise (70% of the maximum HR, HRmax) on a bicycle ergometer (Monark Ergomedic 828 E), followed by a 20 min rest at room temperature in a sitting position (RT-REST). The HRmax was calculated according to Tanaka's formula: HRmax = 208 − 0.7 × age [21]. Session 2 consisted of the same physical exercise test (30 min, 70% of the maximum HR, HRmax) and a 20 min recovery, but immediately after exercise, the participants were subjected to a 3-min immersion in a pool of cold water (8 °C) followed by rest at room temperature in a sitting position (CWI-REST). Volunteers were dressed only in swimming suits and they immersed the whole body with the exception of the head and neck. At both sessions, blood samples were taken from the median cubital vein into polypropylene tubes (6 mL) without anticoagulant to obtain serum at baseline (control, BE), immediately after exercise (AE) and after a 20 min recovery (RT-REST or CWI-REST). The samples were transported to a laboratory in a transport refrigerator at 4 °C and then centrifuged (6000× g for 10 min at 4 °C). Subsequently, serum was separated and stored at −80 °C for further analysis.

2.4. Determination of the Activity of Protease Inhibitor and Lysosomal Enzymes

The activity of AAT was estimated by the Eriksson method [22]. The basis of the assay was a decrease in the enzymatic activity of trypsin due to short incubation with defibrinated blood serum, measured at a wavelength of 410 nm. The activity of AAT was expressed in mg of trypsin-inhibited/mL blood serum. The ASA activity was estimated using the Roy method modified by Błeszyński and Działoszyński [23]. The amount of 4-nitrocatechol (4-NC) released during the enzymatic hydrolysis of 4-p-nitrocatechol sulfate was estimated. The ASA activity was expressed in nmol of 4-NC/mg protein/min. The activity of AcP was measured according to the Bessy method modified by Krawczyński [23]. The amount of p-nitrophenol released during the enzymatic hydrolysis of disodium p-nitrophenylphosphate was estimated and the activity of AcP was expressed in nmol of p-nitrophenol/mg protein/min. The CTS D activity was estimated by Anson's method [24]. The test sample was incubated with 2% denatured hemoglobin as a substrate at 37 °C and the absorbance at a wavelength of 600 nm was measured and compared to the absorbance of the control. The CTS D activity was expressed in nmol of tyrosine/mg protein/min.

2.5. Determination of the Cytokine Concentrations

The concentration of cytokines was estimated using ready-to-use immunoassays: IL-6 (Human IL-6 ELISA KIT, Diaclone SAS, Besancon CEDEX, France), IL-10 (Human IL-10 ELISA KIT, Diaclone SAS, Besancon CEDEX, France), TNF-α (Human TNF-α ELISA KIT, Diaclone SAS, Besancon CEDEX, France), and TGF-β1 (Human TGF-β1 ELISA KIT, Diaclone SAS, Besancon CEDEX, France). The measurements were made according to the manufacturer's instructions. The cytokine concentrations were expressed in pg/mL or in ng/mL. The sensitivity of the methods, depending on the used calibrates, was 2 pg/mL for IL-6, 4.9 pg/mL for IL-10, 8.6 pg/mL for TGF-β1, and 8 pg/mL for TNF-α.

All the studied parameters were analyzed in duplicate, with sample means taken as the result.

2.6. Statistical Analysis

The obtained results underwent univariate analysis of variances (ANOVA) with post hoc statistical analysis (Tukey's HSD test and Tukey's assay for different N). To calculate the sample size, the power of 80% and alpha level of 0.05 were used. In the post hoc analysis, all the assumptions of ANOVA (group equality, Levene's variance homogeneity test, Kolmogorov–Smirnov's normal distribution test, or Shapiro–Wilk's test) were considered. The results are presented as an arithmetic mean ± standard deviation (SD). Differences at the level of significance $p < 0.05$ were accepted as statistically significant. The effect size

(ES: Cohen's d) was used to measure the difference between sessions, using the following formula: Cohen's d = (M2 − M1)/SDpooled, where: SDpooled = $\sqrt{((SD1 + SD2)/2)}$. ES magnitudes were interpreted as follows: <0.2 trivial; 0.2–0.6 small; 0.6–1.2 moderate; 1.2–2.0 large; 2.0–4.0 very large; 4.0 nearly perfect [25].

3. Results

3.1. Basic Characteristics of the Study Group

The characteristics of the studied group is presented in Table 2. The VO_2 max value points to the average aerobic fitness of the subjects [18]. Using the Borg Category Ratio-10 scale, the participants evaluated their physical effort during the experiment as "slightly heavy" [20]. No incidents were recorded during exercise sessions or during recovery.

Table 2. Basic characteristics of the study group (healthy male recreational athletes, $n = 22$).

Parameter	Mean ± S.D.
Age (yr)	25.0 ± 4.8
BH (body height, cm)	179.7 ± 5.0
BM (body mass, kg)	81.4 ± 9.6
BMI (kg/m^2)	25.3 ± 2.7
BF (body fat, %)	15.6 ± 4.3
TBW (total body water, %)	61.5 ± 3.3
VO_2 max (maximum oxygen consumption, mL/kg/min) [1]	40.95 ± 6.6
Borg CR10 (rating of perceived exertion scale) [1]	4.06 ± 0.8
VO_2 max (maximum oxygen consumption, mL/kg/min) [2]	40.67 ± 6.7
Borg CR10 (rating of perceived exertion scale) [2]	4.08 ± 0.6

[1] Session 1, [2] Session 2.

3.2. The Concentration of Cytokines

Statistically significant concentration changes in the investigated cytokines during the session steps were revealed. IL-6 concentration increased more than ten times immediately after exercise (AE) in Session 1 ($p < 0.001$) and was still significantly higher ($p < 0.001$) after 20 min of rest at room temperature (RT-REST) than before exercise (BE) (4.5 ± 1.7, 3.8 ± 1.4, and 0.4 ± 0.1 pg/mL, respectively) (Figure 1a). In Session 2, IL-6 concentration was also nearly ten times higher AE than at baseline ($p < 0.05$), and additionally increased ($p < 0.05$) after 20 min of rest with an initial 3 min cold-water immersion (RT-CWI) (1.8 ± 0.5, 0.2 ± 0.1, and 3.1 ± 1.0 pg/mL, respectively) (Figure 1a). In both sessions, statistically significant increases in IL-10 concentration were found AE ($p < 0.05$) and after 20 min of recovery ($p < 0.001$), when compared to the concentration of this cytokine BE. In Session 1, the concentration of IL-10 was about two-fold higher AE compared to its BE level ($p < 0.05$). Furthermore, the concentration of IL-10 after RT-REST was five-fold higher than AE ($p < 0.001$) and about ten-fold higher than BE ($p < 0.001$) (15.5 ± 5.8, 3.1 ± 1.3, and 1.7 ± 1.1 pg/mL, respectively) (Figure 1b). A similar pattern was observed in Session 2. The concentration of IL-10 was about two-fold higher AE, compared to the BE values ($p < 0.05$). Moreover, the concentration of IL-10 after CWI-REST was five-fold higher than AE ($p < 0.001$) and about eleven-fold higher than BE ($p < 0.001$) (21.5 ± 7.9, 3.7 ± 1.5, and 1.9 ± 1.5 pg/mL, respectively) (Figure 1b). In Session 1, the TNF-α concentration decreased significantly AE ($p < 0.05$). After RT-REST, the concentration of TNF-α statistically increased, as compared to the result obtained AE ($p < 0.05$) (31.1 ± 6.6 and 21.7 ± 9.2 pg/mL, respectively) (Figure 1c). A similar pattern was observed in Session 2. The TNF-α concentration was significantly lower AE, and after CWI-REST, the concentration of this cytokine statistically increased ($p < 0.05$) (24.9 ± 10.7 and 33.1 ± 11.2 pg/mL, respectively) (Figure 1c). No statistically significant changes in TGF-β1 concentration were observed in the course of both sessions (Figure 1d).

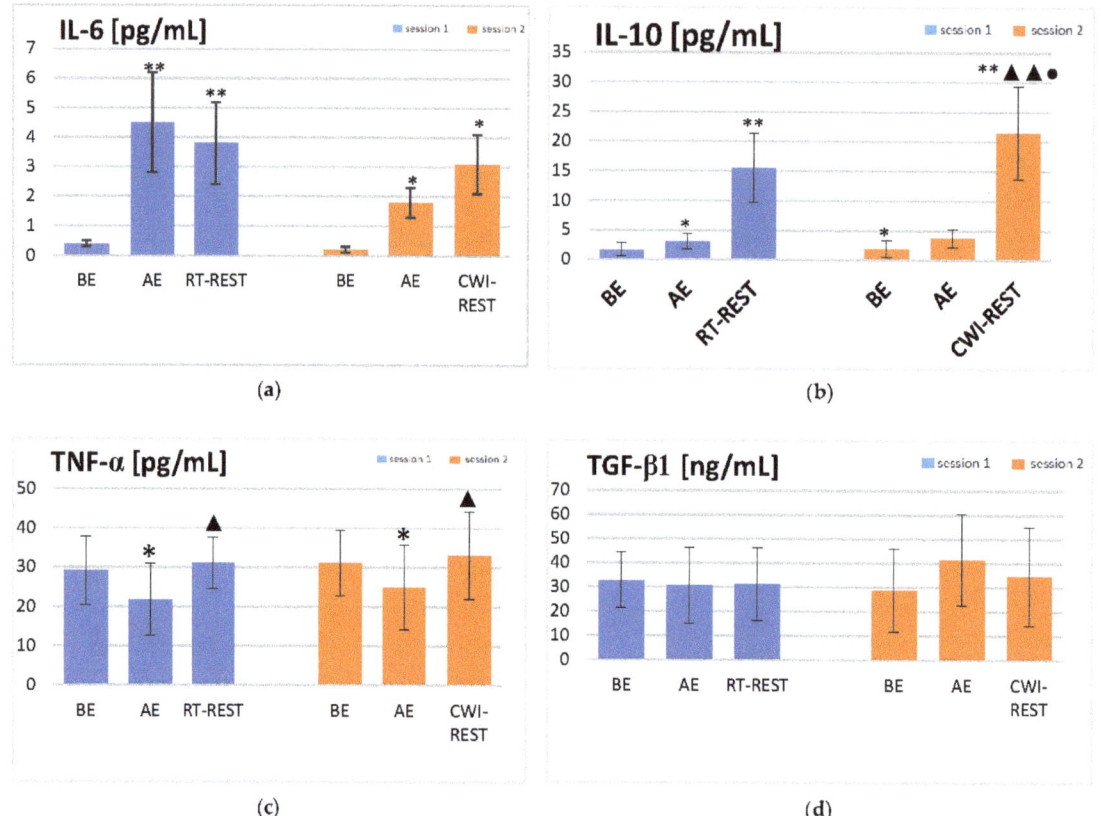

Figure 1. The concentrations of selected cytokines in blood serum of the subjects (young healthy recreational athletes, $n = 22$) during the experiment: (**a**) IL-6 concentration; (**b**) IL-10 concentration; (**c**) TNF-α concentration; (**d**) TGF-β1 concentration. Data are presented as the means ± SD. IL-6—interleukin 6, IL-10—interleukin 10, TNF-α—tumor necrosis factor α, TGF-β1—transforming growth factor β1, BE—before exercise, AF—after exercise, RT-REST—20 min recovery at room temperature, CWI-REST—20 min recovery at room temperature combined with 3 min cold-water immersion, * $p < 0.05$ vs. BE, ** $p < 0.001$ vs. BE, ▲ $p < 0.05$ vs. AE, ▲▲ $p < 0.001$ vs. AE, • $p < 0.001$ vs. RT-REST.

The results obtained in both sessions were compared. The concentration of IL-10 was significantly higher ($p < 0.001$) after CWI-REST than after RT-REST (21.5 ± 7.9 and 15.5 ± 5.8 pg/mL, respectively). The ES between session comparisons of the IL-10 concentration was moderate (0.87). The concentration of other cytokines did not differ in a statistically significant manner, comparing RT-REST and CWI-REST. For IL-6, TNF-a, and TGFβ1, the ESs were small (0.57, 0.22, and 0.18, respectively).

3.3. The Activity of Protease Inhibitor and Lysosomal Enzymes

In Session 1, a statistically significant increase in AAT activity AE was revealed, compared to the activity of this enzyme at baseline ($p < 0.05$). After RT-REST, AAT activity was lower than AE, but it remained higher than BE ($p < 0.05$) (0.75 ± 0.06, 0.80 ± 0.07, and 0.67 ± 0.08 mg inhibited trypsin/mL, respectively) (Figure 2a). In Session 2, the activity of AAT was significantly higher AE than BE ($p < 0.05$) (0.78 ± 0.08 and 0.71 ± 0.08 mg inhibited trypsin/mL, respectively), but decreased to the BE value after CWI-REST (0.72 ± 0.08 mg inhibited trypsin/mL) (Figure 2a). No statistically significant changes in the activities of the lysosomal enzymes were observed in the course of both sessions (Figure 2b–d).

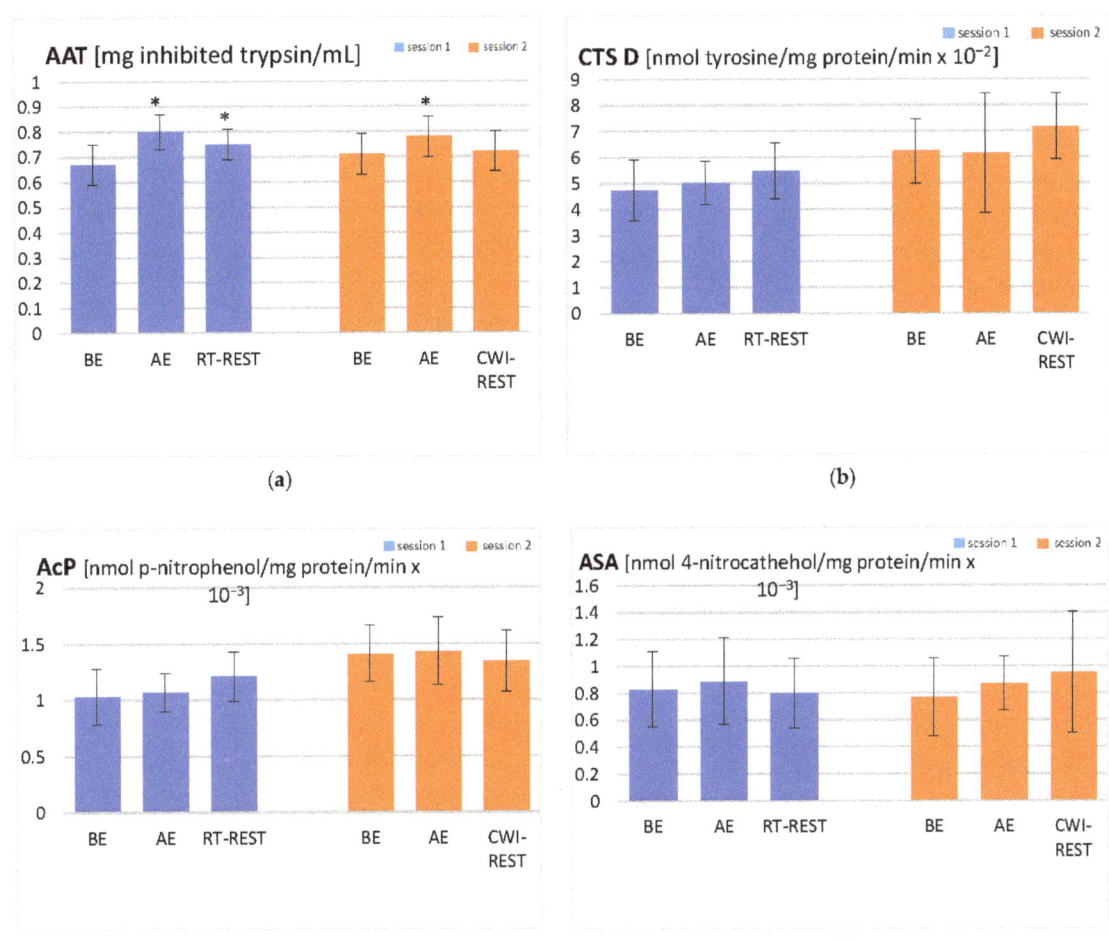

Figure 2. The activities of α1-antytrypsin and lysosomal enzymes in blood serum of the subjects (young healthy recreational athletes, n = 22) during the experiment: (**a**) AAT activity; (**b**) CTS D activity; (**c**) AcP activity; (**d**) ASA activity. Data are presented as the means ± SD. AAT—α1-antytrypsin, CTS D—cathepsin D, AcP—acid phosphatase, ASA—arylsulfatase, BE—before exercise, AE—after exercise, RT-REST—20-min recovery at room temperature, CWI-REST—20-min recovery at room temperature combined with 3-min cold-water immersion, * $p < 0.05$ vs. BE.

The activity of lysosomal enzymes and AAT did not differ in a statistically significant manner, comparing RT-REST and CWI-REST. For AAT, AcP, and ASA, the ESs were small (0.42, 0.53, and 0.37, respectively) and for CTS D, the ES was large (1.44). The large effect size in the case of CTS D with no statistically significant differences between recovery with and without CWI may indicate that the sample size was not big enough.

4. Discussion

The aim of the present study was to determine if a 3 min CWI applied post-exercise is long enough to diminish the level of inflammatory markers in the blood of recreational athletes. Statistically significant increases in IL-6 and IL-10 concentrations were observed in the blood serum of the participants after submaximal exercise. However, a significant post-exercise decrease in TNF-α concentration was observed, followed by a statistically significant increase in the level of this cytokine after RT-REST. Moreover, no statistically significant changes in TGF-β1 concentration were observed. The finding of triggered cytokine production as an effect of physical exercise concurs with many previous studies [26–29]. Zaldivar et al. [26] observed increased levels of both proinflammatory (IL-1α, IL-2, IL-6, TNF-α, TNF-γ) and anti-inflammatory cytokines (IL-10) after 30 min of physical exercise. Santos et al. [27] reported an increase in IL-10 levels in runners after the marathon, which returned to the pre-workout level after 24 h. Mezil et al. [28] found significant increases in IL-6 and TNF-α concentrations 5 min after low-impact, high-intensity interval exercise, and their return to baseline levels 1 h after exercise. A significant rise in the levels of IL-6 and TNF-α after moderate and strenuous exercise was also revealed by Ambarish et al. [29].

The post-exercise increase in IL-6 levels is well documented in existing literature [30–35]. It is worth emphasizing that IL-6 is one of the most rapidly produced myokines as a result of physical exercise, and its levels increase more dramatically than any other cytokine investigated to date [31]. In the present study, the concentration of IL-6 immediately after exercise was as much as 10 times higher than at baseline in either of the studied sessions. What is more, the literature data indicates the stimulating effect of IL-6 on the secretion of IL-10, one of the key anti-inflammatory cytokines [36]. Consistent with these findings, in the present study, an increase in the level of IL-6 was accompanied by an increase in the level of IL-10.

A decrease in TNF-α concentration immediately after exercise, observed in the present study, may indicate that submaximal exercise of the volunteers during the experiment did not cause any significant muscle cell damage. TNF-α concentration is supposed to depend on the secretion of IL-6 as this cytokine inhibits TNF-α expression [36]. However, exercise is likely to suppress TNF-α also via IL-6-independent pathways, as demonstrated by a modest decrease in the level of this cytokine after exercise, found in IL-6 knockout mice [37]. The suppressive effect on TNF-α production may be mediated by β2 adrenergic receptors due to sympatho-adrenergic activation during a single bout of exercise [38]. It may confirm the anti-inflammatory effects of regular exercise. The subjects of the present study were non-professional athletes but they declared a weekly physical activity level ranging from moderate to high. A decrease in the TNFα level as a result of regular moderate exercise was reported by Ambarish et al. [29]. The authors implied that regular moderate exercise optimizes the release of inflammatory cytokines, maintaining them at levels necessary as a buffer to elevate their levels during a sudden burst of exercise.

In the present study, statistically significant post-exercise increases in the AAT activity were observed during both studied sessions. Markovitch et al. [39] demonstrated that the AAT concentration is transiently increased immediately after demanding exercise. An increased activity of AAT after exercise was also reported in the studies of Semple et al. [40] and Schild et al. [41]. The post-exercise increase in the level of IL-6 with a concomitant increase of the AAT activity, found in the present study, may confirm the proposed inflammatory action of IL-6 by stimulation of acute phase protein release [36].

Although many studies have investigated the cytokine response to exercise, only a few of them have validated the anti-inflammatory effects of CWI. A delayed change in the IL-6 level and a decrease in the TNFα level were reported after a 10 min CWI [42] and after a 170 min intermittent CWI [43] in young non-cold-adapted healthy men, but cold exposure was not preceded by exercise. In order to attain the aim of the study, an attempt was made to determine the role of short cold-water immersion, which preceded rest in a sitting position at room temperature, in the modulation of the inflammatory response to submaximal exercise. The beneficial effect of CWI as a post-exercise regeneration method has been presented in many studies [10,11,44]. Several studies report that cold exposure is supposed to aid recovery by attenuating exercise-induced inflammation. However, this mechanism is not well supported in the literature. CWI was found to reduce swelling in athletes subjected to intense exercise [15] and to facilitate the restoration of muscle performance in a stretch–shortening cycle [33]. These effects did not appear to be associated with the modulation of the inflammatory response. Peake et al. [45] suggested that CWI was not more effective than active recovery as far as minimizing inflammation in muscle after exercise is concerned. They observed a post-exercise increase in the intramuscular gene expression of cytokines and neurotrophins. These responses did not differ substantially between cold-water immersion and active recovery. The results obtained in the present study seem to partially confirm the above-mentioned reports. Contrary to our hypothesis, CWI-REST, compared to RT-REST, did not significantly reduce the level of inflammatory markers. Comparing recovery with and without CWI, no statistically significant differences in the level of IL-6, TNF-α, and TGF-β1 were observed. The only statistically significant difference was found in the IL-10 level. The concentration of this cytokine was significantly higher after CWI-REST with moderate ES in comparisons between sessions. IL-10 is considered to be the primary anti-inflammatory agent as it inhibits the production of proinflammatory cytokines by activated monocytes and macrophages [46]. The increased level of IL-10 after CWI-REST, compared to RT-REST, could point to the anti-inflammatory effect of short CWI.

In the present study, the ESs of comparisons between the two recovery methods used were small for most of the measured cytokines. In both sessions, the IL-6 level was statistically higher immediately after exercise. However, a further significant increase in the cytokine concentration was observed only after CWI-REST. This result is in line with the findings of Roberts et al. [32], who revealed an elevated IL-6 level after both CWI and active recovery at 15 and 60 min post-exercise. The up-regulation of IL-6 expression after prolonged cold exposure was also shown by Rhind et al. [47]. Accordingly, CWI following high-intensity sprint exercise did not significantly reduce plasma markers of inflammation in the study of White et al. [33]. The IL-6 level increased significantly immediately after exercise and remained elevated when CWI at both cold (10 °C) and cool (20 °C) temperatures followed the exercise. Moreover, the IL-6 concentration after different CWI modalities was higher than after passive recovery (CON). In the present study, the CWI condition was not associated with reduced cytokine concentrations. However, the up-regulation of the IL-6 level as a consequence of CWI may have a positive aspect. IL-6 acts as a growth factor for skeletal muscle remodeling and regeneration [48]. The increased plasma IL-6 concentration may reflect a sustained release of IL-6 from skeletal muscle in response to CWI-stimulated glycogenolysis [32]. The higher IL-6 level after CWI-REST than after RT-REST may also be due to the modulation of muscle mass as a result of exposure to cold. In contrast, Earp et al. [34] found that the IL-6 level was significantly elevated after 30 min of CON, compared to the CWI session. Differences between the findings described above and in the present study may result from the resistance training status of the participants. In the present study, similar to the research of Peake et al. [49] and Roberts et al. [32], the participants were athletes trained only recreationally, while the participants in the Earp et al. [34] study were resistance trained.

Rhind et al. [47] revealed that, when strenuous exercise preceded exposure to cold, the spontaneous intracellular expression of TNFα was substantially reduced and its serum level was also markedly suppressed in response to cold exposure. The authors suggested that cold-induced changes in the cytokine expression appear to be linked to enhanced catecholamine secretion associated with cold exposure. In non-cold-adapted people, CWI at water temperatures below 15 °C induces a response known as "cold shock", which can be particularly awkward [42]. This stressful physiological reaction is manifested by increased levels of stress hormones, including cortisol, adrenaline, and noradrenaline [42,43]. CWI may benefit recovery after exercise by inducing vasoconstriction and restricting the infiltration of inflammatory cells into muscle [50–52]. According to this mechanism, CWI can reduce clinical signs of inflammation [52]. However, blood plasma levels of cytokines may not be altered at the blood sampling time point. Eimonte et al. [42] observed that although glucocorticoid and catecholamines induce a rapid response, they return to baseline soon after cold exposure. The authors implied that the stress hormones may (re)activate the cytokines gradually, later after CWI. Earp et al. [34] found that the TNFα level after rest with CWI was significantly lower than after CON, but only 15 min post-exercise and not 30 and 60 min after the resistance-exercise bouts. In the present study, the TNF-α level increased significantly to the values observed at baseline after 20 min of both RT-REST and CWI-REST. Both the blood sampling time and the surprisingly lowered TNFα levels after submaximal exercise found in the present study, may explain these discrepancies in the study results. In the study of de Freitas et al. [15], the TNFα levels were comparable between the CWI and placebo groups, but also did not change immediately after exercise, which may suggest that training performed in their study induced no detectable inflammation process in the subjects. It could be assumed that CWI did not reduce the level of TNFα because the exercise load was not sufficient to promote an increase in the level of this inflammatory marker.

In the present study, it was also found that the estimated ES of AAT activity in comparisons between RT-REST and CWI-REST was small. Nevertheless, the AAT activity after CWI-REST was observed to return to the baseline value, while after RT-REST, the AAT activity remained statistically higher than before exercise. It may indicate the beneficial effect of short CWI on the risk of proteolytic tissue damage. The fast response of the AAT activity after different recovery methods, determined in the present study, may confirm its role as an acute phase protein in humans. The primary function of the acute phase response is to protect the organism from further injury and help restore homeostasis [53]. AAT was found to reduce the production of proinflammatory cytokines, inhibit apoptosis, and affect the inhibition of local and systemic inflammatory reactions [54]. It could be inferred that the modulation of cytokine levels might have occurred later than the time points chosen in the present study. Thus, it is highly advisable to extend the blood sampling time point in the experiment protocol to confirm it.

Considering the activities of the lysosomal enzymes, no statistically significant changes were observed in both sessions of the present study. The estimated ESs for ASA and AcP activities were also small. This may indicate that the use of short CWI after physical exercise did not cause lysosomal membrane lability, as the lysosomal enzymes did not leak into the bloodstream. It was proven that lysosomal enzymes are involved in the development of post-exercise muscle fiber damage [7,55]. Lysosomal enzymes in inflammatory infiltrated cells are likely to play a major role in protein catabolism associated with local trauma [56]. The effect of a post-exercise CWI on the lysosomal enzyme activity and the pro- and antioxidant balance in the group of soccer players was determined by Sutkowy et al. [57]. The authors observed that both post-exercise recovery methods, including rest at room temperature and rest at room temperature preceded by CWI, did not significantly affect serum lysosomal enzyme activities, which is in accordance with the results obtained in the present study. No effect on the activity of the lysosomal enzymes was also observed after immersion in a river with a water temperature of 0 °C [58]. As previously mentioned, CWI in water below 15 °C is physiologically stressful and can be particularly hazardous [43]. No changes in the lysosomal enzyme activities in the blood plasma of the participants may suggest that the protocol of using a 3 min CWI in the present study did not cause any disruption of the lysosomal membrane and leakage of the enzymes into the bloodstream.

The limitations of the present study are the small number of the experiment participants and the relatively short duration of cold exposure. Future research should consider extending the cold-water immersion time and collecting blood samples at greater intervals after cold exposure.

5. Conclusions

In conclusion, the results of the present study confirm that aerobic exercise induces the inflammatory response of the organism and add to the existing knowledge of the effects of cold-water immersion after exercise. It is worth emphasizing that the effect of CWI on the natural physiological stress and immune responses remains controversial. An effective protocol for using CWI as a method of post-exercise recovery has not yet been well established. The protocols used so far are largely based on individual experience rather than evidence-based research. Moreover, much research in this area is limited to the study of participants who were experienced (adapted) cold-water swimmers, professional athletes who exercised acutely in the cold, or athletes who were previously immersed in cold water as recovery. In the present experiment, the study group consisted of recreational athletes who had never been subjected to cold exposure before, but CWI limited to 3 min seemed harmless to them. The effect of short CWI on the level of inflammatory markers during post-exercise recovery appeared to be limited. Additionally, a slight beneficial effect of a 3 min CWI on the risk of proteolytic tissue damage was observed. Thus, short exposure to cold might be considered as a widely available and cheap method of recovery improvement in recreational athletes. However, the risk of exposure of the human organism to low temperature, in relation to the expected beneficial effects of recovery, as well as the most appropriate CWI protocols must be verified by further studies, in which the time of CWI or the time of blood collection will be extended.

Author Contributions: Conceptualization, C.M.-K. and A.W.; methodology, C.M.-K. and T.B.; data curation, M.P., C.M.-K. and T.B.; investigation, M.P., T.B., M.B., K.S.-G., R.W. and M.S.; formal analysis, M.P., C.M.-K., K.S.-G. and P.S.; visualization, M.P., C.M.-K., K.S.-G. and R.W.; writing—original draft preparation, M.P., C.M.-K. and K.S.-G.; writing—review and editing, M.P., C.M.-K., K.S.-G. and A.W. All authors have read and agreed to the published version of the manuscript.

Funding: This research received no external funding.

Institutional Review Board Statement: The study was conducted according to the guidelines of the Declaration of Helsinki, and approved by the Bioethics Committee of Collegium Medicum in Bydgoszcz of Nicolaus Copernicus University in Toruń, Poland (protocol code KB 278/2016, date of approval 26 April 2016).

Informed Consent Statement: Written informed consent was obtained from all subjects involved in the study.

Data Availability Statement: The data presented in this study are available on request from the corresponding author. The data are not publicly available due to privacy or ethical restrictions.

Conflicts of Interest: The authors declare no conflict of interest.

References

1. Dishman, R.K. Increasing and maintaining exercise and physical activity. *Behav. Ther.* **1991**, *22*, 345–378. [CrossRef]
2. Nielsen, H.G.; Oktedalen, O.; Opstad, P.K.; Lyberg, T. Plasma cytokine profiles in long-term strenuous exercise. *J. Sports Med.* **2016**, *2016*, 7186137. [CrossRef] [PubMed]
3. Niemela, M.; Kangastupa, P.; Niemela, O.; Bloigu, R.; Juvonen, T. Acute changes in inflammatory biomarker levels in recreational runners participating in a marathon or half-marathon. *Sports Med. Open* **2016**, *2*, 21. [CrossRef] [PubMed]
4. Powers, S.K.; Jackson, M.J. Exercise-induced oxidative stress: Cellular mechanisms and impact on muscle force production. *Physiol. Rev.* **2008**, *88*, 1243–1276. [CrossRef] [PubMed]
5. Powers, S.K.; Deminice, R.; Ozdemir, M.; Yoshihara, T.; Bomkamp, M.P.; Hyatt, H. Exercise-induced oxidative stress: Friend or foe? *J. Sport Health Sci.* **2020**, *9*, 415–425. [CrossRef] [PubMed]
6. Silva, M.A.; Carvalho, T.; Cruz, A.C.; Jesus, L.R.; Silva Neto, L.A.; Trajano, E.T.; Bezerra, F.S. Effect of time-dependent cryotherapy on redox balance of quadriceps injuries. *Cryobiology* **2016**, *72*, 1–6. [CrossRef]
7. Mila-Kierzenkowska, C.; Jurecka, A.; Woźniak, A.; Szpinda, M.; Augustyńska, B.; Woźniak, B. The effect of submaximal exercise preceded by single whole-body cryotherapy on the markers of oxidative stress and inflammation in blood of volleyball players. *Oxid. Med. Cell. Longev.* **2013**, *2013*, 409867. [CrossRef]
8. Woźniak, A.; Woźniak, B.; Drewa, G.; Mila-Kierzenkowska, C.; Rakowski, A. The effect of whole-body cryostimulation on lysosomal enzyme activity in kayakers during training. *Eur. J. Appl. Physiol.* **2007**, *100*, 137–142. [CrossRef]
9. Sutkowy, P.; Woźniak, A.; Mila-Kierzenkowska, C.; Jurecka, A. The activity of lysosomal enzymes in the health men's blood after single Finnish sauna procedure—Preliminary study. *Med. Biol. Sci.* **2012**, *26*, 33–38.
10. Jonak, A.; Skrzek, A. Cryotherapy in athlete's biological regeneration—Review. *Acta Bio-Opt. Inform. Med.* **2009**, *15*, 319–321.
11. Bleakley, C.M.; Bieuzen, F.; Davison, G.W.; Costello, J.T. Whole-body cryotherapy: Empirical evidence and theoretical perspectives. *Open Access J. Sports Med.* **2014**, *5*, 25–36. [CrossRef]
12. Sutkowy, P.; Augustyńska, B.; Woźniak, A.; Rakowski, A. Physical exercise combined with whole-body cryotherapy in evaluating the level of lipid peroxidation products and other oxidant stress indicators in kayakers. *Oxid. Med. Cell. Longev.* **2014**, *2014*, 402631. [CrossRef]
13. Holmes, M.; Willoughby, D.S. The effectiveness of whole body cryotherapy compared to cold water immersion: Implications for sport and exercise recovery. *IJKSS* **2016**, *4*, 32–39. [CrossRef]

14. Bresnahan, R. Cold water immersion and anti-inflammatory response: A systematic review. *ESN Rev.* **2019**, *1*, 1–6.
15. de Freitas, V.H.; Ramos, S.P.; Bara-Filho, M.G.; Freitas, D.G.S.; Coimbra, D.R.; Cecchini, R.; Guarnier, F.A.; Nakamura, F.Y. Effect of cold water immersion performed on successive days on physical performance, muscle damage, and inflammatory, hormonal, and oxidative stress markers in volleyball players. *J. Strength Cond. Res.* **2019**, *33*, 502–513. [CrossRef] [PubMed]
16. International Physical Activity Questionnaire (IPAQ). Available online: https://sites.google.com/site/theipaq/questionnaire_links (accessed on 15 August 2020).
17. Ciechanowska, K.; Weber-Rajek, M.; Sikorska, J.; Bułatowicz, I.; Radzimińska, A.; Strojek, K.; Zukow, W. Biological recovery methods in sport. *J. Health Sci.* **2014**, *4*, 241–252. [CrossRef]
18. Sjostrand, T. Changes in the respiratory organs of workmen at an oresmelting works. *Acta Med. Scand.* **1974**, *196*, 687–699.
19. Astrand, P.O.; Rodahl, K. *Textbook of Work Physiology*; McGraw-Hill: New York, NY, USA, 1986.
20. Borg, E.; Borg, G.; Larsson, K.; Letzter, M.; Sundblad, B.M. An index for breathlessness and leg fatigue. *Scand. J. Med. Sci. Sports* **2010**, *20*, 644–650. [CrossRef] [PubMed]
21. Tanaka, H.; Monahan, K.D.; Seals, D.R. Age-predicted maximal hart rate revisited. *J. Am. Coll. Cardiol.* **2001**, *37*, 153–156. [CrossRef]
22. Błeszyński, W.; Działoszyński, L.M. Purification of soluble arylosulfatase from ox brain. *Biochem. J.* **1965**, *97*, 360–364. [CrossRef]
23. Krawczyński, J. *Diagnostyka Enzymologiczna w Medycynie Praktycznej. Metodyka Badań*; Publikacje Wydawnictwa Lekarskiego PZWL: Warsaw, Poland, 1974.
24. Inkabi, S.E.; Pushpamithran, G.; Richter, P.; Attakora, K. Exercise immunology: Involved components and varieties in different types of physical exercise. *Sci. J. Life Sci.* **2017**, *1*, 31–35.
25. Hopkins, W.G.; Marshall, S.W.; Batterham, A.M.; Hanin, J. Progressive statistics for studies in sports medicine and exercise science. *Med. Sci. Sports Exerc.* **2009**, *41*, 3–13. [CrossRef]
26. Zaldivar, F.; Wang-Rodriguez, J.; Nemet, D.; Schwindt, C.; Galassetti, P.; Mills, P.J.; Wilson, L.D.; Cooper, D.M. Constitutive pro-and anti-inflammatory cytokine and growth factor response to exercise in leukocytes. *J. Appl. Physiol.* **2006**, *100*, 1124–1133. [CrossRef]
27. Santos, V.C.; Sierra, A.P.; Oliveira, R.; Caçula, K.G.; Momesso, C.M.; Sato, F.T.; Silva, M.B.; Oliveira, H.H.; Passos, M.E.; de Souza, D.R.; et al. Marathon race affects neutrophil surface molecules: Role of inflammatory mediators. *PLoS ONE* **2016**, *11*, e0166687. [CrossRef]
28. Mezil, Y.A.; Allison, D.; Kish, K.; Ditor, D.; Ward, W.E.; Tsiani, E.; Klentrou, P. Response of bone turnover markers and cytokines to high-intensity low-impact exercise. *Med. Sci. Sports Exerc.* **2015**, *47*, 1495–1502. [CrossRef]
29. Ambarish, V.; Chandrashekara, S.; Suresh, K.P. Moderate regular exercises reduce inflammatory response for physical stress. *Indian J. Physiol. Pharmacol.* **2012**, *56*, 7–14.
30. Starkie, R.L.; Rolland, J.; Angus, D.J.; Anderson, M.J.; Febbraio, M.A. Circulating monocytes are not the source of elevations in plasma IL-6 and TNF-αlevels after prolonged running. *Am. J. Physiol. Cell Physiol.* **2001**, *280*, 769–774. [CrossRef]
31. Fischer, C.P. Interleukin-6 in acute exercise and training: What is the biological relevance? *Exerc. Immunol. Rev.* **2006**, *12*, 6–33. [PubMed]
32. Roberts, L.A.; Nosaka, K.; Coombes, J.S.; Peake, J.M. Cold water immersion enhances recovery of submaximal muscle function after resistance exercise. *Am. J. Physiol. Regul. Integr. Comp. Physiol.* **2014**, *307*, 998–1008. [CrossRef] [PubMed]
33. White, G.E.; Rhind, S.G.; Wells, G.D. The effect of various cold-water immersion protocols on exercise-induced inflammatory response and functional recovery from high-intensity sprint exercise. *Eur. J. Appl. Physiol.* **2014**, *114*, 2353–2367. [CrossRef] [PubMed]
34. Earp, J.E.; Hatfield, D.L.; Sherman, A.; Lee, E.C.; Kraemer, W.J. Cold-water immersion blunts and delays increases in circulating testosterone and cytokines post-resistance exercise. *Eur. J. Appl. Physiol.* **2019**, *119*, 1901–1907. [CrossRef]
35. Soares, V.; Silveira de Avelar, I.; Espíndola Mota Venâncio, P.; Pires-Oliveira, D.A.A.; de Almeida Silva, P.H.; Rodrigues Borges, A.; Fonseca, G.P.E.F.; Noll, M. Acute changes in interleukin-6 level during four days of long-distance walking. *J. Inflamm. Res.* **2020**, *10*, 871–878. [CrossRef]
36. Van Snick, J. Interleukin-6: An overview. *Annu. Rev. Immunol.* **1990**, *8*, 253–278. [CrossRef]
37. Keller, C.; Keller, P.; Giralt, M.; Hidalgo, J.; Pedersen, B.K. Exercise normalises verexpression of TNF-α in knockout mice. *Biochem. Biophys. Res. Commun.* **2004**, *321*, 179–182.
38. Dimitrov, T.; Hulteng, E.; Hong, S. Inflammation and exercise: Inhibition of monocytic TNF production by acute exercise via β2-adrenergic activation. *Brain Behav. Immun.* **2017**, *61*, 60–66. [CrossRef] [PubMed]
39. Markovitch, D.; Tyrrell, R.M.; Thompson, D. The effect of prior exercise on ex vivo induction of heme oxygenase-1 in human lymphocytes. *Free Radic. Res.* **2007**, *41*, 1125–1134. [CrossRef] [PubMed]
40. Semple, S.J.; Smith, L.L.; McKune, A.J.; Hoyos, J.; Mokgethwa, B.; San Juan, A.F.; Lucia, A.; Wadee, A.A. Serum concentrations of C reactive protein, α1 antitrypsin, and complement (C3, C4, C1 esterase inhibitor) before and during the Vuelta a España. *Br. J. Sports Med.* **2006**, *40*, 124–127. [CrossRef] [PubMed]
41. Schild, M.; Eichner, G.; Beiter, T.; Zügel, M.; Krumholz-Wagner, I.; Hudemann, J.; Pilat, C.; Krüger, K.; Niess, A.M.; Steinacker, J.M.; et al. Effects of acute endurance exercise on plasma protein profiles of endurance-trained and untrained individuals over time. *Mediat. Inflamm.* **2016**, *2016*, 4851935. [CrossRef] [PubMed]

42. Eimonte, M.; Paulauskas, H.; Daniuseviciute, L.; Eimantas, N.; Vitkauskiene, A.; Dauksaite, G.; Solianik, R.; Brazaitis, M. Residual effects of short-term whole-body cold-water immersion on the cytokine profile, white blood cell count, and blood markers of stress. *Int. J. Hyperth.* **2021**, *38*, 696–707. [CrossRef]
43. Eimontea, M.; Eimantasa, N.; Daniuseviciuteb, L.; Paulauskasa, H.; Vitkauskienec, A.; Dauksaitea, G.; Brazaitis, M. Recovering body temperature from acute cold stress is associated with delayed proinflammatory cytokine production in vivo. *Cytokine* **2021**, *143*, 155510. [CrossRef]
44. Klich, S.; Krymski, I.; Michalik, K.; Kawczyński, A. Effect of short-term cold-water immersion on muscle pain sensitivity in elite track cyclists. *Phys. Ther. Sport* **2018**, *32*, 42–47. [CrossRef]
45. Peake, J.M.; Roberts, L.A.; Figueiredo, V.C.; Egner, I.; Krog, S.; Aas, S.N.; Suzuki, K.; Markworth, J.F.; Coombes, J.S.; Cameron-Smith, D.; et al. The effects of cold water immersion and active recovery on inflammation and cell stress responses in human skeletal muscle after resistance exercise. *J. Physiol.* **2017**, *595*, 695–711. [CrossRef] [PubMed]
46. Verbickas, V.; Baranwskiene, N.; Eimantas, N.; Kamandulis, S.; Rutkauskas, S.; Satkunskiene, D.; Sadauskas, S.; Brazaitis, M.; Skurvydas, A. Effects of sprint cycling and stretch-shortering cycle exercises on the neuromuscular, immune and stress indicators in young men. *J. Physiol. Pharmacol.* **2017**, *68*, 125–132. [PubMed]
47. Rhind, S.G.; Castellani, J.W.; Brenner, I.K.; Shephard, R.J.; Zamecnik, J.; Montain, S.J.; Young, A.J.; Shek, P.N. Intracellular monocyte and serum cytokine expression is modulted by exhausting exercise and col exposure. *Am. J. Physiol. Regul. Integr. Comp. Physiol.* **2001**, *281*, R66–R75. [CrossRef]
48. Belizário, J.E.; Fontes-Oliveira, C.C.; Borges, J.P.; Kashiabara, J.A.; Vannier, E. Skeletal muscle wasting and renewal: A pivotal role of myokine IL-6. *SpringerPlus* **2016**, *5*, 1–15. [CrossRef]
49. Peake, J.M.; Neubauer, O.; Della Gatta, P.A.; Nosaka, K. Muscle damage and inflammation during recovery from exercise. *J. Appl. Physiol.* **2017**, *122*, 559–570. [CrossRef]
50. Dhabhar, F.S.; Malarkey, W.B.; Neri, E.; McEwen, B.S. Stress-induced redistribution of immune cells—From barracks to boulevards to battlefields: A tale of three hormones—Curt Richter Award Winner. *Psychoneuroendocrinology* **2012**, *37*, 1345–1368. [CrossRef] [PubMed]
51. White, G.E.; Wells, G.D. Cold-water immersion and other forms of cryotherapy: Physiological changes potentially affecting recovery from high-intensity exercise. *Extrem. Physiol. Med.* **2013**, *2*, 26–37. [CrossRef] [PubMed]
52. Yanagisawa, O.; Kudo, H.; Takahashi, N.; Yoshioka, H. Magnetic resonance imaging evaluation of cooling on blood flow and oedema in skeletal muscles after exercise. *Eur. J. Appl. Physiol.* **2004**, *91*, 737–740. [CrossRef]
53. Wigmore, S.J.; Fearon, K.C.; Ross, J.A.; McNally, S.J.; Welch, W.J.; Garden, O.J. Febrile-range temperature but not heat shock augments the acute phase response to interleukin-6 in human hepatoma cells. *Am. J. Physiol. Gastrointest. Liver Physiol.* **2006**, *290*, G903–G911. [CrossRef]
54. Ehlers, M.R. Immune-modulating effects of alpha-1 antitrypsin. *Biol. Chem.* **2014**, *395*, 1187–1193. [CrossRef]
55. Woźniak, A.; Drewa, T.; Drewa, G.; Woźniak, B.; Malinowski, D.; Rakowski, A. Activity of arylosulphatase, cathepsin D and creatine kinase after submaximal and supermaximal exercise in untrained men and women. *Biol. Sport* **2002**, *19*, 355–364.
56. Farges, M.C.; Balcerzak, D.; Fisher, B.D.; Attaix, D.; Béchet, D.; Ferrara, M.; Baracos, V.E. Increased muscle proteolysis after local trauma mainly reflects macrophage-associated lysosomal proteolysis. *Am. J. Physiol. Endocrinol. Metab.* **2002**, *282*, E326–E335. [CrossRef]
57. Sutkowy, P.; Woźniak, A.; Boraczyński, T.; Boraczyński, M.; Mila-Kierzenkowska, C. The oxidant-antioxidant equilibrium, activities of selected lysosomal enzymes and activity of acute phase protein in peripheral blood of 18-year-old football players after aerobic cycle ergometer test combined with ice-water immersion or recovery at room temperature. *Cryobiology* **2017**, *74*, 126–131. [CrossRef] [PubMed]
58. Mila-Kierzenkowska, C.; Woźniak, A.; Szpinda, M.; Boraczyński, T.; Woźniak, B.; Rajewski, P.; Sutkowy, P. Effects of thermal stress on the activity of selected lysosomal enzymes in blood of experienced and novice winter swimmers. *Scand. J. Clin. Lab. Investig.* **2012**, *72*, 635–641. [CrossRef] [PubMed]

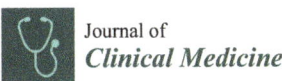

Article

Effects of Acute Psychological and Physiological Stress on Rock Climbers

Pamela Villavicencio [1], Cristina Bravo [2,3,*], Antoni Ibarz [4] and Silvia Solé [2,3]

1. Master Program Integrative Physiology, University of Barcelona, 08028 Barcelona, Spain; pvillasu13@alumnes.ub.edu
2. Department of Nursing and Physiotherapy, University of Lleida, 25198 Lleida, Spain; silvia.sole@udl.cat
3. Research Group of Health Care (GRECS), Institute of Biomedical Research Center, 25198 Lleida, Spain
4. Department of Cellular Biology, Physiology and Immunology, Faculty of Biology, University of Barcelona, 08028 Barcelona, Spain; tibarz@ub.edu
* Correspondence: cristina.bravo@udl.cat

Abstract: Background: The aim of this study was to assess the effects that psychological and physiological stressors have on indoor rock climbers, as well as to identify sex differences. Methods: 14 intermediate rock climbers participated in the study, 10 males and 4 females. Mean age was 31 ± 8 years for males and 21 ± 2 years for females. Day 1 consisted of test familiarization and baseline measurements. Day 2 included two test conditions, startle and fatigue, separated by 20 min. In the startle condition, participants had to lead climb a route, and a loud audio stimulus was presented near the top of the climb. In the fatigue condition, participants were required to climb as fast as they could until muscular failure. The competitive state anxiety inventory second review (CSAI-2R) questionnaire was used to assess somatic anxiety, cognitive anxiety, and self-confidence. The four-square step test (FSST) was used to assess motor control, and cortisol levels were acquired via passive drool (PD). Results: Cortisol concentrations were highest in the pre-startle condition (1.72 µg/dL ± 0.66), and values decreased post-startle (1.67 µg/dL ± 0.74) and post-fatigue (1.42 µg/dL ± 0.72). However, cortisol concentrations increased post-startle in females (1.57 µg/dL ± 0.96). Somatic anxiety in males was significantly higher post-startle (16.36 ± 5.54) than pre-startle (14.23 ± 5.09). Females had significantly higher somatic anxiety post-startle (18.00 ± 8.76), and they had lower self-confidence levels (30.00 ± 5.89) than males. Conclusions: There are differences in the way that males and females prepare and respond to stressful situations. Furthermore, time of day may have had a significant impact on cortisol concentrations.

Keywords: stress; cortisol; saliva; anxiety; rock climbers

Citation: Villavicencio, P.; Bravo, C.; Ibarz, A.; Solé, S. Effects of Acute Psychological and Physiological Stress on Rock Climbers. *J. Clin. Med.* **2021**, *10*, 5013. https://doi.org/10.3390/jcm10215013

Academic Editor: Władysław Jagiełło

Received: 20 August 2021
Accepted: 27 October 2021
Published: 28 October 2021

Publisher's Note: MDPI stays neutral with regard to jurisdictional claims in published maps and institutional affiliations.

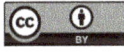

Copyright: © 2021 by the authors. Licensee MDPI, Basel, Switzerland. This article is an open access article distributed under the terms and conditions of the Creative Commons Attribution (CC BY) license (https://creativecommons.org/licenses/by/4.0/).

1. Introduction

Rock climbing is a complex sport that encompasses both psychological and physiological stressors. Indoor rock climbing has two different climbing techniques: lead and top rope climbing [1,2]. In lead climbing, the climber must attend to the safety rope and clip it into anchors as they make their way up the route. If the climber does not clip the safety rope properly, they will generally fall a short distance. On the other hand, in top rope climbing, the safety rope passes through an anchor at the top of the climb, and the climber does not need to manage it. If a climber falls during a top rope climb, they will sag on the rope. Lead climbing has been associated with increased perceived stress because of the increased mental demand and consequence of falling [2]. However, this does not seem to be the case with advanced rock climbers [1].

When the body's homeostasis is disrupted, or perceived to be disrupted, the body initiates a stress response. This response includes the activation of the hypothalamic-pituitary-adrenal (HPA) axis [3]. The HPA axis starts with the secretion of corticotropin-releasing hormone (CRH) from the hypothalamus, followed by the release of adrenocorticotropic hormone (ACTH) from the pituitary gland, and finally the release of glucocorticoids from the adrenal glands. Since cortisol can be used as a biological marker of stress, several studies have measured it either via plasma or salivary samples [2,4,5]. The gold standard for salivary cortisol sampling is the passive drool (PD) method, since the effect of flow rate on saliva composition can be discarded [6].

Rock climbing can quickly induce stress due to the fear and anxiety of falling, as well as the elevated cognitive attention it requires to plan movement sequences, recovery positions, speed of the climb, and timing of clipping the safety rope [2]. The amount of perceived stress can also be influenced by the level of expertise of the climber and whether others are present [7,8]. Studies have found that altering the climbing technique to lead climbing increased both subjective anxiety and plasma cortisol concentrations [2]. The peak plasma cortisol concentration is suggested to occur 15–20 min after the stressor, regardless of the climbing technique [1,5,9]. However, one study found that post-climb salivary concentrations were higher immediately after the climb and not 15 min later [10].

Stress can also influence motor skills. Some studies have found that stress can disrupt the accuracy and coordination of movements, as well as posture [11]. Stress also affects the speed of movement in the fight-or-flight response, causing movements to be quicker at the expense of accuracy [11]. These frantic movements lead to decreased success rates, likely because of altered sensory feedback from the lack of haptic feedback [11]. In stressful situations, there may also be impaired cognitive and visuomotor processes that negatively affect motor skills [11].

When this article was published, there was limited data on the role that stress plays in rock climbers, and even more limited literature on differences between sexes. The purpose of this study was to determine the implications that stress has on motor control and cortisol levels in rock climbers and to bridge the gap between psychological and physiological findings. Our hypothesis is that motor control, measured via dynamic balance and coordination with the four-square step test (FSST), will decrease and that cortisol levels will increase, as has been shown in previous studies [2,10].

2. Materials and Methods

2.1. Participants

A total of 14 participants volunteered to take part in the study, 10 males and 4 females. Mean age, height, and body mass for males was 31 ± 8 years, 176 cm ± 5, and 70 kg ± 6.5, respectively. Mean age, height, and body mass for females was 21 ± 2 years, 166 cm ± 5, and 59 kg ± 2.9, respectively. Participant information is reported in Tables 1 and 2. The study took place at an indoor rock-climbing gym. All participants were intermediate climbers, with a minimum skill level of 6c. They had no injuries or underlying medical conditions and had low to moderate stress levels, as measured by the Perceived Stress Scale (PSS) [12]. Participants completed an informed consent form after a thorough explanation of the study and after completing a physical activity readiness questionnaire (PAR-Q) [13].

Table 1. Male participant information.

Males	N	Min	Max	Mean	SD
Age	10	17	43	30.7	8.49
Height	10	165	180	174.4	4.77
Weight	10	61.6	83.9	70.3	6.52
Years climbing	10	2	25	9.89	8.49
Skill level	10	6b	8c		
Max pull-ups	10	8	29	17	6.89
Bent-arm hang	10	27	76	48.6 s	14.83 s

Table 2. Female participant information.

Females	N	Min	Max	Mean	SD
Age	4	19	24	21	2.45
Height (cm)	4	161	173	165.75	5.5
Weight (kg)	4	55.7	62	59	2.95
Years climbing	4	2	8	4.75	2.5
Skill level	4	6b	7c+		
Max pull-ups	4	7	18	14	4.83
Bent-arm hang	4	30	48	38	8.91 s

2.2. Competitive State Anxiety Inventory Second Review (CSAI-2R) Questionnaire

The CSAI-2R consists of 17 items that are scored on a Likert scale from 1 to 4, and the combined scores result in a final score on each of the 3 subscales (somatic anxiety, cognitive anxiety, and self-confidence). The European Spanish version of the CSAI-2R consists of 18 items [14].

2.3. Four Square Step Test (FSST)

The FSST is a way to measure dynamic balance, stability, and coordination [15]. It requires two sticks to be placed on the floor so that they form a "plus sign", and the participants must step in each square in a set sequence. There are two trials, and the best time is recorded [16].

2.4. Procedure: Day 1

Day 1 of the intervention consisted of anthropometric measurements, procedure familiarization, and strength tests. Participants completed an easy route with the top rope technique. Prior to the climb, they underwent a hand grip test with a Saehan Spring Hand® dynamometer (Saehan Corporation, Changwon 630-728, South Korea) and completed the FSST and the CSAI-2R.

During the climb, participants wore a Polar A300 watch and Polar H10 heart rate monitor (Polar Electro®, Kempele, Finland). They were instructed to climb at their normal pace. After the climb, they completed the hand grip test, the FSST, and the CSAI-2R again.

2.5. Day 1 Strength Tests

The participants finished day 1 with two strength tests: a maximum pull-up test and a bent-arm hang test. These tests were used to assess shoulder power and endurance, which has been shown to be the primary determinant for success in rock climbing [17]. The tests were included to provide objective measurements of participants' physical abilities. The pull-up test was performed with a pronated grip, and 1 repetition was considered as chin over the bar and full elbow extension. The bent-arm hang test was measured as the maximum time the participants could hang with elbows at 90° in the pronated grip position. Results are presented in Tables 1 and 2.

2.6. Day 1 Passive Drool Instructions

At the end of day 1, participants were given 9 Salivette® Cortisol vials (Sarstedt AG & Co., Nümbrecht, Germany) without the synthetic swab, and instructed to take baseline salivary samples for three days at 8:00 a.m., 11:00 a.m., and 2:00 p.m. Participants were given clear written and verbal instructions on the PD method.

2.7. Procedure: Day 2

Day 2 consisted of two different test conditions, separated by a recovery period of 20 min. The first test condition was the startle condition, and it took place at 8:00 a.m. The second condition was the fatigue condition, and it took place at 8:30 a.m. The order of the test conditions was fixed to eliminate the effects of physiological and psychological fatigue in the startle condition. Since the climbing route of the startle condition was more difficult and required a high cognitive, physical, and tactical demand, this condition was performed first. Before climbing, participants had their resting blood pressure taken, and they completed the FSST and CSAI-2R. They provided saliva samples via passive drool, and their 3 min average pre-climb heart rate (Pre-HR_{3min}) was recorded.

The startle condition consisted of a loud stimulus and the added stress of having to lead climb a route that gradually increased in difficulty. There were two possible routes in this condition: either a route that progressed in difficulty from 6b to 6c+ or from 6b to 7b. When the participants were preparing to make a key jump to a more difficult section, an air horn was used to startle them (Goodmark®, Llantarnam, UK). Three of the final participants had an alternate audio stimulus due to lack of gas in the air horn. With these final participants, the investigator hit a pan with a wooden spatula and screamed.

During the climb, the climb duration, success/fail, HR at the start of the climb (HR_{start}), HR average (HR_{avg}), and peak HR (HR_{peak}) were recorded. Immediately after the climb, blood pressure was measured, and participants completed the FSST and CSAI-2R. The climbs were filmed with a Samsung N363 digital camcorder (Samsung Group, Hwaseong, South Korea). Fifteen minutes after the startle, post-climb salivary samples were taken. The time for HR to return to pre-climb levels (Post-$HR_{recovery}$) was also recorded.

In the fatigue condition, participants had to top rope climb a predetermined route as fast as they could and as many times as they could, until muscular failure. There were three routes that varied in difficulty (6b, 6c+, 7b), and the specific route assigned to each participant was based on their self-reported skill level. Time splits of each climb, the number of falls until fatigue, and HR_{start}, HR_{avg}, and HR_{peak} were all recorded. Each climb was filmed. Immediately post-climb, participants had their blood pressure measured, and they completed the FSST and CSAI-2R. Fifteen minutes post-climb, they completed a final salivary sample. Their post-$HR_{recovery}$ time was also recorded.

2.8. Saliva Samples

The PD method requires participants to sit with his or her head flexed forward while saliva passively drips into a container [18]. Participants stored the samples in their refrigerator (4 °C) until day 2, where they brought the samples to the rock-climbing gym. Approximately 3 mL of saliva was collected.

Salivary cortisol samples were stored at −80 °C until analysis. They were then centrifuged at 2500× g for 10 min, and 1.5 mL of the separated samples was placed in Eppendorf microtubes (Starsledt Akhengesellshaft & Co., Nümbrecht, Germany). Salivary cortisol was measured with a Cortisol Saliva Enzyme-Linked Immunosorbent Assay (ELISA) procedure (IBL International GMBH, Hamburg, Germany).

2.9. Statistics

All analyses were performed using the statistical package IBM® SPSS® Statistics Software (SPSS) version 26. Results are expressed as mean ± standard deviation. After verifying that all values were within the normal range, T tests were performed to compare the mean values of different conditions. A one-way ANOVA analysis was used to compare the variables measured between sexes and between test conditions. Pearson's correlation was utilized to analyze the relationship between time to fatigue and body weight, as well as the number of pull-ups and cortisol levels. Differences were considered significant at $p < 0.05$.

3. Results

3.1. Cortisol

No outliers in cortisol concentrations were identified; however, values that were not within the reportable range of 0.015–3.00 µg/dL were discarded, as indicated by the Cortisol Saliva ELISA kit (IBL International GMBH, Germany). Baseline cortisol concentrations were highest at 8:00 a.m., with average values of 0.71 µg/dL ± 0.35. There were significant differences between cortisol concentrations at 8 a.m. for the three baseline measurements in males (0.78 µg/dL ± 0.47, p = 0.00; 0.59 µg/dL ± 0.43, p = 0.002; 0.80 µg/dL ± 0.56, p = 0.003), as well as when compared to pre-startle (1.85 µg/dL ± 0.70, p = 0.000), post-startle (1.73 µg/dL ± 0.67, p = 0.000), and post-fatigue (1.44 µg/dL ± 0.61, p = 0.000). There were no significant differences in cortisol concentrations in males when comparing the three test conditions (1.85 µg/dL ± 0.70, 1.73 µg/dL ± 0.67, 1.44 µg/dL ± 0.61).

Post-startle cortisol concentrations were significant (1.57 µg/dL ± 0.96, p = 0.046) for females when compared with pre-test levels (1.26 µg/dL ± 0.29), and there were also significant differences (p = 0.043) between female pre-startle (1.26 µg/dL ± 0.29) and post-fatigue (1.37 µg/dL ± 1.12). There were significant differences (p = 0.050) in males and females between pre-startle (1.72 µg/dL ± 0.66) and post-fatigue (1.42 µg/dL ± 0.72) cortisol levels. Cortisol baseline concentrations are shown in Figure 1, and concentrations in the different test conditions are shown in Figure 2.

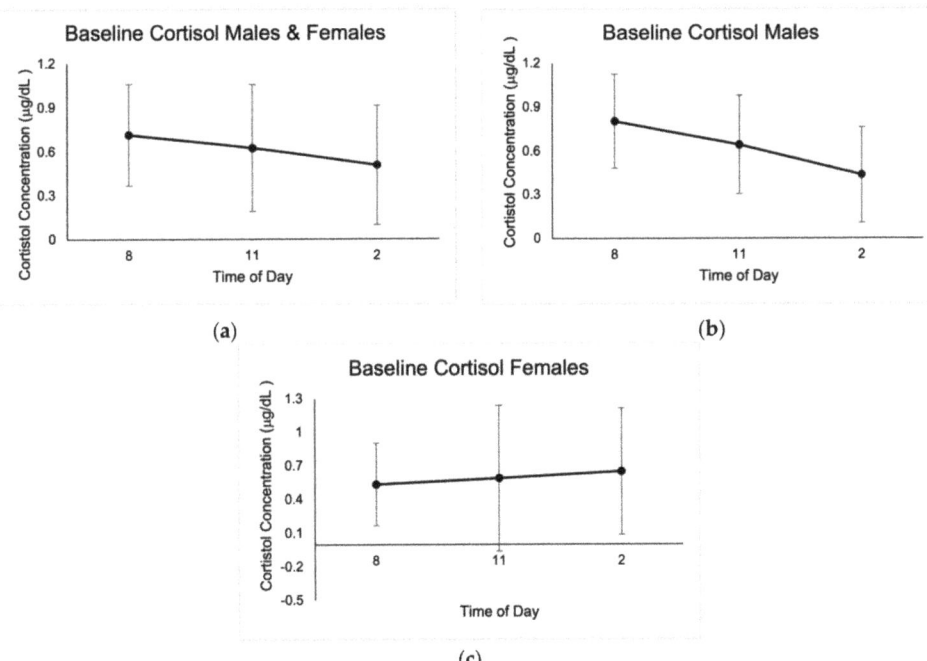

Figure 1. Mean baseline salivary cortisol concentrations expressed in µg/dL ± SD from the three days of sampling at 8:00 a.m., 11:00 a.m., and 2:00 p.m. (**a**) Results for males and females. (**b**) Results for males. (**c**) Results for females.

There were no significant differences between sexes in cortisol concentrations in the pre-startle (1.85 µg/dL ± 0.70, 1.26 µg/dL ± 0.29), post-startle (1.73 µg/dL ± 0.67, 1.57 µg/dL ± 0.96), and post-fatigue (1.44 µg/dL ± 0.61, 1.37 µg/dL ± 1.12) conditions. Based on the ANOVA F analysis, there was a positive correlation between number of pull-ups and pre-test cortisol concentrations (p = 0.008, r = 0.814, R^2 = 0.663, CI = 95%).

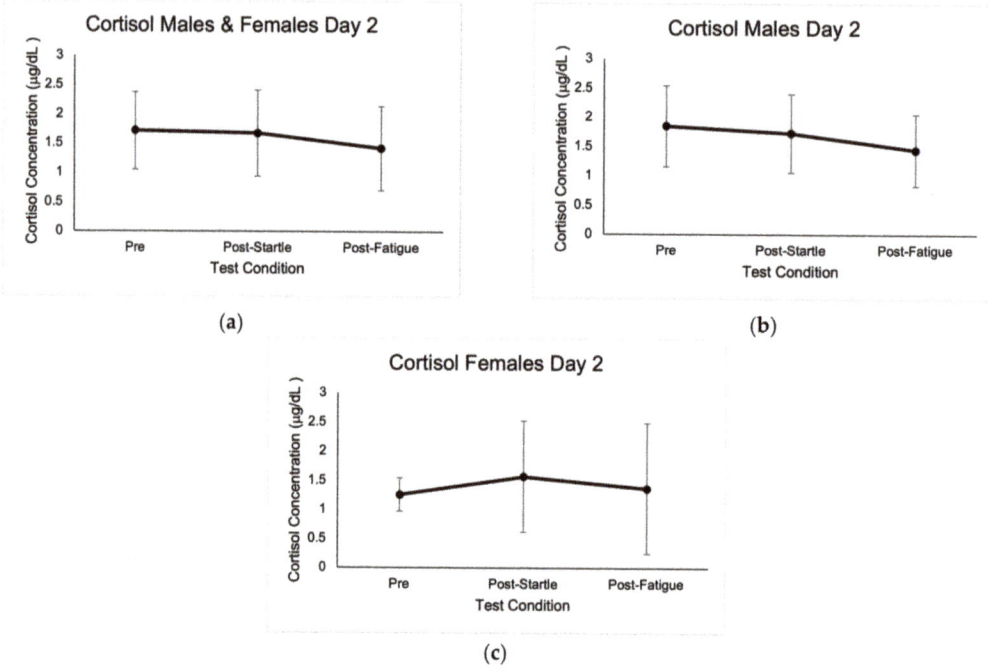

Figure 2. Mean cortisol concentrations expressed in µg/dL ± SD from the three test conditions of day 2. (**a**) Results for males and females. (**b**) Results for males. (**c**) Results for females.

3.2. Heart Rate

Heart rate followed the expected pattern during both climbs. During the startle climb, values increased progressively as the climb went on. During the fatigue climb, heart rate values increased throughout the climb, and the initial heart rate was higher for each subsequent climb.

3.3. FSST

There were no significant differences between FSST values baseline pre-climb day 1 (3.62 s ± 0.75) and post-startle day 2 (3.09 s ± 0.62). There were significant differences ($p = 0.006$) between FSST scores baseline post-climb day 1 (3.45 s ± 0.61) and post-startle day 2 (3.09 s ± 0.62), and significant differences ($p = 0.002$) between males' baseline post-climb day 1 (3.42 s ± 0.53) and post-fatigue day 2 (2.84 s ± 0.43) scores. Results are shown in Tables 3–5.

Table 3. Summary of results for males and females. Significant differences ($p = 0.003$) in somatic anxiety post-startle between males and females. Significant differences ($p = 0.019$) between male and female self-confidence values pre-startle and post-fatigue ($p = 0.02$). Significant differences ($p = 0.006$) in FSST times between baseline post-climb and post-startle. Significant differences ($p = 0.012$) between baseline pre-climb left-hand grip strength and post-fatigue left-hand grip strength.

Variables	Baseline Pre-Climb	Baseline Post-Climb	Pre-Startle	Post-Startle	Pre-Fatigue	Post-Fatigue
Somatic Anxiety	15.50 ± 4.49	17.25 ± 5.64	14.23 ± 5.09	16.36 ± 5.54	15.33 ± 5.03	16.43 ± 5.26
Cognitive Anxiety	16.14 ± 5.68	13.50 ± 4.52	13.54 ± 6.64	13.14 ± 4.69	12.67 ± 4.62	12.00 ± 3.84
Self-Confidence	35.43 ± 5.57	34.50 ± 5.13	35.08 ± 4.94	33.14 ± 7.18	33.33 ± 6.57	34.43 ± 5.88
FSST	3.62 s ± 0.75	3.45 s ± 0.61	3.19 s ± 0.52	3.09 s ± 0.62	2.89 s ± 0.48	2.84 s ± 0.43
Grip Strength Right	46.57 kg ± 10.20	49.90 kg ± 11.38	46.64 kg ± 11.32	46.43 kg ± 10.34	41.15 kg ± 19.18	395.17 kg ± 13.42
Grip Strength Left	48.60 kg ± 9.36	48.03 kg ± 12.17	46.14 kg ± 9.88	44.64 kg ± 9.58	39.74 kg ± 18.51	33.47 kg ± 12.44

Table 4. Summary results for males. Significant differences ($p = 0.019$) in somatic anxiety pre- and post-startle in males. Significant differences ($p = 0.002$) between FSST baseline post-climb and post-fatigue scores. Significant differences ($p = 0.035$) between baseline pre-climb left-hand grip strength and post-fatigue left-hand grip strength. Significant differences ($p = 0.00$) between pre-startle and post-startle right-hand grip strength.

Variables	Baseline Pre-Climb	Baseline Post-Climb	Pre-Startle	Post-Startle	Pre-Fatigue	Post-Fatigue
Somatic Anxiety	14.50 ± 4.35	17.50 ± 6.07	14.23 ± 5.09	16.36 ± 5.54	15.33 ± 5.03	16.43 ± 5.26
Cognitive Anxiety	15.80 ± 6.49	13.75 ± 5.18	13.54 ± 6.64	13.14 ± 4.69	12.67 ± 4.62	12.00 ± 3.84
Self-Confidence	37.20 ± 3.55	36.50 ± 3.96	35.08 ± 4.94	33.14 ± 7.18	33.33 ± 6.57	34.43 ± 5.88
FSST	3.71 s ± 0.82	3.42 s ± 0.53	3.19 s ± 0.52	3.09 s ± 0.62	2.88 s ± 0.48	2.84 s ± 0.43
Grip Strength Right	49.95 kg ± 9.22	53.59 kg ± 10.77	50.55 kg ± 10.48	51.05 kg ± 8.11	46.52 kg ± 18.55	37.91 kg ± 15.31
Grip Strength Left	52.27 kg ± 6.94	51.91 kg ± 11.40	50.40 kg ± 7.99	48.15 kg ± 8.88	45.14 kg ± 17.92	35.35 kg ± 14.74

Table 5. Summary results for females.

Variables	Baseline Pre-Climb	Baseline Post-Climb	Pre-Startle	Post-Startle	Pre-Fatigue	Post-Fatigue
Somatic Anxiety	18.00 ± 4.32	16.75 ± 5.50	15.33 ± 8.39	18.00 ± 8.76	16.25 ± 6.85	17.25 ± 8.46
Cognitive Anxiety	17.00 ± 3.46	13.00 ± 3.46	15.33 ± 9.24	13.50 ± 5.74	13.50 ± 4.73	11.00 ± 1.15
Self-Confidence	31.00 ± 7.75	30.50 ± 5.26	30.00 ± 5.29	30.00 ± 5.89	29.00 ± 5.77	29.00 ± 4.76
FSST	3.41 s ± 0.58	3.52 s ± 0.87	3.34 s ± 0.76	3.60 s ± 0.95	3.09 s ± 0.76	3.13 s ± 0.68
Grip Strength Right	37.25 kg ± 6.65	39.75 kg ± 5.56	36.88 kg ± 6.91	34.88 kg ± 4.13	30.41 kg ± 17.76	29.00 kg ± 4.69
Grip Strength Left	38.50 kg ± 7.94	37.38 kg ± 7.18	35.50 kg ± 4.49	35.88 kg ± 4.17	28.94 kg ± 16.52	29.25 kg ± 2.36

3.4. Anxiety and Self-Confidence

There were significant differences ($p = 0.019$) in somatic anxiety pre-startle (14.23 ± 5.09) and post-startle (16.36 ± 5.54) in males, as well as significant differences ($p = 0.035$) between male and female self-confidence levels pre-startle (35.08 ± 4.94, 30.00 ± 5.29). There were also significant differences ($p = 0.022$) in self-confidence post-fatigue between sexes (34.43 ± 5.88, 29.00 ± 4.76). Results are shown in Tables 3–5.

3.5. Grip Strength

There were significant differences ($p = 0.012$) between baseline left-hand grip strength (48.60 kg ± 9.36) and post-fatigue left-hand grip strength (36.46 kg ± 8.63). Males had significant differences ($p = 0.035$) between baseline left-hand grip strength (52.27 kg ± 6.94) and post-fatigue left-hand grip strength (35.35 ± 14.74). There were differences in female baseline left-hand grip strength (38.50 kg ± 7.94) and post-fatigue left-hand grip strength (29.25 kg ± 2.36), although not significant ($p = 0.058$). Males also had significant ($p = 0.00$) differences in pre-startle (50.55 ± 10.48) and post-startle (51.05 ± 8.11) right–hand grip strength. Results are reported in Tables 3–5.

3.6. Fatigue

There was an inverse correlation between time to fatigue and body weight (CI = 95%, $r = 0.606$, $p = 0.025$). There were significant differences ($p = 0.022$) between sexes: males reached muscular failure after 282.39 s ± 48.20, and females after 367.51 s ± 70.21.

4. Discussion

The results indicate that physical and psychological stress affects males and females in different ways and that cortisol concentrations are strongly affected by time of day. Salivary samples were utilized in this study because since cortisol follows a circadian rhythm, with the highest values occurring 20–40 min after waking, we thought it beneficial to obtain a baseline secretion curve for comparison with the rest of the values [18,19]. Baseline cortisol concentrations followed a normal diurnal pattern, with the highest values occurring at 8:00 a.m.

It is possible that the variations in concentrations between the 8:00 a.m. samples of each day were due to individual error or individual variation in diurnal cortisol slope (DCS). Cortisol concentrations can be easily affected by acute stressors, age, sex, nutrition, sleep, hydration, physical activity, and circadian rhythm [4,9,18]. Salivary composition can also be affected by countless factors, including circadian rhythm, age, sex, smoking, diet, and medications [4]. Since external factors of the participants' day to day were not accounted for, it is possible that variations in these variables altered their DCS. In addition, it is possible that participants did not take the samples at the same time for each of the three baseline days. Although these may have been small variations, it may have been enough to affect the DCS substantially—especially in the waking hours [19,20]. Variations in sampling time may have also been due to difficulty in saliva production. Some participants reported spending 20 min in the PD position to produce sufficient saliva. This may have further delayed the time of day that the sample was obtained, thus influencing cortisol levels. This may have also been a factor on day 2, since some participants took substantially longer to produce enough saliva pre-startle, post-startle, and post-fatigue. Although the pre-startle samples were taken at 8:00 a.m., and the post-startle and post-fatigue samples were taken shortly after, time of day may have profoundly impacted the variance in salivary cortisol levels. Since the fatigue climb was the last test condition, this could explain the decrease in cortisol levels in males and females. Instead of obtaining baseline samples at 8:00 a.m., 11:00 a.m., and 2:00 p.m., perhaps obtaining samples at 8:00 a.m. and 9:00 a.m. would have been a better comparison for this study. Moreover, lead climbing and the auditory stimulus used may not have been strong enough stressors to provoke changes in cortisol levels in males due to their level of experience and more advanced skill level [1].

The 8:00 a.m. pre-startle cortisol levels were higher in both males and females when compared to their respective baseline 8:00 a.m. cortisol levels. This may have been due to an anticipatory cortisol response that primes the central nervous system [21]. This anticipatory response provides some insight into the relationship between psychological stress and physiological responses, as well as highlights the significance of psychobiological processes that occur prior to a stressor. It is possible that this neuroendocrine response was activated when instructions for the startle climb were provided. This would suggest that the stress (and increase in cortisol) that individuals experienced was triggered by their emotional and cognitive representations of what they thought would occur during the climb [21].

Females may have experienced a peak in cortisol levels post-startle because the relative difficulty of the climb may have been higher for them. Female participants were not as comfortable with the lead climbing technique, and this lack of confidence, in addition to the sustained isometric contractions and increasing difficulty of the climb, may have contributed to a peak in cortisol levels post-startle. This is supported by the significant differences in self-confidence between males and females prior to the startle climb.

Increased somatic anxiety post-startle in males may have been due to the added stress of lead climbing. Other studies have had similar findings, noting that participants had increased somatic anxiety when they had to lead climb a route, compared to top rope climbing [2]. Sex differences in somatic anxiety post-startle may be an indicator of differences in male and female responses to stress. There is evidence from functional magnetic resonance imaging (fMRI) that women are more attuned to negative stimuli and that they respond more rapidly to negative stimuli [22]. These sex differences may also explain differences in the self-reported self-confidence post-fatigue climb.

FSST times may have been faster post-startle because of heightened somatic anxiety and focus, due to the fight-or-flight response. It is also possible that the results were influenced by test familiarization and decreased anxiety of social judgment. In day 1, the FSST trials were carried out when the rock-climbing gym was open to the public. Therefore, there were other climbers present that served as an "audience" to the participants in the study. The participants may have also had difficulty focusing on the task at hand because of the various distractions in the gym. The fact that the participants did not know what to expect, that it was their first time performing the FSST, that there was an audience, and that their focus could have been affected, may have all contributed to slower day 1 scores.

It could be that average FSST times did not decrease post-fatigue because the value that was used to indicate fatigue was forearm muscle failure. It may be that although the forearm musculature fatigued to failure, focus and lower limb coordination did not decline.

It is also worth noting that three participants were not able to complete the test post-fatigue, due to poor coordination and unsuccessful execution of the sequence.

5. Conclusions

Our results show that cortisol concentrations follow a normal standard curve, irrespective of the test condition. Cortisol samples were taken 15 min after the stressor, and values were lower post-startle and post-fatigue when compared to the pre-test. It may be that the stressors used in this study were not enough to provoke a stressful situation in the climbers of this study or that higher values were presented immediately after the climb and not 15 min later. Future studies should compare the cortisol response immediately after the stimulus, as well as 15 min later, to determine when the true peak in cortisol occurs. Studies should also look at ways to reduce the amount of time spent in saliva sampling, since extended sampling time may have profoundly affected cortisol levels.

There seem to be differences in the way that males and females psychologically prepare and react to stressful situations. It is difficult to draw conclusions from this sample because a major limitation was the number of participants, especially females. Evidently, there are countless factors that can influence the stress response during climbing, as well as several variables that can serve as indicators of the demand of the climb. Future studies should also take into consideration the biomechanical and strategic changes that occur with increased psychological and physiological stress. This can be done by analyzing video footage and utilizing electromyography (EMG) to determine premotor time and reaction time, as well as changes in muscle activity. Blood samples can also be taken to look at the impact that acute stressors have on biomarkers of oxidative stress, as well as on biomarkers that are suggested to be related to anxiety [4].

Author Contributions: Conceptualization, P.V. and C.B.; methodology, P.V., A.I. and C.B.; formal analysis, C.B.; investigation, P.V. and C.B.; resources, C.B.; writing—original draft preparation, P.V.; writing—review and editing, P.V., C.B. and S.S.; visualization, P.V., C.B. and S.S.; supervision, C.B. and A.I.; project administration, C.B. and A.I.; funding acquisition, C.B. All authors have read and agreed to the published version of the manuscript.

Funding: This research received no external funding.

Institutional Review Board Statement: Ethical review and approval were waived for this study, due to the observational nature of the study.

Informed Consent Statement: Informed consent was obtained from all subjects involved in the study.

Data Availability Statement: Not applicable.

Acknowledgments: The authors would like to thank Carles Ros and Carles Tudela and the team at Ingravita for their support and collaboration on the project. The authors would like to extend their gratitude to Albert Pare for his continued assistance and valuable insights during the investigation, to Sergio Vilches for his contribution in the development of the project and for providing resources for saliva analysis, to Jon González for his help with sample analysis, and to all the climbers that participated in the study, for their cooperation and commitment to the study.

Conflicts of Interest: The authors declare no conflict of interest.

References

1. Fryer, S.; Dickson, T.; Draper, N.; Blackwell, G.; Hillier, S. A Psychophysiological Comparison of On-Sight Lead and Top Rope Ascents in Advanced Rock Climbers. *Scand. J. Med. Sci. Sport* **2013**, *23*, 645–650. [CrossRef]
2. Hodgson, C.I.; Draper, N.; McMorris, T.; Jones, G.; Fryer, S.; Coleman, I. Perceived Anxiety and Plasma Cortisol Concentrations Following Rock Climbing with Differing Safety Rope Protocols. *Br. J. Sports Med.* **2009**, *43*, 531–535. [CrossRef] [PubMed]
3. Nicolaides, N.C.; Kyratzi, E.; Lamprokostopoulou, A.; Chrousos, G.P.; Charmandari, E. Stress, the Stress System and the Role of Glucocorticoids. *Neuroimmunomodulation* **2014**, *22*, 6–19. [CrossRef]
4. Łoś, K.; Waszkiewicz, N. Biological Markers in Anxiety Disorders. *J. Clin. Med.* **2021**, *10*, 1744. [CrossRef] [PubMed]
5. Dickson, T.; Fryer, S.; Draper, N.; Winter, D.; Ellis, G.; Hamlin, M. Comparison of Plasma Cortisol Sampling Sites for Rock Climbing. *J. Sports Med. Phys. Fit.* **2012**, *52*, 688–695.

6. Bellagambi, F.G.; Lomonaco, T.; Salvo, P.; Vivaldi, F.; Hangouët, M.; Ghimenti, S.; Biagini, D.; Di Francesco, F.; Fuoco, R.; Errachid, A. Saliva Sampling: Methods and Devices. An Overview. *TrAC—Trends Anal. Chem.* **2020**, *124*, 115781. [CrossRef]
7. Dickerson, S.S.; Kemeny, M.E. Acute Stressors and Cortisol Responses: A Theoretical Integration and Synthesis of Laboratory Research. *Psychol. Bull.* **2004**, *130*, 355–391. [CrossRef] [PubMed]
8. Whitaker, M.M.; Pointon, G.D.; Tarampi, M.R.; Rand, K.M. Expertise Effects on the Perceptual and Cognitive Tasks of Indoor Rock Climbing. *Mem. Cogn.* **2020**, *48*, 494–510. [CrossRef]
9. Giacomello, G.; Scholten, A.; Parr, M.K. Current Methods for Stress Marker Detection in Saliva. *J. Pharm. Biomed. Anal.* **2020**, *191*, 113604. [CrossRef]
10. Magiera, A.; Roczniok, R.; Sadowska-Krępa, E.; Kempa, K.; Placek, O.; Mostowik, A. The Effect of Physical and Mental Stress on the Heart Rate, Cortisol and Lactate Concentrations in Rock Climbers. *J. Hum. Kinet.* **2018**, *65*, 111–123. [CrossRef]
11. Anderson, G.S.; Di Nota, P.M.; Metz, G.A.S.; Andersen, J.P. The Impact of Acute Stress Physiology on Skilled Motor Performance: Implications for Policing. *Front. Psychol.* **2019**, *10*, 2501. [CrossRef] [PubMed]
12. Remor, E. Psychometric Properties of a European Spanish Version of the Perceived Stress Scale (PSS). *Span. J. Psychol.* **2006**, *9*, 86–93. [CrossRef] [PubMed]
13. Dwyer, G.; Davis, S. *ACSM's Health-Related Physical Fitness Assessment Manual*, 2nd ed.; Wolters Kluwer Health, Lippincott Williams & Wilkins: Baltimore, MD, USA, 2008.
14. Fernández, E.M.A.; Río, G.L.; Fernández, C.A. Propiedades Psicométricas de La Versión Española Del Inventario de Ansiedad Competitiva CSAI-2R En Deportistas. *Psicothema* **2007**, *19*, 150–155.
15. Moore, M.; Barker, K. The Validity and Reliability of the Four Square Step Test in Different Adult Populations: A Systematic Review. *Syst. Rev.* **2017**, *6*, 187. [CrossRef] [PubMed]
16. Dite, W.; Temple, V.A. A Clinical Test of Stepping and Change of Direction to Identify Multiple Falling Older Adults. *Arch. Phys. Med. Rehabil.* **2002**, *83*, 1566–1571. [CrossRef] [PubMed]
17. MacKenzie, R.; Monaghan, L.; Masson, R.A.; Werner, A.K.; Caprez, T.S.; Johnston, L.; Kemi, O.J. Physical and Physiological Determinants of Rock Climbing. *Int. J. Sports Physiol. Perform.* **2020**, *15*, 168–179. [CrossRef]
18. Munro, C.L.; Grap, M.J.; Jablonski, R.; Boyle, A. Oral Health Measurement in Nursing Research: State of the Science. *Biol. Res. Nurs.* **2006**, *8*, 35–42. [CrossRef]
19. Adam, E.K.; Quinn, M.E.; Tavernier, R.; McQuillan, M.T.; Dahlke, K.A.; Gilbert, K.E. Diurnal Cortisol Slopes and Mental and Physical Health Outcomes: A Systematic Review and Meta-Analysis. *Psychoneuroendocrinology* **2017**, *83*, 25–41. [CrossRef] [PubMed]
20. Gallagher, P.; Leitch, M.M.; Massey, A.E.; McAllister-Williams, R.H.; Young, A.H. Assessing Cortisol and Dehydroepiandrosterone (DHEA) in Saliva: Effects of Collection Method. *J. Psychopharmacol.* **2006**, *20*, 643–649. [CrossRef]
21. Aschbacher, K.; O'Donovan, A.; Wolkowitz, O.M.; Dhabhar, F.S.; Su, Y.; Epel, E. Good Stress, Bad Stress and Oxidative Stress: Insights from Anticipatory Cortisol Reactivity. *Psychoneuroendocrinology* **2013**, *38*, 1698–1708. [CrossRef]
22. Bangasser, D.A.; Eck, S.R.; Telenson, A.M.; Salvatore, M. Sex Differences in Stress Regulation of Arousal and Cognition. *Physiol. Behav.* **2018**, *187*, 42–50. [CrossRef] [PubMed]

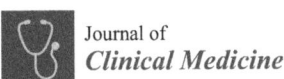

Review

Cardiopulmonary Exercise Test Parameters in Athletic Population: A Review

Reza Mazaheri [1], Christian Schmied [2], David Niederseer [2] and Marco Guazzi [3,*]

1. Department of Sports and Exercise Medicine, Division of Cardiology, Tehran University of Medical Sciences, Tehran 1419733141, Iran; mazaheri_md@tums.ac.ir
2. Department of Cardiology, University Heart Center, University Hospital Zurich, University of Zurich, 8091 Zurich, Switzerland; christian.schmied@usz.ch (C.S.); david.niederseer@usz.ch (D.N.)
3. Department of Health Sciences, San Paolo University Hospital, University of Milano, 20142 Milan, Italy
* Correspondence: marco.guazzi@unimi.it

Abstract: Although still underutilized, cardiopulmonary exercise testing (CPET) allows the most accurate and reproducible measurement of cardiorespiratory fitness and performance in athletes. It provides functional physiologic indices which are key variables in the assessment of athletes in different disciplines. CPET is valuable in clinical and physiological investigation of individuals with loss of performance or minor symptoms that might indicate subclinical cardiovascular, pulmonary or musculoskeletal disorders. Highly trained athletes have improved CPET values, so having just normal values may hide a medical disorder. In the present review, applications of CPET in athletes with special attention on physiological parameters such as VO_2max, ventilatory thresholds, oxygen pulse, and ventilatory equivalent for oxygen and exercise economy in the assessment of athletic performance are discussed. The role of CPET in the evaluation of possible latent diseases and overtraining syndrome, as well as CPET-based exercise prescription, are outlined.

Keywords: athletes; cardiopulmonary exercise test; exercise physiology; sports performance

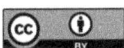

1. Introduction

Cardiopulmonary exercise testing (CPET) provides a full assessment of the physiologic responses of the pulmonary, cardiovascular, muscular, and cellular oxidative systems to exercise [1,2]. Sports physicians and physiologists try to identify the effects of exercise on athletes' organs to figure out their conditioning level and plan training programs to develop elite athletes for the team. Although CPET has become a generally well-accepted method to assess organ system adaptations to chronic regular exercise, its useful applications for more comprehensive assessments in the athletic population are not universally widespread yet.

The proposed indications for CPET in apparently healthy athletes are [3–6]:

- Measurement of baseline fitness and assessment of physiological function of body's systems;
- Evaluation of the integrated cardiopulmonary response in asymptomatic athletes with cardiac diseases;
- Diagnosis of latent disease and/or evaluation of minor nonspecific symptoms;
- Exercise prescription with specific purposes in different sports disciplines.

Athletes mainly recognize CPET assessment just for the measurement of their cardiorespiratory fitness (CRF) that mainly provides aerobic endurance performance expressed as maximal oxygen consumption (VO_2max). VO_2max measured during a graded maximal exercise is the most significant parameter to assess the cardiopulmonary capacity, especially in endurance sports [7], but it should be validated by completing a short constant work rate phase at higher intensities than the VO_2max work rate achieved during the ramp tests [8]. There are additional parameters that extend the number of opportunities to comprehensively study the integrated organ system response to maximal effort. The most remarkable is likely the ventilatory threshold (VT) that indicates aerobic power and is related to the lactate threshold in endurance and even resistance exercises [9]. Moreover, critical power (CP) is a widely used parameter for training that represents threshold intensities associated with the upper limit for prolonged aerobic exercise and signifies high to severe exercise intensity domain [10].

The series of variables are however consistent, and a careful analysis of each one yields to the best information in the time point assessment of physical performance and response to training programs. Oxygen pulse, defined as the ratio between VO_2 and heart rate (HR), indicates stroke volume and peripheral vascular perfusion/extraction response to exercise and reflects the maximal aerobic capacity. Ventilatory efficiency expressed by the relationship between minute ventilation (VE) to carbon dioxide (VCO_2) production (VE/VCO_2 slope) and/or partial pressure of end-tidal carbon dioxide ($PETCO_2$) at rest and during exercise, represents a match of ventilation and perfusion within the pulmonary system [11]. These quite underused parameters require a specific evaluation and interpretation.

Regular exercise has favourable cardiovascular benefits, but competitive athletes usually perform intense training for prolonged periods which exposes their cardiovascular system to increased levels of strain [12]. Intense exercise may trigger adverse cardiac events in an asymptomatic athlete with latent cardiac disease. Moreover, athletes sometimes experience minor symptoms such as dizziness, palpitation, or chest tightness that might indicate some subclinical cardiovascular or pulmonary disorders. In these instances, CPET analysis may be of additional help in clarifying the underlying causes and abnormalities.

In this review, the applications of CPET in athletes with an emphasis on physiological parameters and their implication in the assessment of athletic performance are discussed. Secondly, the role of CPET in the evaluation of minor nonspecific symptoms to determine and/or distinguish cardiac and pulmonary conditions that might limit sports participation is discussed. Finally, recommendations on exercise prescription for athletes based on the CPET results are summarized at the end of the paper.

2. Cardiorespiratory Fitness

2.1. VO_2max

VO_2max is the maximum oxygen uptake of the human body that defines the maximal amount of energy accessible by aerobic metabolism at peak exercise [13]. It is a standard for quantifying CRF [14] and may reflect the limits of the cardiopulmonary system to maximal exercise. The term VO_2max implies an individual's physiological limit that is achieved and sustained for a specified period during maximal effort [15]. Athletes of different sport disciplines present with a wide range of VO_2max, so for better inter-individual comparisons, it is better to express it as percent-predicted value or in millilitres of oxygen per kilogram of body weight per minute (mL/kg/min) [15,16]. Since the ideal body weight could be entirely different between disciplines, it makes sense to use fat-free mass instead of body weight for interdisciplinary comparison of athletes.

Expected values differ between male and female athletes at any given age and on different exercise test modalities. Accurate interpretation of VO_2max should be made with the knowledge of what is expected for an individual athlete. To facilitate sports counselling, it is critical to have validated reference values in target population [14]. Athletes have higher amounts, usually more than 120% of the predicted VO_2max of healthy untrained individuals, therefore, the interpretation of the results have to be done cautiously, as it might mask some latent disorders or potential physiological impairments. The time course of VO_2 recovery after exercise is an essential parameter that must be considered in the athletic population [17]. In highly trained athletes, recovery of VO_2 is more rapid, and just as depicted in Figure 1, the athlete with a higher exercise economy has a faster VO_2 recovery rate than his counterpart with less efficient cardiovascular function.

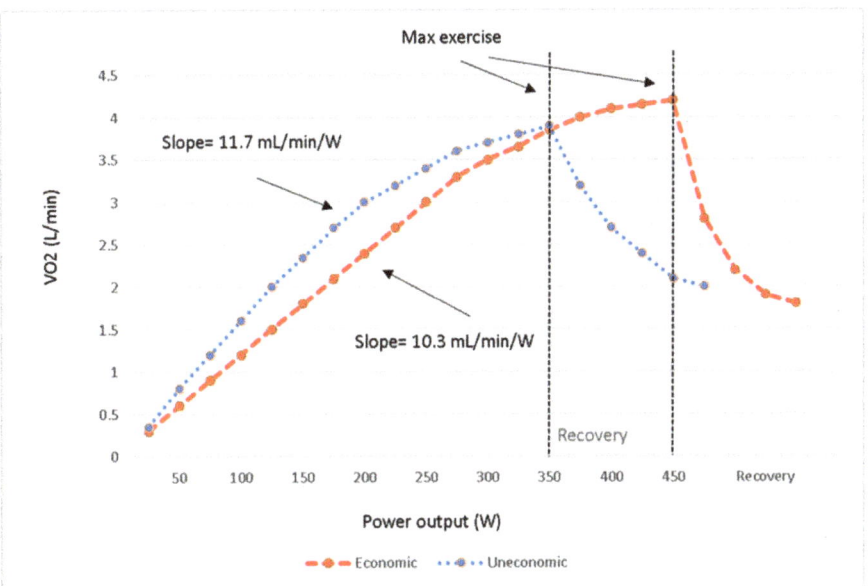

Figure 1. Athletes with different exercise economy as shown by VO_2/workload responses to incremental exercise.

There are considerable differences in the VO_2max of individuals, and numerous genetic variants have been found to be associated with these variations. Studies have reported that genetic components and inheritance account for 44 to 72% of the baseline VO_2max (mL/kg/min) in sedentary subjects [18]. Exercise training improves cardiorespiratory fitness by about 10–25% in previously sedentary individuals [15,19]. This improvement varies greatly between individuals even with a standard exercise training program. Genetic factors determine almost 50% of this VO_2 response to training [19–21]. The presented evidence implies the importance of baseline VO_2max measurements to find talented young athletes and to consult with athletes about their maximum achievable performance in different sport disciplines.

2.2. Ventilatory Threshold (VT)

During incremental exercise, there is a point at which muscles and blood lactate increase due to the rate of lactate production being higher than disposal [22]. The metabolic rate at which excess carbon dioxide (CO_2) develops proportionally to the muscle and blood bicarbonate decreasing rate as a consequence of buffering metabolic acidosis is the ventilatory threshold [22]. This excess CO_2 makes VE increase more steeply relative to the increase in VO_2 [13,15]. Therefore, VT is a point, at which VCO_2/VO_2 slope becomes steeper; the ventilatory equivalent for oxygen (VE/VO_2) begins to increase while the ventilatory equivalent for carbon dioxide (VE/VCO_2) remains stable [23] (Figure 2).

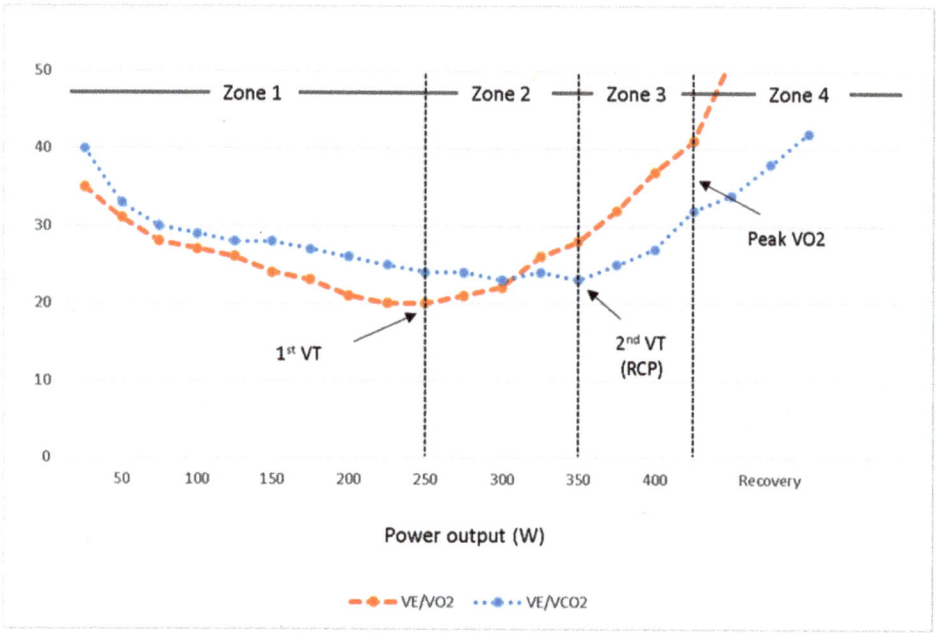

Figure 2. The ventilatory equivalents for oxygen (VE/VO$_2$) and carbon dioxide (VE/VCO$_2$) and their association with first and second VT which form four training zones during an incremental CPET. VT: ventilatory threshold, RCP: respiratory compensation point.

VT is expressed as VO$_2$ (mL/kg/min) or percentage of VO$_2$max and compared with VO$_2$max, is better correlated to athletic endurance performance [24,25]. It usually occurs at 45% to 65% of VO$_2$max in healthy untrained subjects [15,23] and at a higher percentage (close to 90% of VO$_2$max) in highly endurance-trained athletes [25]. It has been shown that after training, there is an increase in VO$_2$ at VT by about 10–25% in sedentary individuals [15]. The weighted mean heritability of submaximal stamina and endurance test performance is 49% and 53% respectively [18]. This evidence shows the importance of genetic predisposition for VT and submaximal endurance performance and its potential application in identifying talents in sports.

It has recently been proposed that the lactate threshold (LT) could be used to set the training load in resistance exercises [9]. Resistance training promotes muscle hypertrophy, strength and power, and the intensity of exercise is the most important component in this way. Studies have identified the LT in strength training exercises at intensities ranging from 27% to 36% of a maximum repetition (1RM) [9]. Exercise at this level of intensity could be optimal training in sports requiring strength and power. To verify the association between LT and VT, investigators identified the VT with positive correlation, agreement and at the same intensity of exercise with LT during an incremental resistance exercise test [26,27]. Although there exists a slight difference between VT and arterial blood lactate accumulation with VT occurs earlier in dynamic exercise [22,28], yet VT can measure both the endurance and resistance performance in athletes.

The modality of exercise test (treadmill or cycle) and the population under investigation potentially influence the VT response to exercise [15]. In trained subjects, VT is significantly higher on the treadmill than cycle ergometer but not in untrained individuals [29]. This difference should be taken into consideration, especially when we want to make comparisons among athletes in different sports disciplines. In a study on 29 male competitive triathletes, Hue O et.al. showed that the VT values on treadmill running were lower than the values reported for elite distance runners [30].

3. Further Key CPET Parameters

3.1. Oxygen Pulse

The oxygen pulse (O_2 pulse) is the ratio of VO_2 in mL/min and HR in beats/min, expressed as mL/beat [23]. According to the Fick equation, $VO_2 = (HR \times SV) \times C(a-v)O_2$, where SV is stroke volume and $C(a-v)O_2$ is the arterio-venous oxygen difference. Thus, the O_2 pulse provides an estimate of stroke volume and peripheral vascular perfusion/extraction response to exercise [15]. Normal values at rest range from 4–6 mL/beat and increase up to 10–20 mL/beat at maximal exercise [23]. Athletes demonstrate a 10%–15% increase in ventricular cavity size and enhanced cardiac filling in diastole that augment their stroke volume (SV) compared with individuals of similar age and size [12,31]. They reveal increased mitochondrial oxidative capacity and capillarity within the skeletal muscle, which results in higher $C(a-v)O_2$ during exercise [32]. As a result, O_2 pulse is higher in trained athletes, but the reference values in this population are yet to be determined.

Central [SV] and peripheral [$C(a-v)O_2$] adaptations to exercise result in higher O_2 pulse in trained subjects. As mentioned earlier, in calculating the O_2 pulse, VO_2 should be in mL/min. So, for making reliable comparisons between athletes, the weight and height of the athletes have to be taken into account. Therefore, the authors of the present paper recommend calculating the O_2 pulse in relation to body surface area (BSA). Since the relative contribution of SV to cardiac output is paramount during the early and intermediate phases of exercise [4,15], the amount of O_2 pulse/BSA at submaximal levels (e.g., 50% or 75% of the VO_2max) demonstrate more central (cardiac, i.e., SV) adaptations and the maximal value shows both central and peripheral (cardiovascular and muscular perfusion/extraction) adaptations to exercise.

Different patterns of adaptations according to O_2 pulse response to incremental exercise are displayed in Table 1. This approach could be a precise manner to compare athletes with different conditioning levels. It guides sports physicians and athletic trainers to distinguish elite athletes and to prescribe the appropriate training program to focus on central (cardio-pulmonary) or peripheral (skeletal muscles) structures based on the standard requirements for any sports discipline.

Table 1. O_2 pulse response of four athletes with different adaptation patterns to incremental exercise in comparison with a reference athlete

	Intensity of Exercise (% VO_2max)		
	50%	75%	100%
Reference athlete O_2 pulse (mL/beat)	14	18	20
Athlete A	↑	↑	↑
Athlete B	↑	↑↔	↓
Athlete C	↓	↓↔	↔↑
Athlete D	↓	↓	↓

Athlete A has a better central and peripheral adaptation to exercise than the reference athlete. Athlete B has better central but lower peripheral adaptation and Athlete C might has better peripheral adaptation than central. Athlete D is worst in both central and peripheral adaptations. Reference athlete: RA, ↑: more than RA, ↑↔: more or equals to RA, ↓↔: less or equals to RA, ↓: less than RA.

3.2. Ventilatory Equivalents (VE/VO_2 and VE/VCO_2)

Athletic performance requires proper integration of cardiovascular, pulmonary, and skeletal muscle physiology. Physiological deficiency of any of these systems diminishes VO_2 and increases ventilatory equivalents [15]. Enhanced mitochondrial function is a result of chronic exercise training [24], and this improvement is valuable for the effective production of adenosine triphosphate (ATP) through oxidative phosphorylation. Inadequate adaptation to exercise reduces the oxidative capacity of skeletal muscles and makes them rely on anaerobic glycolysis for ATP production, which leads to lactic acid accumulation early in exercise. Very deconditioned individuals and patients with mitochondrial myopathy might show the same manifestations but exaggeratedly [33].

Early lactic acidosis is reflected in CPET as a low VT, which is demonstrated by a rapid increase in VE/VO$_2$ and respiratory exchange ratio (RER). Arterio-venous oxygen difference might also be lower in athletes with unfavourable mitochondrial adaptations resulting in a reduced peak O$_2$ pulse. Some studies support the improvement of these parameters in fit individuals by demonstrating a decreased submaximal VE/VO$_2$ and increased peak O$_2$ pulse after exercise training [34,35]. Figure 3 depicts the ventilatory equivalents of two athletes with different mitochondrial adaptations.

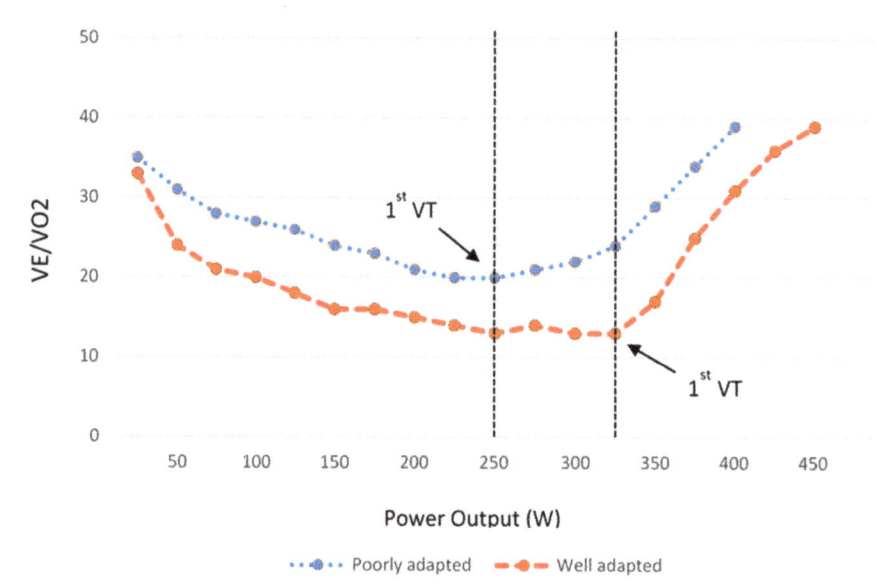

Figure 3. The ventilatory equivalent for O$_2$ in a well-trained athlete compared with a poorly adapted athlete. As it's evident, the ventilatory threshold is at higher workload with lower VE/VO$_2$ values in well-trained athlete than their less fit peer.

The slope of the VE/VCO$_2$ relationship and PETCO$_2$ during an incremental exercise test represent the matching of ventilation and perfusion within the pulmonary system, and they are determinants of ventilatory efficiency in subjects. Studies have revealed a lack of relationship between ventilatory efficiency evaluated by VE/VCO$_2$ slope and sports performance in athletes [36,37].

The relationship between VO$_2$ and the log scale of VE represents the oxygen uptake efficiency slope (OUES) and expresses the ventilatory requirement for O$_2$ [16,23]. Many investigators found it useful in the evaluation of fitness level, and reference values have been proposed [38], but a broadly accepted threshold to define normal response has not been clearly established. Training induced changes in OUES are variable and not sensitive enough to show the improvement of fitness after training [39].

3.3. Exercise Economy (ΔVO$_2$/ΔWorkload)

Exercise economy is defined as the energy expenditure for given absolute exercise intensity and is expressed as VO$_2$ at a given physical work or power output [4,24,40,41]. Remarkable economy means lower VO$_2$ for given power output and is an advantage in endurance performance because it results in the utilisation of a lower percentage of

VO$_2$max for particular exercise intensity. Low VO$_2$max scores can even be compensated by remarkable economy [24].

The importance of exercise economy has been described in different athletes such as runners and soccer players [41,42], and the improvements could be achieved by endurance training through improved muscle oxidative capacity and changes in motor unit recruitment patterns. Researches support the effects of resistance and plyometric exercises and high-intensity interval training (HIIT) on exercise economy [40,41]. Reduction in submaximal VO$_2$ is significantly correlated with the reduced minute ventilation (VE) and heart rate (HR) [24].

The slope of VO$_2$ (mL/min) to workload (Watts) demonstrates the economy of exercise and represents an indirect measure of cardiac output and aerobically generated ATP [23]. Commonly there is a continual rise throughout the exercise with the average slope of 10 mL/min/W with all exercise data [11]. Figure 1 depicts the VO$_2$/workload responses of two athletes with different exercise economy. To evaluate an athlete's exercise economy, it is better to measure it during an incremental test, which is fast enough to continually increase the VO$_2$ similar to the intensities more commonly experienced during sports competition and at supra-LT workloads. In this regard, it is advisable to perform a CPET to measure the VO$_2$ (mL/min) and to use a lower extremity ergometer to quantify the workloads (Watts) for proper measurement of VO$_2$/workload slope.

3.4. Respiratory Compensation Point (RCP)

With increasing exercise intensity above the VT, the lactate production rate gets higher, and a point is reached when bicarbonate is no longer able to counteract exercise-induced metabolic acidosis. In the isocapnic buffering region, bicarbonate is decreasing with no evident hyperventilation. Then, there is an exponential increase in blood lactate concentration and an excess CO$_2$, whereas the increase in VO$_2$ remains linear. The second breakpoint in the ventilation response to exercise is where the peripheral chemoreceptors invoke hyperventilation, which is identified as the second VT or RCP [10,13,43,44].

According to the physiological changes at RCP, there is an inflection of VE versus VCO$_2$ and also VE/VCO$_2$ versus workload, so as depicted in Figure 2, the second VT is identifiable by the nadir of the VE/VCO$_2$ to workload curve [43,44]. Both VE/VO$_2$ and end-tidal O$_2$ pressure (PETO$_2$) increase while there is a deflection point on the PETCO$_2$ trajectory [45]. It is usually achieved at around 70–80% of VO$_2$max or 80–90% of peak HR during incremental exercise [13,43]. In a recent systematic review and meta-analysis, it has been demonstrated that there is a highly significant correlation between RCP and critical power, with the power output at CP being 6% lower than RCP [10,43,45].

The second VT or RCP can be expressed as VO$_2$ (mL/kg/min) or percentage of VO$_2$max. Workload consistent with RCP (Watts) might also provide a scale to compare the ability of different athletes to comply with higher intensities of exercise. Anaerobic capacity is an essential parameter in the performance of athletes, especially those who participate in sports with sudden bursts of high-intensity activity [4]. Therefore, a longer duration of exercise at a constant workload within the CP or at the RCP level (VO$_2$ slow component) could be an advantage for such sportspersons.

Table 2 outlines the effects of training on each CPET variable in well-trained athletes compared to their ordinary counterparts.

Table 2. Key CPET parameters in elite athletes.

	An Elite Athlete Compare to an Ordinary Peer
VO$_2$ max (mL/kg/min)	↑↑
VO$_2$ at VT	↑↑
Watts at VT	↑↑
O$_2$ pulse/BSA	↑
VE/VO$_2$ at VT	↓
VE/VCO$_2$ slope	↔
PETCO$_2$	↔
OUES	↔
ΔVO$_2$/Δworkload	↔↓
VO$_2$ at RCP	↑↑
Watts at RCP	↑↑
Exercise duration at RCP level	↑↑

RCP: respiratory compensation point, VT: ventilatory threshold, OUES: oxygen uptake efficiency slope, ↑↑: quite more, ↑: more, ↔: no difference, ↔↓: equals or less, ↓: less.

4. Role of CPET in Diagnostic Workup

Many athletes experience some occasional vague symptoms such as exertional dyspnea, chest discomfort, and fatigue during their sports career in which the etiology could be cardiovascular, pulmonary, or muscular. Evaluating the physiological response of body organ systems to exercise provides valuable information on potential underlying ailments. In clinical practice, CPET is used to detect latent diseases and can help to differentiate cardiac and pulmonary problems. In elite endurance athletes, expiratory flow limitation (EFL) is assumed to be very frequent, with a prevalence of up to 40% in males and 90% in females [46]. The assessment of the flow-volume loop during CPET would reveal the presence and magnitude of EFL, further clarify a pulmonary mechanism for the symptoms and provide resolution of disease severity [16].

Assessment of ventilatory reserve and efficiency in addition to the standard haemodynamic and ECG monitoring provide insight into probable physiological abnormalities. The ventilatory reserve is the ratio between peak VE on a CPET and the maximum amount of air that can be breathed within one minute by a voluntary effort at rest termed the maximal voluntary ventilation (MVV), which is often measured in 15 s and multiplied by 4 [11,47]. Abnormal ventilatory reserve, which is VE/MVV ≥ 0.8 along with abnormalities in FEV1 and peak expiratory flow (PEF) are indicative of pulmonary limitations [11], but athletes with superior cardiovascular function can demonstrate some degrees of EFL and low ventilatory reserve with normal lung function tests [47]. Since EFL can be a cause of hypoxemia on exertion, pulse oximetry (SPO$_2$) should also be measured throughout the CPET process. Ventilatory efficiency parameters [VE/VCO$_2$ slope and PETCO$_2$], reveal cardiopulmonary coupling and function, and when abnormal, may indicate subclinical ventilation-perfusion abnormalities as a possible mechanism for exertional symptoms [11,16]. Electrocardiographic and/or hemodynamic abnormalities like a hypertensive response to exercise or a slow recovery period might reveal a cardiovascular source for the symptoms.

Excessive training load without adequate recovery period exposes elite athletes to an inability to adjust optimally to the overall load. This process can results in overreaching, or in more severe cases overtraining syndrome (OTS), with different indeterminate signs and symptoms accompanying performance decrements and the development of acute illness [48]. Studies have shown that up to 64% of elite athletes experienced OTS at least once [49]. Parasympathetic alterations with bradycardia in endurance sports, and sympathetic alterations with tachycardia and hypertension in explosive and high intensity sports, have been suggested as various cardiovascular responses [50]. It is been advocated that heart rate and blood lactate concentration variations are the two most discriminating factors between overreached and normal athletes [51]. In an experimental study, Le Meur Y et.al. showed decreased cardiac output at submaximal and maximal exercise intensities with lower VO$_2$max and reduced HR and SV values in triathletes after an overload training period [52]. It, therefore, seems that the CPET of elite athletes should be interpreted more carefully.

5. Exercise Prescription

CPET provides a context for determining a highly individualized training intensity zones for prescribing a structured exercise program. The physiological response to exercise characterizes the first and second VTs and VO$_2$max, which allow for the identification of four intensity zones as it is illustrated in Figure 2 [43]. Heart rate and workload corresponding to each appropriate zone should be used for exercise prescription. Zone 1 consists of all workloads below the first VT, which represents light to moderate-intensity exercise. Zone 2 comprises those workloads between the first and second VT (RCP) equals to moderate to high-intensity exercise. The workloads above the CP that result in VO$_2$max at exhaustion are in Zone 3 constitute high to sever intensity exercise domain. Sprints and all-out efforts above the workloads that allow for the attainment of VO$_2$max are in Zone 4.

Constant workload exercise in Zone 1 brings about a steady-state VO$_2$ that is sustainable for a long duration (>30 min) with only a modest sense of fatigue. It is suitable for the recovery phase of HIIT in athletes. Training in Zone 2 results in VO$_2$ and lactate steady-state conditions and is important in inducing significant improvements in these parameters [24]. The highest workload with steady-state lactate is called critical power (CP), a marker of the upper-limit of sustainable prolonged aerobic exercise [43]. Endurance athletes like marathoners and triathletes benefit from improvements in these parameters.

Exercise training in Zones 3 and 4 might cause VO$_2$ to reach maximum value without steady-state achievement and is better defined by CP concept (Time limit at VO$_2$max). The duration of exercise is variable in these domains and based on the conditioning level of athletes, it would be in the range of 3 to 20 min in Zone 3 and less than that in Zone 4. Given a short exercise duration, these domains can only be used for HIIT programs [53]. There are various HIIT training protocols in the literature [53,54] that precisely characterize the physiological response of the exercise program.

6. Summary and Practical Implications

CPET has extensive practical applications in athletes, and comprehensive knowledge of exercise physiology in connection with various sports disciplines are essential for the interpretation of the results. Measurement of baseline fitness and the assessment of cardiopulmonary function in athletes suspected of having the cardiovascular or pulmonary disease are common indications for CPET. Revealing more talented athletes along with quantifying the physiologic parameters determinant of sports performance could be a reliable guide for team doctors and coaches.

VO$_2$max and VT are the well-known fitness parameters that depend on several factors, including age, sex, genetic predisposition, and exercise training. Athletes need high values for best performance but with varying importance in different sports.

- The critical power (CP) is a beneficial parameter for the assessment of an athlete's endurance status. However, the ventilatory threshold (VT) is a suitable parameter in CPET to set the training loads in a highly individualized manner.
- O$_2$ pulse indicates stroke volume and peripheral vascular perfusion/extraction response to exercise. The values at different levels of exercise demonstrate central and peripheral adaptations to exercise training.
- Ventilatory equivalent for oxygen (VE/VO$_2$) indicates the ventilatory cost for O$_2$ and begins to increase at the VT level. The values are lower at submaximal levels of exercise in well-trained athletes.

- Exercise economy is defined as $\Delta VO_2/\Delta$workload, and the lower amounts are a marker of better endurance performance in elite athletes.
- Respiratory compensation point (RCP) somewhere called the second VT is when there is an exponential increase in VE in response to an excess CO_2 production during incremental exercise. Critical power and, to a lesser extent RCP, represent the high to severe intensity of exercise and are useful in setting up an exercise training program for athletes in specific sport disciplines.

CPET is a well-accepted method to evaluate the function of body organs integrated into exercise. It could be a standard procedure to measure athletic performance in different sport disciplines but is disregarded in this field. Reference values have to be determined in athletes, so the interpretation of the results and performance differences would be accurately quantified. Hereby we call for further research on a large number of athletes in different disciplines to have comprehensive data for each CPET parameter in athletes.

Author Contributions: Conceptualization, all authors; methodology, R.M., C.S. and D.N.; validation, R.M. and M.G.; investigation, R.M., C.S. and D.N.; resources, R.M. and C.S.; data curation, R.M.; writing—original draft preparation, R.M. and D.N.; writing—review and editing, C.S. and M.G.; visualization, all authors; supervision, M.G. All authors have read and agreed to the published version of the manuscript.

Funding: This research received no external funding.

Institutional Review Board Statement: Not applicable.

Informed Consent Statement: Not applicable.

Data Availability Statement: All the data are available in the main text.

Conflicts of Interest: The authors declare no conflict of interest.

References

1. Guazzi, M.; Bandera, F.; Ozemek, C.; Systrom, D.; Arena, R. Cardiopulmonary exercise testing: What is its value? *J. Am. Coll. Cardiol.* **2017**, *70*, 1618–1636. [CrossRef] [PubMed]
2. Sietsema, K.E.; Sue, D.Y.; Stringer, W.W.; Rossiter, H.B.; Ward, S.A. (Eds.) Exercise Testing and Interpretation. In *Wasserman & Whipp's Principles of Exercise Testing and Interpretation: Including Pathophysiology and Clinical Applications*, 6th ed.; Lippincott Williams & Wilkins: Philadelphia, PA, USA, 2020.
3. Albouaini, K.; Egred, M.; Alahmar, A.; Wright, D.J. Cardiopulmonary exercise testing and its application. *Postgrad. Med. J.* **2007**, *83*, 675–682. [CrossRef] [PubMed]
4. Opondo, M.A.; Sarma, S.; Levine, B.D. The Cardiovascular Physiology of Sports and Exercise. *Clin. Sports Med.* **2015**, *34*, 391–404. [CrossRef]
5. Lollgen, H.; Leyk, D. Exercise Testing in Sports Medicine. *Dtsch. Aerzteblatt Online* **2018**, *115*, 409–416. [CrossRef] [PubMed]
6. Myers, J. Applications of cardiopulmonary exercise testing in the management of cardiovascular and pulmonary disease. *Int. J. Sports Med.* **2004**, *26*, S49–S55. [CrossRef] [PubMed]
7. Zinner, C.; Sperlich, B.; Wahl, P.; Mester, J. Classification of selected cardiopulmonary variables of elite athletes of different age, gender, and disciplines during incremental exercise testing. *SpringerPlus* **2015**, *4*, 544. [CrossRef]
8. Poole, D.C.; Jones, A.M. Measurement of the maximum oxygen uptake $\dot{V}o(2max)$: $Vo(2peak)$ is no longer acceptable. *J. Appl. Physiol.* **2017**, *122*, 997–1002. [CrossRef] [PubMed]
9. Dominguez, R.; Mate-Munoz, J.L.; Serra-Paya, N.; Garnacho-Castano, M.V. Lactate Threshold as a Measure of Aerobic Metabolism in Resistance Exercise. *Int. J. Sports Med.* **2017**, *39*, 163–172. [CrossRef] [PubMed]
10. Galán-Rioja, M.; González-Mohíno, F.; Poole, D.C.; González-Ravé, J.M. Relative Proximity of Critical Power and Metabolic/Ventilatory Thresholds: Systematic Review and Meta-Analysis. *Sports Med.* **2020**, *50*, 1771–1783. [CrossRef] [PubMed]
11. Guazzi, M.; Adams, V.; A Conraads, V.M.; Halle, M.; Mezzani, A.; Vanhees, L.; Arena, R.; Fletcher, G.F.; Forman, D.E.; Kitzman, D.W.; et al. EACPR/AHA Joint Scientific Statement. Clinical recommendations for cardiopulmonary exercise testing data assessment in specific patient populations. *Eur. Hear. J.* **2012**, *33*, 2917–2927. [CrossRef]
12. Sharma, S.; Merghani, A.; Mont, L. Exercise and the heart: The good, the bad, and the ugly. *Eur. Hear. J.* **2015**, *36*, 1445–1453. [CrossRef] [PubMed]
13. Mezzani, A. Cardiopulmonary Exercise Testing: Basics of Methodology and Measurements. *Ann. Am. Thorac. Soc.* **2017**, *14*, S3–S11. [CrossRef] [PubMed]

14. Silva, C.G.D.S.E.; A Kaminsky, L.; Arena, R.; Christle, J.; Gil Araujo, C.; Lima, R.; A Ashley, E.; Myers, J. A reference equation for maximal aerobic power for treadmill and cycle ergometer exercise testing: Analysis from the FRIEND registry. *Eur. J. Prev. Cardiol.* **2018**, *25*, 742–750. [CrossRef]
15. Balady, G.J.; Arena, R.; Sietsema, K.; Myers, J.; Coke, L.; Fletcher, G.F.; Forman, D.; Franklin, B.; Guazzi, M.; Gulati, M.; et al. Clinician's Guide to cardiopulmonary exercise testing in adults: A scientific statement from the American Heart Association. *Circulation* **2010**, *122*, 191–225. [CrossRef] [PubMed]
16. Guazzi, M.; Arena, R.; Halle, M.; Piepoli, M.F.; Myers, J.; Lavie, C.J. 2016 focused update: Clinical recommendations for cardiopulmonary exercise testing data assessment in specific patient populations. *Eur. Hear. J.* **2016**, *39*, 1144–1161. [CrossRef]
17. Sietsema, K.E. Approaches to Data Summary and Interpretation. In *Wasserman & Whipp's Principles of Exercise Testing and Interpretation: Including Pathophysiology and Clinical Applications*, 6th ed.; Sietsema, K.E., Sue, D.Y., Stringer, W.W., Rossiter, H.B., Ward, S.A., Eds.; Lippincott Williams & Wilkins: Philadelphia, PA, USA, 2020.
18. Miyamoto-Mikami, E.; Zempo, H.; Fuku, N.; Kikuchi, N.; Miyachi, M.; Murakami, H. Heritability estimates of endurance-related phenotypes: A systematic review and meta-analysis. *Scand. J. Med. Sci. Sports* **2017**, *28*, 834–845. [CrossRef] [PubMed]
19. Schutte, N.M.; Nederend, I.; Hudziak, J.J.; Bartels, M.; de Geus, E.J. Twin-sibling study and meta-analysis on the heritability of maximal oxygen consumption. *Physiol. Genom.* **2016**, *48*, 210–219. [CrossRef] [PubMed]
20. Williams, C.J.; Williams, M.G.; Eynon, N.; Ashton, K.J.; Little, J.P.; Wisloff, U.; Coombes, J.S. Genes to predict VO2max trainability: A systematic review. *BMC Genom.* **2017**, *18*, 81–110. [CrossRef]
21. Sarzynski, M.A.; Ghosh, S.; Bouchard, C. Genomic and transcriptomic predictors of response levels to endurance exercise training. *J. Physiol.* **2016**, *595*, 2931–2939. [CrossRef] [PubMed]
22. Poole, D.C.; Rossiter, H.B.; Brooks, G.A.; Gladden, L.B. The anaerobic threshold: 50+ years of controversy. *J. Physiol.* **2020**, *599*, 737–767. [CrossRef] [PubMed]
23. Myers, J.; Arena, R.; Cahalin, L.P.; Labate, V.; Guazzi, M. Cardiopulmonary Exercise Testing in Heart Failure. *Curr. Probl. Cardiol.* **2015**, *40*, 322–372. [CrossRef]
24. Jones, A.M.; Carter, H. The effect of endurance training on parameters of aerobic fitness. *Sports Med.* **2000**, *29*, 373–386. [CrossRef] [PubMed]
25. Sarma, S.; Levine, B.D. Beyond the Bruce Protocol: Advanced Exercise Testing for the Sports Cardiologist. *Cardiol. Clin.* **2016**, *34*, 603–608. [CrossRef] [PubMed]
26. de Sousa, N.M.F.; Magosso, R.F.; Pereira, G.B.; Souza, M.C.; Vieira, A.; Marine, D.A.; Perez, S.A.; Baldissera, V. Acute cardiorespiratory and metabolic responses during resistance exercise in the lactate threshold intensity. *Int. J. Sports Med.* **2012**, *33*, 108–113. [CrossRef] [PubMed]
27. Mate-Munoz, J.L.; Dominguez, R.; Lougedo, J.H.; Garnacho-Castano, M.V. The lactate and ventilatory thresholds in resistance training. *Clin. Physiol. Funct. Imaging* **2016**, *37*, 518–524. [CrossRef] [PubMed]
28. Hughes, E.F.; Turner, S.C.; Brooks, G.A. Effects of glycogen depletion and pedaling speed on "anaerobic threshold". *J. Appl. Physiol.* **1982**, *52*, 1598–1607. [CrossRef]
29. Hansen, D.; Dendale, P.; Berger, J.; Meeusen, R. Low agreement of ventilatory threshold between training modes in cardiac patients. *Graefe's Arch. Clin. Exp. Ophthalmol.* **2007**, *101*, 547–554. [CrossRef]
30. Hue, O.; Le Gallais, D.; Chollet, D.; Prefaut, C. Ventilatory threshold and maximal oxygen uptake in present triathletes. *Can. J. Appl. Physiol.* **2000**, *25*, 102–113. [CrossRef]
31. La Gerche, A.; Burns, A.T.; Taylor, A.J.; Macisaac, A.I.; Heidbuchel, H.; Prior, D.L. Maximal oxygen consumption is best predicted by measures of cardiac size rather than function in healthy adults. *Graefe's Arch. Clin. Exp. Ophthalmol.* **2012**, *112*, 2139–2147. [CrossRef] [PubMed]
32. Roca, J.; Agusti, A.G.; Alonso, A.; Poole, D.C.; Viegas, C.; Barbera, J.A.; Rodriguez-Roisin, R.; Ferrer, A.; Wagner, P.D. Effects of training on muscle O2 transport at VO2max. *J. Appl. Physiol.* **1992**, *73*, 1067–1076. [CrossRef] [PubMed]
33. Riley, M.S.; Nicholls, D.P.; Cooper, C.B. Cardiopulmonary Exercise Testing and Metabolic Myopathies. *Ann. Am. Thorac. Soc.* **2017**, *14*, S129–S139. [CrossRef] [PubMed]
34. Bhambhani, Y.; Singh, M. The effects of three training intensities on VO2 max and VE/VO2 ratio. *Can. J. Appl. Sport Sci. J. Can. Sci. Appl. Sport* **1985**, *10*, 44–51.
35. di Paco, A.; Dube, B.P.; Laveneziana, P. Changes in Ventilatory Response to Exercise in Trained Athletes: Respiratory Physiological Benefits Beyond Cardiovascular Performance. *Arch. Bronconeumol.* **2017**, *53*, 237–244. [CrossRef]
36. Salazar-Martinez, E.; de Matos, T.R.; Arrans, P.; Santalla, A.; Orellana, J.N. Ventilatory efficiency response is unaffected by fitness level, ergometer type, age or body mass index in male athletes. *Biol. Sport* **2018**, *35*, 393–398. [CrossRef] [PubMed]
37. Salazar-Martinez, E.; Santalla, A.; Orellana, J.N.; Strobl, J.; Burtscher, M.; Menz, V. Influence of high-intensity interval training on ventilatory efficiency in trained athletes. *Respir. Physiol. Neurobiol.* **2018**, *250*, 19–23. [CrossRef] [PubMed]
38. Sun, X.G.; Hansen, J.E.; Stringer, W.W. Oxygen uptake efficiency plateau: Physiology and reference values. *Graefe's Arch. Clin. Exp. Ophthalmol.* **2012**, *112*, 919–928. [CrossRef]
39. Mourot, L.; Perrey, S.; Tordi, N.; Rouillon, J.D. Evaluation of fitness level by the oxygen uptake efficiency slope after a short-term intermittent endurance training. *Int. J. Sports Med.* **2004**, *25*, 85–91. [CrossRef]
40. Beattie, K.; Kenny, I.C.; Lyons, M.; Carson, B.P. The effect of strength training on performance in endurance athletes. *Sports Med.* **2014**, *44*, 845–865. [CrossRef] [PubMed]

41. Barnes, K.R.; Kilding, A.E. Strategies to improve running economy. *Sports Med.* **2014**, *45*, 37–56. [CrossRef] [PubMed]
42. Dolci, F.; Hart, N.H.; Kilding, A.; Chivers, P.; Piggott, B.; Spiteri, T. Movement Economy in Soccer: Current Data and Limitations. *Sports* **2018**, *6*, 124. [CrossRef] [PubMed]
43. Mezzani, A.; Hamm, L.F.; Jones, A.M.; E McBride, P.; Moholdt, T.; A Stone, J.; Urhausen, A.; A Williams, M. Aerobic exercise intensity assessment and prescription in cardiac rehabilitation: A joint position statement of the European Association for Cardiovascular Prevention and Rehabilitation, the American Association of Cardiovascular and Pulmonary Rehabilitation and the Canadian Association of Cardiac Rehabilitation. *Eur. J. Prev. Cardiol.* **2013**, *20*, 442–467. [CrossRef]
44. Binder, R.K.; Wonisch, M.; Corra, U.; Cohen-Solal, A.; Vanhees, L.; Saner, H.; Schmid, J.-P. Methodological approach to the first and second lactate threshold in incremental cardiopulmonary exercise testing. *Eur. J. Cardiovasc. Prev. Rehabil.* **2008**, *15*, 726–734. [CrossRef]
45. Palermo, P.; Corra, U. Exercise Prescriptions for Training and Rehabilitation in Patients with Heart and Lung Disease. *Ann. Am. Thorac. Soc.* **2017**, *14*, S59–S66. [CrossRef] [PubMed]
46. Bussotti, M.; Di Marco, S.; Marchese, G. Respiratory disorders in endurance athletes—how much do they really have to endure? *Open Access J. Sports Med.* **2014**, *5*, 47–63. [CrossRef]
47. Stickland, M.K.; Butcher, S.J.; Marciniuk, D.D.; Bhutani, M. Assessing exercise limitation using cardiopulmonary exercise testing. *Pulm. Med.* **2012**, *2012*, 1–13. [CrossRef] [PubMed]
48. Schwellnus, M.; Soligard, T.; Alonso, J.-M.; Bahr, R.; Clarsen, B.; Dijkstra, H.P.; Gabbett, T.J.; Gleeson, M.; Hägglund, M.; Hutchinson, M.R.; et al. How much is too much? (Part 2) International Olympic Committee consensus statement on load in sport and risk of illness. *Br. J. Sports Med.* **2016**, *50*, 1043–1052. [CrossRef] [PubMed]
49. Carfagno, D.G.; Hendrix, J.C., 3rd. Overtraining syndrome in the athlete: Current clinical practice. *Curr. Sports Med. Rep.* **2014**, *13*, 45–51. [CrossRef] [PubMed]
50. Kreher, J.B.; Schwartz, J.B. Overtraining syndrome: A practical guide. *Sports Health* **2012**, *4*, 128–138. [CrossRef]
51. Le Meur, Y.; Hausswirth, C.; Natta, F.; Couturier, A.; Bignet, F.; Vidal, P.P. A multidisciplinary approach to overreaching detection in endurance trained athletes. *J. Appl. Physiol.* **2013**, *114*, 411–420. [CrossRef] [PubMed]
52. Le Meur, Y.; Louis, J.; Aubry, A.; Guéneron, J.; Pichon, A.; Schaal, K.; Corcuff, J.-B.; Hatem, S.; Isnard, R.; Hausswirth, C. Maximal exercise limitation in functionally overreached triathletes: Role of cardiac adrenergic stimulation. *J. Appl. Physiol.* **2014**, *117*, 214–222. [CrossRef] [PubMed]
53. Buchheit, M.; Laursen, P.B. High-intensity interval training, solutions to the programming puzzle: Part I: Cardiopulmonary emphasis. *Sports Med.* **2013**, *43*, 313–338. [CrossRef] [PubMed]
54. Buchheit, M.; Laursen, P.B. High-intensity interval training, solutions to the programming puzzle. Part II: Anaerobic energy, neuromuscular load and practical applications. *Sports Med.* **2013**, *43*, 927–954. [CrossRef] [PubMed]

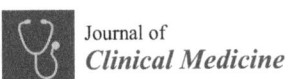

Journal of Clinical Medicine

Article

Blood Biomarkers Variations across the Pre-Season and Interactions with Training Load: A Study in Professional Soccer Players

Filipe Manuel Clemente [1,2,*], Francisco Tomás González-Fernández [3,4], Halil Ibrahim Ceylan [5], Rui Silva [1], Saeid Younesi [6], Yung-Sheng Chen [7], Georgian Badicu [8], Paweł Wolański [9] and Eugenia Murawska-Ciałowicz [10]

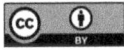

Citation: Clemente, F.M.; González-Fernández, F.T.; Ceylan, H.I.; Silva, R.; Younesi, S.; Chen, Y.-S.; Badicu, G.; Wolański, P.; Murawska-Ciałowicz, E. Blood Biomarkers Variations across the Pre-Season and Interactions with Training Load: A Study in Professional Soccer Players. *J. Clin. Med.* **2021**, *10*, 5576. https://doi.org/10.3390/jcm10235576

Academic Editor: David Rodríguez-Sanz

Received: 3 October 2021
Accepted: 24 November 2021
Published: 27 November 2021

Publisher's Note: MDPI stays neutral with regard to jurisdictional claims in published maps and institutional affiliations.

Copyright: © 2021 by the authors. Licensee MDPI, Basel, Switzerland. This article is an open access article distributed under the terms and conditions of the Creative Commons Attribution (CC BY) license (https://creativecommons.org/licenses/by/4.0/).

[1] Escola Superior Desporto e Lazer, Instituto Politécnico de Viana do Castelo, Rua Escola Industrial e Comercial de Nun'Álvares, 4900-347 Viana do Castelo, Portugal; rui.s@ipvc.pt
[2] Instituto de Telecomunicações, Delegação da Covilhã, 1049-001 Lisboa, Portugal
[3] Department of Physical Activity and Sport Sciences, Pontifical University of Comillas, 07013 Palma, Spain; francis.gonzalez.fernandez@gmail.com
[4] SER Research Group, Pontifical University of Comillas, 07013 Palma, Spain
[5] Physical Education and Sports Teaching Department, Kazim Karabekir Faculty of Education, Ataturk University, Erzurum 25240, Turkey; halil.ibrahimceylan60@gmail.com
[6] Research Unit for Sport and Physical Activity, Faculty of Sport Sciences and Physical Education, University of Coimbra, 3004-531 Coimbra, Portugal; saeidyounesi78@yahoo.com
[7] Department of Exercise and Health Sciences, University of Taipei, Taipei 11153, Taiwan; yschen@utaipei.edu.tw
[8] Department of Physical Education and Special Motricity, University Transilvania of Brasov, 500068 Brasov, Romania; georgian.badicu@unitbv.ro
[9] Department of Physiology, Gdansk University of Physical Education and Sport, 80-336 Gdansk, Poland; pawel.wolanski@awf.gda.pl
[10] Department of Physiology and Biochemistry, University School of Physical Education, 51-612 Wrocław, Poland; eugenia.murawska-cialowicz@awf.wroc.pl
* Correspondence: filipeclemente@esdl.ipvc.pt

Simple Summary: Sports training may impact the variations of biomarkers in soccer players. Twenty-five professional soccer players were assessed twice in the season for their hematology and biochemical status, while training loads were monitored over the season. Relationships between changes in biomarkers and accumulated training loads were tested. Results revealed that that intense training in the pre-season period leads to decreases and increases in different hematological and biochemical markers.

Abstract: Background: Pre-season training in soccer can induce changes in biological markers in the circulation. However, relationships between chosen hematological and biochemical blood parameters and training load have not been measured. **Objective:** Analyze the blood measures changes and their relationships with training loads changes after pre-season training. **Methodology:** Twenty-five professional soccer players were assessed by training load measures (derived from rate of perceived exertion- known as RPE) during the pre-season period. Additionally, blood samples were collected for hematological and biochemical analyses. **Results:** For hematological parameters, significant increases were found for platelets (PLT) (dif: 6.42; $p = 0.006$; d = −0.36), while significant decreases were found for absolute neutrophils count (ANC) (dif: −3.98; $p = 0.006$; d = 0.11), and absolute monocytes count (AMC) (dif: −16.98; $p = 0.001$; d = 0.78) after the pre-season period. For biochemical parameters, there were significant increases in creatinine (dif: 5.15; $p = 0.001$; d = −0.46), alkaline phosphatase (ALP) (dif: 12.55; $p = 0.001$; d = −0.84), C-reactive protein (CRP) (dif: 15.15; $p = 0.001$; d = −0.67), cortisol (dif: 2.85; $p = 0.001$; d = −0.28), and testosterone (dif: 5.38; $p = 0.001$; d = −0.52), whereas there were significant decreases in calcium (dif: −1.31; $p = 0.007$; d = 0.49) and calcium corrected (dif: −2.18; $p = 0.015$; d = 0.82) after the pre-season period. Moreover, the Hooper Index (dif: 13.22; $p = 0.01$; d = 0.78), and all derived RPE measures increased after pre-season period. Moderate-to-very large positive and negative correlations (r range: 0.50–0.73) were found between the training load and hematological measures percentage of changes. Moderate-to-large positive and negative correlations (*r* range: 0.50–0.60) were found between training load and biochemical measures percentage of changes. **Conclusions:** The results indicated heavy physical loads during the pre-season, leading to a decrease in immune functions. Given the significant relationships between blood and training load measures, monitoring hematological and biochemical measures allow coaches to minimize injury risk, overreaching, and overtraining.

Keywords: soccer; performance; biology; workload

1. Introduction

Elite soccer has intermittent characteristics that require players to frequently engage in a high level of aerobic and anaerobic capacity [1]. Average VO_2max values achieved by soccer athletes can reach up to approximately 63 mL/kg/min. While, maximal aerobic speed (MAS) can reach up to 17 km/h [2]. Professional soccer players have to perform low-intensity activities interspersed with high-intensity short explosive actions during training and matches [3].

Indeed, modern soccer is characterized by increasingly demanding physical activities during both training sessions and matches [4]. In fact, professional players can cover up to 7000 m of total distances (TD) in a single training session, and approximately 13,000 m during a match [5]. From the above-mentioned TD volume, players are required to cover significant distances in different high-intensity velocity thresholds, such as high-intensity running (HIR), high-speed running (HSR), sprints, and accelerations and decelerations [6,7]. Furthermore, different positions in the field require different physical demands. Therefore, it is essential to consider not only the biological individuality of each player, but also the physical demands of each position on the field [8].

As mentioned above, the pre-season is considered a critical period as, overall, players need to improve their fitness levels after the offseason period [9]. The detraining effects of the offseason period are accompanied by impairments in both physical and skills performance, that may be more pronounced if there is no individualized training program during the offseason [9,10]. Despite that, a study conducted on 23 elite soccer players showed improvements of approximately 8% in their aerobic and anaerobic performance after a pre-season period [11]. Furthermore, physical and physiological changes during the in-season can be dependent on the physical and physiological status observed at the beginning of the season [12]. However, a recent study showed that improvements in aerobic fitness after a pre-season period may not happen in a linear fashion as the authors found that fitness changes after the pre-season have a great variability between different seasons [13].

For such reasons, it is of paramount importance to monitor internal load measures on a daily basis. There are several psychometric measures, including fatigue, stress, soreness, quality of sleep factors, and their respective Hooper Index score (sum of the four factors), to monitor the well-being status of each player on a daily basis [14,15]. The Hooper Index score has been associated with the training load in soccer, showing its usefulness for practice [16]. In fact, a recent study conducted on nine professional soccer players revealed that the Hooper Index score had lower typical errors than the heart rate variability [17]. Thus, its usefulness seems to be promising in monitoring player's fatigue during a soccer season. Furthermore, the load monitoring can be daily applied using subjective measures. Those measure are based on the rate of perceived exertion (RPE) scales to obtain an indicator of global internal load of soccer training sessions, such as the session-rate of perceived exertion (s-RPE) [18]. In addition, other authors have started to use other RPE measures in their investigations, such as the sRPE general, sRPE breath, and sRPE neuromuscular [19,20]. These new s-RPE measures can determine the subjective perception of exertion on different body structures [20]. However, Los Arcos et al. [21], revealed no relationships between sRPE general, sRPE breath, and sRPE neuromuscular with changes in aerobic fitness.

Besides the common influencers of aerobic fitness (e.g., ventilatory kinetics, cardiac process, neuromuscular status), other hematological and biochemical parameters assume a preponderant role in athletes' performance [22]. However, there is incongruent evidence regarding the effects of acute and/or chronic training stimulus on hematological parameters, such as hemoglobin (Hb), red blood cells (RBC), and hematocrit (Ht) [23]. It seems that there is a trend to observe increases in the above-mentioned hematological parameters after a period of soccer training, especially during the preparation phase [24]. The Hb, RBC, and Ht are important hematological parameters since they are linked to the player's aerobic capacity, which is one of the physical aspects most trained during the pre-season [23,25]. In the case of biochemical parameters, they represent an important role for the monitoring of an athlete's responses to the training loads imposed [26]. For instance, cortisol and testosterone levels represent good markers of training stress, with cortisol being associated to catabolic processes and testosterone to anabolic processes [27]. In fact, a study conducted on 25 soccer players affirmed that the high training volumes during the pre-season period causes a decrease in testosterone levels and an increase in cortisol levels [28]. Thus, in consequence of high training loads imposed, the athletes enter in a catabolic state that impairs physical performance [29].

These facts reinforce the need to be aware of other possible biochemical associations with the imposed training loads on athletes, especially during the pre-season period, where higher loads are imposed to athletes. Moreover, considering the injury rate during a soccer season, the neutrophils, monocytes, and eosinophils have an important role in the reaction to inflammation, acting as a defense through the process of phagocytosis. Lymphocytes and basophils also constitute a major importance in the immune system and in the defense against acute viral and bacterial infections [30], given that their relationships with training loads can be useful in relation to primary prevention of injuries. To the best of our knowledge, there is no study addressing different blood biomarkers variations and their interactions with different external load measures during the pre-season period. For those reasons, the purpose of this study is twofold: (i) Analyze the variations of chosen biological markers before and after the pre-season period and (ii) analyze the relationships between variations of biological markers and workload imposed on the players.

2. Materials and Methods

The article reported according to STROBE (the Strengthening the Reporting of Observational Studies in Epidemiology) guidelines for cohort designs [31].

2.1. Study Design and Setting

The present study followed an observational analytic cohort design with a quasi-experimental (pre-post) design. The period of data collection occurred between 2 June (beginning of the pre-season) and 19 September (after pre-season) of 2019. On 2 June and 19 September, players were assessed for their biological markers. Between the periods, the players were daily assessed for the training load parameters and wellbeing. From the blood samples collected to measure the biological markers, hematological and biochemical parameters were analyzed. All players were internally monitored in all training sessions during the pre-season period. All internal loads were monitored using subjective measures. For the quantification of subjective internal loads, the rate of perceived exertion (RPE) and the session-rate of perceived exertion (s-RPE) for general, breath, and neuromuscular perceived exertions were applied.

2.2. Participants and Study Size

Twenty-five professional soccer players (mean ± SD; age 28.1 ± 4.6 years old, height 176.7 ± 4.9 cm, body mass 72.0 ± 7.8 kg, and body fat percentage 10.3 ± 3.8%; body mass index using Quetelet equation: 23.4 kg/m^2), from a professional club competing in the first league of Qatar (2019/2020 season), participated in this study. The inclusion criteria were (i) completed blood samples collections before and after pre-season period;

(ii) no history of any neuropsychological impairments that could affect the results of the experiment (iii) absence of injuries, physical constraints, or illnesses during study period; (iv) absence of fatigue or illness during the blood samples collections of before and after the pre-season period; (v) participating in a minimum of 80% training sessions during the study period; and (vi) not have taken drugs such as pain killers or others that may influence the biochemical status during the two weeks before assessments. Technical staff and professional soccer players were informed regarding the study design and its related benefits and risks, as well as the main aims of the current investigation. All players signed an informed consent form to voluntarily participate in this study. All the professional soccer players in this study were treated according to the American Psychological Association (APA) guidelines, which ensure the anonymity of participants' responses. The study protocol was approved by the Scientific Committee of School of Sport and Leisure (Melgaço, Portugal) with the code number CTC-ESDL-CE00118. The study followed the ethical standards of the Declaration of Helsinki.

2.3. Variables, Data Sources, and Quantitative Variables

2.3.1. Anthropometry

Anthropometric measures were performed before and after the pre-season period, at the same time of the day. Body mass was measured using a body composition monitor (HD-351, Tanita, Arlington Heights, IL, USA) to the nearest 0.1 kg. While, the height was measured using a stadiometer to the nearest 0.1 cm (Seca 217, Ham- burg, Germany). Fat mass was also estimated using the body composition monitor. All measurements were performed by the same professional with a level 2 certification from the International Society for the Advancement of Kinanthropometry (ISAK). The experienced professional was considered mainly for the case of ensuring accuracy and precision in anthropometric measures related to height. Moreover, this professional also ensured the reproducibility conditions for the case of body composition analysis using bioimpedance. Those conditions were related to the protocol of cleaning the machine every time a player was measured, waiting the same time between players and after cleaning, and ensuring the same player's position during the measurement.

2.3.2. Biological Markers

Hematological Parameters

Laboratory blood samples were collected from players' antecubital vein in a seated position. Blood samples (15 mL) were collected between 8:00 and 10:00 am, before and after the pre-season period. The blood samples were collected with all players in fasting, and with at least 12 h of rest (the time between the last training session, and the second blood draw) before the laboratory blood tests. All blood samples were centrifuged at 2500 rpm for 10 min, and the serum of each sample was immediately frozen at $-80\ °C$ for later biochemical analysis. Furthermore, 3 mL of blood were collected into vacutainer tubes containing ethylenediaminetetraacetic acid (EDTA). The blood samples were analyzed through flow cytometry, using a flow cytometer (FACSCalibur^{TM}, BD Biosciences, San Jose, CA, USA) and using an automated hematology analyzer (Sysmex kx-21N Kobe, JAPAN). This method allowed to obtain hematological variables as follow: WBC: White blood cells; RBC: Red blood cells; Hb: Hemoglobin; Ht: Hematocrit; MCV: Mean corpuscular volume; MCHb: Mean corpuscular hemoglobin; MCHbC: Mean corpuscular hemoglobin concentration; RCDW: Red cells distribution width; PLT: Platelets; MPLTV: Mean platelets volume; NEUT: Neutrophils; LYMP: Lymphocytes; MNC: Monocytes; EOS: Eosinophils; BSO: Basophils; ANC: Absolute neutrophils count; AMC: Absolute monocytes count; ALC: Absolute lymphocytes count; and AEC: Absolute eosinophils count.

Biochemical Parameters

From the 15 mL of each blood sample, 7 mL of the original blood samples were placed into vacutainer tubes containing gelose for biochemical analysis. The blood serum was used to determine the following biochemical measures: Sodium, potassium, calcium, creatinine, alkaline phosphatase (ALP), albumin, ferritin, C-reactive protein (CRP), total cholesterol (TC), high-density lipoprotein cholesterol (C-HDL), low-density lipoprotein cholesterol (C-LDL), triglycerides (TG), cortisol, testosterone, and testosterone/cortisol ratio. All biochemical measures were analyzed using an Auto Chemistry Analyzer BM-100 (BioMaxima S.A., Lublin, Poland). The analyzer used was maintained by regular quality control procedures according to the manufacturer's instruction to avoid any inconvenience during the procedures. The C-LDL was calculated based on the Friedewald Equation, i.e., TC-(TG/5)–C-HDL.

2.3.3. Training Load Monitoring

Internal Loads

Regarding internal loads, subjective measures were used. The CR-10 scale was used to quantify each player rate of perceived exertion (RPE) [32]. Based on the CR-10 scale, a value of 1 means "very light activity" and a value of 10 means "maximal exertion". Approximately 10 to 30 min after each training session, the RPE was individually collected and without the influence of others [33]. All players were familiarized with the RPE scale. Furthermore, to obtain the session-rate of perceived exertion (s-RPE), the RPE value attributed by each player was multiplied by the duration in minutes of each training session [34]. Thus, the s-RPE (expressed in arbitrary units [A.U.]), was used as the final outcome of subjective internal load measure to be analyzed in the present study. sRPE general, sRPE breath, and sRPE neuromuscular were also monitored as recommended elsewhere, for professional soccer players [19].

Well-Being Measures

For quantifying the well-being status of each player, a self-reported questionnaire comprised of a 7-point scale was used on a daily basis [15]. The questionnaire included questions involving stress, fatigue, delayed onset muscle soreness (DOMS), and sleep quality perceived levels. After the players answered the questions, the Hooper Index was used for analysis based on the scale, being calculated based on the sum of points from the four categories. This latter measure is the sum of the four question ratings. The questionnaire was sent to each player approximately 30-min before the training or match session.

Urine Color

The urine color chart [35] was implemented to the players before and after the preseason period. At both times, urine was collected in a clear container and compared by the same observer with urine color chart. In this scale, the score varies between 1 (lightest) and 8 (darkest). The color "yellow", "pale yellow", or "straw yellow" indicates euhydration, while "dark" represents hypohydration [35]. The scale was previously confirmed as valid [36] to assess hydration.

2.3.4. Statistical Procedures

Statistical analyses were carried out using the software Statistica (version 13.1; Statsoft, Inc., Tulsa, OK, USA). For all analyses, significance was accepted at $p < 0.05$. Descriptive statistics are represented as mean ± standard deviation (SD) with standard mean difference data. Tests of normal distribution and homogeneity (Kolmogorov–Smirnov and Levene's, respectively) were conducted on all data before analysis. Paired sample t-test was used for determining differences as a repeated measures analysis (pre–post). Cohen d was the effect size indicator. To interpret the magnitude of the effect size, we adopted the following criteria: d = 0.20, small; d = 0.50, medium; and d = 0.80, large [37]. A Pearson's correlation coefficient r was used to examine the relationship between the percentage of change of all biological mark [100 − (post × 100)/pre] and the training load (urine, sleep quality, stress, fatigue, soreness, Hooper Index, RPE general, RPE breath, RPE neuromuscular, sRPE general, sRPE breath, and sRPE neuromuscular [100 − (post × 100)/pre]). To interpret the magnitude of these correlations, we adopted the following criteria [37]: $r \leq 0.1$, trivial; $0.1 < r \leq 0.3$, small; $0.3 < r \leq 0.5$, moderate; $0.5 < r \leq 0.7$, large; $0.7 < r \leq 0.9$, very large; and $r > 0.9$, almost perfect. Regression analysis was used to model the prediction of SMD blood biomarkers from remaining variables with positive correlation.

3. Results

First, a paired measure *t*-test with hematological parameters (WBC, RBC, RCDW, Hb, MCV, MCHb, MCHbC, MPLTV, EOS%, BASO%, NEUT%, LYMP%, MNC%, ALC, and AEC) showed no significant differences between before and after the pre-season period. There was a significant increase in PLT, while a significant decrease in AMC and ANC after the pre-season period (see Table 1, for more information).

Table 1. Before and after pre-season data (mean ± SD) of anthropometric and hematological parameters (HP).

	Before Pre-season	After Preseason	% Change	t-Test (p)
Antropometric measures				
Body Mass (kg)	72.00 ± 6.37	69.92 ± 6.44	2.77	$p = 0.001$ ** |d = 0.32
Body Fat (%)	10.30 ± 3.15	8.10 ± 2.49	19.79	$p = 0.001$ ** |d = 0.77
Hematological parameteres				
WBC (10^9/L)	5.38 ± 1.02	5.20 ± 1.21	−3.35	$p = 0.10$ |d = 0.16
RBC (10^{12}/L)	4.94 ± 0.27	4.94 ± 0.34	0.00	$p = 1.00$ |d = 0.00
Hb (g/L)	14.63 ± 0.73	14.67 ± 0.65	0.27	$p = 0.61$ |d = −0.05
Ht (%)	43.03 ±1.44	42.93 ± 1.67	−0.23	$p = 0.79$ |d = 0.06
MCV (fL)	86.98 ± 4.58	87.64 ± 4.40	0.76	$p = 0.34$ |d = −0.14
MCHb (pg)	29.84 ± 1.58	29.92 ± 1.79	0.27	$p = 0.26$ |d = 0.16
MCHbC (g/dL)	33.91 ± 0.81	33.93 ± 0.85	0.06	$p = 0.87$ |d = −0.02
RCDW (%)	13.40 ± 0.83	13.49 ± 0.91	0.67	$p = 0.28$ |d = −0.10
PLT (10^3/μL)	217.00 ± 38.41	230.94 ± 38.57	6.42	$p = 0.006$ * |d = −0.36
MPLTV (fL)	8.82 ± 0.90	8.68 ± 0.78	−1.59	$p = 0.06$ |d = 0.16
NEUT (%)	43.01 ± 9.83	42.99 ± 10.84	−0.05	$p = 0.98$ |d = 0.001
LYMP (%)	42.91 ± 9.55	44.36 ± 10.10	3.38	$p = 0.24$ |d = −0.14
MNC (%)	9.49 ± 1.97	9.04 ± 1.71	−4.74	$p = 0.09$ |d = 0.24
EOS (%)	3.46 ±1.26	3.44 ± 1.11	−0.58	$p = 0.88$ |d = 0.01
BASO (%)	0.70 ± 0.28	0.68 ± 0.26	−2.86	$p = 0.35$ |d = 0.07
ANC (10^9/L)	2.26 ± 0.81	2.17 ± 0.79	−3.98	$p = 0.006$ * |d = 0.11
ALC (10^9/L)	2.34 ± 0.50	2.26 ± 2.97	−3.42	$p = 0.26$ |d = 0.03
AMC (10^9/L)	0.53 ± 0.11	0.44 ± 0.12	−16.98	$p = 0.001$ * |d = 0.78
AEC (10^9/L)	0.19 ± 0.11	0.19 ± 0.11	0.00	$p = 0.86$ |d = 0.00

HP: Hematological parameters; WBC: White blood cells; RBC: Red blood cells; Hb: Hemoglobin; Ht: Hematocrits; MCV: Mean corpuscular volume; MCHb: Mean corpuscular hemoglobin; MCHbC: Mean corpuscular hemoglobin concentration; RCDW: Red cell distribution width; PLT: Platelets; MPLTV: Mean platelets volume; NEUT: Neutrophils; LYMP: Lymphocytes; MNC: Monocytes; EOS: Eosinophils; BASO: Basophils; ANC: Absolute neutrophils count; ALC: Absolute lymphocytes count; AMC: Absolute monocytes count; AEC: Absolute eosinophils count; * Denotes significance at $p < 0.05$, and ** denotes significance at $p < 0.01$.

A new paired measures *t*-test with biochemical parameters including, potassium, albumin, ferritin level, TC, TG, C-HDL, and, C-LDL, showed no significant differences between before and after the pre-season period. There was a significant increase in creatinine, ALP, CRP, cortisol, and testosterone, while a significant decrease in calcium and calcium corrected after the pre-season period (see Table 2, for more information).

Table 2. Before and after pre-season data (mean ± SD) of biochemical parameters (BcP).

	Before Pre-Season	After Pre-Season	% Change	t-Test (p)
Sodium (mmol/L)	140.68 ± 1.22	140.76 ± 1.07	0.06	$p = 0.70$ | d = −0.06
Potassium (mmol/L)	4.01 ± 0.28	4.09 ± 0.35	2.00	$p = 0.08$ | d = −0.25
Creatinine (µmol/L);	83.55 ± 9.59	87.85 ± 8.75	5.15	$p = 0.001$ ** | d = −0.46
Calcium (mmol/L)	2.29 ± 0.07	2.26 ± 0.05	−1.31	$p = 0.007$ ** | d = 0.49
Calcium Corr. (mmol/L)	2.29 ± 0.07	2.24 ± 0.05	−2.18	$p = 0.015$ * | d = 0.82
ALP (IU/L)	65.75 ± 11.40	75.13 ± 10.79	12.55	$p = 0.001$ ** | d = −0.84
Albumin (g/L)	40.95 ± 2.53	40.41 ± 2.51	−1.32	$p = 0.94$ | d = 0.21
Ferritin (µg/L)	97.81 ± 59.15	101.69 ± 65.53	3.97	$p = 0.16$ | d = −0.06
CRP (mcg/mL)	2.64 ±0.55	3.04 ±0.63	15.15	$p = 0.001$ ** | d = −0.67
TC (mmol/L)	4.35 ± 0.85	4.45 ± 0.69	2.30	$p = 0.30$ | d = −0.12
TG (mmol/L)	1.34 ± 0.96	1.23 ± 0.78	−8.21	$p = 0.14$ | d = 0.12
C-HDL (mmol/L)	1.27 ± 0.35	1.33 ± 0.38	4.72	$p = 0.09$ | d = −0.16
C-LDL (mmol/L)	2.70 ± 0.64	2.54 ± 0.61	−5.93	$p = 0.24$ | d = 0.25
Cortisol (mcg/dL)	20.72 ± 2.16	21.31 ± 1.95	2.85	$p = 0.001$ ** | d = −0.28
Testosterone (mcg/dL)	6.51 ± 0.63	6.86 ± 0.69	5.38	$p = 0.001$ ** | d = −0.52

BcP: Biochemical parameters; ALP: Alkaline phosphatase; CRP: C-reactive protein; TC: Total cholesterol; TG: Triglycerides; C-HDL: High-density lipoprotein cholesterol; C-LDL: Low-density lipoprotein cholesterol; * Denotes significance at $p < 0.05$, and ** denotes significance at $p < 0.01$.

At this point, testosterone/cortisol ratio (T/C ratio) was calculated. In fact, the T/C ratio has been considered as an important physiologicaal variable to gauge individual condition and responses. In this sense, a t-test with data form the T/C ratio showed the same values before (0.317 ± 0.05) and after (0.324 ± 0.04) pre-season period [$t(25) = 2.13$, $p = 0.07$, d = 0]. Testosterone/cortisol ratio over the period can be found in Figure 1.

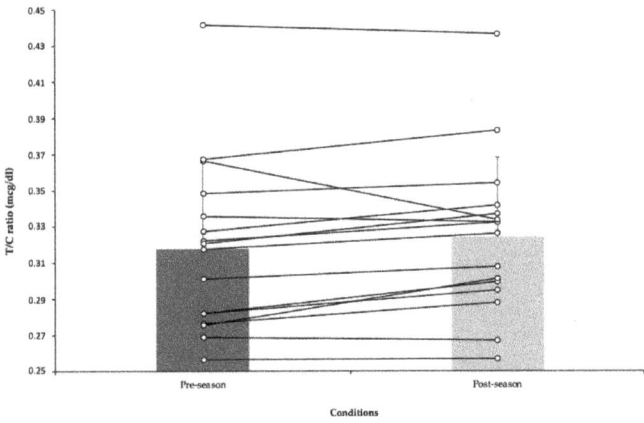

Figure 1. Before and after pre-season data (mean ± SD) of testosterone/cortisol ratio.

Regarding training load data, a paired measures t-test revealed no significant differences between before and after the pre-season period for urine color, stress, fatigue, sleep quality, and soreness measures. There was a significant increase in the Hooper Index, RPE (general), RPE (breath), RPE (neuromuscular), sRPE (general), sRPE (breath), and sRPE (neuromuscular) after pre-season compared to before pre-season (see Table 3, for more information).

Table 3. Before and after pre-season data of training loads (mean ± SD).

	Before Pre-Season	After Pre-Season	% Change	t-Test (p)
Urine color (A.U.)	2.43 ± 0.28	2.39 ± 0.20	−1.65	$p = 0.65$ | d = 0.16
Sleep Quality (A.U.)	2.75 ± 0.48	2.62 ± 0.39	−4.73	$p = 0.30$ | d = 0.29
Stress (A.U.)	2.33 ± 0.82	2.23 ± 0.31	−4.29	$p = 0.58$ | d = 0.16
Fatigue (A.U.)	2.88 ± 0.64	2.81 ± 0.62	−2.43	$p = 0.64$ | d = 0.11
Soreness (A.U.)	2.99 ± 0.66	2.74 ± 0.54	−8.36	$p = 0.14$ | d = 0.41
Hooper index (A.U.)	9.15 ± 1.63	10.36 ± 1.49	13.22	$p = 0.01$ * | d = 0.78
RPE (General) (A.U.)	3.23 ± 0.58	3.63 ± 0.44	12.38	$p = 0.03$ * | d = −0.77
RPE (Breath) (A.U.)	2.65 ± 0.28	3.11 ± 0.31	17.36	$p = 0.006$ ** | d = −1.55
RPE (Neuromuscular) (A.U.)	3.29 ± 0.50	3.05 ± 0.40	−7.29	$p = 0.04$ * | d = 0.53
sRPE (General) (A.U.)	217.81 ± 52.69	295.79 ± 46.84	35.80	$p = 0.001$ ** d = −1.56
sRPE (Breath) (A.U.)	179.46 ± 25.92	251.58 ± 31.89	40.19	$p = 0.001$ ** | d = −2.48
sRPE (Neuromuscular) (A.U.)	174.65 ± 44.05	287.65 ± 40.08	64.70	$p = 0.001$ ** | d = −2.56

RPE: Rate of perceived exertion; sRPE: Session rate of perceived exertion; A.U.: Arbitrary units * Denotes significance at $p < 0.05$, and ** denotes significance at $p < 0.01$.

Table 4 shows the relationships between percentage change of training load and the percentage of changes in hematological parameters. Very large positive correlations between RPE (general) and MCN% ($r = 0.73$; $p = 0.001$), and very large negative correlations between RPE (neuromuscular) and NEUT% ($r = -0.71$; $p = 0.002$) were found. Large positive correlations were found for the Hooper Index ($r = 0.67$; $p = 0.004$), soreness ($r = 0.61$; $p = 0.01$), and fatigue ($r = 0.57$; $p = 0.02$) with ALC percentage of changes. In addition, large positive correlations between sRPE (general) ($r = 0.60$; $p = 0.012$), RPE (neuromuscular) ($r = 0.53$; $p = 0.03$), and MNC percentage of changes were found. While, moderate negative correlations were found between stress and EOS ($r = -0.50$; $p = 0.04$) percentage of changes.

The associations between the percentage of change of training load and the percentage of changes of biochemical parameters can be seen in Table 5. Large negative correlations between sRPE (general) and sodium ($r = -0.60$; $p = 0.013$), between sleep quality ($r = -0.58$; $p = 0.01$), stress ($r = -0.53$; $p = 0.033$) and albumin, and between urine ($r = -0.51$; $p = 0.04$) and creatinine percentage of changes were found. On the other hand, large positive correlations between sRPE (breath) ($r = 0.60$; $p = 0.014$) and testosterone, and between RPE (general) ($r = 0.56$; $p = 0.02$) and C-HDL percentage of changes were found. While, moderate positive correlations between RPE (neuromuscular) ($r = 0.50$; $p = 0.04$) and ALP percentage of changes were found.

Table 4. Pearson correlations between percentage change of HP (before and after the pre-season) and percentage change of training loads (before and after the pre-season).

	Urine	Sleep Quality	Stress	Fatigue	Soreness	Hooper Index	RPE (General)	RPE (Breath)	RPE (Neuromuscular)	sRPE (General)	sRPE (Breath)	sRPE (Neuromuscular)
WBC (10⁹/L)	r = 0.10 | p = 0.69	r = −0.03 | p = 0.90	r = 0.37 | p = 0.15	r = 0.28 | p = 0.28	r = 0.38 | p = 0.13	r = 0.37 | p = 0.15	r = 0.11 | p = 0.679	r = 0.2209 | p = 0.41	r = 0.05 | p = 0.83	r = 0.12 | p = 0.65	r = 0.20 | p = 0.45	r = 0.26 | p = 0.32
RBC (10¹²/L)	r = 0.25 | p = 0.34	r = −0.33 | p = 0.20	r = −0.06 | p = 0.79	r = 0.03 | p = 0.89	r = 0.04 | p = 0.98	r = 0.07 | p = 0.78	r = 0.38 | p = 0.137	r = −0.2644 | p = 0.32	r = −0.08 | p = 0.75	r = 0.40 | p = 0.11	r = 0.02 | p = 0.99	r = −0.20 | p = 0.45
Hb (g/dL)	r = 0.37 | p = 0.15	r = −0.24 | p = 0.35	r = −0.15 | p = 0.55	r = −0.17 | p = 0.52	r = −0.20 | p = 0.45	r = −0.11 | p = 0.67	r = 0.19 | p = 0.471	r = −0.4672 | p = 0.06	r = −0.28 | p = 0.28	r = −0.16 | p = 0.55	r = −0.26 | p = 0.33	r = −0.20 | p = 0.45
Ht (%)	r = 0.09 | p = 0.71	r = −0.20 | p = 0.45	r = −0.26 | p = 0.31	r = 0.03 | p = 0.89	r = −0.04 | p = 0.88	r = 0.01 | p = 0.96	r = 0.04 | p = 0.858	r = −0.3453 | p = 0.19	r = −0.28 | p = 0.29	r = 0.10 | p = 0.69	r = −0.17 | p = 0.52	r = −0.34 | p = 0.19
MCV (fL)	r = −0.20 | p = 0.44	r = 0.07 | p = 0.79	r = −0.05 | p = 0.82	r = 0.29 | p = 0.27	r = 0.25 | p = 0.34	r = −0.26 | p = 0.32	r = −0.15 | p = 0.56	r = −0.08 | p = 0.75	r = −0.26 | p = 0.32	r = −0.10 | p = 0.71	r = −0.05 | p = 0.84	r = −0.24 | p = 0.36
MCHb (pg)	r = −0.16 | p = 0.54	r = 0.04 | p = 0.86	r = 0.03 | p = 0.90	r = −0.09 | p = 0.73	r = −0.19 | p = 0.46	r = −0.25 | p = 0.34	r = −0.03 | p = 0.90	r = −0.11 | p = 0.68	r = −0.20 | p = 0.43	r = −0.15 | p = 0.56	r = −0.23 | p = 0.38	r = −0.09 | p = 0.73
MCHbC (g/dL)	r = −0.20 | p = 0.45	r = −0.30 | p = 0.25	r = 0.01 | p = 0.96	r = −0.25 | p = 0.33	r = −0.31 | p = 0.22	r = −0.40 | p = 0.12	r = 0.12 | p = 0.63	r = 0.07 | p = 0.79	r = −0.18 | p = 0.4	r = −0.05 | p = 0.83	r = −0.18 | p = 0.49	r = −0.20 | p = 0.45
RCDW (%)	r = 0.02 | p = 0.92	r = −0.23 | p = 0.37	r = −0.28 | p = 0.28	r = −0.12 | p = 0.64	r = −0.06 | p = 0.80	r = −0.16 | p = 0.55	r = 0.15 | p = 0.57	r = 0.23 | p = 0.39	r = −0.00 | p = 0.97	r = 0.07 | p = 0.77	r = 0.13 | p = 0.61	r = 0.11 | p = 0.67
PLT (10³/μL)	r = 0.14 | p = 0.60	r = 0.04 | p = 0.86	r = −0.02 | p = 0.93	r = −0.24 | p = 0.35	r = −0.37 | p = 0.15	r = −0.17 | p = 0.52	r = −0.42 | p = 0.10	r = −0.41 | p = 0.10	r = −0.36 | p = 0.16	r = −0.24 | p = 0.35	r = −0.31 | p = 0.22	r = 0.07 | p = 0.77
MPLTV (fL)	r = 0.06 | p = 0.81	r = −0.06 | p = 0.79	r = −0.03 | p = 0.90	r = 0.24 | p = 0.36	r = 0.23 | p = 0.38	r = 0.33 | p = 0.20	r = 0.05 | p = 0.83	r = −0.25 | p = 0.34	r = 0.13 | p = 0.61	r = 0.24 | p = 0.35	r = 0.12 | p = 0.64	r = −0.02 | p = 0.93
NEUT (%)	r = −0.17 | p = 0.52	r = −0.39 | p = 0.13	r = 0.12 | p = 0.64	r = −0.35 | p = 0.17	r = −0.30 | p = 0.25	r = −0.25 | p = 0.38	r = −0.04 | p = 0.87	r = −0.39 | p = 0.13	r = −0.71 | p = 0.002 *	r = −0.11 | p = 0.66	r = −0.42 | p = 0.10	r = −0.02 | p = 0.93
LYMP (%)	r = 0.02 | p = 0.93	r = 0.14 | p = 0.60	r = 0.03 | p = 0.88	r = 0.03 | p = 0.90	r = 0.07 | p = 0.77	r = 0.07 | p = 0.79	r = 0.04 | p = 0.87	r = 0.34 | p = 0.19	r = 0.32 | p = 0.22	r = 0.03 | p = 0.90	r = 0.28 | p = 0.29	r = −0.03 | p = 0.89
MNC (%)	r = 0.09 | p = 0.73	r = −0.41 | p = 0.11	r = −0.21 | p = 0.43	r = −0.021 | p = 0.93	r = −0.01 | p = 0.95	r = −0.16 | p = 0.54	r = 0.73 | p = 0.001 *	r = 0.31 | p = 0.23	r = 0.53 | p = 0.03 *	r = 0.60 | p = 0.012 *	r = 0.37 | p = 0.15	r = 0.05 | p = 0.82
EOS (%)	r = 0.04 | p = 0.86	r = −0.30 | p = 0.25	r = −0.50 | p = 0.04 *	r = −0.08 | p = 0.75	r = −0.04 | p = 0.87	r = −0.13 | p = 0.60	r = 0.17 | p = 0.52	r = −0.20 | p = 0.44	r = −0.09 | p = 0.72	r = 0.16 | p = 0.54	r = −0.09 | p = 0.73	r = −0.21 | p = 0.43
BASO (%)	r = 0.12 | p = 0.63	r = −0.21 | p = 0.41	r = −0.13 | p = 0.63	r = 0.29 | p = 0.26	r = 0.26 | p = 0.32	r = 0.11 | p = 0.67	r = 0.47 | p = 0.06	r = 0.35 | p = 0.17	r = 0.29 | p = 0.26	r = 0.34 | p = 0.18	r = 0.29 | p = 0.27	r = −0.08 | p = 0.74
ANC (10⁹/L)	r = 0.08 | p = 0.76	r = −0.28 | p = 0.28	r = 0.18 | p = 0.48	r = −0.20 | p = 0.44	r = −0.13 | p = 0.61	r = −0.02 | p = 0.93	r = −0.07 | p = 0.78	r = −0.40 | p = 0.12	r = −0.46 | p = 0.07	r = −0.01 | p = 0.96	r = −0.28 | p = 0.29	r = 0.06 | p = 0.81
ALC (10⁹/L)	r = −0.09 | p = 0.72	r = 0.36 | p = 0.17	r = 0.40 | p = 0.11	r = 0.57 | p = 0.02 *	r = 0.61 | p = 0.01 *	r = 0.67 | p = 0.004 *	r = 0.07 | p = 0.97	r = 0.33 | p = 0.20	r = 0.23 | p = 0.38	r = 0.13 | p = 0.62	r = 0.41 | p = 0.10	r = 0.03 | p = 0.89
AMC (10⁹/L)	r = 0.11 | p = 0.66	r = −0.13 | p = 0.62	r = −0.11 | p = 0.61	r = −0.25 | p = 0.34	r = −0.15 | p = 0.57	r = −0.20 | p = 0.45	r = 0.01 | p = 0.95	r = 0.04 | p = 0.86	r = 0.19 | p = 0.46	r = −0.06 | p = 0.79	r = −0.11 | p = 0.65	r = −0.16 | p = 0.53
AEC (10⁹/L)	r = 0.23 | p = 0.38	r = −0.23 | p = 0.37	r = −0.48 | p = 0.05	r = −0.21 | p = 0.42	r = −0.20 | p = 0.43	r = −0.28 | p = 0.29	r = 0.16 | p = 0.54	r = −0.10 | p = 0.69	r = 0.11 | p = 0.67	r = 0.18 | p = 0.48	r = −0.06 | p = 0.80	r = 0.06 | p = 0.80

HP: Hematological parameters; WBC: White blood cells; RBC: Red blood cells; Hb: Hemoglobin; Ht: Hematocrits; MCV: Mean corpuscular volume; MCHb: Mean corpuscular hemoglobin; MCHbC: Mean corpuscular hemoglobin concentration; RCDW: Red cell distribution width; PLT: Platelets; MPLTV: Mean platelets volume; NEUT: Neutrophils; LYMP: Lymphocytes; MNC: Monocytes; EOS: Eosinophils; BASO: Basophils; ANC: Absolute neutrophils count; ALC: Absolute lymphocytes count; AMC: Absolute monocytes count; AEC: Absolute eosinophils count; * Denotes significance at $p < 0.05$.

Table 5. Pearson correlations between percentage change of BcP (before and after the pre-season and percentage change of training loads (before and after the pre-season).

	Urine	Sleep Quality	Stress	Fatigue	Soreness	Hooper Index	RPE (General)	RPE (Breath)	RPE (Neuromuscular)	sRPE (General)	sRPE (Breath)	sRPE (Neuro-muscular)
Sodium (mmol/L)	r = −0.17|p = 0.51	r = 0.08|p = 0.75	r = 0.16|p = 0.53	r = −0.31|p = 0.23	r = −0.35|p = 0.18	r = −0.44|p = 0.08	r = −0.46|p = 0.07	r = −0.01|p = 0.94	r = 0.04|p = 0.86	r = −0.60|p = 0.013 *	r = −0.44|p = 0.08	r = −0.05|p = 0.98
Potassium (mmol/L)	r = −0.02|p = 0.91	r = −0.35|p = 0.18	r = −0.38|p = 0.14	r = 0.06|p = 0.80	r = 0.05|p = 0.98	r = −0.11|p = 0.65	r = 0.38|p = 0.14	r = 0.04|p = 0.86	r = 0.40|p = 0.12	r = 0.34|p = 0.18	r = 0.21|p = 0.43	r = −0.13|p = 0.62
Creatinine (µmol/L);	|p = 0.04 *	r = 0.12|p = 0.65	r = 0.15|p = 0.55	r = −0.04|p = 0.99	r = −0.11|p = 0.67	r = −0.09|p = 0.73	r = 0.27|p = 0.30	r = 0.20|p = 0.43	r = 0.20|p = 0.45	r = 0.25|p = 0.34	r = 0.26|p = 0.32	r = 0.38|p = 0.14
Calcium (mmol/L)	r = 0.31|p = 0.24	r = −0.43|p = 0.09	r = 0.05|p = 0.84	r = −0.29|p = 0.26	r = −0.23|p = 0.38	r = −0.07|p = 0.78	r = 0.14|p = 0.58	r = −0.45|p = 0.07	r = −0.48|p = 0.05	r = 0.24|p = 0.36	r = −0.20|p = 0.45	r = 0.13|p = 0.61
Calcium Corr.	0.82	r = 0.10|p = 0.69	r = 0.36|p = 0.17	r = −0.02|p = 0.92	r = −0.06|p = 0.98	r = 0.27|p = 0.30	r = −0.19|p = 0.45	r = −0.46|p = 0.07	r = −0.38|p = 0.13	r = −0.02|p = 0.93	r = −0.19|p = 0.46	r = −0.05|p = 0.83
ALP (IU/L)	r = −0.22 |p = 0.40	r = −0.09|p = 0.71	r = −0.23|p = 0.376	r = −0.05|p = 0.98	r = −0.08|p = 0.76	r = −0.17|p = 0.52	r = 0.38|p = 0.14	r = 0.19|p = 0.47	r = 0.50|p = 0.04 *	r = 0.36|p = 0.17	r = 0.26|p = 0.31	r = 0.09|p = 0.72
Albumin (g/L)	r = 0.24 |p = 0.35	r = −0.58|p = 0.01 *	r = −0.53|p = 0.033 *	r = −0.25|p = 0.33	r = −0.17|p = 0.52	r = −0.22|p = 0.39	r = 0.38|p = 0.14	r = −0.15|p = 0.57	r = 0.13|p = 0.63	r = 0.37|p = 0.15	r = 0.03|p = 0.89	r = −0.07|p = 0.77
Ferritin (µg/L)	r = 0.39 |p = 0.13	r = 0.26|p = 0.32	r = 0.07|p = 0.796	r = 0.05|p = 0.84	r = 0.15|p = 0.56	r = 0.18|p = 0.49	r = −0.33|p = 0.20	r = −0.05|p = 0.83	r = 0.14|p = 0.58	r = −0.27|p = 0.30	r = −0.09|p = 0.73	r = −0.04|p = 0.85
CRP (mcg/mL)	r = 0.09 |p = 0.71	r = −0.22|p = 0.40	r = −0.19|p = 0.465	r = −0.05|p = 0.83	r = −0.04|p = 0.85	r = −0.19|p = 0.46	r = −0.18|p = 0.49	r = −0.10|p = 0.69	r = −0.06|p = 0.80	r = −0.22|p = 0.40	r = −0.25|p = 0.33	r = −0.35|p = 0.17
TC (mmol/L)	r = 0.09|p = 0.73	r = 0.23|p = 0.37	r = −0.15|p = 0.559	r = −0.12|p = 0.64	r = −0.16|p = 0.53	r = −0.09|p = 0.73	r = −0.06|p = 0.80	r = −0.13|p = 0.61	r = −0.21|p = 0.42	r = −0.09|p = 0.71	r = −0.15|p = 0.55	r = −0.31|p = 0.23
TG (mmol/L)	r = 0.26|p = 0.31	r = 0.15|p = 0.56	r = −0.23|p = 0.377	r = 0.14|p = 0.58	r = 0.08|p = 0.75	r = 0.05|p = 0.84	r = −0.14|p = 0.59	r = 0.09|p = 0.71	r = 0.49|p = 0.05	r = −0.08|p = 0.76	r = 0.10|p = 0.68	r = −0.10|p = 0.69
C-HDL (mmol/L)	r = 0.11|p = 0.68	r = −0.46|p = 0.07	r = −0.34|p = 0.195	r = 0.07|p = 0.79	r = 0.06|p = 0.81	r = −0.08|p = 0.75	r = 0.56|p = 0.02 *	r = 0.21|p = 0.43	r = 0.12|p = 0.65	r = 0.4135|p = 0.111	r = 0.24|p = 0.35	r = −0.44|p = 0.08
C-LDL (mmol/L)	r = 0.06|p = 0.82	r = 0.1752|p = 0.516	r = 0.050|p = 0.854	r = −0.03|p = 0.88	r = −0.12|p = 0.63	r = −0.08|p = 0.74	r = 0.14|p = 0.58	r = 0.14|p = 0.59	r = 0.07|p = 0.97	r = 0.0588|p = 0.829	r = 0.05|p = 0.85	r = −0.04|p = 0.86
Cortisol (mcg/dL)	r = 0.32 |p = 0.21	r = 0.2735|p = 0.305	r = −0.06|p = 0.812	r = 0.14|p = 0.60	r = 0.14|p = 0.59	r = 0.25|p = 0.34	r = −0.43|p = 0.09	r = −0.21|p = 0.41	r = 0.04|p = 0.87	r = −0.2787|p = 0.296	r = −0.07|p = 0.77	r = −0.04|p = 0.86
Testosterone (mcg/dL)	r = −0.18 |p = 0.49	r = −0.2311|p = 0.389	r = 0.013|p = 0.959	r = 0.41|p = 0.11	r = 0.47|p = 0.06	r = 0.43|p = 0.09	r = 0.25|p = 0.34	r = 0.46|p = 0.07	r = 0.10|p = 0.69	r = 0.3913|p = 0.134	r = 0.60|p = 0.014 *	r = 0.05|p = 0.84

BcP: Biochemical parameters; ALP: Alkaline phosphatase; CRP: C-reactive protein; TC: Total cholesterol; TG: Triglycerides; C-HDL: High-density lipoprotein cholesterol; C-LDL: Low-density lipoprotein cholesterol; * Denotes significance at $p < 0.05$.

A multilinear regression analysis was performed to verify which variable of percentage of change of training load (agreement with the correlation analysis) could be used to better explain the percentage of change of hematological and/or biochemical parameters.

The percentage of change of urine color was a predictor of the percentage of change of creatine ($r = -0.51$). The percentage of change of sleep quality was a predictor of the percentage of change of albumin ($r = 0.58$). The percentage of change of stress was a predictor of the percentage of change of EOS and albumin ($r = -0.50$ and $r = -0.53$). The percentage of change of fatigue was a predictor of the percentage of change of ALC ($r = -0.57$). The percentage of change of soreness and hooper index were predictors of the percentage of change of ALC ($r = 0.61$ and $r = 0.67$), respectively. The percentage of change of RPE (general) was a predictor of the percentage of change of MNC and C-HDL ($r = 0.73$ and $r = 0.56$), respectively. The percentage of change of RPE (neuromuscular) was a predictor of the percentage of change of NEUT, MNC and ALP ($r = -0.71, r = 0.53$, and $r = 0.50$), respectively. The percentage of change of sRPE (general) was a predictor of the percentage of change of MNC and sodium ($r = 0.60$ and $r = -0.60$), respectively. The percentage of change of sRPE (breath) was a predictor variable of the percentage of change of testosterone ($r = 0.60$) (see Table 6. for more information).

Table 6. Regression analysis for the percentage change of training loads based on percentage change on the remaining blood biomarkers.

Training Load	Biomarkers	b *	SE of B *	R^2	Adjusted R^2	F	p
% change of urine color	% change of creatine	−0.51	0.22	0.26	0.21	5.10	0.04
% change of sleep quality	% change of albumin	−0.58	0.21	0.34	0.30	7.44	0.01
% change of stress	% change of EOS	−0.50	0.23	0.25	0.20	4.86	0.04
	% change of albumin	−0.53	0.22	0.28	0.23	5.63	0.03
% change of fatigue	% change of ALC	0.57	0.21	0.32	0.27	6.80	0.02
% change of soreness	% change of ALC	0.61	0.21	0.37	0.33	8.40	0.01
% change of hooper index	% change of ALC	0.67	0.19	0.45	0.41	11.57	0.004
% change of RPE general	% change of MNC	0.73	0.18	0.53	0.50	16.02	0.001
	% change of C-HDL	0.56	0.21	0.32	0.27	6.70.	0.02
% change of RPE neuromuscular	% change of NEUT	−0.71	0.18	0.50	0.47	14.41	0.001
	% change of MNC	0.53	0.22	0.28	0.23	5.49	0.03
	% change of ALP	0.50	0.23	0.25	0.19	4.72	0.04
% change of sRPE general	% change of MNC	0.60	0.21	0.37	0.32	8.28	0.01
	% change of sodium	−0.60	0.21	0.36	0.31	8.05	0.01
% change of sRPE breath	% change of testosterone	0.60	0.21	0.36	0.31	7.90	0.01

* Denotes significance at $p < 0.05$.

4. Discussion

The purpose of this study was twofold: (i) Analyze the variations of biological markers before and after the pre-season period and (ii) analyze the relationships between variations of biological markers and workload imposed on the players. To the best of our knowledge, there is no study that addresses different blood biomarkers variations and their interactions with different internal load measures during the pre-season period. The major findings of the present study indicate that the Hooper Index, RPE (general, breath, and neuromuscular), and sRPE (general, breath, and neuromuscular) increased progressively after the pre-season. Likewise, PLT, creatinine, CRP, ALP, cortisol, and testosterone increased, whereas ANC, AMC, calcium, and calcium corrected decreased significantly after the pre-season period. Furthermore, several significant relationships were found between blood biomarkers, training load parameters (RPE and sRPE), and psychometric variables (the Hooper Index, fatigue, stress, soreness, and quality of sleep).

The pre-season is widely accepted to be the period with a high training load [38,39], and concomitant augmented risk of sustaining injuries [40]. High-quality pre-season soccer training plays a role not only in improving physical fitness (aerobic capacity), but also in injury prevention [41]. The monitoring of blood biomarkers before and after pre-season plays a role in increasing positive adaptation, and reducing the risk of injuries, illness, and overreaching caused by stress factors that occur during soccer matches over a season [42]. In our study, significant increases were found in training load parameters, the Hooper Index, RPE (general), RPE (breath), RPE (neuromuscular), sRPE (general), sRPE (breath), and sRPE (neuromuscular) after pre-season compared to before pre-season. Recent studies have frequently shown that internal or external workload indices [43]. In addition, the Hooper Index parameters were found to be higher during the pre-season period compared to other periods of the season [44,45]. The increase in training load parameters in the pre-season is usually due to the progressive overload principle of training, to prepare the players to meet the physical demands of the upcoming season [39].

Furthermore, the present study revealed a significant increase in PLT after the pre-season period. In the literature, there are studies with different results regarding the decrease [22], increase [46–48], or lack of changes [42] in PLT after long-term intensive soccer or different kinds of exercises. Michail et al. [46] revealed a similar conclusion to the results of the present study, as they found a significant increase from $231 \times 10^3/\mu L$ to $244 \times 10^3/\mu L$ of the PLT amount after the soccer intensive exercise intervention program. Moreover, a study conducted on 13 male soccer players, with significant augment in PLT levels (209.76 ± 33.83 to $249.76 \pm 61.09 \times 10^3/\mu L$) was noted following 2 weeks of pre-tournament moderate-to-high intensity training period [49]. Contrary to our study, Ozen et al. [50] found an increase in PLT after the pre-season training period in well-trained young soccer players. However, their reported increase (pre: 205.57 ± 54.94, post: 214.85 ± 23.12) was not significant.

The reason for a high number of circulating PLT in the blood (thrombocytosis) after intense soccer exercise can be explained by epinephrine hormone secration, which has the ability to cause a strong contraction of the spleen (the storage area of one-third of the body's PLT), and may play a role in the increase in PLT after exercise [51]. Likewise, it was declared that the mechanisms related to the increase in PLT after high intensity exercises were not clear [48]. However, those increases might be due to increased PLT production by cells in the bone marrow, and decreased removal of PLT from the blood, which was one of the functions of the spleen [48]. Another possible mechanism is shear and oxidative stress, which can activate PLT. Exercise-activated PLT contribute in growth factors liberation and proinflammatory mediators [52]. As in this study, an increase in PLT after intense exercise may also be associated with an improvement in performance. It was previously reported that hyperactive PLT have some pleiotropic effects on endurance sport performance, both by releasing ergogenic mediators and triggering an increase in performance-enhancing substances, such as nitric oxide into the circulation [53].

Regarding hematological parameters, our study revealed that the ANC and AMC significantly decreased after the pre-season period. Consistent with our findings, Heisterberg et al. [54] indicated that the numbers of circulating monocytes decreased at the end of a training season. In other study, it was noted that there was an increase in neutrophils and a decrease in lymphocytes after short periods of pre-tournament training [49]. Ozen et al. [50] reported no significant differences in subpopulations of leukocytes (lymphocytes, neutrophil, monocyte, and basophil percentage) after the pre-season period in young male football players. In a previous study, which was not consistent with the findings of our study in terms of neutrophil, an increase in neutrophil counts was found after regular and vigorous soccer exercises, and it was suggested that this situation was associated with minor inflammatory events [22]. In addition, contrary to our study, Dias et al. [55] notified an increase in total leukocyte, neutrophil, and monocyte counts, whereas lymphocytes reduced by the end of the season in volleyball athletes, and they also claimed that the increase in total neutrophils and monocytes might be due to muscle tissue remodeling, resulting from potential damage induced by training load and competition.

Furthermore, the present study revealed that decreases in ANC and AMC after the pre-season period may be related to the timing of blood collection after the last exercise session. In our study, there was a time of 12 h between the last training session, and the second blood draw (after the pre-season). This may have caused a short-term temporary suppression of the immune system in soccer players after the last training session, i.e., the previous day's acute high-intensity exercise. This situation is defined as "open window" immunological phenomenon in the literature [56–58]. Moreover, previous studies showed that high-intensity exercises could lead to a short-term, acute inflammatory response [59–62]. Another study also supports the findings of the present study, in which the authors alleged that intense endurance activities decreased neutrophils, and monocytes in athletes, and this condition was related to the depression of the immune systems, which triggered an increased the risk of disease or infection, especially the pre-season period [63]. Lastly, regarding the leukocyte count and subpopulations in the pre-season period, the present study shows that there is no pathological condition, only the decreases in ANC and AMC may be associated with timing of blood collections. It can also be suggested that training in pre-season do not produce chronic effects on immune function and susceptibility to infection.

Creatinine is a metabolic product of a creatine breakdown during energy metabolism. The serum creatinine level is a known parameter for evaluating renal function in clinical medicine, and is used as an indicator of general health status and water-electrolyte balance in sports medicine [64]. The present study revealed that there was a significant increase in creatinine after the pre-season period. Our results are not consistent with some studies. For instance, Meyer & Meister [65] found only minor changes in creatinine levels in professional football players over a season. Another study revealed that there was no significant change in the serum creatinine level of rugby players before and after the training camp [66]. Furthermore, Andelković et al. [22] affirmed that serum creatinine levels in soccer players decreased significantly throughout the study, which might be related to the increase in training and competition workloads during the half competitive season. Prior studies on soccer player demonstrated that creatinine levels were higher in players with greater training and match loads (cumulative match-time) throughout the season [64], and also increased post-match in comparison with pre-match values due to the high intensity of the performance during the match [67]. Regarding creatinine as a by-product of muscle contraction, its rise after a match or higher training load, especially the pre-season period, could be due to the deterioration of muscle tissue [67]. Additionally, another study asserted that the increase in plasma creatinine after intense soccer exercise stemmed from the creatinine release from working muscles, dehydration, and/or reduction in renal blood flow and glomerular filtration rate [68]. In our study, there were negative large correlations between the percentage of change of urine color and percentage of change of creatinine. After creatinine is used by the muscles, it is filtered by the kidneys, and excreted in the urine, based on this information, this study reveals that urine is the determinant of the percentage change in creatinine.

Increased levels of oxidative stress are closely associated with markers of muscle damage with high inflammation [59]. CRP is the most common inflammation molecule of the body's acute phase response, and it increases the inflammatory response to various stimuli that initiate the acute phase response [47,69,70]. In our study, significant increases were found in CRP values after post-pre-season compared to pre-pre-season. The CRP level has been found to increase during the inflamed state, that is, after intense exercise [71,72]. Significant increases in CRP after a soccer match in amateur soccer athletes was previously shown [47]. Mohr et al. [73] also found CRP values before (0.9 ± 0.1 mg/L), and after (1.3 ± 0.0 mg/L) the preparation period in professional soccer players. The studies mentioned above support the results of our study. However, these results differ from the study published by Radzimiński et al. [70], where it was found that elevated CRP values were not detected in soccer players during a pre-season sports camp (pre: 1.44 ± 0.7 mg/L, post: 0.83 ± 0.34 mg/L), i.e., above the reference range (<5.0 mg/L).

It was recently determined that decreases in CRP levels of futsal players, also asserted that reductions in the CRP level indicated that players adapt to the training load applied throughout the competitive season [59]. Radzimiński et al. [70], emphasized that inflammation in the bodies of pre-season soccer players might be the result of misuse of high-intensity training loads in a short time. On the other hand, a previous study stated that GPS variables associated with high-intensity activities, such as running speeds, accelerations, and decelerations were useful markers for detecting muscle damage or inflammation [74]. Similarly, Coppalle et al. [69] found a significant and very large correlation between total distance covered (>20 km/h) and CRP after the pre-season period in professional soccer players. The increment in CRP after the pre-season may be related to the frequent use of high-intensity activities in training during this period. However, the present study exhibited that this increase in CRP does not seem to reflect a pathological condition. Finally, it was pointed out that the rise in CRP after intensive exercise could be the result of mechanisms, such as the inflammatory response to injuries or agents (interleukin-6, i.e., the main stimulator of CRP secretion) that might be associated with elevated inflammation in athletes [47].

Moreover, the present study showed that alkaline phosphatase (ALP) significantly increased after the pre-season period. In the literature, some studies showed that ALP increased after intense soccer exercise [68,75], while some studies showed that no significant change in the ALP level of players with a higher training load over a season [64]. As in our study, the increase in ALP after intense soccer exercises might be associated with the result of some leakage from skeletal muscles of enzymes that play a role in the sustained release of ATP, and catabolize amino acids during exercises [68]. In addition, the increase in ALP after the pre-season period in our study may be explained by another study [76], as the authors suggested that the elevation in ALP levels reflected liver increased activity for gluconeogenesis, lipid peroxidation, and increased bone turnover triggered by the duration and intensity of exercise. Considering the CRP and ALP parameters related to inflammation, the physiological increase in CRP and ALP may be the result of acute high-intensity exercise [61] performed the day before blood collections. However, the present study demonstrated that pre-season intense soccer training does not cause any chronic effect on susceptibility to inflammation.

Calcium is a necessary mineral for proper growth, maintenance, and repair of bone tissue, nerve conduction, blood coagulation, and regulation of muscle contraction. Serum calcium level is tightly arranged by calcitonin and parathyroid hormone, independent of acute calcium intake [77–79]. In our study, statistically significant reductions were found in the calcium and calcium corrected after the pre-season period. The study of Mashiko et al. [66] does not coincide with our results, as they reported that there was no significant difference in the serum calcium level of rugby players after 20 days of pre-season intensive training. In our study, the decrease in calcium after an intense pre-season period can be explained as follows; calcium may leak into the tissue to create muscle contractions during exercise, so blood levels may decrease after intense exercises. In the report published by the UEFA expert group on nutrition in elite soccer, a daily calcium intake of 1300–1500 mg/dL is recommended for professional soccer players to optimize bone health in cases of relative energy deficiency in sports [77]. Accordingly, a recent study determined that soccer players did not meet their daily calcium needs in the pre-season period [79]. Given the importance of calcium for bone health, reductions in calcium concentration may result in decreases in bone mineral density, which can elevate the risk of injury to players throughout the season.

Cortisol and testosterone hormones play a role in catabolic and anabolic processes [80], are frequently used in studies as training stress markers, and these markers are closely associated with overreaching and overtraining syndromes [28,81]. The results found in the present study demonstrated that both cortisol and testosterone were significantly augmented in response to a soccer pre-season period. Di Luigi et al. [82] reported that salivary cortisol and testosterone level increased after an acute response to soccer exercise in young soccer player. Similarly, Muscella et al. [83] observed increases in both testosterone and cortisol levels after an intense training period in soccer referees. Nogueira et al. [84] remarked that testosterone increased, while the cortisol hormone decreased in futsal players after 4-weeks of pre-season. The same authors [84], noted that these results promoted an anabolic environment, which is also consistent with the finding of the study conducted by Perroni et al. [81]. Nevertheless, there are studies showing the formation of a catabolic environment (increases in cortisol, and decreases in testosterone levels) due to a high training load in the pre-season period [28,29,39,42]. It was reported that such a catabolic physiological environment could adversely affect various physical performance-related parameters such as speed, vertical jump height, and muscle strength throughout the season [28]. The T/C ratio is used to evaluate the balance between anabolic and catabolic activity [85,86], and represents a beneficial tool in the early detection of overtraining [87]. The present study revealed that there were no significant changes in the T/C ratio after the pre-season training period. This result was supported by a previous study that showed that no significant changes in the T/C ratio after intense pre-season traninig in soccer players [88], and non-athletic men [83]. Contrary to our findings, recent studies observed significant reductions in the T/C ratio in response to a high volume of training sessions [39,89], and a period of congested match play [86,89] in professional soccer players. Similarly, another study demonstrated that a decrease equal or higher than 30% in the T/C ratio reflected state of catabolism, which resulted in a prolonged recovery time, fatigue, and deterioration of competitive soccer performance [90]. Additionally, our result was not similar to previous studies that reported that the T/C ratio increased significantly in team sports athletes after the pre-season period [81,84,85,89]. As in the present study, Botelho et al. [88] stated that a significantly unchanged T/C ratio after the pre-season period was associated with a favorable response to the training load, and adequate coping with training stresses. The current study revealed that the T/C ratio, which did not change significantly, and the conversely significant increases in cortisol and testosterone, after the pre-season could be explained by an environment that reflects a dynamic hemostatic balance between an anabolic and catabolic process in muscle [81,83]. This is very important in terms of both the prevention of the risk of injury of the players, and the quality of their physical performance during the training and competition season. Nonetheless, considering the testosterone, cortisol, and T/C ratio, the training load distribution and the load-rest relationship are well adjusted during the pre-season period, and the players have responded adequately to the training load without the accumulation of fatigue. Additionally, they probably have not experienced overreaching and overtraining. Moreover, the current study showed that the percentage of change of sRPE breath was a predictor variable of percentage of change of testosterone. Consistent with the present study, Peñailillo et al. [91] reported that the rate of perceived exertion was positively related to the change in testosterone levels. Accordingly, another study found that a higher internal training load (RPE-based) triggered anabolic stimulus (that is increases testosterone secretion) which positively affected performance in professional soccer players [92].

The present study indicated that negative large correlations were observed between a percentage of change of sleep quality and percentage of change of albumin, and also a percentage of sleep quality was a predictor variable of percentage of change of albumin. Sleep needs and rest are important for rapid recovery, and preventing the risk of illness, injury, and bad-overreaching in the pre-season period [93]. The deterioration in sleep quality due to a higher training load can be observed in the pre-season period, which may negatively affect biochemical parameters, especially albumin [30,42]. A previous study showed that that high-volume running exercises, which were frequently performed during pre-season training, caused a high sweating rate, which led to blood thickening, and as a result, it triggered an increase in the amount of albumin in the blood. Furthermore, in our study, blood measurements were performed in the morning hours (08.00–10.00 a.m.).

Moreover, it was indicated that the augment in serum albumin levels in morning hours was closely related to the fact that normal blood thickening was not restored by overnight rest after exercise [66].

In the literature, there are limited studies examining the relationship between internal load indices (RPE, sRPE), wellness parameters (hooper index), and blood biomarkers. This is the first study to examine the relationship between pre-season training load (RPE, sRPE, and the Hooper Index) and blood biomarkers. Still, regarding the relationships between blood biomarkers, training load parameters (RPE and sRPE), and psychometric variables found in the present study, it is suggested that the internal load and Hooper Index parameters are associated with markers of inflammation and muscle damage. Interestingly, Dias et al. [55] reported that immune variables, such as total leukocytes, neutrophils, and lymphocytes might be modulated by training loads and by tactical and physical components. Indeed, Coppalle et al. [69] indicated that muscle damage or inflammation indicators, such as lactate dehydrogenase were correlated to RPE values, and suggested that the fatigue-related muscle damage enzyme increased at high perceived exertion levels. The same findings were also observed in our study. However, further research is needed to generalize the results from this study.

The present study contains some limitations that should be emphasized. First, the number of participants in our study was not very large. Considering the relationship between nutrition and hematological/biochemical parameters, no determination was made regarding the nutritional status of players in the pre-season period. In other words, the food consumption of players was not followed nor were there even supplements taken in the period. Furthermore, no measurements were made regarding the injury rate of the players. The relationship between pre-season training load parameters and injury rate could be examined. Despite the limitations mentioned above, the present study is to first examine different blood biomarkers variations and their interactions with different internal load measures during the pre-season period. In the future, by elevating the number of participants, it is recommended to increase the number of studies to compare blood biomarkers taking into account the gender and age factor in teams in different leagues according to player positions during the pre-season or the entire season, and to examine the relationships between these biomarkers, training load, and injury rate.

5. Conclusions

The present study revealed that intense training in the preseason period leads to decreases (ANC, AMC, calcium, and calcium corrected), and increases (PLT, creatinine, CRP, ALP, cortisol, and testosterone) in different hematological and biochemical markers. The present study also showed several significant relationships between blood biomarkers, training load parameters, and wellness variables. Given that, training load distribution is of critical importance in the optimization of blood biomarkers, especially during the pre-season period. In addition, ensuring a balance between the training load and blood biomarkers in the pre-season period contributes to the maintenance of high level physical performance of players during the entire season, and to prevent the risk of injury, bad-overreaching, and overtraining. Moreover, comprehensive monitoring of blood biomarkers in terms of hematological, nutritional, biochemical, muscle damage, and hormonal markers along with internal load indices and wellness measures can provide clearer insights into the mechanisms underlying players' performance throughout the season.

Author Contributions: Conceptualization, F.M.C.; methodology, F.M.C. and F.T.G.-F.; data collection: S.Y.; formal analysis, F.T.G.-F. and R.S.; writing—original draft preparation, F.M.C., F.T.G.-F., H.I.C., R.S., S.Y., Y.-S.C., G.B., P.W. and E.M.-C.; writing—review and editing, F.M.C., F.T.G.-F., H.I.C., R.S., S.Y., Y.-S.C., G.B., P.W. and E.M.-C.; supervision, F.M.C. All authors have read and agreed to the published version of the manuscript.

Funding: This work is funded by Fundação para a Ciência e Tecnologia/Ministério da Ciência, Tecnologia e Ensino Superior through national funds and when applicable, co-funded EU funds under project UIDB/EEA/50008/2020.

Institutional Review Board Statement: The study protocol was approved by the Scientific Committee of School of Sport and Leisure (Melgaço, Portugal) with code number CTC-ESDL-CE00118. The study followed the ethical standards of the Declaration of Helsinki.

Informed Consent Statement: Informed consent was obtained from all subjects involved in the study.

Acknowledgments: This study made is a part of one curricular unit of Master in Sports Training at Escola Superior de Desporto e Lazer, Instituto Politécnico de Viana do Castelo, Portugal.

Conflicts of Interest: The authors declare no conflict of interest.

References

1. Dolci, F.; Hart, N.H.; Kilding, A.; Chivers, P.; Piggott, B.; Spiteri, T. Movement Economy in Soccer: Current Data and Limitations. *Sports* **2018**, *6*, 124. [CrossRef] [PubMed]
2. Slimani, M.; Znazen, H.; Miarka, B.; Bragazzi, N.L. Maximum Oxygen Uptake of Male Soccer Players According to their Competitive Level, Playing Position and Age Group: Implication from a Network Meta-Analysis. *J. Hum. Kinet.* **2019**, *66*, 233–245. [CrossRef] [PubMed]
3. Andrzejewski, M.; Konarski, J.M.; Chmura, J.; Pluta, B. Changes in the activity profiles of soccer players over a three-match training micro cycle. *Int. J. Perform. Anal. Sport* **2014**, *14*, 814–828. [CrossRef]
4. Saeidi, A.; Khodamoradi, A. Physical and Physiological Demand of Soccer Player Based on Scientific Research. *Int. J. App. Sci. Physic. Edu* **2017**, *1*, 1–12.
5. Dolci, F.; Hart, N.H.; Kilding, A.E.; Chivers, P.; Piggott, B.; Spiteri, T. Physical and Energetic Demand of Soccer: A Brief Review. *Strength Cond. J.* **2020**, *42*, 70–77. [CrossRef]
6. Harper, D.J.; Carling, C.; Kiely, J. High-Intensity Acceleration and Deceleration Demands in Elite Team Sports Competitive Match Play: A Systematic Review and Meta-Analysis of Observational Studies. *Sport. Med.* **2019**, *49*, 1923–1947. [CrossRef]
7. Clemente, F.M.; Silva, R.; Castillo, D.; Los Arcos, A.; Mendes, B.; Afonso, J. Weekly Load Variations of Distance-Based Variables in Professional Soccer Players: A Full-Season Study. *Int. J. Environ. Res. Public Health* **2020**, *17*, 3300. [CrossRef]
8. Martín-García, A.; Casamichana, D.; Gómez Díaz, A.; Cos, F.; Gabbett, T.J. Positional differences in the most demanding passages of play in football competition. *J. Sport. Sci. Med.* **2018**, *17*, 563–570.
9. Clemente, F. Detrimental Effects of the Off-Season in Soccer Players: A Systematic Review and Meta-analysis. *Sport. Med.* **2021**, *51*, 795–814. [CrossRef]
10. Silva, J.R.; Brito, J.; Akenhead, R.; Nassis, G.P. The Transition Period in Soccer: A Window of Opportunity. *Sport. Med.* **2016**, *46*, 305–313. [CrossRef]
11. Meckel, Y.; Doron, O.; Eliakim, E.; Eliakim, A. Seasonal Variations in Physical Fitness and Performance Indices of Elite Soccer Players. *Sports* **2018**, *6*, 14. [CrossRef]
12. Silva, R.; Lima, R.; Camões, M.; Leão, C.; Matos, S.; Pereira, J.; Bezerra, P.; Clemente, F.M. Physical fitness changes among amateur soccer players: Effects of the pre-season period. *Biomed. Hum. Kinet.* **2021**, *13*, 63–72. [CrossRef]
13. Los Arcos, A.; Castillo, D.; Martínez-Santos, R. Influence of initial performance level and tactical position on the aerobic fitness in soccer players after preseason period. *Sci. Med. Footb.* **2018**, *2*, 294–298. [CrossRef]
14. Nobari, H.; Alves, A.R.; Haghighi, H.; Clemente, F.M.; Carlos-Vivas, J.; Pérez-Gómez, J.; Ardigò, L.P. Association between training load and well-being measures in young soccer players during a season. *Int. J. Environ. Res. Public Health* **2021**, *18*, 4451. [CrossRef] [PubMed]
15. Hooper, S.L.; Mackinnon, L.T. Monitoring Overtraining in Athletes. *Sport. Med.* **1995**, *20*, 321–327. [CrossRef] [PubMed]
16. Clemente, F.M.; Mendes, B.; Nikolaidis, P.T.; Calvete, F.; Carriço, S.; Owen, A.L. Internal training load and its longitudinal relationship with seasonal player wellness in elite professional soccer. *Physiol. Behav.* **2017**, *179*, 262–267. [CrossRef]
17. Rabbani, A.; Clemente, F.M.; Kargarfard, M.; Chamari, K. Match Fatigue Time-Course Assessment Over Four Days: Usefulness of the Hooper Index and Heart Rate Variability in Professional Soccer Players. *Front. Physiol.* **2019**, *10*. [CrossRef] [PubMed]
18. Impellizzeri, F.M.; Rampinini, E.; Coutts, A.J.; Sassi, A.; Marcora, S.M. Use of RPE-based training load in soccer. *Med. Sci. Sports Exerc.* **2004**, *36*, 1042–1047. [CrossRef] [PubMed]
19. Arcos, A.L.; Yanci, J.; Mendiguchia, J.; Gorostiaga, E.M. Rating of Muscular and Respiratory Perceived Exertion in Professional Soccer Players. *J. Strength Cond. Res.* **2014**, *28*, 3280–3288. [CrossRef]
20. Borg, E.; Borg, G.; Larsson, K.; Letzter, M.; Sundblad, B.-M. An index for breathlessness and leg fatigue. *Scand. J. Med. Sci. Sports* **2010**, *20*, 644–650. [CrossRef]
21. Los Arcos, A.; Martínez-Santos, R.; Yanci, J.; Mendiguchia, J.; Méndez-Villanueva, A. Negative Associations between Perceived Training Load, Volume and Changes in Physical Fitness in Professional Soccer Players. *J. Sports Sci. Med.* **2015**, *14*, 394.
22. Andelkovic, M.; Baralic, I.; Dordevic, B.; Stevuljevic, J.K.; Radivojevic, N.; Dikic, N.; Škodric, S.R.; Stojkovic, M. Hematological and Biochemical Parameters in Elite Soccer Players during A Competitive Half Season. *J. Med. Biochem.* **2015**, *34*, 460–466. [CrossRef] [PubMed]
23. Bekris, E.; Gioldasis, A.; Gissis, I.; Anagnostakos, K.; Eleftherios, M. From Preparation to Competitive Period in Soccer: Hematological Changes. *Sport Sci. Rev.* **2015**, *24*, 103–114. [CrossRef]

24. Silva, A.S.R.; Santhiago, V.; Papoti, M.; Gobatto, C.A. Hematological parameters and anaerobic threshold in Brazilian soccer players throughout a training program. *Int. J. Lab. Hematol.* **2008**, *30*, 158–166. [CrossRef]
25. Requena, B.; García, I.; Suárez-Arrones, L.; Sáez De Villarreal, E.; Naranjo Orellana, J.; Santalla, A. Off-Season Effects on Functional Performance, Body Composition, and Blood Parameters in Top-Level Professional Soccer Players. *J. Strength Cond. Res.* **2017**, *31*, 939–946. [CrossRef]
26. Hader, K.; Rumpf, M.C.; Hertzog, M.; Kilduff, L.P.; Girard, O.; Silva, J.R. Monitoring the Athlete Match Response: Can External Load Variables Predict Post-match Acute and Residual Fatigue in Soccer? A Systematic Review with Meta-analysis. *Sport. Med.-Open* **2019**, *5*, 48. [CrossRef]
27. Rowell, A.E.; Aughey, R.J.; Hopkins, W.G.; Stewart, A.M.; Cormack, S.J. Identification of sensitive measures of recovery after external load from football match play. *Int. J. Sports Physiol. Perform.* **2017**, *12*, 969–976. [CrossRef]
28. Kraemer, W.J.; French, D.N.; Paxton, N.J.; Häkkinen, K.; Volek, J.S.; Sebastianelli, W.J.; Putukian, M.; Newton, R.U.; Rubin, M.R.; Gómez, A.L.; et al. Changes in exercise performance and hormonal concentrations over a big ten soccer season in starters and nonstarters. *J. Strength Cond. Res.* **2004**, *18*, 121–128. [PubMed]
29. Cormack, S.J.; Newton, R.U.; McGuigan, M.R.; Cormie, P. Neuromuscular and endocrine responses of elite players during an Australian rules football season. *Int. J. Sports Physiol. Perform.* **2008**, *3*, 439–453. [CrossRef] [PubMed]
30. Pedlar, C.R.; Newell, J.; Lewis, N.A. Blood Biomarker Profiling and Monitoring for High-Performance Physiology and Nutrition: Current Perspectives, Limitations and Recommendations. *Sport. Med.* **2019**, *49*, 185–198. [CrossRef] [PubMed]
31. von Elm, E.; Altman, D.G.; Egger, M.; Pocock, S.J.; Gøtzsche, P.C.; Vandenbroucke, J.P. The Strengthening the Reporting of Observational Studies in Epidemiology (STROBE) Statement: Guidelines for Reporting Observational Studies. *Int. J. Surg.* **2014**, *12*, 1495–1499. [CrossRef]
32. Borg, G. *Perceived Exertion and Pain Scales*; Human Kinetics: Champaign, IL, USA, 1998; ISBN 0880116234.
33. Foster, C.; Florhaug, J.A.; Franklin, J.; Gottschall, L.; Hrovatin, L.A.; Parker, S.; Doleshal, P.; Dodge, C. A new approach to monitoring exercise training. *J. Strength Cond. Res.* **2001**, *15*, 109–115.
34. Foster, C. Monitoring training in athletes with reference to overtraining syndrome. *Med. Sci. Sports Exerc.* **1998**, *30*, 1164–1168. [CrossRef]
35. Armstrong, L.E.; Maresh, C.M.; Castellani, J.W.; Bergeron, M.F.; Kenefick, R.W.; LaGasse, K.E.; Riebe, D. Urinary Indices of Hydration Status. *Int. J. Sport Nutr.* **1994**, *4*, 265–279. [CrossRef]
36. Kavouras, S.A.; Johnson, E.C.; Bougatsas, D.; Arnaoutis, G.; Panagiotakos, D.B.; Perrier, E.; Klein, A. Validation of a urine color scale for assessment of urine osmolality in healthy children. *Eur. J. Nutr.* **2016**, *55*, 907–915. [CrossRef] [PubMed]
37. Batterham, A.M.; Hopkins, W.G. Making Meaningful Inferences about Magnitudes. *Int. J. Sports Physiol. Perform.* **2006**, *1*, 50–57. [CrossRef] [PubMed]
38. Djaoui, L.; Haddad, M.; Chamari, K.; Dellal, A. Monitoring training load and fatigue in soccer players with physiological markers. *Physiol. Behav.* **2017**, *181*, 86–94. [CrossRef]
39. Selmi, O.; Ouergui, I.; Levitt, E.D.; Marzouki, H.; Knechtle, B.; Nikolaidis, P.T.; Bouassida, A. Training, psychometric status, biological markers and neuromuscular fatigue in soccer. *Biol. Sport* **2022**, *39*, 319–327. [CrossRef]
40. Jones, C.M.; Griffiths, P.C.; Mellalieu, S.D. Training Load and Fatigue Marker Associations with Injury and Illness: A Systematic Review of Longitudinal Studies. *Sport. Med.* **2017**, *47*, 943–974. [CrossRef]
41. Eliakim, E.; Doron, O.; Meckel, Y.; Nemet, D.; Eliakim, A. Pre-season Fitness Level and Injury Rate in Professional Soccer—A Prospective Study. *Sport. Med. Int. Open* **2018**, *02*, 84–90. [CrossRef] [PubMed]
42. Huggins, R.A.; Fortunati, A.R.; Curtis, R.M.; Looney, D.P.; West, C.A.; Lee, E.C.; Fragala, M.S.; Hall, M.L.; Casa, D.J. Monitoring Blood Biomarkers and Training Load Throughout a Collegiate Soccer Season. *J. Strength Cond. Res.* **2019**, *33*, 3065–3077. [CrossRef] [PubMed]
43. Clemente, F.; Silva, R.; Ramirez-Campillo, R.; Afonso, J.; Mendes, B.; Chen, Y.-S. Accelerometry-based variables in professional soccer players: Comparisons between periods of the season and playing positions. *Biol. Sport* **2020**, *37*, 389–403. [CrossRef]
44. Ferreira, M.; Camões, M.; Lima, R.F.; Silva, R.; Castro, H.D.O.; Mendes, B.; Bezerra, P.; Clemente, F.M. Variations of workload and well-being measures across a professional basketball season. *Rev. Bras. Cineantropometria Desempenho Hum.* **2021**, *23*, e75863. [CrossRef]
45. Fessi, M.S.; Nouira, S.; Dellal, A.; Owen, A.; Elloumi, M.; Moalla, W. Changes of the psychophysical state and feeling of wellness of professional soccer players during pre-season and in-season periods. *Res. Sport. Med.* **2016**, *24*, 375–386. [CrossRef] [PubMed]
46. Michail, M.; Athanasios, S.; Ioannis, I.; Aristotelis, G.; Konstantinos, M.; Alexandros, I.; Georgios, A. Effects of small-sided games on the haematological profile of soccer players. *J. Phys. Educ. Sport* **2021**, *21*, 1860–1870.
47. Souglis, A.; Antonios, T.K. The influence of competitive activity on selected biochemical and haematological parameters of amateur soccer athletes. *J. Phys. Educ. Sport* **2015**, *15*, 24–31.
48. Younesian, A.; Rahnama, N. Haematology of professional soccer players before and after 90 min match. *Cell. Mol. Biol. Lett.* **2015**, *9*, 133–136.
49. Osei, F.; Moses, M.O.; Pambo, P.; Baffour-Awuah, B.; Asamoah, B.; Afrifa, D.; Appiah, E.J.; Akwa, L.G.; Obour, A. Changes in cardiovascular parameters of a-university football athletes associated with short duration pre-tournament training. *Sci. Afr.* **2020**, *8*, 1–6. [CrossRef]

50. Özen, G.; Atar, Ö.; Yurdakul, H.; Pehlivan, B.; Koç, H. The effect of pre-season football training on hematological parameters of well-trained young male football players. *Pedagog. Phys. Cult. Sport.* **2020**, *24*, 303–309. [CrossRef]
51. Zar, A.; Ahmadi, F.; Krustrup, P.; Fernandes, R.J. Effect of high-intensity interval exercise in the morning and evening on platelet indices and exercise-induced thrombocytosis. *Middle East J. Rehabil. Heal. Stud.* **2020**, *7*, e104417. [CrossRef]
52. Heber, S.; Volf, I. Effects of Physical (In)activity on Platelet Function. *Biomed Res. Int.* **2015**, *2015*, 1–11. [CrossRef]
53. Lippi, G.; Salvagno, G.L.; Danese, E.; Skafidas, S.; Tarperi, C.; Guidi, G.C.; Schena, F. Mean platelet volume (MPV) predicts middle distance running performance. *PLoS ONE* **2014**, *9*, e0112892. [CrossRef]
54. Heisterberg, M.F.; Fahrenkrug, J.; Krustrup, P.; Storskov, A.; Kjær, M.; Andersen, J.L. Extensive monitoring through multiple blood samples in professional soccer players. *J. Strength Cond. Res.* **2013**, *27*, 1260–1271. [CrossRef] [PubMed]
55. Dias, R.; Frollini, A.B.; Brunelli, D.T.; Yamada, A.K.; Leite, R.D.; Simões, R.A.; Cavaglieri, C.R. Immune parameters, symptoms of upper respiratory tract infections, and training-load indicators in volleyball athletes. *Int. J. Gen. Med.* **2011**, *4*, 837–844.
56. Gonçalves, C.A.M.; Dantas, P.M.S.; dos Santos, I.K.; Dantas, M.; da Silva, D.C.P.; Cabral, B.G.D.A.T.; Guerra, R.O.; Júnior, G.B.C. Effect of Acute and Chronic Aerobic Exercise on Immunological Markers: A Systematic Review. *Front. Physiol.* **2020**, *10*, 1602. [CrossRef] [PubMed]
57. Kakanis, M.W.; Peake, J.; Brenu, E.W.; Simmonds, M.; Gray, B.; Hooper, S.L.; Marshall-Gradisnik, S.M. The open window of susceptibility to infection after acute exercise in healthy young male elite athletes. *Exerc. Immunol. Rev.* **2010**, *16*, 119–137. [CrossRef]
58. Suzuki, K.; Hayashida, H. Effect of Exercise Intensity on Cell-Mediated Immunity. *Sports* **2021**, *9*, 8. [CrossRef] [PubMed]
59. Barcelos, R.P.; Tocchetto, G.L.; Lima, F.D.; Stefanello, S.T.; Rodrigues, H.F.M.; Sangoi, M.B.; Moresco, R.N.; Royes, L.F.F.; Soares, F.A.A.; Bresciani, G. Functional and biochemical adaptations of elite level futsal players from Brazil along a training season. *Medicina* **2017**, *53*, 285–293. [CrossRef]
60. Cerqueira, É.; Marinho, D.A.; Neiva, H.P.; Lourenço, O. Inflammatory Effects of High and Moderate Intensity Exercise—A Systematic Review. *Front. Physiol.* **2020**, *10*, 1550. [CrossRef]
61. Kasapis, C.; Thompson, P.D. The effects of physical activity on serum C-reactive protein and inflammatory markers: A systematic review. *J. Am. Coll. Cardiol.* **2005**, *45*, 1563–1569. [CrossRef]
62. Malm, C.; Sjödin, B.; Sjöberg, B.; Lenkei, R.; Renström, P.; Lundberg, I.E.; Ekblom, B. Leukocytes, cytokines, growth factors and hormones in human skeletal muscle and blood after uphill or downhill running. *J. Physiol.* **2004**, *556*, 983–1000. [CrossRef]
63. Bachero-Mena, B.; Pareja-Blanco, F.; González-Badillo, J.J. Enhanced Strength and Sprint Levels, and Changes in Blood Parameters during a Complete Athletics Season in 800 m High-Level Athletes. *Front. Physiol.* **2017**, *8*, 637. [CrossRef]
64. Nowakowska, A.; Kostrzewa-Nowak, D.; Buryta, R.; Nowak, R. Blood biomarkers of recovery efficiency in soccer players. *Int. J. Environ. Res. Public Health* **2019**, *16*, 3279. [CrossRef] [PubMed]
65. Meyer, T.; Meister, S. Routine blood parameters in elite soccer players. *Int. J. Sports Med.* **2011**, *32*, 875–881. [CrossRef] [PubMed]
66. Mashiko, T.; Umeda, T.; Nakaji, S.; Sugawara, K. Effects of exercise on the physical condition of college rugby players during summer training camp. *Br. J. Sports Med.* **2004**, *38*, 186–190. [CrossRef] [PubMed]
67. Colombini, A.; Machado, M.; Lombardi, G.; Lanteri, P.; Banfi, G. Modifications of biochemical parameters related to protein metabolism and renal function in male soccer players after a match. *J. Sports Med. Phys. Fitness* **2014**, *54*, 658–664.
68. Ekun, O.A.; Emiabata, A.F.; Abiodun, O.C.; Ogidi, N.O.; Adefolaju, F.O.; Ekun, O.O. Effects of football sporting activity on renal and liver functions among young undergraduate students of a Nigerian tertiary institution. *BMJ Open Sport Exerc. Med.* **2017**, *3*, e000223. [CrossRef]
69. Coppalle, S.; Rave, G.; Ben Abderrahman, A.; Ali, A.; Salhi, I.; Zouita, S.; Zouita, A.; Brughelli, M.; Granacher, U.; Zouhal, H. Relationship of pre-season training load with in-season biochemical markers, injuries and performance in professional soccer players. *Front. Physiol.* **2019**, *10*, 409. [CrossRef]
70. Radzimiński, Ł.; Jastrzębski, Z.; López-Sánchez, G.F.; Szwarc, A.; Duda, H.; Stuła, A.; Paszulewicz, J.; Dragos, P. Relationships between training loads and selected blood parameters in professional soccer players during a 12-day sports camp. *Int. J. Environ. Res. Public Health* **2020**, *17*, 8580. [CrossRef]
71. Margeli, A.; Skenderi, K.; Tsironi, M.; Hantzi, E.; Matalas, A.L.; Vrettou, C.; Kanavakis, E.; Chrousos, G.; Papassotiriou, I. Dramatic elevations of interleukin-6 and acute-phase reactants in athletes participating in the ultradistance foot race Spartathlon: Severe systemic inflammation and lipid and lipoprotein changes in protracted exercise. *J. Clin. Endocrinol. Metab.* **2005**, *90*, 3914–3918. [CrossRef]
72. Martín-Sánchez, F.J.; Villalón, J.M.; Zamorano-León, J.J.; Rosas, L.F.; Proietti, R.; Mateos-Caceres, P.J.; González-Armengol, J.J.; Villarroel, P.; Macaya, C.; López-Farré, A.J. Functional status and inflammation after preseason training program in professional and recreational soccer players: A proteomic approach. *J. Sport. Sci. Med.* **2011**, *10*, 45–51.
73. Mohr, M.; Draganidis, D.; Chatzinikolaou, A.; Barbero-Álvarez, J.C.; Castagna, C.; Douroudos, I.; Avloniti, A.; Margeli, A.; Papassotiriou, I.; Flouris, A.D.; et al. Muscle damage, inflammatory, immune and performance responses to three football games in 1 week in competitive male players. *Eur. J. Appl. Physiol.* **2016**, *116*, 179–193. [CrossRef]
74. Young, W.B.; Hepner, J.; Robbins, D.W. Movement demands in Australian Rules football as indicators of muscle damage. *J. Strength Cond. Res.* **2012**, *26*, 492–496. [CrossRef] [PubMed]
75. Ghorbani, P.; Gaeini, A. The effect of one bout high intensity interval training on liver enzymes level in elite soccer players. *J. Basic Appl. Sci.* **2013**, *5*, 1191–1194.

76. Bürger-Mendonça, M.; Bielavsky, M.; Barbosa, F.C.R. Liver overload in Brazilian triathletes after half-ironman competition is related muscle fatigue. *Ann. Hepatol.* **2008**, *7*, 245–248. [CrossRef]
77. Collins, J.; Maughan, R.J.; Gleeson, M.; Bilsborough, J.; Jeukendrup, A.; Morton, J.P.; Phillips, S.M.; Armstrong, L.; Burke, L.M.; Close, G.L.; et al. UEFA expert group statement on nutrition in elite football. Current evidence to inform practical recommendations and guide future research. *Br. J. Sports Med.* **2021**, *55*, 416. [CrossRef] [PubMed]
78. Goolsby, M.A.; Boniquit, N. Bone Health in Athletes: The Role of Exercise, Nutrition, and Hormones. *Sports Health* **2017**, *9*, 108–117. [CrossRef] [PubMed]
79. Książek, A.; Zagrodna, A.; Słowińska-Lisowska, M. Assessment of the dietary intake of high-rank professional male football players during a preseason training week. *Int. J. Environ. Res. Public Health* **2020**, *17*, 8567. [CrossRef]
80. Fragala, M.S.; Kraemer, W.J.; Denegar, C.R.; Maresh, C.M.; Mastro, A.M.; Volek, J.S. Neuroendocrine-immune interactions and responses to exercise. *Sport. Med.* **2011**, *41*, 621–639. [CrossRef]
81. Perroni, F.; Fittipaldi, S.; Falcioni, L.; Ghizzoni, L.; Borrione, P.; Vetrano, M.; Del Vescovo, R.; Migliaccio, S.; Guidetti, L.; Baldari, C. Effect of pre-season training phase on anthropometric, hormonal and fitness parameters in young soccer players. *PLoS ONE* **2019**, *14*, e0225471. [CrossRef]
82. Di Luigi, L.; Baldari, C.; Gallotta, M.C.; Perroni, F.; Romanelli, F.; Lenzi, A.; Guidetti, L. Salivary steroids at rest and after a training load in young male athletes: Relationship with chronological age and pubertal development. *Int. J. Sports Med.* **2006**, *27*, 709–717. [CrossRef]
83. Muscella, A.; Stefàno, E.; Marsigliante, S. The effects of training on hormonal concentrations and physical performance of football referees. *Physiol. Rep.* **2021**, *9*, e14740. [CrossRef]
84. Nogueira, F.C.D.A.; de Freitas, V.H.; Nogueira, R.A.; Miloski, B.; Werneck, F.Z.; Bara-Filho, M.G. Improvement of physical performance, hormonal profile, recovery-stress balance and increase of muscle damage in a specific futsal pre-season planning. *Rev. Andaluza Med. Del Deport.* **2018**, *11*, 63–68. [CrossRef]
85. Michailidis, Y. Stress hormonal analysis in elite soccer players during a season. *J. Sport Heal. Sci.* **2014**, *3*, 279–283. [CrossRef]
86. Saidi, K.; Ben Abderrahman, A.; Boullosa, D.; Dupont, G.; Hackney, A.C.; Bideau, B.; Pavillon, T.; Granacher, U.; Zouhal, H. The Interplay Between Plasma Hormonal Concentrations, Physical Fitness, Workload and Mood State Changes to Periods of Congested Match Play in Professional Soccer Players. *Front. Physiol.* **2020**, *11*, 835. [CrossRef]
87. Roli, L.; De Vincentis, S.; Rocchi, M.B.L.; Trenti, T.; De Santis, M.C.; Savino, G. Testosterone, cortisol, hGH, and IGF-1 levels in an Italian female elite volleyball team. *Health Sci. Reports* **2018**, *1*, e32. [CrossRef] [PubMed]
88. Botelho, R.; Abad, C.C.C.; Spadari, R.C.; Winckler, C.; Garcia, M.C.; Guerra, R.L.F. Psychophysiological Stress Markers During Preseason Among Elite Female Soccer Players. *J. Strength Cond. Res.* **2020**. Publish Ahead. [CrossRef]
89. Coelho, D.B.; Pimenta, E.M.; da Paixão, R.C.; Morandi, R.F.; Becker, L.K.; Ferreira-Júnior, J.B.; Coelho, L.G.M.; Silami-Garcia, E. Análise da demanda fisiológica crônica de uma temporada anual de futebol. *Rev. Bras. Cineantropometria Desempenho Hum.* **2015**, *17*, 400–408. [CrossRef]
90. Filaire, E.; Bernain, X.; Sagnol, M.; & Lac, G. Preliminary results on mood state, salivary testosterone:cortisol ratio and team performance in a professional soccer team. *Eur. J. Appl. Physiol.* **2001**, *86*, 179–184.
91. Peñailillo, L.E.; Escanilla, F.A.; Jury, E.R.; Castro-Sepulveda, M.A.; Deldicque, L.; Zbinden-Foncea, H.P. Differences in salivary hormones and perception of exertion in elite women and men volleyball players during tournament. *J. Sports Med. Phys. Fitness* **2018**, *58*, 1688–1694. [CrossRef]
92. Rowell, A.E.; Aughey, R.J.; Hopkins, W.G.; Esmaeili, A.; Lazarus, B.H.; Cormack, S.J. Effects of training and competition load on neuromuscular recovery, testosterone, cortisol, and match performance during a season of professional football. *Front. Physiol.* **2018**, *9*, 668. [CrossRef] [PubMed]
93. Nédélec, M.; McCall, A.; Carling, C.; Legall, F.; Berthoin, S.; Dupont, G. Recovery in soccer: Part II-recovery strategies. *Sport. Med.* **2013**, *43*, 9–22. [CrossRef] [PubMed]

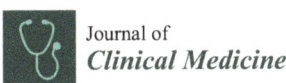

Article

Postural Stability in Single-Leg Quiet Stance in Highly Trained Athletes: Sex and Sport Differences

Nebojša Trajković [1], Darjan Smajla [2,3], Žiga Kozinc [2,4] and Nejc Šarabon [2,3,4,5,*]

1. Faculty of Sport and Physical Education, University of Niš, Čarnojevićeva 10a, 18000 Nis, Serbia; nele_trajce@yahoo.com
2. Faculty of Health Sciences, University of Primorska, Polje 42, SI-6310 Izola, Slovenia; darjan.smajla@fvz.upr.si (D.S.); ziga.kozinc@fvz.upr.si (Ž.K.)
3. Human Health Department, InnoRenew CoE, Livade 6, SI-6310 Izola, Slovenia
4. Andrej Marušič Institute, University of Primorska, Muzejski trg 2, SI-6000 Koper, Slovenia
5. Laboratory for Motor Control and Motor Behavior, S2P, Science to Practice, Ltd., Tehnološki Park 19, SI-1000 Ljubljana, Slovenia
* Correspondence: nejc.sarabon@fvz.upr.si

Abstract: This study aimed to determine if there is a difference in postural stability in highly trained adolescents and young adult athletes regarding sex and sport. The participants were young athletes (n = 464) from seven different sports. We considered the center of pressure (CoP) velocity (total, anterior–posterior (AP) and medial–lateral (ML)), CoP amplitude (AP and ML), and CoP frequency (AP and ML), as assessed by single-leg quiet stance test. Significant interactions were found between sex and sport for all CoP variables ($p < 0.02$). Additionally, a significant main effect of sport was also found in all CoP variables ($p = 0.01$). Regarding sex, significant effects were found for all CoP amplitude variables ($p = 0.01$), as well as for CoP velocity variables, except for CoP ML ($p = 0.06$). Moreover, there was no sex effect for CoP frequency AP ($p = 0.18$). The results of the current study confirm the claim that the criteria for optimal postural strategies for elite athletes likely depend on a given sport.

Keywords: postural sway; balance; equilibrium; elite athletes; gender effect

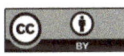

1. Introduction

Postural stability is considered a very important factor for athletes in different sports [1]. Due to its potential role in mitigating risk for injuries, postural stability has been the subject of interest of researchers. Postural stability evaluated through assessment of body sway enables quantifying the function of maintaining equilibrium during periods of standing still, locomotion, and any activities requiring a high degree of balance performance [2]. Evidence from a systematic review [3] suggests that athletes sway less than nonathletes and that highly trained elite athletes sway less than low-level athletes. The importance of good stability in some sports, (i.e., ballet, dance, gymnastics) is obvious. Previous comparisons of body sway among athletes from different sports have shown that gymnasts have better postural stability than football players, swimmers, and basketball players [4,5]. Negahban et al. [6] suggested that elite athletes may be more efficient in conditions consistent with their main experience and process of training. Accordingly, recent evidence suggests that sport-specific expertise induces alterations in sensory integration that underpins spatial referencing and postural control [7].

Novel research indicates that postural stability in athletes is not influenced by sex [8]. However, some studies noted better postural stability in females, which was suggested to be related to earlier physical and psychological maturation processes [9] and superior sensory integration [10]. Previous research has documented that female athletes have different anatomical characteristics, which could explain lower postural sway [11]. The development of proprioception and vestibular functions in females is also one factor that could interact with the improvement of the postural stability system [12]. These sex differences and inconsistency during childhood and adulthood were confirmed in several studies [13–16], indicating that girls tend to have better postural stability during childhood, while during adulthood, the situation is reversed. Therefore, improving the understanding of sport-specific patterns in postural stability and its interaction with sex is important, in order to develop better injury prevention programs and decrease injury risk.

Single-leg body sway parameters can be used for analyzing the static performance of stabilization in the condition of unilateral distribution of body weight, which is usual in sports activities. Good single-leg stabilization characteristic reflects on the smaller increase in vertical force and the shorter weight transfer in different movement tasks [17,18]. The single-leg stance test is also recommended for clinicians as a useful tool for a brief assessment of the risk of falling [19]. Therefore, evaluation of postural sway in single-leg tests presents an important stability evaluation tool. The importance of postural stability in sport and everyday life has been well recognized and confirmed. However, only a few studies investigated postural stability considering sport and sex using different tests [20,21]. Moreover, most studies were conducted on children or older adults [9,11–13,15,17]. Having in mind that single-leg stance measurement has more applications in clinical and sport medicine settings [22] and that most injurious falls occurred in activities that involved single-leg stance [23], it is of great importance to understand the possible sport-specific characteristics of postural stability. Accordingly, there is a widespread call to identify a postural stability measure that can best distinguish between different sports and sex in highly trained young athletes.

In light of the aforementioned evidence, we used a previously collected database containing more than 400 participants, who all performed single-leg body sway assessments with open eyes. We chose the single-leg stance test because of its similarity with the movements in sports that require balancing on a single leg and the fact that athletes must be able to maintain good postural stability before any kind of motor action, in order to act efficiently [24]. The aim of the study was to assess the postural stability during single-leg quiet stance in highly trained male and female young athletes from different sports. We expected to observe differences in center of pressure (CoP) characteristics between sex and sports in highly trained young athletes.

2. Materials and Methods

2.1. Participants

The participants in the present study were young athletes (n = 464) from 7 different sports. The sample was taken from the database of a larger project, exploring interlimb asymmetries and performance in athletes [25,26]. All sports groups that performed postural sway assessments and involved both male and female participants were considered. Details of the sample sizes for each group, along with baseline demographic data, are presented in Table 1. Exclusion criteria included lower leg injuries in the past 6 months and possible neurological or noncommunicable diseases self-reported by participants. Participants were given detailed information about the testing procedures and were required to sign a written informed consent form prior to the measurements. For minor participants, parents or guardians were also notified and signed an informed consent form on their behalf. The National Committee for Medical Ethics of the Republic of Slovenia approved the experimental protocol (Approval Number 0120-99/2018/5) and was conducted in accordance with the latest revision of the Declaration of Helsinki.

2.2. Procedures

Body sway was assessed in a single-leg stance position without footwear. Participants performed three 30 s repetitions with each leg in the single-leg position, with 60 s long breaks between repetitions. The experimenter began the acquisition after stabilization (1–2 s). The postural sway was analyzed on the preferred leg, which was determined as the leg that the participant would use to kick a ball. The hip of the opposite leg (i.e., non-standing leg) was in a neutral position (0°), and the thigh was parallel to the standing leg, while the knee was flexed at 90° and was not allowed to touch the standing leg. The standing leg's knee was in the extended position but not hyperextended (locked). The hands were placed on the hips.

Table 1. Basic participant data.

	n	Age (years)	Body Height (cm)	Body Mass (kg)	Weekly Training	Years of Training
Basketball—M	107	17.4 (2.2)	189.3 (8.2)	81.4 (12.9)	6.4 (1.9)	6.9 (2.4)
Basketball—F	58	16.7 (1.6)	175.2 (5.6)	70.2 (11.2)	5.5 (1.3)	6.4 (2.5)
Dance—M	23	24.2 (5.9)	179.0 (4.9)	71.7 (6.6)	5.9 (2.2)	12.0 (4.4)
Dance—F	54	22.3 (7.0)	166.9 (5.3)	55.3 (6.1)	6.6 (2.6)	9.9 (4.0)
Track and Field—M	21	17.8 (2.6)	180.5 (5.8)	73.8 (7.9)	5.4 (1.6)	6.5 (3.1)
Track and Field—M	8	17.7 (3.0)	167.2 (3.7)	60.3 (5.8)	5.4 (1.1)	6.3 (2.2)
Running—M	31	29.2 (8.8)	181.2 (5.6)	77.2 (6.8)	5.2 (2.5)	11.0 (8.8)
Running—F	18	36.9 (10.9)	166.0 (8.1)	60.9 (7.6)	4.0 (1.7)	7.7 (4.5)
Tennis—M	68	17.2 (10.4)	175.0 (11.1)	65.2 (12.1)	6.1 (2.8)	8.9 (3.6)
Tennis—F	42	15.9 (3.0)	168.5 (8.4)	60.0 (9.9)	6.3 (3.2)	8.2 (3.9)
Martial arts—M	18	19.9 (3.1)	180.3 (6.0)	75.5 (8.9)	5.6 (1.3)	7.7 (2.5)
Martial arts—F	17	19.7 (3.4)	169.1 (6.6)	60.1 (5.1)	5.1 (1.4)	7.7 (2.8)
Speed skating—M	12	16.8 (5.1)	169.5 (15.5)	61.3 (16.5)	5.3 (1.9)	6.9 (3.4)
Speed skating—M	7	16.9 (3.4)	161.1 (8.4)	57.3 (10.9)	4.9 (2.0)	6.0 (3.9)

M—male; F—female.

A piezoelectric platform (model 9260AA, Kistler, Winterthur, Switzerland) was used to acquire ground reaction force data at a sampling rate of 1000 Hz. The data were automatically filtered (low-pass Butterworth, 2nd order, 10 Hz) in the software MARS (version 4.0, Kistler, Winterthur, Switzerland). Additionally, data were automatically processed in MARS to obtain outcome variables of interest. For further analysis, an average of three replicates was used for all outcome variables. We considered mean CoP velocity (total, anterior–posterior (AP) and medial–lateral (ML)), CoP amplitude (AP and ML) and CoP frequency (AP and ML). CoP amplitude was determined as the average CoP sway in the AP or ML direction, calculated as the total length of the COP sway path in a given direction only, divided by the number of directional changes. CoP frequency was defined as the frequency of CoP oscillations, calculated as the number of peaks in the AP or ML direction (i.e., changes in the direction of CoP motion) divided by the measurement time [27].

2.3. Statistical Analysis

Statistical analysis was performed in SPSS (version 25.0; SPSS Inc., Chicago, IL, USA). Descriptive statistics were calculated and reported as mean ± standard deviation. The normality of the data distribution was checked with Shapiro–Wilk tests ($p \leq 0.121$). A 2 × 7 MANCOVA was used to examine the interaction effect between sex and sport on a multivariate level. We used a 2 × 7 ANCOVA (between-subject design) to evaluate the sex and sports effects on body sway measures after controlling their effect for age (mean centered), body height (mean centered), and BMI (mean centered). The main effects of sex and sports estimated mean differences between men and women, and various sports players, respectively. The sex × sport interaction effect was employed to determine whether various sports players on average differ in body sway measures depending on the sex of sports players. For comparison of the sports included, the post hoc test was used. The effect sizes (ES) pertaining to ANOVA were expressed as partial eta squared ($\eta2$) and interpreted as small (<0.13), medium (0.13–0.26), and large (>0.26) [28].

3. Results

CoP variables, velocity, amplitude and frequency for preferred leg by sex and sports are presented in Table 2. Figure 1 represents the data for both sexes combined. A 2 × 7 MANCOVA showed that all studied variables significantly depend on sex (F = 5.936, p = 0.001, η2 = 0.087), sport (F = 14.614, p = 0.001, η2 = 0.185), and sport × sex interaction (F = 2.561, p = 0.001, η2 = 0.039). A 2 × 7 ANCOVA followed and showed significant interaction between sex and sport for all CoP velocity variables (p = 0.01) with small effect size (η2 = 0.046–0.073).There were significant main effects for sex (p < 0.001) and sport participation (p < 0.001). Concerning sex, females reported lower scores for CoP velocity than males (p = 0.01; η2 = 0.027–0.079, small ES), except for CoP velocity ML, where no significant effect of sex was found (p = 0.06; η2 = 0.08, small ES). Similarly, there was a significant effect of sports (p = 0.01), with small ES ranging from η2 = 0.062 to η2 = 0.093.

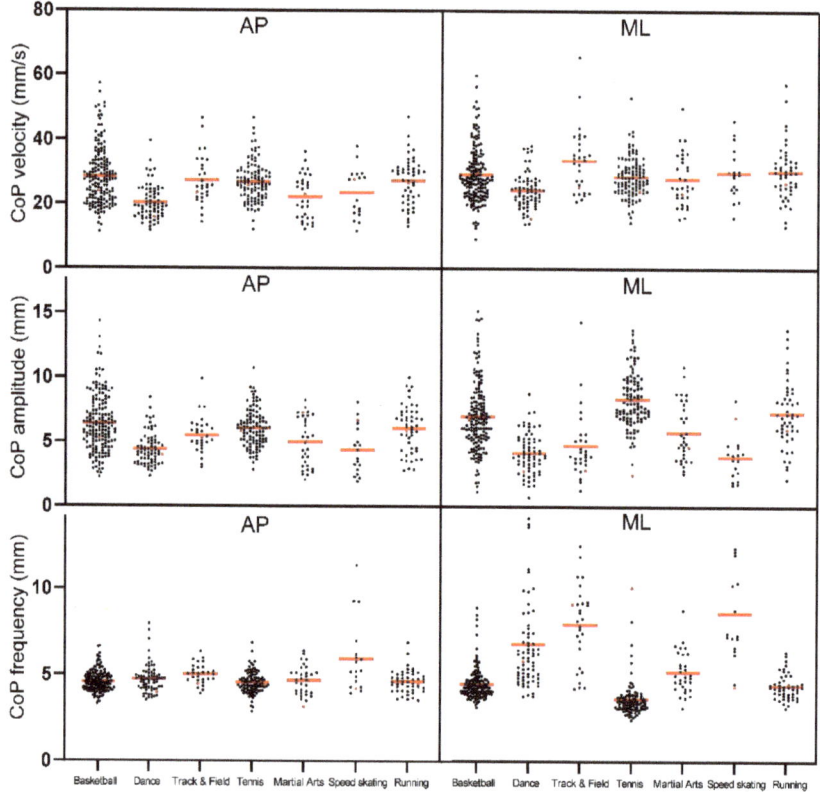

Figure 1. Representation of body sway data across sports (anterior–posterior direction, left panel; medial–lateral direction, right panel). Horizontal lines represent the mean of the groups). Statistical values are included in Table 2.

There were significant sex × sport interactions found for CoP frequency (CoP AP F = 4.51; p = 0.01; CoP ML F = 2.45; p = 0.02). Moreover, there was no main effect of sex for CoP AP frequency (p > 0.05). Regarding sport modality, there was a significant main effect for CoP AP and ML frequency (p = 0.01; η2 = 0.143–0.400).

Table 2. Comparison of CoP velocity, amplitude, and frequency according to sex and sport; values are mean ± SD. Statistically significant effect are in bold.

		Basketball	Dance	Track and Field	Tennis	Martial Arts	Speed Skating	Running	Sport × Sex F; p Value	Sport F; p Value	Sex F; p Value
CoP velocity (mm/s)											
Total	male	49.8 ± 12.8 b	37.2 ± 10.6 ac	49.1 ± 13.9 b	45.1 ± 8.8	47.1 ± 8.9	44.1 ± 9.7	44.4 ± 9.5	**5.01; 0.01**	**5.58; 0.01**	**12.31; 0.01**
	female	36.3 ± 8.0	34.4 ± 6.3 g	45.2 ± 10.2 be	41.3 ± 8.8 b	31.6 ± 6.8 g	38.5 ± 13.4	45.6 ± 14.8 be			
AP	male	31.5 ± 8.7 be	21.2 ± 6.9 acd	28.9 ± 7.9 b	27.7 ± 6.1 ab	27.4 ± 4.4	26.2 ± 7.1	26.9 ± 6.1	**5.85; 0.01**	**7.67; 0.01**	**24.44; 0.01**
	female	22.1 ± 19.9	19.9 ± 4.5 dg	22.9 ± 4.3 b	25.2 ± 6.0 be	16.9 ± 4.1 dg	19.2 ± 6.7	27.6 ± 8.9 be			
ML	male	32.2 ± 8.6	26.1 ± 7.1 c	33.6 ± 10.5 b	29.7 ± 6.1	32.8 ± 7.5	30.2 ± 5.9	30.1 ± 6.9	**3.94; 0.01**	**5.62; 0.01**	3.68; 0.06
	female	24.2 ± 5.8 c	24.0 ± 4.6 c	34.1 ± 9.4 abe	27.4 ± 5.7	23.1 ± 5.2 c	29.6 ± 10.7	31.0 ± 10.1			
CoP amplitude (mm)											
AP	male	7.1 ± 2.1 bcf	4.5 ± 1.2 adeg	5.6 ± 1.5 a	6.2 ± 1.5 b	6.3 ± 1.2 b	5.1 ± 1.8 a	6.3 ± 1.7 b	**5.97; 0.01**	**8.17; 0.01**	**21.43; 0.01**
	female	4.8 ± 1.3	4.3 ± 1.3 d	5.0 ± 1.1	5.6 ± 1.3 bef	3.6 ± 1.3 d	3.0 ± 0.8 d	5.5 ± 1.9			
ML	male	7.9 ± 2.6 bcf	4.7 ± 1.6 adeg	4.6 ± 2.8 adeg	8.4 ± 2.1 bcf	7.3 ± 1.9 bcf	4.3 ± 1.8 ade	7.5 ± 1.6 bc	**3.86; 0.01**	**26.37; 0.01**	**7.01; 0.01**
	female	5.2 ± 1.7 bdf	3.8 ± 1.4 adg	4.7 ± 2.0 d	7.9 ± 2.1 abcefg	4.1 ± 1.1 d	2.9 ± 1.2 adg	6.7 ± 2.8 bdf			
CoP Frequency (Hz)											
AP	male	4.5 ± 0.5 cf	4.7 ± 0.9	5.1 ± 0.4 ad	4.5 ± 0.6 cf	4.3 ± 0.6 f	5.4 ± 1.5 ad	4.3 ± 0.4 f	**4.51; 0.01**	**10.36; 0.01**	1.82; 0.18
	female	4.7 ± 0.6 f	4.7 ± 0.7 f	4.6 ± 0.6 f	4.4 ± 0.5 fg	4.9 ± 0.9 f	6.6 ± 2.6 abcdeg	5.1 ± 0.6 df			
ML	male	4.2 ± 0.6 bcf	5.8 ± 1.5 acdg	8.0 ± 2.3 abdeg	3.7 ± 1.1 bcf	4.6 ± 0.7 cf	7.7 ± 2.5 adeg	4.2 ± 0.6 bcf	2.45; 0.02	**46.42; 0.01**	**8.22; 0.01**
	female	5.0 ± 1.1 bcdf	7.2 ± 3.5 adfg	7.8 ± 2.4 adg	3.5 ± 0.9 abcef	5.8 ± 1.2 df	10.2 ± 3.4 abdeg	4.8 ± 0.7 bcg			

a—significant differences from basketball; b—significant differences from dance; c—significant differences from track and field; d—significant differences from tennis; e—significant differences from martial arts; f—significant differences from speed skating; g—significant differences from running; AP—anterior-posterior; ML—medial-lateral; statistically significant sex × sport interactions were found for CoP AP amplitude ($p = 0.01$), as well as in CoP ML amplitude ($p = 0.01$), although the effect sizes were all small (η2 = 0.023–0.078). There was a significant main effect of sex and sport for both CoP AP and CoP ML amplitude ($p = 0.01$). Effect size ranged from small (η2 = 0.087) to large (η2 = 0.263) regarding sport, and from 0.022 to 0.082 regarding sex.

4. Discussion

This study aimed to analyze characteristics of single-leg quiet stance body sway in a highly trained athletic population and to explore the effects of sex and sport. The major findings in the current study point to sport-specific characteristics regarding postural stability in single-leg stance. Results for CoP velocity and amplitude clearly show that dancers are better able to maintain a stable single-leg stance than athletes from other sports. Moreover, the results of the present study show that, when comparing highly trained athletes of both sexes, there were differences in almost all CoP variables. Male athletes presented higher values of CoP velocity and amplitude but also for CoP frequency during single-leg stance.

The single-leg upright stance represents a challenging part of human locomotion because, compared with bipedal stance, it requires keeping the center of body mass within the smaller area of the support [13], which leads to more corrective movements by the postural control system in order to maintain balance [29]. Female athletes in the current study reported lower scores ($p = 0.01$) for CoP velocity ($\eta2 = 0.030$–0.079) and amplitude ($\eta2 = 0.055$–0.082), compared with male athletes. Studies investigating postural control between sexes showed inconsistent results depending on the age group. Boys aged nine years showed significantly poorer single-leg postural stability than the girls of the same age [13], and similar was for participants in adolescent age [14]. On the contrary, female young adults seem to have lower postural stability, as shown by higher CoP velocities, compared with males [16]. The differences remain through adulthood as well in older adults—women tend to be less stable than men during single stance [15]. The main predictor that could influence this inconsistency in the results is the visual system, which was found to be the primary sensory system involved in maintaining postural stability in a broad range of age groups [30]. One more factor that could change the variability in postural stability is physical activity. This was confirmed in a study conducted on healthy young adults, in which no differences between sexes were detected when participants were physically active [31]. Female athletes in the current study showed better postural stability, compared with males with the difference being most pronounced for CoP velocity and amplitude, while the difference in CoP frequency was noted in the medial–lateral direction only ($p < 0.05$). Reduced CoP sway area and velocity in females of similar age were also noted in the recent study [21]. Possible reasons for better postural stability in this age are the maturation process [32] lower body weight [13], as well as better proprioception and control due to smaller absolute muscle mass and strength [33]. Additionally, it was stated that sex differences exist in children and adolescents due to the significantly lower body height in girls [13]. However, the participants in the abovementioned study were untrained children that were younger than participants in the current study, which may account for the discrepancies in some studies. Therefore, reasons for better postural control in younger age, as well as the reasons for the decline in later ages, should be investigated further.

It was stated that the postural balance of elite athletes should be always monitored, due to the establishment of sport-specific imbalances that could affect their performance [34]. The results of the current study suggest that dancers have better postural stability during single-leg stance than athletes from other sports, in all measured CoP characteristics. The differences are probably the result of adaptive balance strategies used by dancers in training, in which both abilities, cognitive and physical, are coordinated [35]. Additionally, their continuous training that uses balance control could minimize the effect of external perturbations [36] and thus improve postural control. However, the increase in body sway in the absence of vision in ballet dancers was previously reported by Bruyneel et al. [37]. Matsuda et al. [20] showed that soccer players make greater use of the somatosensory system during single-leg stance, compared with basketball players, swimmers, and nonathletes. However, highly trained female volleyball players showed higher CoP fractal dimensions, compared with controls, which is probably due to the adoption of certain habits. [38]. According to the authors, these high values show evidence for flexible and variable strategies of maintaining balance by highly trained athletes. This was confirmed in the current study among young highly trained athletes in that dancers were better able to maintain a stable, single-leg stance, compared with athletes from other sports. Only martial arts showed similar results to those of dance for CoP velocity and amplitude but also higher. The mechanism behind the best postural stability in dancers may be associated with the development of a motor skill for voluntary stabilization of important muscle groups, as well as better sensorimotor solutions for posture control [39]. The importance of dance exercise in maintaining good postural stability was well documented in adolescent females [40].

Some limitations of the present study need to be acknowledged. Across sports, the sample sizes varied considerably and were relatively small for some of the sports. Moreover, the samples were not sex balanced (e.g., dancers. Despite taking sexes into account as a factor in analyses, some main effects could still be driven by a larger representation of one sex in the sample (e.g., females in dancing). However, having in mind that, in some sports, it is hard to find highly trained athletes on an elite level, and since we included a considerable number of different sports, it was of great importance to conduct and analyze body sway because of important clinical implications in young athletes. Moreover, we did not include a healthy control group, which could have strengthened our interpretations. One more limitation is the fact that measures were assessed only during static conditions. Most of the selected sports rely more on dynamic conditions demands than static postures. Therefore, future studies should use both dynamic and static postural tests, in order to provide an overall assessment of balance in different sports. Nevertheless, the greatest strength of this study is encompassing a large number of sports and highly trained athletes compared at this age.

5. Conclusions

According to our findings, postural stability in highly trained adolescents and young adult athletes was influenced by sex and sport. Female athletes showed better postural stability than male athletes. The athletes engaged in dance showed the highest postural control, compared with other sports. The results of the current study confirm the claim that the criteria for optimal postural strategies for elite athletes likely depend on a given sport. This is of great importance in providing additional information about postural control abilities in highly trained athletes from different sports.

Author Contributions: Conceptualization, all authors; methodology, N.Š.; software, N.Š.; validation, N.Š. and D.S.; formal analysis, N.T.; investigation, Ž.K. and D.S.; resources, N.Š.; data curation, N.T., D.S. and Ž.K.; writing—original draft preparation, N.T. and Ž.K.; writing—review and editing, D.S. and N.Š.; visualization, all authors.; supervision, N.Š.; project administration, D.S. and N.Š.; funding acquisition, N.Š. All authors have read and agreed to the published version of the manuscript.

Funding: This study was supported by the Slovenian Research Agency through a project entitled "Body asymmetries as a risk factor in musculoskeletal injury development: studying aetiological mechanisms and designing corrective interventions for primary and tertiary preventive care" (TELASI-PREVENT (L5-1845)). The agency played no role in the conceptualization of the study, data acquisition, data analysis, or manuscript writing. Žiga Kozinc acknowledges the support of the Rectors Fund of the University of Primorska (internal post-doctoral project RAVOTEZ: Assessing Balance with Quantifying Transient Behavior of Postural Sway: From Validation To Practical Application; Grant Number: 2991-3-2/21). The fund played no role in the conceptualization of the study, data acquisition, data analysis, or manuscript writing.

Institutional Review Board Statement: The National Committee for Medical Ethics of the Republic of Slovenia approved the experimental protocol (Approval Number 0120-99/2018/5). The protocol was conducted in accordance with the latest revision of the Declaration of Helsinki.

Informed Consent Statement: Informed consent was obtained from all subjects involved in the study.

Data Availability Statement: The data presented in this study are available on request from the corresponding author.

Conflicts of Interest: The authors declare no conflict of interest.

References

1. Hrysomallis, C. Balance Ability and Athletic Performance. *Sports Med.* **2011**, *41*, 221–232. [CrossRef] [PubMed]
2. Assaiante, C.; Mallau, S.; Viel, S.; Jover, M.; Schmitz, C. Development of postural control in healthy children: A functional approach. *Neural Plast.* **2005**, *12*, 109–118. [CrossRef] [PubMed]
3. Kiers, H.; Van Dieën, J.; Dekkers, H.; Wittink, H.; Vanhees, L. A systematic review of the relationship between physical activities in sports or daily life and postural sway in upright stance. *Sports Med.* **2013**, *43*, 1171–1189. [CrossRef] [PubMed]
4. Bressel, E.; Yonker, J.C.; Kras, J.; Heath, E.M. Comparison of static and dynamic balance in female collegiate soccer, basketball, and gymnastics athletes. *J. Athl. Train.* **2007**, *42*, 42.
5. Davlin, C.D. Dynamic balance in high level athletes. *Percept. Mot. Skills* **2004**, *98*, 1171–1176. [CrossRef]
6. Negahban, H.; Aryan, N.; Mazaheri, M.; Norasteh, A.A.; Sanjari, M.A. Effect of expertise in shooting and Taekwondo on bipedal and unipedal postural control isolated or concurrent with a reaction-time task. *Gait Posture* **2013**, *38*, 226–230. [CrossRef]
7. Thalassinos, M.; Fotiadis, G.; Arabatzi, F.; Isableu, B.; Hatzitaki, V. Sport Skill—Specific expertise biases sensory integration for spatial referencing and postural control. *J. Mot. Behav.* **2018**, *50*, 426–435. [CrossRef]
8. Jastrzębska, A.D. Gender differences in postural stability among 13-year-old alpine skiers. *Int. J. Environ. Res. Public Health* **2020**, *17*, 3859. [CrossRef]
9. Butz, S.M.; Sweeney, J.K.; Roberts, P.L.; Rauh, M.J. Relationships among age, gender, anthropometric characteristics, and dynamic balance in children 5 to 12 years old. *Pediatr. Phys. Ther.* **2015**, *27*, 126–133. [CrossRef]
10. Steindl, R.; Kunz, K.; Schrott-Fischer, A.; Scholtz, A.W. Effect of age and sex on maturation of sensory systems and balance control. *Dev. Med. Child Neurol.* **2006**, *48*, 477–482. [CrossRef]
11. Dorneles, P.P.; Pranke, G.I.; Mota, C.B. Comparison of postural balance between female and male adolescents. *Fisioter. Pesq.* **2013**, *20*, 210–214. [CrossRef]
12. Smith, A.; Ulmer, F.; Wong, D. Gender differences in postural stability among children. *J. Hum. Kinet.* **2012**, *33*, 25–32. [CrossRef] [PubMed]
13. Lee, A.J.Y.; Lin, W.-H. The influence of gender and somatotype on single-leg upright standing postural stability in children. *J. Appl. Biomech.* **2007**, *23*, 173–179. [CrossRef] [PubMed]
14. Schedler, S.; Kiss, R.; Muehlbauer, T. Age and sex differences in human balance performance from 6–18 years of age: A systematic review and meta-analysis. *PLoS ONE* **2019**, *14*, e0214434. [CrossRef] [PubMed]
15. Riva, D.; Mamo, C.; Fanì, M.; Saccavino, P.; Rocca, F.; Momenté, M.; Fratta, M. Single stance stability and proprioceptive control in older adults living at home: Gender and age differences. *J. Aging Res.* **2013**, *2013*, 561695. [CrossRef] [PubMed]
16. Błaszczyk, J.W.; Beck, M.; Sadowska, D. Assessment of postural stability in young healthy subjects based on directional features of posturographic data: Vision and gender effects. *Acta Neurobiol. Exp.* **2014**, *74*, 433–442.
17. Roemer, K.; Raisbeck, L. Temporal dependency of sway during single leg stance changes with age. *Clin. Biomech.* **2015**, *30*, 66–70. [CrossRef]
18. Huurnink, A.; Fransz, D.P.; Kingma, I.; de Boode, V.A.; van Dieën, J.H. The assessment of single-leg drop jump landing performance by means of ground reaction forces: A methodological study. *Gait Posture* **2019**, *73*, 80–85. [CrossRef]
19. Kozinc, Ž.; Löfler, S.; Hofer, C.; Carraro, U.; Šarabon, N. Diagnostic balance tests for assessing risk of falls and distinguishing older adult fallers and non-fallers: A systematic review with meta-analysis. *Diagnostics* **2020**, *10*, 667. [CrossRef]
20. Matsuda, S.; Demura, S.; Uchiyama, M. Centre of pressure sway characteristics during static one-legged stance of athletes from different sports. *J. Sports Sci.* **2008**, *26*, 775–779. [CrossRef]
21. Andreeva, A.; Melnikov, A.; Skvortsov, D.; Akhmerova, K.; Vavaev, A.; Golov, A.; Draugelite, V.; Nikolaev, R.; Chechelnickaia, S.; Zhuk, D. Postural Stability in Athletes: The Role of Age, Sex, Performance Level, and Athlete Shoe Features. *Sports* **2020**, *8*, 89. [CrossRef]
22. Riemann, B.L.; Schmitz, R. The relationship between various modes of single leg postural control assessment. *Int. J. Sports Phys. Ther.* **2012**, *7*, 257–266. [PubMed]
23. Nevitt, M.C.; Cummings, S.R.; Hudes, E.S. Risk Factors for Injurious Falls: A Prospective Study. *J. Gerontol.* **1991**, *46*, M164–M170. [CrossRef] [PubMed]
24. Paillard, T.; Noé, F.; Rivière, T.; Marion, V.; Montoya, R.; Dupui, P. Postural performance and strategy in the unipedal stance of soccer players at different levels of competition. *J. Athl. Train.* **2006**, *41*, 172–176. [PubMed]
25. Kozinc, Ž.; Žitnik, J.; Smajla, D.; Šarabon, N. The difference between squat jump and countermovement jump in 770 male and female participants from different sports. *Eur. J. Sport Sci.* **2021**, 1–24. [CrossRef]
26. Kozinc, Ž.; Šarabon, N. Bilateral deficit in countermovement jump and its association with change of direction performance in basketball and tennis players. *Sport. Biomech.* **2021**, 1–14. [CrossRef]
27. Sarabon, N.; Kern, H.; Loefler, S.; Jernej, R. Selection of body sway parameters according to their sensitivity and repeatability. *Eur. J. Transl. Myol.* **2010**, *20*, 5. [CrossRef]
28. Bakeman, R. Recommended effect size statistics for repeated measures designs. *Behav. Res. Methods* **2005**, *37*, 379–384. [CrossRef]
29. Hertel, J.; Olmsted-Kramer, L.C.; Challis, J.H. Time-to-boundary measures of postural control during single leg quiet standing. *J. Appl. Biomech.* **2006**, *22*, 67–73. [CrossRef]
30. Grace Gaerlan, M.; Alpert, P.T.; Cross, C.; Louis, M.; Kowalski, S. Postural balance in young adults: The role of visual, vestibular and somatosensory systems. *J. Am. Acad. Nurse Pract.* **2012**, *24*, 375–381. [CrossRef]

31. Torres, S.F.; Reis, J.G.; de Abreu, D.C.C. Influence of gender and physical exercise on balance of healthy young adults. *Fisioter. Mov.* **2014**, *27*, 399–406. [CrossRef]
32. Nolan, L.; Grigorenko, A.; Thorstensson, A. Balance control: Sex and age differences in 9- to 16-year-olds. *Dev. Med. Child Neurol.* **2005**, *47*, 449–454. [CrossRef] [PubMed]
33. Duzgun, I.; Kanbur, N.O.; Baltaci, G.; Aydin, T. Effect of Tanner stage on proprioception accuracy. *J. Foot Ankle Surg.* **2011**, *50*, 11–15. [CrossRef] [PubMed]
34. Gobbi, G.; Galli, D.; Carubbi, C.; Pelosi, A.; Lillia, M.; Gatti, R.; Queirolo, V.; Costantino, C.; Vitale, M.; Saccavini, M. Assessment of body plantar pressure in elite athletes: An observational study. *Sport Sci. Health* **2013**, *9*, 13–18. [CrossRef]
35. Crotts, D.; Thompson, B.; Nahom, M.; Ryan, S.; Newton, R.A. Balance abilities of professional dancers on select balance tests. *J. Orthop. Sport. Phys. Ther.* **1996**, *23*, 12–17. [CrossRef] [PubMed]
36. Maki, B.E.; McIlroy, W.E. The role of limb movements in maintaining upright stance: The "change-in-support" strategy. *Phys. Ther.* **1997**, *77*, 488–507. [CrossRef]
37. Bruyneel, A.V.; Mesure, S.; Paré, J.C.; Bertrand, M. Organization of postural equilibrium in several planes in ballet dancers. *Neurosci. Lett.* **2010**, *485*, 228–232. [CrossRef]
38. Borzucka, D.; Kręcisz, K.; Rektor, Z.; Kuczyński, M. Postural control in top-level female volleyball players. *BMC Sports Sci. Med. Rehabil.* **2020**, *12*, 65. [CrossRef]
39. Horak, F.B.; Henry, S.M.; Shumway-Cook, A. Postural perturbations: New insights for treatment of balance disorders. *Phys. Ther.* **1997**, *77*, 517–533. [CrossRef]
40. Cheng, H.; Law, C.; Pan, H.; Hsiao, Y.; Hu, J.; Chuang, F.; Huang, M. Preliminary results of dancing exercise on postural stability in adolescent females. *Kaohsiung J. Med. Sci.* **2011**, *27*, 566–572. [CrossRef]

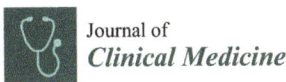

Article

Anatomical and Neuromuscular Factors Associated to Non-Contact Anterior Cruciate Ligament Injury

Marc Dauty [1,2,3,4], Vincent Crenn [5], Bastien Louguet [2,4], Jérôme Grondin [1,2], Pierre Menu [1,2,3,4] and Alban Fouasson-Chailloux [1,2,3,4,*]

1. CHU Nantes, Service de Médecine Physique et Réadaptation Locomotrice, University Hospital of Nantes, Hôpital St. Jacques, 85 rue Saint Jacques, 44093 Nantes, France; marc.dauty@chu-nantes.fr (M.D.); jerome.grondin@chu-nantes.fr (J.G.); pierre.menu@chu-nantes.fr (P.M.)
2. CHU Nantes, Service de Médecine du Sport, University Hospital of Nantes, Hôpital St. Jacques, 85 rue Saint Jacques, 44093 Nantes, France; bastien.louguet@chu-nantes.fr
3. INSERM UMR U1229 Regenerative Medicine and Skeleton, RMeS, Nantes University, 44035 Nantes, France
4. IRMS—Institut Régional de Médecine du Sport, Hôpital St. Jacques, 85 rue Saint Jacques, 44093 Nantes, France
5. CHU Nantes, Clinique Chirurgicale Orthopédique et Traumatologique, Hôtel-Dieu, 44000 Nantes, France; vincent.crenn@chu-nantes.fr
* Correspondence: alban.fouassonchailloux@chu-nantes.fr

Abstract: The majority of anterior cruciate ligament (ACL) injuries occur during non-contact mechanisms. Knowledge of the risk factors would be relevant to help prevent athletes' injuries. We aimed to study risk factors associated with non-contact ACL injuries in a population of athletes after ACL reconstruction. From a cohort of 307 athletes, two populations were compared according to the non-contact or contact mechanism of ACL injury. Gender, age and body mass index (BMI) were reported. Passive knee alignment (valgus and extension), knee laxity (KT-1000 test), and isokinetic knee strength were measured on the non-injured limb. The relationship between these factors and the non-contact sport mechanism was established with models using logistic regression analysis for the population and after selection of gender and cut-offs of age, BMI and knee laxity calculated from Receiver Operating Characteristics curve area and Youden index. Age, BMI, antero-posterior laxity, isokinetic knee strength, passive knee valgus and passive knee extension were associated with non-contact ACL injury. According to the multivariate model, a non-contact ACL injury was associated with non-modifiable factors, age (OR: 1.05; $p = 0.001$), passive knee extension (OR: 1.14; $p = 0.001$), and with one modifiable factor (Hamstring strength: OR: 0.27; $p = 0.01$). For women, only passive knee valgus was reported (OR: 1.27; $p = 0.01$). Age, passive knee extension and weak Hamstring strength were associated with a non-contact ACL injury. Hamstring strengthening could be proposed to prevent ACL injury in young male athletes or in case of knee laxity.

Keywords: knee; ACL injury; sport; hamstring; strength; laxity

1. Introduction

Every year, several hundred thousand ACL reconstructions following a sports injury are performed in the world [1–3]. The mechanism of ACL rupture is the most frequent non-contact injury in 70% to 75% of the cases, particularly during pivot contact sport practice [4,5]. Several risk factors have been identified to explain non-contact ACL injuries [6–11]. These risk factors are classified into two distinct categories: extrinsic or environmental (weather condition, playing surface, sport level . . .), and intrinsic, inherent to the individual (anatomic, neuromuscular, biomechanical, physiological, psychological and genetic factors) [4,8,10]. In this latter category, some risk factors are modifiable (e.g., body weight or muscle strength) or not (e.g., anatomical knee structure, joint laxity) because they can or cannot be controlled by the individual to reduce the ACL injury risk [10]. In the non-modifiable intrinsic risk factors, female gender and youth age (>14 or ≤20 years old)

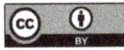

are identified as risk factors of non-contact ACL rupture [12–16]. Knee anatomy measured by X-ray or Magnetic Resonance Imaging, such as a decreased femoral intercondylar Notch width or an increased medial or lateral tibial plateau slopes are known as risk factors of non-contact mechanisms of ACL injury [8,17–20]. General joint laxity, passive knee extension (recurvatum) and anterior-posterior knee laxity seem to be risk factors for the occurrence of a non-contact ACL injury, especially in women [13,21–25].

Depending on modifiable intrinsic risk factors, an increase in Body Mass Index (BMI) seems to be a questionable risk factor for non-contact ACL rupture [9,11,16,21] Biomechanical and neuromuscular factors would be impaired [26]. Dynamic knee valgus would be poorly controlled in women during a non-contact ACL rupture, due to an increase in hip varus, knee valgus and Hamstring strength deficit (or an imbalance of Hamstring/Quadriceps ratio) [11,27–32]. However, the links between dynamic knee valgus and static knee valgus (non-modifiable factor) are poorly known [33–35].

Therefore, a better understanding of these risk factors seems necessary in order to avoid non-contact ACL ruptures during sport practice. These risk factors should be easily measurable to be useful in clinical practice [30]. The objective of this study was to investigate the association between intrinsic factors considered at risk (age, BMI, passive knee alignment, antero-posterior laxity and isokinetic strength knee) and the non-contact ACL injury. Gender has to be particularly taken into consideration because women athletes suffer ACL injury at a 2- to 6-fold greater rate than male [14,36,37]. Methodologically, it was hypothesized that the two knees were identical in a same athlete before injury and that patients who had a non-contact ACL injury had more frequently predisposing associated factors than patients with contact ACL injury. This particular method had been used because of the difficulty for many years in tracking down athletes who had not had knee surgery, pending the occurrence of a primary ACL rupture [38,39].

2. Materials and Methods

2.1. Population

All athletes over the age of 14 who had performed an isokinetic knee evaluation as part of the usual 6-month follow-up of an ACL surgical reconstruction were included from 2 January 2018 to 17 March 2020 (French COVID 19 confinement). Patients were excluded if they had undergone bilateral ACL reconstruction, a second ACL reconstruction of the same knee, an LCP reconstruction and/or multiple peripheral ligaments reconstruction, or a modification of the knee alignment by bone surgical correction. Patients were also excluded if they refused to participate in the study. Finally, three hundred and seven patients were included, 206 men and 101 women (age: 26 ± 9 years, weight: 71 ± 12 kg, height: 173 ± 8 cm, BMI: 23.4 ± 3.2 kg/m^2). Thirty patients were excluded because of bilateral ACL reconstruction, 27 because of a second ACL reconstruction, 10 because of LCP reconstruction, 10 because of multiple ligaments reconstruction and 5 because of an operated knee axis modification. No patient refused to participate to the study.

2.2. Anthrometric Parameters

Age, weight and height were measured and the Body Mass Index (BMI) was calculated using the weight-related formula for square height [9].

2.3. Knee Anatomic Parameters

Knee anatomical parameters were measured on the contralateral healthy knee and on the knee with ACL reconstruction by the same observer (MD). The 7 days test–retest reliability of the clinical knee measurements was assessed in the first 30 subjects included, using the intra-class correlation coefficient. Knee alignment was measured in the frontal plane in a standing position according to knee morphotypes [4,6]. Passive knee valgus was quantified by measuring the inter-malleolar distance using a ruler to the nearest millimeter. The intra-examiner reliability of measurements was excellent (ICC: 0.97 (0.95–0.98)). Passive knee extension was evaluated in degrees in the sagittal plane in dorsal decubitus with a goniometer when passively extending the knee [6,40]. The intra-examiner reliability of measurements was excellent (ICC: 0.97 (0.94–0.98)).

Knee laxity was measured in millimetres by the same experimented physician using a KT-1000® arthrometer (MEDmetric™ Corp., San Diego, CA, USA) [11,22,40]. A cut-off ≥ 3 mm corresponds to the threshold of pathological laxity [22,41,42]. The intra-examiner reliability is good for 134 Newton [43].

2.4. Isokinetic Knee Parameters

Muscle strength was assessed using an isokinetic dynamometer CYBEX NORM® (Lumex Inc., Ronkonkoma, NY, USA) according to an identical protocol for each subject. Knee quadriceps (extensors) and hamstrings (flexors) strength of the healthy knee were assessed in concentric mode at 60 and 180°/s angular velocities. The knee range of motion was limited to 100 degrees (from the full extension to 100 degrees of flexion). Gravity correction was used for all tests. Three repetitions at 60°/s and then 5 repetitions at 180°/s were performed. The relative isokinetic strength was calculated by reporting maximum peak torque to the bodyweight. The hamstring-to-quadriceps ratio (H/Q) was calculated for 60°/s angular speed. The reliability of quadriceps strength measurement (ICC between 0.95 and 0.98) and hamstrings strength measurement (ICC between 0.93 and 0.97) is excellent at 60 and 180°/s angular speed [44]. The reliability of H/Q ratio is good only for the 60°/s angular speed (ICC between 0.65 and 0.79) [44].

2.5. Definition of Non-Contact and Contact ACL Rupture

Non-contact ACL injury was defined by a knee twisting mechanism (the foot usually remained fixed to the ground while the leg rotated overstretching knee ligaments). that occurred without collision and without high kinetic reception (high-impact rotation landing).

Contact ACL injury was defined by a knee twisting mechanism that occurred when the subject came into contact with another subject on the knee or body or if there was a high kinetic reception as it is the case with a high-speed skiing fall, for example [45].

Non-contact or contact mechanism of ACL injury during sport practice and anthropometric parameters were reported by the orthopedic surgeon before ACL reconstruction. Anatomic and isokinetic evaluations were realized blindly by an independent physician.

2.6. Statistical Analysis

Two populations were identified according to the occurrence of the non-contact or contact ACL injury. The statistical analyses were performed using SPSS 23.0 software (Armonk, NY, USA, IBM Corp.). Quantitative parameters were presented as mean and standard deviation and qualitative parameters in frequency. Univariate analysis (independent Student t-test) and a χ^2 test or Fisher's exact test were used to compare quantitative and qualitative data of the non-contact and contact groups. The results were considered statistically significant at the 5% critical level ($p < 0.05$).

To confirm associations, 10 events per analyzed variable are recommended [46]. Since the objective was to analyze 8 potential intrinsic risk factors as gender, age, BMI, passive knee valgus, passive knee extension, anterior-posterior laxity and hamstring or quadriceps knee strength, more than 80 subjects were necessary. Due to a known incidence of 75% of ACL rupture without contact in the general population [5] and an incidence of 63.5% (195 of 307) of ACL rupture without contact found in our studied population, a minimum of 170 subjects were required at the end point to conduct the analysis at 0.05 type I error rate and at 0.10 type II error rate.

Multivariate analysis was assessed using the binary step by step ascendant logistic Wald regression (inclusion probability < 0.10 for associated risk factors). Logistic regression function was used to model the probability of non-contact ACL injury. Because of continuous quantitative parameters, the ORs were estimated from the exponential of the coefficient B of the logistic regression [47]. The Hosmer–Lemeshow test was used to describe if the data fitted the model well. The R-squares of Cox-Snell and Nagelkerke (% of the variance explained by the predictors) were used to know if the model was well adjusted.

Different models were shown in accordance to gender and after selection of cut-offs of variables identified by Youden index and ROC (Receiver Operating Characteristics) curve area to know how well this cut-off could distinguish the different non-contact groups [48]. The ROC curve area was interpreted as excellent (0.9–1), good (0.8–0.9), fair (0.7–0.8), poor (0.6–0.7), or failed (0.5–0.6) [49,50].

3. Results

Out of the 307 patients, 195 reported having had a non-contact ACL injury (63.5%) and 112 a contact injury during sports practice prior to ACL reconstruction (Table 1). A significant difference was found between the 2 groups for the following qualitative variables: age, weight, BMI, quadriceps and hamstring strength at 60 and 180°/s, passive knee valgus, passive knee extension and knee laxity, and they were included in the binary logistic regression model (Table 2). The overall accuracy or diagnosis efficiency of non-contact ACL injury was 63.5% from three parameters: age, Hamstring strength at 180°/s, and passive knee extension (Table 3). The data fitted the model well (Hosmer–Lemeshow test; $p = 0.499$), and the model was well adjusted (R-squares of Cox-Snell and Nagelkerke of 0.12 and 0.16, respectively). Only 1 case was not well classified.

Table 1. Sport participation and mechanisms of ACL injury before ACL reconstruction.

Sports	Noncontact Group (n = 195)	Contact Group (n = 112)
Soccer, n (%)	79 (40.5%)	56 (50%)
Basketball, n (%)	38 (19.5%)	12 (10.7%)
Ski, n (%)	29 (14.9%)	8 (7.1%)
Handball, n (%)	16 (8.2%)	6 (5.4%)
Rugby, n (%)	5 (2.6%)	7 (6.3%)
Other sports, n (%)	23 (20.5%)	28 (14.4%)

Table 2. Comparison of associated factors according to the mechanism of ACL injury in all population (Univariate analysis).

	Non Contact Group (n = 195)	Contact Group (n = 112)	OR	95%CI	p
Gender male (n = 206)	61.2%	38.8%	0.73	0.44–1.20	0.22
Gender female (n = 101)	70.7%	29.3%	1.50	0.87–2.58	0.17
Age (years)	27 ± 9	24 ± 8	1.04	1.01–1.07	0.002
Weight (kg)	72 ± 13	69 ± 10	1.02	1.00–1.04	0.04
Height (cm)	174 ± 8	173 ± 8	1.01	0.98–1.04	0.41
BMI (kg/m^2)	23.7 ± 3.6	22.9 ± 2.5	1.08	1.00–1.17	0.04
Q60 (Nm/kg)	2.49 ± 0.50	2.64 ± 0.45	0.53	0.33–0.87	0.01
Q180 (Nm/kg)	1.60 ± 0.31	1.71 ± 0.31	0.34	0.16–0.73	0.006
H60 (Nm/kg)	1.30 ± 0.29	1.42 ± 0.29	0.25	0.11–0.56	0.001
H180 (Nm/kg)	0.98 ± 0.22	1.07 ± 0.22	0.17	0.06–0.49	0.001
H/Q60 (%)	52.5 ± 8.1	54.1 ± 8.2	0.09	0.006–1.70	0.11
H/Q180 (%)	61.6 ± 10.5	63.1 ± 9.6	0.23	0.02–2.3	0.21
P K VL (mm)	1.8 ± 2.8	0.7 ± 1.7	1.24	1.09–1.40	0.001
P K E (°)	6.2 ± 4.4	4.0 ± 4.1	1.13	1.06–1.19	0.001
Knee Laxity (mm)	3.8 ± 1.6	3.3 ± 1.6	1.19	1.03–1.37	0.01

Abbreviations: BMI: Body Mass Index; Q60: Isokinetic quadriceps strength at 60°/s; H/Q: Hamstring-to-Quadriceps ratio; P K VL: Passive Knee Valgus; P K E: Passive Knee Extension; OR: Odd Ratio; 95%CI: Confidence Interval at 95%.

The different cut-offs for our population are presented in Table 3. However, ROC curve areas are poor (0.6–0.7) for passive knee extension, passive knee valgus and age, and failed (0.5–0.6) for BMI and knee laxity (Table 4). Considering male gender, we found that passive knee extension and age (non-modifiable factors) and Hamstring strength (modifiable factor) were associated with the non-contact ACL injury. Considering female gender, only passive knee valgus was associated with non-contact ACL injury (Table 3). Only hamstring isokinetic strength was a modifiable and protective factor after selection of cut-offs of age $\leq$ 23.5 year, or of knee laxity $\geq$ 4.5 mm (Table 3).

Table 3. Multivariate models of noncontact ACL injury in all population and after gender or cut-offs variables selection (gender; age $\leq$ 23.5 year; BMI $\geq$ 22.5 kg/m^2 and Knee Laxity $\geq$ 4.5mm).

	B	Wald	OR	95%CI	p
All population					
Age	0.049	10.0	1.05	1.02–1.08	0.001
H strength at 180°/s	−1.30	5.4	0.27	0.09–0.80	0.01
P K E	0.135	19.1	1.14	1.07–1.21	0.001
Constant	−0.055	0.005	0.15		
Men (n = 206)					
Age	0.054	7.76	1.01	1.01–1.09	0.005
H strength at 180°/s	−1.56	3.89	0.04	0.04–0.98	0.048
P K E	0.136	14.0	1.06	1.06–1.23	0.001
Constant	0.065	0.003	1.06		
Women (n = 101)					
P K VL	0.244	6.66	1.27	1.06–1.53	0.01
Constant	0.238	0.72	1.18		
Age $\leq$ 23.5 year (n = 145)					
P K E	0.088	4.37	1.09	1.01–1.18	0.03
H strength at 60°/s	−1.26	4.74	0.28	0.09–0.88	0.02
Constant	1.55	3.00	4.75		
BMI $\geq$ 22.5 kg/m^2 (n = 180)					
P K VL	0.193	5.89	1.21	1.03–1.41	0.01
P K E	0.152	11.4	1.16	1.06–1.27	0.001
Age	0.056	8.26	1.05	1.01–1.09	0.004
Constant	−1.98	9.1	0.13		
KT1000 $\geq$ 4.5 mm (n = 109)					
H strength at 180°/s	−2.51	5.93	0.08	0.01–0.61	0.01
Constant	3.46	10.4	31		

Abbreviations: OR: Odd Ratio; 95%CI: Confidence Interval at 95%. H: Hamstring; P K E: Passive Knee Extension; P K VL: Passive Knee Valgus.

Table 4. Cut-offs of associated factors with noncontact ACL rupture identified by ROC curve area and Youden index.

	ROC Curve Area	95%CI	Se (%)	Sp (%)	LR+	LR−
P K E = 4 degrees	0.643	0.579–0.708	61	58.9	1.48	0.66
P K VL = 15 mm	0.605	0.542–0.669	41	79.5	2	0.74
Age = 23.5 years	0.602	0.538–0.667	67.2	47.3	1.27	0.69
BMI = 22.5 Kg/m^2	0.556	0.491–0.621	60	46.4	1.12	0.86
Knee Laxity = 4.5 mm	0.585	0.519–0.650	40.5	73.2	1.51	0.81

Abbreviations: ROC: Receiver Operating Characteristics; 95%CI: 95% confident interval; Se: Sensitivity; Sp: Specificity; LR+: positive likelihood ratio; LR−: negative likelihood ratio.

4. Discussion

The interest of identifying associated factors with a non-contact ACL injury is to set up subsequently preventive strategies to decrease the incidence of this type of injury [51]. Because non-contact ACL injury occurrence is multifactorial, multivariate analysis was necessary to analyze the combination of factors to identify groups at risk of non-contact ACL injury. When the whole population had been studied, age and passive knee extension presented a significant association with the non-contact ACL injury. This result is interesting to advise an individual before practicing a sport at risk for the knees. However, no preventive intervention can be proposed because these two factors are not modifiable. On the contrary, the association with weak hamstring strength, considered as a protective factor (OR: 0.27), is very interesting because this factor can be improved by strengthening.

The comparison with prospective studies which proposed multivariate risk factor models is not easy because the same parameters have not been studied. However, the presence of a passive knee extension has often been found to be a risk factor for ACL knee injury, especially in female soccer or basketball players (OR from 3.8 to 4.7) [28,40]. However, the relationship with non-contact ACL injury is debatable for all athletes when this factor is evaluated individually (non-adjusted univariate model). Vauhnik et al. have shown no significant relationship (OR: 1.00 (0.93–1.16); $p = 0.44$) in women [21] and more recently, Amraee et al. have considered passive knee extension to be a non-associated factor after comparison with a non-injured population [6]. However, when this parameter is part of the general laxity, it is associated with non-contact ACL injury, whatever the gender (OR: 3.1 for men and 2.7 for women) [11]. From our results, this parameter was associated only 1.14 times with a non-contact knee injury. The difference of association can be explained by the fact that a small passive knee extension does not have the same meaning as a large passive knee extension. Thus, the presence of passive knee extension does not sufficiently reflect the risk, probably because the link is all the stronger as the passive knee extension is great. Determining a cut-off of the passive knee extension is therefore more specific than using this variable in a dichotomic way. From our population, this cut-off was of 4 degrees with a sensitivity of 61% and specificity of 58.9%. From a mechanical point of view, a knee hyperextension stresses the ACL by increasing the anterior tibial translation, which may occur at the end of a jump or during a running deceleration. In such cases, an ACL impingement on the intercondylar notch width can occur until the ligament rupture [23,24,31,32].

Passive knee valgus had already been studied as a risk factor of non-contact ACL injury but according to the Q angle method (angle between the anterior superior iliac spine-center of the patella-tibial tubercle). Knee valgus corresponds to an excessive Q angle [24]. With this parameter, no relationship was found with non-contact ACL injury [6,24]. The controversy could be explained by the Q angle method expressed in degrees, which is different from the present knee valgus measurement method expressed in millimeters. The association was 1.27 times in our population, but only in women. The best cut-off was 15 mm with a poor sensitivity of 41% and a good specificity of 79%. From a mechanical point of view, knee valgus is associated with a greater coxa vara with concurrent increase in tibio-femoral rotation force and dynamic anterior tibial translation, thus imposing greater stress on the ACL [52]. Dynamically, knee valgus, assessed by 3D motion analysis at landing, predicts ACL injury in women [37]. The fact that passive knee valgus was the only founding factor associated with non-contact ACL injury in women in our study may confirm a relationship between passive and dynamic valgus.

Body Mass Index was considered a risk factor but only in women athletes [11,16]. We have found a relationship with this parameter only in univariate analysis, but no association was confirmed after multivariate analysis in the whole population or only in the women population. In the same way, weight was identified an associated factor only in univariate analysis. After selection of the men population, no association was found after multivariate analysis. Evans et al. have shown a relationship but only in a military population different from our sport population [9]. Yet, we have shown that patients with non-contact ACL injury were at risk of injury in case of Body Mass Index ≥ 22.5 kg/m^2. Passive knee valgus and passive knee extension increased this risk of 1.21 and 1.16 times, respectively. In this particular population, the Body Mass Index is the only modifiable factor.

In our study, the age of the non-contact ACL group was older (mean: 27 years old) than those of the contact ACL injury group (mean: 24 years old). This parameter is debatable because age was not considered a risk factor in prospective study [11,28,29]. Only Hagglund et al., have described a cut-off superior to 14 years old in a retrospective study of very young female soccer players, aged between 12 to 17 years old [16]. In contrast, age was not associated with non-contact ACL injury in two other populations aged 18 and 33 years old [15,21]. However, when the population under 23.5 years old was taken into consideration, passive knee extension and a poor Hamstring isokinetic strength were associated with non-contact ACL injury. Because hamstring isokinetic strength was a protective factor (OR from 0.09 to 0.88), strengthening this muscle group would be interesting for ACL injury prevention. Some authors have already described knee muscle strength as the objective neuromuscular risk factor of non-contact ACL injury with controversial results [11,28,29]. Myer et al. have shown weak hamstring isokinetic strength with relative great quadriceps isokinetic strength in women with ACL injury [29]. On the contrary, Uhorchak et al. have not found a particular knee strength risk of non-contact ACL injury [11]. However, the strength normalized to body weight was questionable in this study because this parameter was expressed in an unusual unit in % of the bodyweight and not in Nm/kg [11]. Therefore, the values were very different from ours and may explain the absence of the possibility to identify isokinetic knee strength as a risk factor. Soderman and al. have used bilateral knee strength symmetry index and hamstring-to-quadriceps ratio as strength parameters [28]. Bilateral symmetry indexes were not different between traumatic and non-traumatic injuries groups. However, the mean of the hamstring-to-quadriceps ratio of the two legs was lower in the traumatic group (OR: 0.93 (0.88–0.99); $p = 0.02$) [28]. We have not confirmed this result, maybe because we have only studied the hamstring-to-quadriceps ratio of the healthy knee and not the mean of the two knees.

Antero-posterior knee laxity is known to be associated with noncontact ACL rupture particularly in women and in young athletes [11,21,22,40]. From our results, this relationship can be extended to a large population whatever gender or age when this parameter is analyzed alone. However, in multivariate model, this parameter was not powerful enough to be taken into consideration to improve the diagnosis accuracy of noncontact ACL injury.

From our results, non-contact ACL injury prevention could be proposed by hamstring strengthening, particularly in a population under the age of 23.5 years, or in case of knee laxity ≥ 4.5 mm. An increased of the relative hamstring co-contraction with the quadriceps may lead to an increased knee flexion, a reduced knee abduction and a reduced anterior tibial shear during dynamic motion [29]. In addition, hamstring knee strength should control knee rotation when a dynamic knee valgus is combined in closed kinetic chain to avoid ACL impingement [37].

One limitation of the present study was to use a method focusing on many intrinsic factors, without studying all factors such as knee geometrical morphology using MRI while many results had been published on this subject [20]. This choice was made so as to study factors easy to measure in clinical practice in order to propose a "predictive approach" of ACL injury without expensive medical means. In addition, MRI measurements have the limit of not performing the knee in support, which may explain some controversies [35]. However, radiological or posturometric examinations could be of greater value. A second limitation was to consider that both limbs of a patient were symmetrical before injury. Indeed, we cannot exclude that some patients might have differences between the injured limb and the non-injured one. The ACL injury risk factors of the non-injured limb may be not exactly the same as those of the injured limb [38,39]. Nevertheless, our cross-sectional method made it possible to be certain of ACL injury of one of the two knees considered identical. At last, the studied population was an athlete population who practice sports involving knee injury risks. The conclusions of this work are therefore probably not applicable to all populations, especially to non-sports populations.

5. Conclusions

Non-contact ACL injury was associated with age, passive knee extension and weak hamstring knee strength in an ACL reconstruction population whatever gender. Passive knee valgus is strongly associated with the female population. Unfortunately, all these factors are not changeable. Only hamstring isokinetic strength could be improved by strengthening. These modifiable intrinsic factors are also associated with different sub-populations particularly in men, but also in young athletes under 23.5 years old and in populations with an anteroposterior knee laxity upper 4.5 mm. According to these results, hamstring strengthening could be achieved especially in these populations. However, this preventive attitude needs to be confirmed by prospective comparative studies in future.

Author Contributions: Conceptualization, M.D. and A.F.-C.; formal analysis, M.D.; investigation, M.D., J.G., P.M., V.C., B.L. and A.F.-C.; methodology, A.F.-C and M.D.; project administration, A.F.-C.; resources, M.D.; software, M.D.; supervision, A.F.-C.; validation, P.M.; writing—original draft, M.D. and A.F.-C.; writing—review and editing, A.F.-C., P.M., V.C., B.L., J.G., and M.D. All authors have read and agreed to the published version of the manuscript.

Funding: This research received no external funding.

Institutional Review Board Statement: The study was performed according to the World Medical Association Declaration of Helsinki and according to the French legislation (articles L.1121-1 paragraph 1 and R1121-2, Public health code), with the agreement of the local Ethics Committee (Groupe Nantais d'Ethique dans le Domaine de la Santé (GNEDS)) on 19 February 2020.

Informed Consent Statement: The patients gave their written consent to participate in the study.

Data Availability Statement: The data presented in this study are available on request from the corresponding author. The data are not publicly available due to ethical reasons.

Conflicts of Interest: The authors declare no conflict of interest.

References

1. Kim, M.K.; Baek, K.H.; Song, K.H.; Kwon, H.S.; Lee, J.M.; Kang, M.I.; Yoon, K.H.; Cha, B.Y.; Son, H.Y.; Lee, K.W. Exercise Treadmill Test in Detecting Asymptomatic Coronary Artery Disease in Type 2 Diabetes Mellitus. *Diabetes Metab. J.* **2011**, *35*, 34. [CrossRef]
2. Rahr-Wagner, L.; Lind, M. The Danish Knee Ligament Reconstruction Registry. *Clin. Epidemiol.* **2016**, *8*, 531–535. [CrossRef] [PubMed]
3. Mall, N.A.; Chalmers, P.N.; Moric, M.; Tanaka, M.J.; Cole, B.J.; Bach, B.R.; Paletta, G.A. Incidence and Trends of Anterior Cruciate Ligament Reconstruction in the United States. *Am. J. Sports Med.* **2014**, *42*, 2363–2370. [CrossRef] [PubMed]
4. Griffin, L.Y.; Agel, J.; Albohm, M.J.; Arendt, E.A.; Dick, R.W.; Garrett, W.E.; Garrick, J.G.; Hewett, T.E.; Huston, L.; Ireland, M.L.; et al. Noncontact Anterior Cruciate Ligament Injuries: Risk Factors and Prevention Strategies. *J. Am. Acad. Orthop. Surg.* **2000**, *8*, 141–150. [CrossRef] [PubMed]
5. Wetters, N.; Weber, A.E.; Wuerz, T.H.; Schub, D.L.; Mandelbaum, B.R. Mechanism of Injury and Risk Factors for Anterior Cruciate Ligament Injury. *Oper. Tech. Sports Med.* **2016**, *24*, 2–6. [CrossRef]
6. Amraee, D.; Alizadeh, M.H.; Minoonejhad, H.; Razi, M.; Amraee, G.H. Predictor Factors for Lower Extremity Malalignment and Non-Contact Anterior Cruciate Ligament Injuries in Male Athletes. *Knee Surg. Sports Traumatol. Arthrosc. Off. J. ESSKA* **2017**, *25*, 1625–1631. [CrossRef] [PubMed]
7. Hohmann, E.; Tetsworth, K.; Glatt, V.; Ngcelwane, M.; Keough, N. Medial and Lateral Posterior Tibial Slope Are Independent Risk Factors for Noncontact ACL Injury in Both Men and Women. *Orthop. J. Sports Med.* **2021**, *9*, 23259671211015940. [CrossRef]
8. Pfeifer, C.E.; Beattie, P.F.; Sacko, R.S.; Hand, A. Risk factors associated with non-contact anterior cruciate ligament injury: A systematic review. *Int. J. Sports Phys. Ther.* **2018**, *13*, 575–587. [CrossRef] [PubMed]
9. Evans, K.N.; Kilcoyne, K.G.; Dickens, J.F.; Rue, J.-P.; Giuliani, J.; Gwinn, D.; Wilckens, J.H. Predisposing Risk Factors for Non-Contact ACL Injuries in Military Subjects. *Knee Surg. Sports Traumatol. Arthrosc. Off. J. ESSKA* **2012**, *20*, 1554–1559. [CrossRef]
10. Smith, H.C.; Vacek, P.; Johnson, R.J.; Slauterbeck, J.R.; Hashemi, J.; Shultz, S.; Beynnon, B.D. Risk Factors for Anterior Cruciate Ligament Injury: A Review of the Literature-Part 1: Neuromuscular and Anatomic Risk. *Sports Health* **2012**, *4*, 69–78. [CrossRef]
11. Uhorchak, J.M.; Scoville, C.R.; Williams, G.N.; Arciero, R.A.; St Pierre, P.; Taylor, D.C. Risk Factors Associated with Noncontact Injury of the Anterior Cruciate Ligament: A Prospective Four-Year Evaluation of 859 West Point Cadets. *Am. J. Sports Med.* **2003**, *31*, 831–842. [CrossRef]

12. Hughes, G.; Watkins, J. A Risk-Factor Model for Anterior Cruciate Ligament Injury. *Sports Med. Auckl. NZ* **2006**, *36*, 411–428. [CrossRef] [PubMed]
13. Myer, G.D.; Paterno, M.V.; Ford, K.R.; Quatman, C.E.; Hewett, T.E. Rehabilitation after Anterior Cruciate Ligament Reconstruction: Criteria-Based Progression through the Return-to-Sport Phase. *J. Orthop. Sports Phys. Ther.* **2006**, *36*, 385–402. [CrossRef]
14. Beynnon, B.D.; Vacek, P.M.; Newell, M.K.; Tourville, T.W.; Smith, H.C.; Shultz, S.J.; Slauterbeck, J.R.; Johnson, R.J. The Effects of Level of Competition, Sport, and Sex on the Incidence of First-Time Noncontact Anterior Cruciate Ligament Injury. *Am. J. Sports Med.* **2014**, *42*, 1806–1812. [CrossRef] [PubMed]
15. Fernández-Jaén, T.; López-Alcorocho, J.M.; Rodriguez-Iñigo, E.; Castellán, F.; Hernández, J.C.; Guillén-García, P. The Importance of the Intercondylar Notch in Anterior Cruciate Ligament Tears. *Orthop. J. Sports Med.* **2015**, *3*, 2325967115597882. [CrossRef] [PubMed]
16. Hägglund, M.; Waldén, M. Risk Factors for Acute Knee Injury in Female Youth Football. *Knee Surg. Sports Traumatol. Arthrosc. Off. J. ESSKA* **2016**, *24*, 737–746. [CrossRef] [PubMed]
17. Jeon, N.; Choi, N.-H.; Hwangbo, B.-H.; Victoroff, B.N. An Increased Lateral Femoral Condyle Ratio in Addition to Increased Posterior Tibial Slope and Narrower Notch Index Is a Risk Factor for Female Anterior Cruciate Ligament Injury. *Arthrosc. J. Arthrosc. Relat. Surg. Off. Publ. Arthrosc. Assoc. N. Am. Int. Arthrosc. Assoc.* **2021**, in press. [CrossRef]
18. Bayer, S.; Meredith, S.J.; Wilson, K.W.; de Sa, D.; Pauyo, T.; Byrne, K.; McDonough, C.M.; Musahl, V. Knee Morphological Risk Factors for Anterior Cruciate Ligament Injury: A Systematic Review. *J. Bone Jt. Surg. Am.* **2020**, *102*, 703–718. [CrossRef] [PubMed]
19. Kızılgöz, V.; Sivrioğlu, A.K.; Ulusoy, G.R.; Aydın, H.; Karayol, S.S.; Menderes, U. Analysis of the Risk Factors for Anterior Cruciate Ligament Injury: An Investigation of Structural Tendencies. *Clin. Imaging* **2018**, *50*, 20–30. [CrossRef] [PubMed]
20. Shen, L.; Jin, Z.-G.; Dong, Q.-R.; Li, L.-B. Anatomical Risk Factors of Anterior Cruciate Ligament Injury. *Chin. Med. J.* **2018**, *131*, 2960–2967. [CrossRef] [PubMed]
21. Vauhnik, R.; Morrissey, M.C.; Rutherford, O.M.; Turk, Z.; Pilih, I.A.; Pohar, M. Knee Anterior Laxity: A Risk Factor for Traumatic Knee Injury among Sportswomen? *Knee Surg. Sports Traumatol. Arthrosc. Off. J. ESSKA* **2008**, *16*, 823–833. [CrossRef]
22. Woodford-Rogers, B.; Cyphert, L.; Denegar, C.R. Risk Factors for Anterior Cruciate Ligament Injury in High School and College Athletes. *J. Athl. Train.* **1994**, *29*, 343–346. [PubMed]
23. Ramesh, R.; Von Arx, O.; Azzopardi, T.; Schranz, P.J. The Risk of Anterior Cruciate Ligament Rupture with Generalised Joint Laxity. *J. Bone Jt. Surg. Br.* **2005**, *87*, 800–803. [CrossRef]
24. Loudon, J.K.; Jenkins, W.; Loudon, K.L. The Relationship between Static Posture and ACL Injury in Female Athletes. *J. Orthop. Sports Phys. Ther.* **1996**, *24*, 91–97. [CrossRef] [PubMed]
25. Kramer, L.C.; Denegar, C.R.; Buckley, W.E.; Hertel, J. Factors Associated with Anterior Cruciate Ligament Injury: History in Female Athletes. *J. Sports Med. Phys. Fit.* **2007**, *47*, 446–454.
26. Rafeeuddin, R.; Sharir, R.; Staes, F.; Dingenen, B.; George, K.; Robinson, M.A.; Vanrenterghem, J. Mapping Current Research Trends on Neuromuscular Risk Factors of Non-Contact ACL Injury. *Phys. Ther. Sport Off. J. Assoc. Chart. Physiother. Sports Med.* **2016**, *22*, 101–113. [CrossRef]
27. Konishi, Y.; Aihara, Y.; Sakai, M.; Ogawa, G.; Fukubayashi, T. Gamma Loop Dysfunction in the Quadriceps Femoris of Patients Who Underwent Anterior Cruciate Ligament Reconstruction Remains Bilaterally. *Scand. J. Med. Sci. Sports* **2007**, *17*, 393–399. [CrossRef] [PubMed]
28. Söderman, K.; Alfredson, H.; Pietilä, T.; Werner, S. Risk Factors for Leg Injuries in Female Soccer Players: A Prospective Investigation during One out-Door Season. *Knee Surg. Sports Traumatol. Arthrosc. Off. J. ESSKA* **2001**, *9*, 313–321. [CrossRef] [PubMed]
29. Myer, G.D.; Ford, K.R.; Foss, K.D.B.; Liu, C.; Nick, T.G.; Hewett, T.E. The Relationship of Hamstrings and Quadriceps Strength to Anterior Cruciate Ligament Injury in Female Athletes. *Clin. J. Sport Med. Off. J. Can. Acad. Sport Med.* **2009**, *19*, 3–8. [CrossRef] [PubMed]
30. Hewett, T.E.; Myer, G.D.; Ford, K.R.; Heidt, R.S.; Colosimo, A.J.; McLean, S.G.; van den Bogert, A.J.; Paterno, M.V.; Succop, P. Biomechanical Measures of Neuromuscular Control and Valgus Loading of the Knee Predict Anterior Cruciate Ligament Injury Risk in Female Athletes: A Prospective Study. *Am. J. Sports Med.* **2005**, *33*, 492–501. [CrossRef]
31. Boden, B.P.; Sheehan, F.T.; Torg, J.S.; Hewett, T.E. Noncontact Anterior Cruciate Ligament Injuries: Mechanisms and Risk Factors. *J. Am. Acad. Orthop. Surg.* **2010**, *18*, 520–527. [CrossRef]
32. Shimokochi, Y.; Shultz, S.J. Mechanisms of Noncontact Anterior Cruciate Ligament Injury. *J. Athl. Train.* **2008**, *43*, 396–408. [CrossRef]
33. Alentorn-Geli, E.; Myer, G.D.; Silvers, H.J.; Samitier, G.; Romero, D.; Lázaro-Haro, C.; Cugat, R. Prevention of Non-Contact Anterior Cruciate Ligament Injuries in Soccer Players. Part 1: Mechanisms of Injury and Underlying Risk Factors. *Knee Surg. Sports Traumatol. Arthrosc. Off. J. ESSKA* **2009**, *17*, 705–729. [CrossRef]
34. Pantano, K.J.; White, S.C.; Gilchrist, L.A.; Leddy, J. Differences in Peak Knee Valgus Angles between Individuals with High and Low Q-Angles during a Single Limb Squat. *Clin. Biomech. Bristol Avon* **2005**, *20*, 966–972. [CrossRef]
35. Pangaud, C.; Laumonerie, P.; Dagneaux, L.; LiArno, S.; Wellings, P.; Faizan, A.; Sharma, A.; Ollivier, M. Measurement of the Posterior Tibial Slope Depends on Ethnicity, Sex, and Lower Limb Alignment: A Computed Tomography Analysis of 378 Healthy Participants. *Orthop. J. Sports Med.* **2020**, *8*, 2325967119895258. [CrossRef]

36. Arendt, E.; Dick, R. Knee Injury Patterns among Men and Women in Collegiate Basketball and Soccer. NCAA Data and Review of Literature. *Am. J. Sports Med.* **1995**, *23*, 694–701. [CrossRef]
37. Hewett, T.E.; Myer, G.D.; Ford, K.R.; Paterno, M.V.; Quatman, C.E. Mechanisms, Prediction, and Prevention of ACL Injuries: Cut Risk with Three Sharpened and Validated Tools. *J. Orthop. Res. Off. Publ. Orthop. Res. Soc.* **2016**, *34*, 1843–1855. [CrossRef]
38. Paterno, M.V.; Rauh, M.J.; Schmitt, L.C.; Ford, K.R.; Hewett, T.E. Incidence of Second ACL Injuries 2 Years After Primary ACL Reconstruction and Return to Sport. *Am. J. Sports Med.* **2014**, *42*, 1567–1573. [CrossRef]
39. Swärd, P.; Kostogiannis, I.; Roos, H. Risk Factors for a Contralateral Anterior Cruciate Ligament Injury. *Knee Surg. Sports Traumatol. Arthrosc. Off. J. ESSKA* **2010**, *18*, 277–291. [CrossRef]
40. Myer, G.D.; Ford, K.R.; Paterno, M.V.; Nick, T.G.; Hewett, T.E. The Effects of Generalized Joint Laxity on Risk of Anterior Cruciate Ligament Injury in Young Female Athletes. *Am. J. Sports Med.* **2008**, *36*, 1073–1080. [CrossRef]
41. Jardin, C.; Chantelot, C.; Migaud, H.; Gougeon, F.; Debroucker, M.J.; Duquennoy, A. Reliability of the KT-1000 arthrometer in measuring anterior laxity of the knee: Comparative analysis with Telos of 48 reconstructions of the anterior cruciate ligament and intra- and interobserver reproducibility. *Rev. Chir. Orthop. Reparatrice Appar. Mot.* **1999**, *85*, 698–707.
42. Robert, H.; Nouveau, S.; Gageot, S.; Gagnière, B. A New Knee Arthrometer, the GNRB: Experience in ACL Complete and Partial Tears. *Orthop. Traumatol. Surg. Res. OTSR* **2009**, *95*, 171–176. [CrossRef]
43. Boyer, P.; Djian, P.; Christel, P.; Paoletti, X.; Degeorges, R. Reliability of the KT-1000 arthrometer (Medmetric) for measuring anterior knee laxity: Comparison with Telos in 147 knees. *Rev. Chir. Orthop. Reparatrice Appar. Mot.* **2004**, *90*, 757–764. [CrossRef]
44. Impellizzeri, F.M.; Bizzini, M.; Rampinini, E.; Cereda, F.; Maffiuletti, N.A. Reliability of Isokinetic Strength Imbalance Ratios Measured Using the Cybex NORM Dynamometer. *Clin. Physiol. Funct. Imaging* **2008**, *28*, 113–119. [CrossRef]
45. Montalvo, A.M.; Schneider, D.K.; Webster, K.E.; Yut, L.; Galloway, M.T.; Heidt, R.S.; Kaeding, C.C.; Kremcheck, T.E.; Magnussen, R.A.; Parikh, S.N.; et al. Anterior Cruciate Ligament Injury Risk in Sport: A Systematic Review and Meta-Analysis of Injury Incidence by Sex and Sport Classification. *J. Athl. Train.* **2019**, *54*, 472–482. [CrossRef]
46. Peduzzi, P.; Concato, J.; Kemper, E.; Holford, T.R.; Feinstein, A.R. A Simulation Study of the Number of Events per Variable in Logistic Regression Analysis. *J. Clin. Epidemiol.* **1996**, *49*, 1373–1379. [CrossRef]
47. Bahr, R.; Holme, I. Risk Factors for Sports Injuries–a Methodological Approach. *Br. J. Sports Med.* **2003**, *37*, 384–392. [CrossRef]
48. Ruopp, M.D.; Perkins, N.J.; Whitcomb, B.W.; Schisterman, E.F. Youden Index and Optimal Cut-Point Estimated from Observations Affected by a Lower Limit of Detection. *Biom. J. Biom. Z.* **2008**, *50*, 419–430. [CrossRef] [PubMed]
49. Altman, D.G.; Bland, J.M. Diagnostic Tests 3: Receiver Operating Characteristic Plots. *BMJ* **1994**, *309*, 188. [CrossRef] [PubMed]
50. Deeks, J. When Can Odds Ratios Mislead? Odds Ratios Should Be Used Only in Case-Control Studies and Logistic Regression Analyses. *BMJ* **1998**, *317*, 1155–1156; author reply 1156–1157. [CrossRef] [PubMed]
51. Van Tiggelen, D.; Wickes, S.; Stevens, V.; Roosen, P.; Witvrouw, E. Effective Prevention of Sports Injuries: A Model Integrating Efficacy, Efficiency, Compliance and Risk-Taking Behaviour. *Br. J. Sports Med.* **2008**, *42*, 648–652. [CrossRef] [PubMed]
52. Mohamed, E.E.; Useh, U.; Mtshali, B.F. Q-Angle, Pelvic Width, and Intercondylar Notch Width as Predictors of Knee Injuries in Women Soccer Players in South Africa. *Afr. Health Sci.* **2012**, *12*, 174–180. [CrossRef] [PubMed]

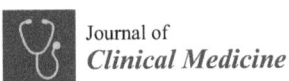

Article

Mechanical Hyperalgesia but Not Forward Shoulder Posture Is Associated with Shoulder Pain in Volleyball Players: A Cross-Sectional Study

Daniel Pecos-Martín [1], Sergio Patiño-Núñez [2], Jessica Quintero-Pérez [3], Gema Cruz-Riesco [4], Cintia Quevedo-Socas [4], Tomás Gallego-Izquierdo [1], Hector Beltran-Alacreu [5,*] and Josué Fernández-Carnero [6,7,8,9,10]

1 Physiotherapy and Pain Group, Department of Physical Therapy, University of Alcalá, 28871 Madrid, Spain; daniel.pecos@uah.es (D.P.-M.); tomas.gallego@uah.es (T.G.-I.)
2 Departamento de Fisioterapia, Medicina y Ciencias Biomédicas, Universidad de A Coruña, Campus de Oza s/n, 15006 A Coruña, Spain; sergio.patino@udc.es
3 Licenciatura de Fisioterapia, Facultad de Medicina, Benemérita Universidad Autónoma de Puebla, Puebla 72410, Mexico; jessquin09@hotmail.com
4 Research Institute of Physiotherapy and Pain, University of Alcalá, 28805 Madrid, Spain; gemcruz44@gmail.es (G.C.-R.); cintiaquevedo1999@gmail.com (C.Q.-S.)
5 Toledo Physiotherapy Research Group (GIFTO), Faculty of Physical Therapy and Nursing, Universidad de Castilla-La Mancha, 45071 Toledo, Spain
6 Department of Physical Therapy, Occupational Therapy, Rehabilitation and Physical Medicine, Rey Juan Carlos University, 28922 Alcorcón, Spain; josue.fernandez@urjc.es
7 La Paz Hospital Institute for Health Research (IdiPAZ), 28029 Madrid, Spain
8 Grupo Multidisciplinar de Investigación y Tratamiento del Dolor, Grupo de Excelencia Investigadora, URJC-Banco de Santander, 28922 Madrid, Spain
9 Motion in Brains Research Group, Institute of Neuroscience and Movement Sciences (INCIMOV), Centro Superior de Estudios Universitarios La Salle, Universidad Autonóma de Madrid, 28023 Madrid, Spain
10 Grupo de Investigación de Dolor Musculoesquelético y Control Motor, Universidad Europea de Madrid, 28670 Villaviciosa de Odón, Spain
* Correspondence: hector.beltran@uclm.es; Tel.: +34-926-051-556

Abstract: Shoulder antepulsion, altered scapular kinematics and imbalance of muscle activity are commonly associated with shoulder pain. This study aimed to observe if there is an association between the forward shoulder angle (FSA) and the pectoralis minor length index (PMI) in volleyball players with and without shoulder pain. Furthermore, this study observed if there is an association between shoulder posture and upper limb mechanical hyperalgesia in volleyball players with and without shoulder pain. Methods: a cross-sectional study was conducted in the Physiotherapy and Pain Research Center in Alcalá de Henares (Spain). A total of 56 volleyball players met the inclusion criteria and agreed to enter the study. Subjects were divided into two groups: shoulder pain group (SPG) and control group (without pain). The following measurements of the dominant sides of the players were collected: FSA, PMI, and pressure pain threshold (PPT) in serratus anterior, lower trapezius, infraspinatus, teres minor, upper trapezius, levator scapulae, pectoralis major, radial nerve, cubital nerve, and median nerve. Results: The Spearman's Rho revealed no significant correlations were found between FSA and PMI. Moreover, Spearman's Rho test revealed in the SPG a negative moderate correlation between FSA and Infraspinatus-PPT (Rho = −0.43; $p = 0.02$); FSA and levator scapulae-PPT (Rho = −0.55; $p < 0.01$); FSA and pectoralis major-PPT (Rho = −0.41; $p = 0.02$); PMI and cubital nerve-PPT (Rho = −0.44; $p = 0.01$). Conclusions: No association was found between the forward shoulder angle and the pectoralis minor index in volleyball players with and without shoulder pain. There is a moderate negative association between shoulder forward angle and muscle mechanical hyperalgesia in volleyball players with shoulder pain, but no such associations were found in volleyball players without shoulder pain. Treatment of the infraspinatus, levator scapulae, pectoralis major, and pectoralis minor muscles could improve shoulder pain and ulnar nerve mechanosensitivity.

Citation: Pecos-Martín, D.; Patiño-Núñez, S.; Quintero-Pérez, J.; Cruz-Riesco, G.; Quevedo-Socas, C.; Gallego-Izquierdo, T.; Beltran-Alacreu, H.; Fernández-Carnero, J. Mechanical Hyperalgesia but Not Forward Shoulder Posture Is Associated with Shoulder Pain in Volleyball Players: A Cross-Sectional Study. J. Clin. Med. 2022, 11, 1472. https://doi.org/10.3390/jcm11061472

Academic Editor: David Rodríguez-Sanz

Received: 4 January 2022
Accepted: 5 March 2022
Published: 8 March 2022

Publisher's Note: MDPI stays neutral with regard to jurisdictional claims in published maps and institutional affiliations.

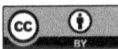

Copyright: © 2022 by the authors. Licensee MDPI, Basel, Switzerland. This article is an open access article distributed under the terms and conditions of the Creative Commons Attribution (CC BY) license (https://creativecommons.org/licenses/by/4.0/).

Keywords: forward shoulder angle; pectoralis minor length; mechanical hyperalgesia; volleyball

1. Introduction

Overuse or repetitive motion injuries are very common in sports [1]. This type of injury can be a major source of disability and pain and can leave players unable to engage in physical activity or competition. There is little evidence on the real impact and severity in sport, due to the methodological difficulties involved in recording them [1]. Volleyball is one of the sports affected by overuse injuries [2–4]. The biomechanics of the different movements involved in volleyball, in particular the spike and serve, together with the anatomy of volleyball players coincide with the most prevalent overuse injuries, the shoulder region (19.0 ± 11.2%) and the spine (16.8 ± 9.7%) [3,4]. These structures are subjected not only to repetition of movement but also to high torsional values and amplitude of movement in short periods of time [3].

The assessment of posture and biomechanics is a useful clinical tool in shoulder pain. Shoulder antepulsion, also known as "rounded shoulder", is characterized by a position in which the scapula rotates downwards and remains tilted forward, increasing cervical lordosis and upper thoracic kyphosis [5]. It has been previously published that postural or biomechanical alterations such as forward head position, shoulder antepulsion, altered scapular kinematics, and imbalance of muscle activity are associated with shoulder pain [6]. This could lead to the development of pain depending on the tolerance and adaptive capacity of the central nervous system [7]. In addition, there is evidence that a high percentage of patients with non-specific arm pain have their shoulders in antepulsion and head forward (78% and 71%, respectively) [6,8].

Loss of activity of the lower trapezius and serratus anterior, a marked thoracic kyphosis and the anatomy of the scapula itself can cause the shoulder antepulsion. In addition, tension of the pectoralis minor [5], which, together with the downward displacement of the coracoid process, may affect the gliding of the brachial plexus cords. Complete scapular protraction (due to its junctions with soft tissues and surrounding structures) may reduce the space between the clavicle and the first rib, restricting nerve gliding, and as a result of a combination of movements of structures of the shoulder girdle itself, anterior displacement of the humeral head may occur [9]. This can lead to some postural alterations such as an antepulsion of the shoulder can alter the mechanosensitivity of different tissues, thus decreasing their tolerance to mechanical stress even if it does not provoke a nociceptive response [10]. A recent study adds data on this association by concluding that individuals with shoulder impingement syndrome had a greater thoracic kyphosis and less extension movement than age- and gender-matched healthy controls [11]. For all these reasons, more studies are needed in the sports population to observe whether these types of associations or relationships exist and what clinical implications they may have.

Currently there are no studies that correlate the forward shoulder position with photometry with the shortening of the pectoralis minor in any type of population. Nor has it been studied whether these postural alterations are related to pain and mechanical hyperalgesia in volleyball players.

For the above reasons, the objectives of this study are as follows:

1. To observe the differences in upper limb posture and mechanical hyperalgesia between volleyball players with and without shoulder pain;
2. To observe if there is an association between the forward shoulder angle and the pectoralis minor index in volleyball players with and without shoulder pain;
3. To observe if there is an association between shoulder posture and upper limb mechanical hyperalgesia in volleyball players with and without shoulder pain.

2. Materials and Methods

This research was a cross-sectional study conducted according to the Strengthening the Reporting of Observational studies in Epidemiology (STROBE) statement [12], and following the declaration of Helsinki. The study protocol received approval from the Research Ethics Committee of University CEU Cardenal Herrera from Valencia (CEI16/0112). All the participants agreed to participate and signed an informed consent form. The study was conducted at the Physiotherapy and Pain Research Center in Alcalá de Henares (Spain).

2.1. Participants

Recruitment was carried out through an invitation to participate in the study was sent to the different volleyball sports clubs in the local area. Eligible participants were women and men from the age of 18 onwards and being a regular volleyball player (3 or more hours per week). Exclusion criteria included participants who has previous neck and shoulder injuries or surgery and were unable to read or speak in Spanish.

2.2. Procedure

Shoulder position was assessed in volleyball players with and without shoulder pain by determining the position of the humeral head and the length of the pectoralis minor muscle [6,13]. In addition, the mechanosensitivity of neuromuscular structures related to the upper quadrant of the evaluated subjects was assessed [14].

The assessments were performed by three physiotherapists independently and none of them knew the subject's condition in relation to shoulder pain, this was done to ensure the simple blind. Study participants were randomly assigned to each assessment by choosing a ballot with a number on it. Subjects who selected number 1 were first assessed for shoulder position, subjects who selected number 2 were assessed for mechanosensitivity of the musculature, and subjects who selected number 3 were assessed for mechanosensitivity in the nerve trunks.

2.3. Outcome Measures

2.3.1. Forward Shoulder Angle (Forward Shoulder Position)

Posture was assessed using a postural analysis software [14,15]. Markers were placed on the acromion and the spinous process of C7. Participants were placed in a standing position, sideways 40 cm from the wall, and instructed to maintain a natural resting position. A reflex camera (Nikon Model D5300 SLR, Tokyo, Japan) was placed on a tripod one meter high and three meters from the wall. One photograph was taken from the right side and one photograph from the left side.

The forward shoulder angle (FSA) was determined by calculating the angle formed by a vertical line passing posterior to the marker at C7 and a line connecting C7 and the acromion marker. Those participants who showed values equal to or greater than 52° were considered a forward shoulder position (FSP) [6]. This procedure has shown good reliability with an very high intraclass correlation coefficient (ICC) (0.89) [6]. The photographs were taken by a physiotherapist with more than 10 years of experience in the management of musculoskeletal pain and was blinded to the values obtained from the other assessments.

2.3.2. Pectoralis Minor Length Measurements

Pectoralis minor (PM) length is expressed as the pectoralis minor index (PMI) which is calculated as PM length (cm)/subject height × 100. This normalization index is used to allow for the variety of soft tissue and body structure between subjects [16]. To measure the length of the PM muscle the reference points were the inferior medial angles of the coracoid process, and lateral to the sternocostal junction of the fourth rib on its underside. These landmarks have shown an ICC of 0.96 [16]. A digital caliper (Mitutoyo/200 mm, Kawasaki, Japan) was used to measure the distance between these two points. Measurement using a caliper has shown an ICC of 0.83 to 0.87 [17].

Participants were placed supine with both hands on the abdomen, with the shoulders slightly abducted, and in a relaxed elbow flexion position. The elbows were flexed to eliminate the passive influence of the biceps brachii muscle [18]. PMI assessment was performed by a second evaluator blinded to the other assessments values and with more than 10 years of experience in the management of musculoskeletal problems.

2.3.3. Tissue Mechanosensitivity (Muscle and Nerve Trunks)

The degree of tissue mechanosensitivity was assessed by determining the pressure pain threshold (PPT) with algometry, i.e., quantitative assessment of the sensory perception of the mechanical stimulus [19]. The PPT was measured with a manual algometer (Wagner Force Dial, Model FDK20) which has a head of 1 cm^2 and determines the pressure in kg/cm^2 [19]. The pressure was increased by 1 kg per second until the subject indicated changes in pressure sensation. The assessor stopped applying pressure when the participant expressed pain. Three measurements were made at each location with a 30-s rest period in between. The mean value of the three measurements was used for statistical analysis. A third evaluator blinded to the other assessments measured the PPT of the following muscles: serratus anterior, lower trapezius, infraspinatus, teres minor, upper trapezius, levator scapulae, pectoralis major. The muscle was palpated to locate the most mechanosensitive point and perform the PPT measurement. Measurement of the PPT with an algometer has been shown to have good reliability with an ICC of 0.87 to 0.89 [19].

A fourth evaluator performed bilateral PPT measurements of the nerve trunks of the upper extremity: median nerve, radial nerve, and ulnar nerve. The nerves were evaluated at the locations described by Sterling et al. [19], which have shown good reliability with an ICC of 0.92 to 0.97. The median nerve identified in the ulnar fossa inside the tendon of the biceps muscle. The radial nerve was located in the lateral intermuscular septum between the medial and lateral head of the triceps brachii muscle, and the ulnar nerve was located in the ulnar canal of the elbow. Both evaluators had more than 10 years of experience in the management of musculoskeletal system alterations.

2.3.4. Pain Intensity

Shoulder pain was assessed using a visual analog scale (VAS). The subject with pain indicated what their pain was on a 10-cm line where 0 represented no pain and 10 the worst pain imaginable. This tool has been shown to be reliable with an ICC of 0.94 [20]. The VAS measure was expressed in cm. Participants with more than 0 cm in the VAS were placed in the shoulder pain group (SPG), the rest of participants were placed in the control group (CG).

2.4. Sample Size

Sample size and power calculations were performed with an appropriate software (G*Power 3.1) [21]. This study was based on a model of correlations, and the FSA was the primary outcome, with an effect size of 0.75. Given an alpha level of 0.05 and a power of 0.80, two groups were generated with a total sample size of 50. The groups included shoulder pain and without pain (control) with a minimum of 25 participants per group.

2.5. Data Analysis

Statistical analysis was performed with the Statistical Package for the Social Sciences, version 28 (IBM Corporation, Armonk, NY, USA). The normality of the study variables was tested using the Shapiro–Wilk test. A normal distribution of the variables was not obtained in the Shapiro–Wilk test ($p < 0.05$). Qualitative variables are presented as an absolute value and the percentage of the relative frequency [n (%)]. Continuous variables are represented as median (1st and 3rd quartiles). All statistical tests were interpreted at a significance level of 5% ($p < 0.05$). To test the differences between groups for FSA, PMI, muscle PPT, and nerve PPT, the Mann–Whitney U test was performed to verify which ones entailed statistically significant differences. Finally, the correlations between the study variables were analyzed for each group with the Spearman's Rho test considering the results as 0.01 to 0.19 very low correlation, 0.2 to 0.39 low correlation, 0.4 to 0.69 moderate correlation, 0.7 to 0.89 high correlation, 0.9 to 0.99 very high correlation, and 1 large or perfect correlation.

3. Results

3.1. Participants and Descriptive Data

A total of 56 volleyball players met the inclusion criteria and agreed to enter the study, leaving a sample of 28 in the SPG group and 28 in the CG. The median age of the sample was 22.5 (19 and 24), with most of them being female $n = 33$ (58.9%). No statistically significant differences were found in the descriptive characteristics measured in both groups ($p > 0.05$). The descriptive data of the participants are shown in Table 1.

Table 1. Characteristics of the groups. Values are median (first and third quartiles) and n (%).

	Shoulder Pain Group ($n = 28$)	Control Group ($n = 28$)	p Value
Age (years)	21.5 (20 and 23.75)	21.5 (18 and 26)	0.74
Sex (female n, [%])	19 [67.9%]	14 [50%]	-
Weight (kg)	63.5 (57 and 71.75)	67.5 (57.25 and 76.75)	0.66
Height (cm)	170 (166.25 and 183.25)	178 (167.75 and 180.75)	0.25
BMI	22.57 (20.44 and 23.71)	21.85 (20.83 and 23.32)	0.49
Dominant side (right n, [%])	26 [92.9%]	21 [75%]	-
VAS (0–10 cm)	6.25 (6 and 7)	-	-
Pain duration (months)	1 (0 and 6.75)	-	-
FSP (yes n, [%])	15 [53.6%]	15 [53.6%]	-

VAS, visual analogue scale; FSP, forward shoulder position.

3.2. Comparison between Groups

The Mann–Whitney U test revealed no statistical differences between groups for FSA ($p = 0.33$) and for PMI ($p = 0.29$), see Table 2. On the other hand, significant statistical differences between groups for muscle PPT in Lower Trapezius ($p = 0.019$), Infraspinatus ($p < 0.01$), Teres Minor ($p < 0.01$), Upper Trapezius ($p = 0.019$), Pectoralis Major ($p = 0.02$), and for radial nerve PPT ($p = 0.04$), see Table 2.

Table 2. Measurements of the study. Values are median (first and third quartiles) and n (%).

		Shoulder Pain Group ($n = 28$)	Control Group ($n = 28$)	Mann–Whitney U Test (p Value)
FSA (degrees)		49 (42.25 and 56.5)	50.5 (48 and 57.5)	0.33
PMI (cm)		13 (11.88 and 13.98)	13.83 (12.25 and 14.51)	0.29
PPT (kg/cm^2)				
	Serratus Anterior	2.35 (1.6 and 3.07)	2.72 (2.26 and 3.37)	0.059
	Lower Trapezious	2.52 (2.21 and 3.1)	3 (2.72 and 3.8)	0.019 *
	Infraspinatus	2.3 (2.02 and 2.85)	3 (2.6 and 4)	<0.01 **
	Teres Minor	2.25 (1.92 and 2.73)	2.7 (2.3 and 4)	<0.01 **
	Levator scapulae	2.2 (1.62 and 2.73)	2.75 (1.8 and 3.37)	0.06
	Upper Trapezius	2.12 (1.6 and 2.43)	2.42 (2.1 and 3.46)	0.019 *
	Pectoralis Major	2.15 (1.55 and 2.57)	2.7 (2 and 3.58)	0.02 *
	Median Nerve	2.4 (2.1 and 3.13)	2.77 (2.21 and 3.17)	0.4
	Radial Nerve	3 (2.18 and 3.67)	3.62 (2.61 and 4.03)	0.04 *
	Cubital Nerve	2.65 (2.46 and 3.47)	3.32 (2.52 and 4)	0.27

* $p < 0.05$, ** $p < 0.01$. FSA, forward shoulder angle; PMI, pectoralis minor index; PPT, pain pressure threshold.

3.3. Correlations

The Spearman's Rho test revealed in the SPG a negative moderate correlations between FSA and Infraspinatus-PPT (Rho = −0.43; $p = 0.02$); FSA and Levator Scapulae-PPT (Rho = −0.55; $p < 0.01$); FSA and Pectoralis Major-PPT (Rho = −0.41; $p = 0.02$); PMI and

Cubital Nerve-PPT (Rho = −0.44; p = 0.01); VAS and Upper Trapezius-PPT (Rho = −0.41; p = 0.02); VAS and Median Nerve-PPT (Rho = −0.51; p < 0.01). No significant correlations were found between posture measurements (FSA and PMI) and VAS, see Table 3.

Table 3. Spearman's Rho correlations in Shoulder pain Group.

	PMI	VAS	Serratus Anterior	Lower Trapezius	Infraspinatus	Teres Minor	Levator Scapulae	Upper Trapezius	Pectoralis Major	Median Nerve	Radial Nerve	Cubital Nerve
FSA	0.12	−0.21	−0.36	−0.21	−0.43 *	−0.33	−0.55 *	−0.24	−0.41 *	−0.2	−0.14	−0.13
PMI	1	−0.002	−0.12	0.2	−0.02	−0.03	−0.11	0.14	−0.17	−0.09	−0.16	−0.44 *

* p < 0.05; FSA, forward shoulder angle; PMI, pectoralis minor index; VAS, visual analogue scale.

No significant correlations were found according to the Spearman's Rho test in the CG, see Table 4.

Table 4. Spearman's Rho correlations in Control Group.

	PMI	VAS	Serratus Anterior	Lower Trapezius	Infraspinatus	Teres Minor	Levator Scapulae	Upper Trapezius	Pectoralis Major	Median Nerve	Radial Nerve	Cubital Nerve
FSA	−0.29	-	0.01	0.98	0.11	−0.08	−0.02	0.21	−0.2	0.06	0.05	0.02
PMI	1	-	0.11	−0.12	−0.03	−0.06	−0.27	−0.1	0.03	−0.11	0	−0.08

FSA, forward shoulder angle; PMI, pectoralis minor index; VAS, visual analogue scale.

4. Discussion

This study is the first one that had explored the association of the forward shoulder angle and the pectoralis minor index in volleyball players. To summarize, the two main principal findings of this study are as follows:

1. No association was found between the forward shoulder angle and the pectoralis minor index in volleyball players with and without shoulder pain;
2. Results show that mechanical hyperalgesia is increased in players with shoulder pain versus those without, but there are no differences in forward shoulder posture or shortening of the pectoralis minor;
3. There is a moderate negative association between shoulder forward angle with muscle mechanical hyperalgesia (Infraspinatus, Levator Scapulae and Pectoralis Major); and the pectoralis minor index with the mechanical hyperalgesia of the cubital nerve in volleyball players with shoulder pain. No such associations were found in volleyball players without shoulder pain.

4.1. Posture

The results of this study appeals to the fact that shoulder position is not a key factor or a clear contributor to shoulder pain [11,22]. These results are in agreement with the findings of Ozunlu et al. [23] and Ribeiro et al. [23] Ozunlu et al. [23] showed that asymmetric scapular posture in volleyball players might be normal and not necessarily related to injury and Ribeiro A et al. [23] reported that scapular asymmetry may be normal and it should not be automatically considered as a pathological sign in throwing athletes. This situation has also been related to other areas of the body, such as the low back region, where there is no correlation between imaging tests and pain [24].

Precisely and related to PMI, several recently conducted studies concluded that there is no association between shoulder pain and function with the length of the pectoralis minor in patients with chronic shoulder pain [25,26]. This is consistent with our results although they are not performed in a sports population.

Although it has been found in another study that patients with forward shoulders have greater scapular internal rotation and less serratus anterior activity, these alterations are not associated with shoulder pain [6]. Therefore, although it has been proposed that the round shoulder posture may be related to shoulder pain and dysfunction because it alters the kinematics and muscle activity generating stressful situations in the shoulder, it seems that this relationship cannot always be established [27]. Perhaps clinical reasoning should be based more on dynamic observation of posture rather than static observation of posture [28].

It has been suggested that in the assessment of shoulder posture in patients with shoulder pain it could be interesting to observe how the change in shoulder posture affects the signs and symptoms of the patient with shoulder pain [29]. Lewis JS et al. showed that changing posture in patients with shoulder pain had positive effects on mobility and pain in these subjects [29]. A cohort study investigated people with shoulder pain and concluded that the best prognostic factor for these patients was the change of symptoms during the modification of scapula posture in the arm elevation movement [30]. Therefore, postural alteration would be clinically relevant when postural modification during the assessment of the patient with shoulder pain also modifies the patient's signs and symptoms [28]. On the other hand, demonstrating to a patient that symptoms are modifiable could give the individual confidence to move and better adherence to treatment [31].

4.2. Mechanical Hyperalgesia

The relationship between posture and tissue mechanosensitivity has been studied previously. Although the mechanical stress suffered by the structures involved in a poor posture could produce an alteration of the sensitivity of these structures, it seems that the presence of pain plays an important role in the degree of mechanosensitization [7,32,33]. Martinez-Merinero P et al. [7], Rojas VEA et al. [32], and Pacheco J et al. [33], showed that mechanosensitivity of neck muscles and upper extremity nerve trunks is related to neck pain more than to forward head position. Similarly, a study conducted by Haik M et al. [34] in which they found that subjects with shoulder pain demonstrated mechanical hyperalgesia compared with healthy controls.

The results obtained in our study have shown that the mechanosensitivity of the assessed muscles is related to shoulder pain and not with rounded shoulder posture. The infraspinatus, levator scapulae, and pectoralis major muscles were shown to have greater mechanical hyperalgesia in volleyball players with shoulder pain. These data are consistent with the results of Hidalgo-Lozano et al. reporting that elite swimmers with shoulder pain showed significant lower PPT in levator scapulae, sternocleidomastoid, upper trapezius, and infraspinatus compared with healthy athletes [35]. Pain and altered mechanosensitivity could be a consequence of repetitive overhead movements. The infraspinatus, levator scapulae, and pectoralis major muscles can produce shoulder pain [36]. In particular, the infraspinatus muscle has been shown to be important in shoulder problems [37,38]. It is a structure involved in functional problems and shoulder pain [37,38]. During a sports competition, volleyball players with shoulder pain were treated for the infraspinatus muscle and the players were able to continue in the competition [37].

On the other hand, another interesting finding of this study was the relationship the pectoralis minor index with mechanical hyperalgesia of the ulnar nerve. The pectoralis minor index expresses the length of the pectoralis minor muscle [16]. The association between a decrease in pectoralis minor length and shoulder pain has been described in athletes [39]. And pectoral shortening as a factor associated with volleyball-related shoulder pain and dysfuntion [40]. During arm elevation, subjects with shortened pectoralis minor showed decreased external rotation/retraction and posterior tilting of the scapula [40]. Limitation of scapular movements could compromise the pectoralis minor space and increase mechanical stress on the ulnar nerve [40]. Increased mechanical stress on the ulnar nerve could lead to pain and other neurogenic alterations in the upper extremity [41].

Although the relationship between the pectoralis minor muscle and the ulnar nerve has not been studied to our knowledge, it could be a cause of shoulder pain in all overhead activities.

4.3. Clinical Implications

Establishing a definitive structural diagnosis for an athlete presenting with shoulder pain is a difficult process. There appears to be a poor correlation between orthopedic and imaging tests and symptoms related to shoulder pain. In this regard, postural deviations have been frequently cited as a cause of shoulder pain and disability. This study, like others, challenges this approach. Therefore, the importance of postural disturbances during the assessment of a subject with shoulder pain should be approached differently. The shoulder forward posture may not be related to shoulder pain.

On the other hand, it seems that the shoulder musculature could be one of the causes of pain in these patients. During spiking in volleyball there is a significant increase in activity and stress on the shoulder musculature [42]. Probably, repeated overhead movements may produce an increase in mechanical muscle hyperalgesia. The mechanical muscle hyperalgesia could translate into increased tension and onset of shoulder pain.

Treatment of the infraspinatus, levator scapulae, pectoralis major, and pectoralis minor muscles could improve shoulder pain and ulnar nerve mechanosensitivity.

The literature suggests that mechanical hyperalgesia is related to poorer muscle function, and this leads to poorer motor control recruitment [35,43–45]. In sport medicine, this can be key factor in both prevention and injury recovery. Therefore, the results of this study suggest that the shoulder forward posture or the pectoralis minor index does not appear to be associated with shoulder pain, but yes, the mechanical hyperalgesia of the shoulder complex musculature. Therefore, an assessment of mechanical hyperalgesia in athlete patients with shoulder pain is suggested before posture. We can therefore suggest that in the examination of these patients it would be advisable to pay attention to the signs and symptoms of pain processing rather than to assessing shoulder posture.

4.4. Limitations

One of the main limitations of this study is that it is a cross-sectional study can only demonstrate association and not causation. Longitudinal studies are now needed to determine the role of mechanical hyperalgesia and posture in the development of shoulder pain in volleyball players. In addition, one of the limitations due to the small sample size and high effect size established, is that smaller correlations may exist. The population size was small. Future studies with larger samples are needed to further confirm the current results.

5. Conclusions

No association was found between the forward shoulder angle and the pectoralis minor index in volleyball players with and without shoulder pain. There is a moderate negative association between shoulder forward angle and muscle mechanical hyperalgesia in volleyball players with shoulder pain, but no such associations were found in volleyball players without shoulder pain. Treatment of the infraspinatus, levator scapulae, pectoralis major, and pectoralis minor muscles could improve shoulder pain and ulnar nerve mechanosensitivity.

Author Contributions: Conceptualization, D.P.-M., S.P.-N., J.Q.-P. and T.G.-I.; methodology D.P.-M., H.B.-A. and J.F.-C.; validation, all authors; formal analysis, H.B.-A. and J.F.-C.; investigation, all authors; resources, D.P.-M and T.G.-I.; data acquisition, G.C.-R. and C.Q.-S.; writing—original draft preparation, D.P.-M., H.B.-A. and J.F.-C.; writing—review and editing, all authors; supervision, all authors; project administration, D.P.-M.; funding acquisition, D.P.-M. All authors have read and agreed to the published version of the manuscript.

Funding: Part of Hector Beltran-Alacreu's salary is financed by the European Regional Development Fund (2020/5154).

Institutional Review Board Statement: The Research Ethics Committee of University CEU Cardenal Herrera from Valencia (CEI16/0112).

Informed Consent Statement: Informed consent was obtained from all subjects involved in the study. Written informed consent has been obtained from the patient(s) to publish this paper.

Data Availability Statement: Data available on request due to privacy and ethical restrictions.

Conflicts of Interest: The authors certify that they have no affiliations with or financial involvement in any organization or entity with a direct financial interest in the subject matter or materials discussed in the article.

References

1. Clarsen, B.; Bahr, R.; Heymans, M.; Engedahl, M.; Midtsundstad, G.; Rosenlund, L.; Thorsen, G.; Myklebust, G. The prevalence and impact of overuse injuries in five Norwegian sports: Application of a new surveillance method. *Scand. J. Med. Sci. Sports* **2014**, *25*, 323–330. [CrossRef]
2. Bahr, R.; Reeser, J.C.; Fédération Internationale de Volleyball. Injuries among world-class professional beach volleyball players. The Fédération Internationale de Volleyball beach volleyball injury study. *Am. J. Sports Med.* **2003**, *31*, 119–125. [CrossRef]
3. Seminati, E.; Minetti, A.E. Overuse in volleyball training/practice: A review on shoulder and spine-related injuries. *Eur. J. Sport Sci.* **2013**, *13*, 732–743. [CrossRef]
4. Frisch, K.E.; Clark, J.; Hanson, C.; Fagerness, C.; Conway, A.; Hoogendoorn, L. High Prevalence of Nontraumatic Shoulder Pain in a Regional Sample of Female High School Volleyball Athletes. *Orthop. J. Sports Med.* **2017**, *5*, 2325967117712236. [CrossRef]
5. Lee, J.; Cynn, H.; Yoon, T.; Ko, C.; Choi, W.; Choi, S.; Choi, B. The effect of scapular posterior tilt exercise, pectoralis minor stretching, and shoulder brace on scapular alignment and muscles activity in subjects with round-shoulder posture. *J. Electromyogr. Kinesiol.* **2015**, *25*, 107–114. [CrossRef]
6. Thigpen, C.A.; Padua, D.A.; Michener, L.A.; Guskiewicz, K.; Giuliani, C.; Keener, J.D.; Stergiou, N. Head and shoulder posture affect scapular mechanics and muscle activity in overhead tasks. *J. Electromyogr. Kinesiol.* **2010**, *20*, 701–709. [CrossRef]
7. Martinez-Merinero, P.; Nuñez-Nagy, S.; Achalandabaso-Ochoa, A.; Fernandez-Matias, R.; Pecos-Martin, D.; Gallego-Izquierdo, T. Relationship between Forward Head Posture and Tissue Mechanosensitivity: A Cross-Sectional Study. *J. Clin. Med.* **2020**, *9*, 634. [CrossRef]
8. Kang, J.-H.; Park, R.-Y.; Lee, S.-J.; Kim, J.-Y.; Yoon, S.-R.; Jung, K.-I. The Effect of The Forward Head Posture on Postural Balance in Long Time Computer Based Worker. *Ann. Rehabil. Med.* **2012**, *36*, 98–104. [CrossRef]
9. Julius, A.; Lees, R.; Dilley, A.; Lynn, B. Shoulder posture and median nerve sliding. *BMC Musculoskelet. Disord.* **2004**, *5*, 23. [CrossRef]
10. Martínez-Merinero, P.; Lluch, E.; Gallezo-Izquierdo, T.; Pecos-Martin, D.; Manzano, G.P.; Nuñez-Nagy, S.; Falla, D. The influence of a depressed scapular alignment on upper limb neural tissue mechanosensitivity and local pressure pain sensitivity. *Musculoskelet. Sci. Pract.* **2017**, *29*, 60–65. [CrossRef]
11. Hunter, D.J.; A Rivett, D.; McKeirnan, S.; Smith, L.; Snodgrass, S.J. Relationship between Shoulder Impingement Syndrome and Thoracic Posture. *Phys. Ther.* **2019**, *100*, 677–686. [CrossRef]
12. Vandenbroucke, J.P.; von Elm, E.; Altman, D.G.; Gøtzsche, P.C.; Mulrow, C.D.; Pocock, S.J.; Poole, C.; Schlesselman, J.J.; Egger, M. Strengthening the Reporting of Observational Studies in Epidemiology (STROBE): Explanation and elaboration. *Int. J. Surg.* **2014**, *12*, 1500–1524. [CrossRef]
13. Borstad, J.D.; Ludewig, P.M. The effect of long versus short pectoralis minor resting length on scapular kinematics in healthy individuals. *J. Orthop. Sports Phys. Ther.* **2005**, *35*, 227–238. [CrossRef]
14. Weber, P.; Corrêa, E.C.R.; Milanesi, J.M.; Soares, J.C.; Trevisan, M.E. Craniocervical posture: Cephalometric and biophotogrammetric analysis. *Braz. J. Oral Sci.* **2012**, *11*, 416–421.
15. Ruivo, R.M.; Pezarat-Correia, P.; Carita, A.I. Cervical and shoulder postural assessment of adolescents between 15 and 17 years old and association with upper quadrant pain. *Braz. J. Phys. Ther.* **2014**, *18*, 364–371. [CrossRef]
16. Borstad, J.D. Measurement of Pectoralis Minor Muscle Length: Validation and Clinical Application. *J. Orthop. Sports Phys. Ther.* **2008**, *38*, 169–174. [CrossRef]
17. Lewis, J.S.; Valentine, R.E. The pectoralis minor length test: A study of the intra-rater reliability and diagnostic accuracy in subjects with and without shoulder symptoms. *BMC Musculoskelet. Disord.* **2007**, *8*, 64. [CrossRef]
18. Walton, D.M.; MacDermid, J.C.; Nielson, W.; Teasell, R.W.; Chiasson, M.; Brown, L. Reliability, Standard Error, and Minimum Detectable Change of Clinical Pressure Pain Threshold Testing in People With and Without Acute Neck Pain. *J. Orthop. Sports Phys. Ther.* **2011**, *41*, 644–650. [CrossRef]
19. Sterling, M.; Treleaven, J.; Edwards, S.; Jull, G. Pressure pain thresholds of upper limb peripheral nerve trunks in asymptomatic subjects. *Physiother. Res. Int. J. Res. Clin. Phys. Ther.* **2000**, *5*, 220–229. [CrossRef]
20. Hawker, G.A.; Mian, S.; Kendzerska, T.; French, M. Measures of adult pain: Visual Analog Scale for Pain (VAS Pain), Numeric Rating Scale for Pain (NRS Pain), McGill Pain Questionnaire (MPQ), Short-Form McGill Pain Questionnaire (SF-MPQ), Chronic Pain Grade Scale (CPGS), Short Form-36 Bodily Pain Scale (SF-36 BPS), and Measure of Intermittent and Constant Osteoarthritis Pain (ICOAP). *Arthritis Care Res.* **2011**, *63* (Suppl. 11), S240–S252.
21. Faul, F.; Erdfelder, E.; Buchner, A.; Lang, A.-G. Statistical power analyses using G*Power 3.1: Tests for correlation and regression analyses. *Behav. Res. Methods* **2009**, *41*, 1149–1160. [CrossRef]

22. Barrett, E.; O'Keeffe, M.; O'Sullivan, K.; Lewis, J.; McCreesh, K. Is thoracic spine posture associated with shoulder pain, range of motion and function? A systematic review. *Man. Ther.* **2016**, *26*, 38–46. [CrossRef]
23. Ozunlu, N.; Tekeli, H.; Baltaci, G. Lateral Scapular Slide Test and Scapular Mobility in Volleyball Players. *J. Athl. Train.* **2011**, *46*, 438–444. [CrossRef]
24. Brinjikji, W.; Luetmer, P.; Comstock, B.; Bresnahan, B.; Chen, L.; Deyo, R.; Halabi, S.; Turner, J.; Avins, A.; James, K.; et al. Systematic Literature Review of Imaging Features of Spinal Degeneration in Asymptomatic Populations. *Am. J. Neuroradiol.* **2014**, *36*, 811–816. [CrossRef]
25. Navarro-Ledesma, S.; Fernandez-Sanchez, M.; Struyf, F.; Suarez, A.L. Association of Both Scapular Upward Rotation and Scapulothoracic Muscle Lengths with Shoulder Pain, Function, and Range of Movement. *J. Manip. Physiol. Ther.* **2020**, *43*, 824–831. [CrossRef]
26. Navarro-Ledesma, S.; Fernandez-Sanchez, M.; Luque-Suarez, A. Does the pectoralis minor length influence acromiohumeral distance, shoulder pain-function, and range of movement? *Phys. Ther. Sport* **2018**, *34*, 43–48. [CrossRef]
27. Fathollahnejad, K.; Letafatkar, A.; Hadadnezhad, M. The effect of manual therapy and stabilizing exercises on forward head and rounded shoulder postures: A six-week intervention with a one-month follow-up study. *BMC Musculoskelet. Disord.* **2019**, *20*, 86. [CrossRef]
28. Lewis, J.S.; McCreesh, K.; Barratt, E.; Hegedus, E.J.; Sim, J. Inter-rater reliability of the Shoulder Symptom Modification Procedure in people with shoulder pain. *BMJ Open Sport Exerc. Med.* **2016**, *2*, e000181. [CrossRef]
29. Lewis, J.S.; Wright, C.; Green, A. Subacromial Impingement Syndrome: The Effect of Changing Posture on Shoulder Range of Movement. *J. Orthop. Sports Phys. Ther.* **2005**, *35*, 72–87. [CrossRef]
30. Chester, R.; Jerosch-Herold, C.; Lewis, J.; Shepstone, L. Psychological factors are associated with the outcome of physiotherapy for people with shoulder pain: A multicentre longitudinal cohort study. *Br. J. Sports Med.* **2016**, *52*, 269–275. [CrossRef]
31. Atreja, A.; Bellam, N.; Levy, S.R. Strategies to enhance patient adherence: Making it simple. *MedGenMed Medscape Gen. Med.* **2005**, *7*, 4.
32. Rojas, V.; Pluma, A.; Pecos-Martín, D.; Achalandabaso-Ochoa, A.; Fernández-Matías, R.; Martinez-Merinero, P.; Nuñez-Nagy, S.; Gallego-Izquierdo, T. Relationship between Neuromuscular Mechanosensitivity and Chronic Neck Pain in Guitarists: A Cross-Sectional Study. *Int. J. Environ. Res. Public Health* **2021**, *18*, 2673. [CrossRef]
33. Pacheco, J.; Raimundo, J.; Santos, F.; Ferreira, M.; Lopes, T.; Ramos, L.; Silva, A.G. Forward head posture is associated with pressure pain threshold and neck pain duration in university students with subclinical neck pain. *Somatosens. Mot. Res.* **2018**, *35*, 103–108. [CrossRef]
34. Haik, M.N.; Evans, K.; Smith, A.; Henríquez, L.; Bisset, L. People with musculoskeletal shoulder pain demonstrate no signs of altered pain processing. *Musculoskelet. Sci. Pract.* **2018**, *39*, 32–38. [CrossRef]
35. Hidalgo-Lozano, A.; Fernandez-De-Las-Penas, C.; Calderón-Soto, C.; Domingo-Camara, A.; Madeleine, P.; Arroyo-Morales, M. Elite swimmers with and without unilateral shoulder pain: Mechanical hyperalgesia and active/latent muscle trigger points in neck-shoulder muscles. *Scand. J. Med. Sci. Sports* **2011**, *23*, 66–73. [CrossRef]
36. Simons, G.S.; Travell, J. *Myofascial Pain and Dysfunction: Trigger Points Manual: Volume 1: Upper Half of Body*, 2nd ed.; Williams & Wilkins: Philadelphia, PA, USA, 1999.
37. Osborne, N.J.; Gatt, I.T. Management of shoulder injuries using dry needling in elite volleyball players. *Acupunct. Med. J. Br. Med. Acupunct. Soc.* **2010**, *28*, 42–45. [CrossRef]
38. Leong, H.T.; Ng, G.Y.-F.; Chan, S.C.; Fu, S.N. Rotator cuff tendinopathy alters the muscle activity onset and kinematics of scapula. *J. Electromyogr. Kinesiol.* **2017**, *35*, 40–46. [CrossRef]
39. Harrington, S.; Meisel, C.; Tate, A. A Cross-Sectional Study Examining Shoulder Pain and Disability in Division I Female Swimmers. *J. Sport Rehabil.* **2014**, *23*, 65–75. [CrossRef]
40. Reeser, J.C.; Joy, E.A.; Porucznik, C.A.; Berg, R.L.; Colliver, E.B.; Willick, S.E. Risk Factors for Volleyball-Related Shoulder Pain and Dysfunction. *PMR* **2010**, *2*, 27–36. [CrossRef]
41. Sanders, R.J.; Annest, S.J. Pectoralis Minor Syndrome: Subclavicular Brachial Plexus Compression. *Diagnostics* **2017**, *7*, 46. [CrossRef]
42. Miura, K.; Tsuda, E.; Kogawa, M.; Ishibashi, Y. The effects of ball impact position on shoulder muscle activation during spiking in male volleyball players. *JSES Int.* **2020**, *4*, 302–309. [CrossRef]
43. Jorge, J.G.; Moreira, V.M.; Hattori, W.T.; Dionisio, V.C. Hyperalgesia affects muscle activity and knee range of motion during a single-limb mini squat in individuals with knee osteoarthritis: A cross-sectional study. *BMC Musculoskelet. Disord.* **2021**, *22*, 45. [CrossRef]
44. Bron, C.; Dommerholt, J.; Stegenga, B.; Wensing, M.; AB Oostendorp, R. High prevalence of shoulder girdle muscles with myofascial trigger points in patients with shoulder pain. *BMC Musculoskelet. Disord.* **2011**, *12*, 139. [CrossRef]
45. Hidalgo-Lozano, A.; Fernández-De-Las-Peñas, C.; Alonso-Blanco, M.C.; Ge, H.-Y.; Arendt-Nielsen, L.; Arroyo-Morales, M. Muscle trigger points and pressure pain hyperalgesia in the shoulder muscles in patients with unilateral shoulder impingement: A blinded, controlled study. *Exp. Brain Res.* **2010**, *202*, 915–925. [CrossRef]

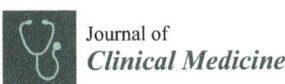

Article

Blood Pressure and Heart Rate Responses to an Isokinetic Testing Protocol in Professional Soccer Players

Arturo Pérez-Gosalvez, Francisco García-Muro San José *, Ofelia Carrión-Otero, Tomás Pérez-Fernández and Luis Fernández-Rosa

Facultad de Medicina, Universidad San Pablo-CEU, CEU Universities, Urbanización Montepríncipe, Boadilla del Monte, Boadilla, 28660 Madrid, Spain; apgosalvez@ceu.es (A.P.-G.); o.carrion@ceu.es (O.C.-O.); tpfernan@ceu.es (T.P.-F.); luferro@ceu.es (L.F.-R.)
* Correspondence: fgarciamuro@ceu.es

Abstract: The aim of this study was to determine blood pressure (BP) and heart rate (HR) responses triggered during an isokinetic testing protocol in professional soccer players and compare cardiovascular parameters at completion of this isokinetic protocol with those during a treadmill test. Using purposive sampling, 63 professional soccer players were recruited. Cardiovascular responses were measured noninvasively during a bilateral testing protocol of knee flexion and extension. Treadmill ergospirometry following an incremental speed protocol was performed to analyze the same cardiovascular parameters at rest and at completion of this test. There were significant differences in diastolic blood pressure (DBP) and HR according to field position. The parameters presented high homogeneity at both competitive levels. Systolic blood pressure, mean arterial pressure, HR, and rate pressure product at completion of the treadmill test were significantly higher than those at completion of the isokinetic protocol. Intermittent isokinetic testing protocol of the knee triggers normal and safe BP and HR responses in healthy professional soccer players. The HR of the defenders was higher than those of the forwards and midfielders but was independent of the competitive level. The values of cardiovascular parameters at isokinetic protocol completion were lower than those during the treadmill test.

Keywords: soccer; blood pressure; heart rate; isokinetic dynamometry; testing; treadmill test

Citation: Pérez-Gosalvez, A.; García-Muro San José, F.; Carrión-Otero, O.; Pérez-Fernández, T.; Fernández-Rosa, L. Blood Pressure and Heart Rate Responses to an Isokinetic Testing Protocol in Professional Soccer Players. *J. Clin. Med.* **2022**, *11*, 1539. https://doi.org/10.3390/jcm11061539

Academic Editor: David Rodríguez-Sanz

Received: 19 January 2022
Accepted: 8 March 2022
Published: 11 March 2022

Publisher's Note: MDPI stays neutral with regard to jurisdictional claims in published maps and institutional affiliations.

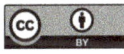

Copyright: © 2022 by the authors. Licensee MDPI, Basel, Switzerland. This article is an open access article distributed under the terms and conditions of the Creative Commons Attribution (CC BY) license (https://creativecommons.org/licenses/by/4.0/).

1. Introduction

Soccer is the most practiced sport worldwide today, with approximately 265 million players across five continents, which is equivalent to 4% of the world's population [1]. Traditionally considered [2,3] a discontinuous and intermittent physical exercise that encompasses low-, medium-, and high-intensity activities, soccer generates physiological and metabolic demands [4] that have increased with the physical demands necessitated by the professionalization of this sport.

Researchers have studied the physiological variables of professional soccer players during matches, such as distance covered (10–13 km), [5] mean heart rate (HR; 165–170 bpm, equivalent to 85% of the maximum HR), or oxygen uptake (45–65% of VO_2 max with telemetric controls) [6,7]. These variables are used to analyze energy metabolism, with some researchers reporting 70–85% aerobic metabolism use and the remainder as anaerobic metabolism [8]. However, this measurement is difficult because it depends on the duration of the high-intensity phases and the recovery period [9,10].

These physiological parameters have become more relevant as the requirements of professional soccer players have increased, and several cases of soccer players experiencing cardiovascular events during matches have been reported in recent years [11], with "sudden death" being the most remarkable both clinically and socially. In fact, between 25% and 49% of athletes who experienced sudden death in Spain were practicing soccer [12,13].

Therefore, many researchers have performed various functional assessment tests in the laboratory and controlled field tests that attempt to reproduce the conditions that a soccer player is subjected to during a match [8,14–16]. The most widely used field tests are categorized as aerobic, anaerobic, and specific, and the most referenced laboratory tests are ergospirometry, anaerobic tests, isometric/isotonic contractions, and isokinetic dynamometry [17].

Many researchers have conducted different functional assessment tests in the laboratory and controlled field tests that try to mimic, in as standardized and objective a manner as possible, the conditions that a football player is subjected to during a match [8,14,15,18]. Among all these tests, isokinetic dynamometry allows for an objective assessment of a football player's muscle function as well as his response to maximum intensity requirements [19,20]. Thus, isokinetic dynamometric systems have been used to perform specific strength training, rehabilitate postsurgical musculoskeletal processes [21,22], prevent muscle imbalances that are a risk factor against muscle injuries [23–25], and evaluate the muscle strength and power of the lower extremities in soccer players [26,27]. For this, isokinetic dynamometry has been considered the gold standard among the strength tests that can be performed on a soccer player [28].

The maximum requirement of this test is an adequate musculoskeletal state and a sufficient cardiorespiratory condition to satisfy the requirements; thus, it would be interesting to evaluate a soccer player's cardiovascular response during a usual isokinetic protocol. This protocol constitutes a controlled laboratory test, which is part of the usual physical assessment of soccer players, and generates metabolic, muscular, and cardiovascular demands that differ from those generated during maximal aerobic exercise. This cardiovascular response has previously been studied in incremental dynamic exercise in soccer players, with the treadmill test used to evaluate cardiorespiratory fitness; this method has also been used to detect possible cardiovascular functional risks [29]. Although the isokinetic assessment test is an indispensable requirement in the evaluation of the physical fitness of soccer players, there are no previous studies assessing the cardiac and blood pressure risk in these athletes.

However, to date, no reliable published studies with an adequate sample size have described how soccer players' BP and HR respond to the demands of an isokinetic testing protocol of the lower extremity musculature. Studies describing the cardiovascular response to isokinetic exercise in healthy or old adults are scarce [30,31] and possess high sample variability [32–35], which prevents the extrapolation of their results to a highly trained population capable of developing high levels of muscle strength and power in the lower extremities.

This study aimed to describe the BP and HR responses triggered by an isokinetic testing protocol in professional soccer players and compare cardiovascular parameters at completion of this isokinetic protocol with those during a treadmill test.

2. Materials and Methods

2.1. Participants

A minimum sample size of 46 was deemed to be representative of the adult population using GRANMO version 7.12 [36], assuming a reference population of 1000, a 95% confidence interval level, an estimate of the standard deviation of 20, a precision of 6, and a 10% replacement rate. A total of 63 professional male outfield soccer players (age 22.6 ± 1.2 years; height: 179.2 ± 5.2 cm; weight: 72.9 ± 5.5 kg), including 23 defenders (age 22.3 ± 3.5 years; height 181.5 ± 4.4 cm; weight: 74.6 ± 4.1 kg), 25 midfielders (age 20.9 ± 2.5 years; height: 178.6 ± 4.7 cm; weight: 73.4 ± 5.1 kg), and 15 forwards (age: 19.7 ± 1.9 years; height: 176.8 ± 5.9 cm; weight: 70.2 ± 6.6 kg), participated in this study. They belonged to a professional soccer team during the measurement period, with 20 on the first-division team and 43 on the second-division team.

This study was performed during preseason, and players were recruited using purposive sampling. Prior to the study, the players were evaluated by a sports medicine specialist who performed an anamnesis and clinical examination following the Union of European Football Associations recommendations [37] to confirm that the players met the conditions for professional sports practice. Subsequently, electrocardiogram, echocardiography, and spirometry were performed to rule out possible contraindications in performing the tests [38]. None of the participating players showed warning signs that contraindicated their inclusion in the study.

All players who had a current federation record as a professional soccer player and who were physically and medically fit to start the season were included. Players who had undergone surgery in the previous 12 months of any pathology in the lower extremities or who had suffered an injury in the lower extremities that would have forced them to suspend sports activity for at least 1 month were excluded. Players undergoing medical treatment with a drug that interfered with physical capacity and those who suffered from acute systemic diseases were also excluded.

All participants were fully informed about the protocol prior to participation and provided informed consent in accordance with the principles of the Declaration of Helsinki. The study was approved by the ethics committee of CEU San Pablo University (approval code, 238/17/18).

A repeated-measures design involving active soccer players was used to determine the BP and HR responses triggered by the isokinetic testing protocol. Then, we compared the HR and BP values at completion of this isokinetic protocol with those achieved during a treadmill test.

Both tests (isokinetic and treadmill) were performed during the preseason of the soccer teams; the usual schedule followed in the medical and functional examinations of the soccer players' sports club was respected. These athletes are evaluated annually using isokinetic assessment and treadmill ergospirometry of the lower extremities.

Once their medical history was recorded, the soccer players performed an isokinetic strength test in the Research Unit in the Physical Therapies Laboratory of the Faculty of Medicine of CEU San Pablo University. After completion, the data were collected, and the second test was conducted within 3 days. The treadmill test was performed in the exercise physiology laboratory of the School of Sports Medicine in Complutense University of Madrid in the recommended environment [39]. Each player's information was encrypted to guarantee anonymity.

2.2. Isokinetic Testing Protocol Description

The isokinetic test was selected, as it is a test included in the functional assessment of elite football players worldwide and validated by UEFA [33] and Spanish Association of Football Team Doctors [40]. For this reason, this population group must face this test as a regular evaluation element of their physical condition.

Initially, with the participant sitting with their feet on the ground, baseline measurements of BP and HR were recorded using a BTL-08 ABPM II portable and digital sphygmomanometer (BTL Industries Ltd. Hertfordshire, United Kingdom). Subsequently, without removing the BP cuff from the participant's upper limb, the device was placed inside a sheath that was attached to an adjustable strap placed around the waist of the participant; thus, the following measurements could be performed without replacing the sphygmomanometer.

The participants performed a general 10 min warm-up exercise on a Monark cycle ergometer (model 818E) at a moderate pace and resistance, immediately after which BP, HR, systolic blood pressure (SBP), diastolic blood pressure (DBP), rate pressure product (RPP) (RPP = HR × SBP), and mean arterial pressure (MAP) (MAP = DBP + (0.333 × [SBP − DBP])) were recorded.

The participants were then asked to remove their shoes and sit on the IsoMed2000 strength-testing system (D&R Ferstl GmbH, Hemau, Germany) in an upright position, with 85° flexion at the hip. The participants were secured by straps around the chest, waist, and right thigh. The dynamometer lever arm was aligned with the participant's tibial spine, 2.5 cm proximal to the right medial malleolus; after ensuring it was comfortable for the participant, it was fixed using a Velcro strap. The rotating axis of the dynamometer was aligned with the knee joint's axis of rotation (lateral epicondyle of the femur). After checking the strap tension, the participant was instructed to hold on to the hand grips on the side of the seat during the efforts [41], and the isokinetic testing protocol was initiated (Figure 1).

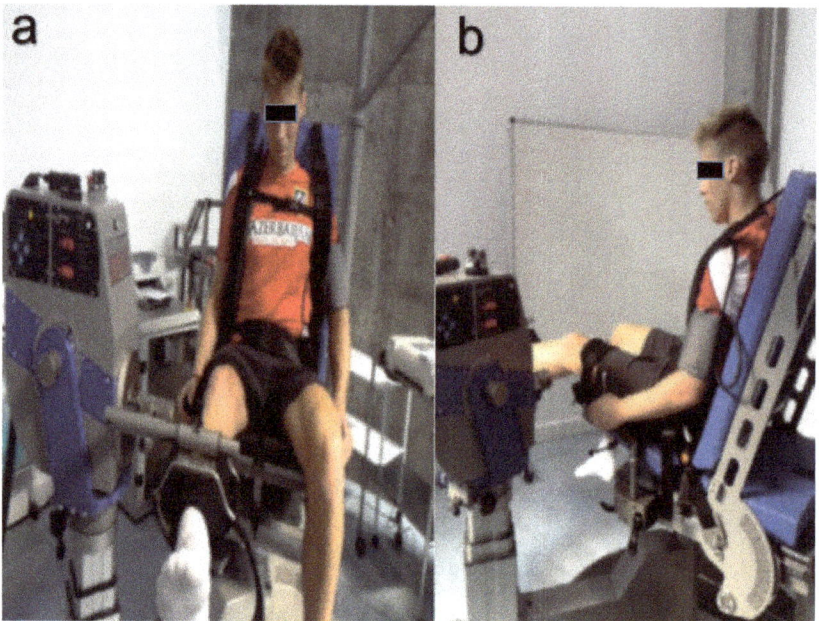

Figure 1. Positioning of a subject before starting the isokinetic testing protocol (**a**) and prior to the beginning of the contraction series with the left lower extremity (**b**).

Before starting the protocol, the right lower extremity (RLE) was weighed using the automatic limb weighing system of the dynamometer to adjust for the gravitational effect on torque.

A bilateral study protocol of continuous concentric/concentric contraction was followed at low (60°/s), medium (180°/s), and high velocities (240°/s) of knee flexion and extension through the knee's range of motion, from 0° (full extension) to 90° (flexed), as recommended by the Spanish Association of Football Teams Physicians in its protocol for professional soccer players [40].

Prior to assessment at each angular velocity, the participants performed three to five submaximal contractions of increasing intensity (25%, 50%, and 80%), completing the established range of motion with both knee flexion and extension, to adapt the musculature to the effort requested later [42,43]. The participants were oriented to avoid the Valsalva maneuver and to breathe spontaneously throughout the movement [44].

The protocol series required the performance of 5 repetitions of flexion and extension at 60°/s, 10 repetitions at 180°/s, and 25 repetitions at 240°/s, all at maximum intensity and always starting with the right leg. During the protocol, encouragements by verbal coaching and visual feedback were provided to all participants to help them concentrate on the quality and maximum intensity of their movements [45,46].

Immediately after completing each of the six established series of contractions, the investigator activated the BP monitor and asked the participant to rest and without speaking to check BP, HR, SBP, DBP, RPP, and MAP (approximately 30–40 s). After verifying that the device had recorded the measurements, muscle warm-up/adaptation contractions were started in the next series of protocol contractions. Between the third (right leg at 240°/s) and fourth (left leg at 60°/s) series, the time for measuring BP and HR was used to move the dynamometer lever to the opposite side of the participant. This procedure lasted 30–40 s to homogenize the rest time with that of the series performed in the right leg [47,48].

Once the final BP and HR measurements were recorded and checked (after the sixth series), the straps, attachment to the mobile arm, and sphygmomanometer cuff were removed, and the athlete was recommended to spend 5–10 min passively stretching the lower extremity musculature before leaving the investigation unit.

2.3. Treadmill Ergospirometry Test Description

Treadmill ergospirometry test was performed after the isokinetic test. The "incremental speed protocol" for ergospirometry commonly used in the School of Sports Medicine of Complutense University was followed in the functional assessment of the participants [49,50]. For this, a treadmill (H.P. Cosmos), gas analyzer (model Vmax, Sensor Medics), and electrocardiograph (Quest Exercise Stress System, Burdick Inc; Milton, WI, USA) were used. After checking the BP and HR of the participants at rest, they performed a 2 min warm-up exercise on the treadmill at 4 km/h following the usual protocol [51,52], with electrocardiographic control but no respiratory control.

The maximum treadmill test was started at an initial speed of 6 km/h for all participants. Every 2 min, the speed was increased by 2 km/h until the participant was exhausted, with the slope constant at 1% as in the warm-up exercise. BP and HR were measured within 30 s after completion of the exhaustion test. Recovery started at 5 km/h, and this speed was maintained until the participant's complete recovery.

2.4. Statistical Analyses

We used the Kolmogorov–Smirnov and Levene tests to assess the normality of the values and the equality of variances, respectively. We then performed univariate repeated-measures analysis of variance (ANOVA) to determine differences among SBP, DBP, MAP, HR, and RPP values. Finally, we used Student's paired t-test to assess possible differences between phases. Bonferroni's post hoc tests were applied for comparative analyses of between-group differences when a significant interaction was found. SPSS version 24.0 for Windows was used for statistical analysis (Statistical Package for the Social Sciences, Chicago, IL, USA). The results are expressed as the mean ± standard error, and the significance level was $p < 0.05$.

3. Results

Descriptive

A global descriptive analysis of the cohort (n = 63) including the different cardiovascular parameters at the different measurement times is shown in Table 1.

During the isokinetic protocol, the maximum SBP value was 207 mmHg (at the fourth measurement), maximum DBP was 103 mmHg (at the third measurement), and maximum HR was 148 bpm (at the final measurement). The minimum SBP, DBP, and HR values were 102 mmHg, 44 mmHg, and 39 bpm. Intra-subject differences in DBP with respect to the measurement at rest never exceeded 13 mmHg.

Because all the parameters described followed normal distribution in the cohort (n = 63), repeated-measures ANOVA was performed to compare each parameter among the different measurement points and to assess the effect of time on the obtained means (Figure 2).

ANOVA revealed an effect of measurement time on SBP ($F_{5.363} = 52.91$; $p < 0.001$; $\eta p2 = 0.5$). When comparing pairs of measurements, a significant effect was produced at rest and after 10 min warm-up exercise compared with that at the other measurements ($p < 0.001$). There were no significant differences between the third measurement (post RLE 60°/s) and the other measurements or between any of them ($p > 0.05$). DBP was also affected by different measurement times (F = 9.30; $p < 0.001$; $\eta p2 = 0.149$). The pairwise comparison showed statistically significant differences between the measurement at baseline and those at rest except for the sixth ($p = 0.313$) and final ($p > 0.5$) measurements. There were also significant differences between the third and fourth measurements (post RLE 60°/s and post RLE 180°/s) with respect to the sixth measurement ($p = 0.045$ and $p = 0.016$, respectively) and between the fourth and final measurements ($p = 0.03$). HR was also affected by different measurement times ($F_{3.521} = 188.37$; $p < 0.001$; $\eta p2 = 0.780$). HR resulted in highly significant differences ($p < 0.001$) among all the measurements except between the fifth (post RLE 240°/s) and seventh (post LLE 180°/s) measurements.

Table 1. Description of the cardiovascular parameters during the isokinetic protocol at different measurements. Means and standard deviations obtained for the global sample (n = 63) and according to the field position and competition level of the soccer players are shown.

	Rest	Post-Bike	RLE 60°/s	RLE 180°/s	RLE 240°/s	LLE 60°/s	LLE 180°/s	LLE 240°/s
General (n = 63)								
SBP	127.8 ± 10.5 (152–102)	143.6 ± 12.4 * (181–127)	149.1 ± 14.7 *† (191–127)	155.2 ± 15.7 *† (207–119)	154.7 ± 14.3 *† (187–129)	155.2 ± 13.7 *† (189–128)	127.8 ± 10.5 (152–102)	127.8 ± 10.5 (152–102)
DBP	71.2 ± 8.4 (90–47)	79.3 ± 8.6 * (101–61)	79.1 ± 9.9 *∥ (103–57)	79.5 ± 10.1 ‡§ (102–58)	76.4 ± 9.8 ‡ (96–54)	75.5 ± 10.6 (96–50)	77.5 ± 10.3 ‡ (94–57)	74.9 ± 9.9 (93–44)
MAP	90.3 ± 7.4 (108.5–76.5)	100.7 ± 8.4 * (127.6–82)	102.4 ± 9.4 * (121.3–85.6)	104.5 ± 9.4 *† (122–86)	102.4 ± 8.8 * (125–84.6)	102 ± 9.7 * (123–78.3)	102.5 ± 10 * (124–80.3)	101.2 ± 10 * (127.6–72.3)
HR	61.3 ± 10.4 (92–39)	74.5 ± 13 ƕ (103–45)	84.1 ± 17.5 ƕ (121–48)	91.2 ± 18.4 ƕ (126–49)	104.3 ± 18.7 ƕ (139–65)	97 ± 19.5 ⨳ (141–51)	102.3 ± 18.3 ↻ (138–51)	112.9 ± 18.9 ƕ (148–61)
RPP	7860.9 (11,088–4641)	10,786.1 ƕ (16.109–66.72)	12,602.5 ƕ (19.656–6.419)	14,189.6 ƕ (21.452–7.301)	16,123.6 ƕ (25.993–9.417)	15,140.5 ⨳ (24.150–7.191)	15,798.1 ↻ (23.046–7.089)	17,442.3 ƕ (26.069–8.784)
By Field Position								
Forwards (n = 15)								
SBP	125.4 ± 8.4	142.6 ± 12	146.1 ± 13.3	151 ± 14.6	152.3 ± 12.4	150.1 ± 8.9	151.8 ± 13.5	153.3 ± 14.8
DBP	69.3 ± 8.3	76 ± 8.7	77.2 ± 8.7	74.5 ± 10	71.7 ± 8.8	72.8 ± 11	78.6 ± 9.4	74.3 ± 8.8
MAP	87.8 ± 7.4	98.2 ± 8	100.1 ± 8.8	99.8 ± 8	98.5 ± 8.1	98.6 ± 8.5	102.9 ± 9.7	100.6 ± 10
HR	61.1 ± 14	78.3 ± 17	86.9 ± 19.6	90.9 ± 17.9	106.4 ± 18.3	97.1 ± 20.2	101.2 ± 21.8	109.5 ± 23.1
RPP	7683.8	11,219	12,822	13,781	16,255	14,612	15,505	16,854
Midfielders (n = 25)								
SBP	130.8 ± 9.5	146.7 ± 12.4	153.7 ± 17	156.3 ± 15.1	156.2 ± 16.2	156.2 ± 13.7	152.9 ± 18	158 ± 16.3
DBP	73.3 ± 7.1	79.7 ± 8.6	79.1 ± 10.2	80.1 ± 9.9	77.4 ± 10.8	72.9 ± 10.1	74.7 ± 10.6	72.1 ± 8.4
MAP	92.3 ± 6.6	102 ± 9.2	103.4 ± 11.1	105.5 ± 9.6	103.7 ± 10.8	100.6 ± 10.5	100.7 ± 11.8	100.7 ± 9.9
HR	59.5 ± 9.2	73.6 ± 14.7	80.5 ± 15.3	87.8 ± 20	98.1 ± 20.2	90.2 ± 18.4	98.3 ± 18.3	108.4 ± 19.2
RPP	7815	10,854	12,458	13,779	15,425	14,151	15,075	17,148
Defenders (n = 23)								
SBP	126.4 ± 12.2	139.8 ± 12.5	145.2 ± 12.6	154.3 ± 13.7	152.2 ± 12.3	157.6 ± 16	154.3 ± 15.5	151.4 ± 15.8
DBP	71.2 ± 8.4	80.3 ± 8.6	80.4 ± 11.1	83 ± 8.8 Ω	77.9 ± 9.2	78.8 ± 10.2	77.5 ± 8.8	77.4 ± 11.2
MAP	89.4 ± 7.8	100.1 ± 7.8	102 ± 8.3	106.7 ± 8.6	102.6 ± 6.6	105.1 ± 9	103.1 ± 8.7	101.7 ± 10.7
HR	63.2 ± 8.9	74.7 ± 9.7	87.5 ± 17.8	96.5 ± 16.5	110.2 ± 16.1	105.5 ± 17.7 #	107.3 ± 14.8	119.1 ± 13.8
RPP	8019.6	10,436	12,731	14,855	16,705	16,605	16,503	17,925
By Competition Level								
1st team (n = 20)								
SBP	127.1 ± 12.1	144 ± 14.4	149.4 ± 15.1	154.1 ± 15.3	153 ± 16.3	153.3 ± 16.3	151.6 ± 16.1	153.9 ± 15.8
DBP	70.8 ± 8.7	78 ± 9.9	79.4 ± 12.2	81.8 ± 8.6	78 ± 9.2	75.8 ± 9.9	75.6 ± 10	76.6 ± 9.6
MAP	89.4 ± 8.2	100 ± 9.6	102.7 ± 12.5	105.9 ± 7.8	101.5 ± 9.3	101.5 ± 9.6	101.9 ± 9.9	102.4 ± 10.3
HR	64.2 ± 12.5	76.4 ± 13.4	85.8 ± 17.2	92.1 ± 19.4	102.8 ± 20.3	96.6 ± 21	101.2 ± 16.6	103 ± 19.1
RPP	8127.2 ± 1598.7	10,996.7 ± 2353.8	12,801.6 ± 2753.5	14,123.5 ± 3005.2	15,723.7 ± 3608.7	14,804.7 ± 3643.6	15,329.4 ± 2978.4	15,908.8 ± 3509.4
2nd Team (n = 43)								
SBP	127.7 ± 9.9	142.2 ± 11.7	148.2 ± 14.9	154.3 ± 14.1	154.1 ± 12.6	156.1 ± 12.4	154.9 ± 16.5	154.1 ± 15.6
DBP	71.6 ± 7.6	79.5 ± 8.1	79 ± 9	78.7 ± 10.5	76.3 ± 10	74.8 ± 11.1	75.2 ± 8.5	74.4 ± 10.4
MAP	90.1 ± 7	100.5 ± 7.8	102 ± 9.1	103.8 ± 9.8	102.2 ± 8.7	101.9 ± 9.8	101.7 ± 9.1	100.8 ± 10.7
HR	59.9 ± 9.5	74.7 ± 13.7	84.2 ± 17.7	91.7 ± 18.1	105.7 ± 18.2	98.2 ± 18.9	112.7 ± 16.6	112.6 ± 20.2
RPP	7691.3 ± 1570.9	10,694.5 ± 2353.9	12,580.1 ± 3309	14,206.1 ± 3299.6	16,309.9 ± 3132.8	15,367.6 ± 3370.7	17,419.8 ± 3002.9	17,330.1 ± 3429.1

Data presented as mean +/− SD. Max, maximum value obtained by a sample subject; Min, minimum value obtained by a subject in the sample. Abbreviations: RLE, right lower extremity; LLE, left lower extremity; HR, heart rate; SBP, systolic blood pressure; DBP, diastolic blood pressure; MAP, mean arterial pressure; RPP, rate pressure product. * significantly higher than the resting measurement $p < 0.001$; † significantly higher than post-bike measurement $p < 0.001$; ‡ significantly higher than the measurement at rest $p = 0.001$. ∥ significantly higher than the 6th measurement (LLE 60°/s) $p < 0.05$. § significantly higher than the 8th measurement (LLE 60°/s) $p < 0.05$. ƕ significantly higher than all previous measurements $p < 0.001$. ⨳ significantly higher than all previous measurements $p < 0.001$, except the 5th. ↻ significantly higher than previous measurements $p < 0.001$, except for the 5th and 6th. Ω significantly higher than Forwards in the same measurement $p < 0.05$.

Finally, the effect of the different measurement times on MAP ($F_{5.538} = 29.47$; $p < 0.001$; $\eta p2 = 0.357$) and RPP ($F_{4.577} = 168.55$; $p < 0.001$; $\eta p2 = 0.761$) were observed. There were significant differences in MAP between the baseline measurement with respect to the rest measurement ($p < 0.001$) and between the second and fourth measurements ($p < 0.01$). There were differences in RPP among all measurements except among the fifth, sixth, and seventh measurements ($p > 0.05$) and between the fourth and sixth measurements ($p = 0.086$).

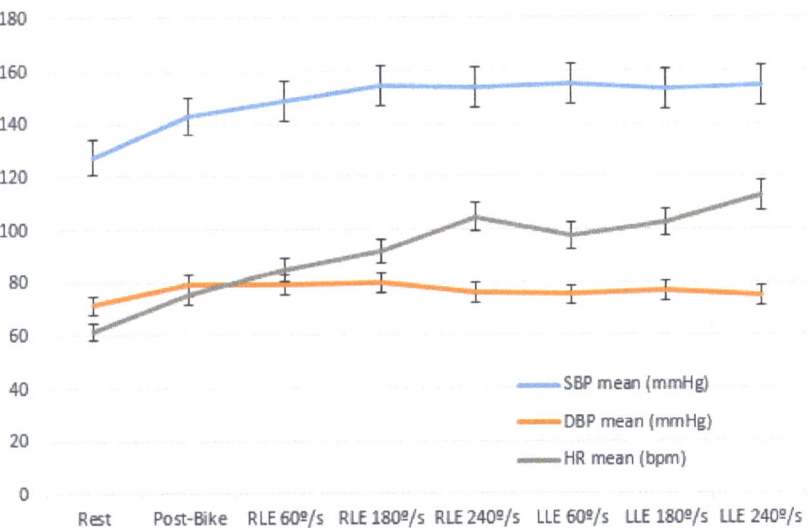

Figure 2. Heart rate (HR), systolic blood pressure (SBP), diastolic blood pressure (DBP) response of the global sample (n = 63) during the proposed isokinetic testing protocol (error bars show the SD of the mean in each measurement). Abbreviations: RLE, right lower extremity; LLE, left lower extremity.

Repeated-measures ANOVA was performed to assess the effect of time on cardiovascular parameters in the participants according to their field position (defenders, midfielders, and forwards) as well as the interaction of this effect with field position.

The changes in SBP ($F_{10.745}$ = 1.02; p = 0.463) and RPP ($F_{9.252}$ = 1.66; p = 0.096) with respect to the measurement points followed the same profile as that in the global sample. There was no interaction of the effect "time" and the factor "field position" when comparing the means of the different measurement points. An interaction of the effect of time with respect to field position was obtained for DBP (F = 2.1; p = 0.012; $\eta p2$ = 0.076), with a significant difference at the fourth measurement (180°/s RLE) between the defenders and forwards (p = 0.043). Although there were no significant differences among the field positions in the other measurements, the DBP response at the fifth measurement differed among the groups. In turn, an interaction effect of "time–field position" was found for HR ($F_{7.086}$ = 1.76; p = 0.042; $\eta p2$ = 0.065) during the isokinetic protocol measurements. The mean HR values of the defenders were higher than those of the forwards and midfielders, with significant differences at the sixth measurement (p = 0.037); the other measurements displayed homogeneous HR response in all groups. Finally, there was an interaction effect of "time–field position" in MAP (F_{14} = 1.96; p = 0.02; $\eta p2$ = 0.072), although when performing pairwise comparison, no significant differences were found among the groups at any of the measurements. MAP in the forwards changed with respect to that in the defenders and midfielders, without significant differences.

When the participants were categorized according to competitive level (first- and second-division teams), the cardiovascular parameters during the isokinetic protocol followed a normal distribution. No interaction of "time effect" and "category factor" in the cardiovascular parameters was recorded in the comparison of the means at the different measurement points. SBP ($F_{5.361}$ = 0.31; p = 0.914), DBP (F = 0.48; p = 0.84), HR ($F_{3.559}$ = 0.78; p = 0.520), MAP ($F_{5.507}$ = 0.34; p = 0.9), and RPP ($F_{4.601}$ = 0.67; p = 0.62) showed high homogeneity in their response in both categories.

Table 2 shows the mean values of the cardiovascular parameters analyzed at the end of both tests and the significance of the comparisons.

Table 2. Comparison of the cardiovascular values achieved by the global sample (n = 63) at the end of the isokinetic protocol and treadmill ergospirometry.

Variable	Rest			Final		
	Isokinetic	Ergospirometry	p-Value	Isokinetic	Ergospirometry	p-Value
SBP	127.8 ± 10.5 (152–102)	117.4 ± 8.5 (138–95)	<0.001 *	154.6 ± 14.5 (199–119)	172.4 ± 19.1 (220–120)	<0.001 *
DBP	71.2 ± 8.4 (90–47)	70.8 ± 8.2 (90–50)	0.529	74.8 ± 10.2 (93–44)	72.1 ± 12.8 (100–50)	0.279
MAP	90.3 ± 7.4 (108.5–76.5)	86.3 ± 6.8 (101.6–70)	0.814	101.2 ± 10 (127.6–72.3)	105.5 ± 11.8 (126.6–73.3)	0.044 *
HR	61.3 ± 10.4 (92–39)	60.9 ± 10.4 (92–39)	0.820	113.7 ± 19.2 (148–61)	191.5 ± 7.9 (205–173)	<0.001 *
RPP	7860.9 (11,088–4641)	7137 ± 1473 (11,960–4410)	<0.001 *	17,504 ± 3230 (26,069–8784)	33,143 ± 3852 (22,080–44,000)	<0.001 *

Data presented as mean +/− SD. HR, heart rate; SBP, systolic blood pressure; DBP, diastolic blood pressure; MAP, mean arterial pressure; RPP, rate pressure product. * Signification $p < 0.05$.

There were significant differences in the final SBP, MAP, HR, and RPP values of both assessment tests, with all parameters significantly higher at the end of the treadmill ergospirometry.

4. Discussion

Notably, none of the participants presented complications or abnormal BP or HR responses to the exercises [53]. The cardiovascular reference values used to determine abnormal responses were those used for dynamic incremental exercise (treadmill test) [38,54,55] because no study in the literature has established non-physiological BP and HR responses for isokinetic exercises. Therefore, because "normal" cardiovascular response values during an isokinetic testing protocol have not been established, it is advisable to use those established for stress tests as a fundamental reference when studying cardiovascular responses during maximum exercise.

The novelty of this study lies in describing the behavior of BP and HR in the group of professional soccer players not because they are just another population group but because they will be subjected to this assessment test on a regular basis during the seasons in which they compete. This means that there is a high prevalence of this test in this specific population group. Furthermore, this test could be used in the future to obtain more global and detailed information on the AT and HR of a soccer player to these physical demands and prevent possible future undesirable or pathological clinical events.

There were no players in whom SBP decreased in relation to that at rest, which is recommended [56]. This is considered a normotensive response to the effort because maximum SBP and DBP values of up to 240 and 115 mmHg, respectively, have been established in highly trained participants [57,58], with an increase in DBP of up to 15 mmHg considered normal during maximum-intensity exercise [54,59]. The maximum HR recorded was clearly below the cardiovascular safety limits as expected from intense exercise with limited duration.

4.1. Heart Rate

The mean HR of all participants showed a practically linear significant increase throughout the assessment protocol except between the fifth and sixth measurements, with differences between each consecutive recording time of approximately 7–13 bpm, and the mean HRmax was 112.9 ± 18.9 bpm at completion of the protocol. It is evident that the interruption in the linear increase in HR at the sixth measurement (LLE 60°/s) is related to the change in the LE made by muscular effort, subsequently continuing the progressive increase in HR with the same profile as before the change of LE. In fact, it is probable that if the six series of isokinetic testing were performed with the same LE, higher maximum values than those obtained in this study would be achieved.

On analyzing the variations in HR between each proposed angular velocity, we observed that the greatest increases occurred after warming up on an exercise bike (13.4 bpm) and in the series at high angular velocity (240°/s), where it increased by 13.1 bpm (RLE 240°/s) and 11.6 bpm (LLE 240°/s) compared with that in the immediately previous series measurement. In these series at 240°/s, 25 repetitions of knee flexion/extension were performed, leading to a longer effort time than that in the series at 60°/s (5 repetitions) and 180°/s (10 repetitions). This finding corroborates the results of other studies, in which the increase in HR depends more on the duration than on the intensity of the exercise [31,60–62]. Because isokinetic testing protocol is designed with consecutive series and little recovery time [30,60], it results in higher HR responses than those to isolated series at a given angular velocity or at rest intervals greater than 90 s between each series [35,63]. In fact, in a continuous isokinetic testing protocol, the mean HR increased to values close to those obtained in maximum stress tests until the participant reaches exhaustion [64].

However, in the usual isokinetic tests of the knee musculature in soccer players [27,65,66], no more than three or four series are performed at different velocities, so the effort of each series does not exceed 1 min; therefore, HRmax values are not attained. Studies that report greater increases in HR in adults after a series of isokinetic exercises generally have longer durations of the said series [30,67].

On comparison of the HR response of our sample during the isokinetic testing protocol with that in the studies, it is evident that HR in soccer players is much lower than that in untrained adults [30,31,34,62,68]. This suggests that cardiovascular adaptations to soccer players' training trigger a smaller increase in HR during isokinetic exercises despite our sample having a lower mean age than that of samples in other studies. Given that higher HR values are obtained during isokinetic exercises in young individuals [30,35,68], the adaptations to training by this population group are more significant than the participants' age.

This reflection seems to be confirmed by the absence of differences in the HR response during isokinetic exercises between the first-division team (24.5 years) and second-division team (19.9 years) players. In fact, the behavior of HR between both groups was very similar at all measurements, indicating the limited influence of age and competitive level in the HR response.

4.2. Blood Pressure

The SBP values of the global sample increased progressively until the fourth measurement (RLE 180°/s), when, after reaching a mean value of 155.2 ± 15.7 mmHg, it remained practically unchanged at the subsequent measurements. It even decreased slightly at the seventh and eighth measurements until completion of the isokinetic testing protocol, with a mean value of 154.3 ± 15.3 mmHg. After the third and fourth measurements, there were no significant differences in the increase in SBP, resulting in an incremental curve that reached a plateau (fourth measurement), and it remained stable until completion of the protocol. This SBP response is like that described in healthy adults performing compared to incremental dynamic exercises [69,70] although the mean values in our study were lower. Similarly, no decrease in SBP was observed after changing LE between the fifth and sixth measurements as in HR, so this change did not influence the overall response to the protocol.

We did not identify an influence of angular velocity on the BP response because the increases occurred during the first two series, and SBP subsequently remained unchanged. Some researchers who assessed the SBP response in isokinetic exercise series at different velocities recorded higher SBP at low angular velocities [32,34,67,71], whereas others did not report significant differences between knee flexion–extension series at different angular velocities, as in our case [60,62]. Therefore, it appears logical that in consecutive series of exercise protocols with limited recovery time, angular velocity is not a relevant element in the SBP response.

The SBP values in this study are hardly comparable with those in other studies because no similar designs were found that measured cardiovascular parameters during an isokinetic testing protocol, and no studies assessed professional soccer players [34,72]. Thus, the lower SBP values in our participants are likely related to better cardiovascular adaptations to exercise by soccer players; the BP response profile may follow a similar pattern in healthy adults. It is evident that an isokinetic protocol with a series of contractions established at different velocities cannot generate excessive increases in SBP as reported during protocols performed to exhaustion [32] or with heavy-resistance exercises involving large muscle groups [73,74].

The position of the soccer players was not associated with differences in the SBP response although the midfielders had higher baseline values (130.8 mmHg) and maintained them during essentially all measurements compared with the other players, with a non-significant increase in final SBP of 5 and 7 mmHg compared with that in forwards and defenders, respectively. However, these small differences do not follow a stable pattern that justifies an influence of the field position on the SBP response. These differences are even smaller when comparing players based on their competitive level, in which both the SBP response and the mean values obtained by the two groups are very similar and not significantly different.

The DBP value increased by 8 mmHg after warming up and remained almost unchanged until the fourth measurement (RLE 180°/s), after which it gradually decreased except for a slight increase in the seventh measurement, reaching a mean value of 74.9 ± 9.9 mmHg at protocol completion. This slight increase in DBP is lower than that reported in other isokinetic (non-exhausting) exercise designs in untrained participants [75,76] and clearly lower than that in studies with isometric exercise protocols for HR or percentage of VO_2 max [77–79]. Thus, the adaptation to exercise by individuals with a high level of training seems to trigger lower values of DBP response during isokinetic exercises. Notably, the expected DBP response to non-exhausting isokinetic exercise protocols is a slight increase of ≤15 mmHg in highly trained participants. This behavior differs from that to dynamic incremental exercises [50] but is very similar to that to non-incremental exercises [80]; therefore, the duration and particularly the progressive intensity of the exercise seem to be key elements in the behavior of this parameter.

The greatest increase in DBP occurs after warming up, and it remains largely unchanged thereafter. Therefore, it is evident that the possible hypertensive effect related to isokinetic exercise would only be associated with exhausting isokinetic exercise designs [32,64] as in the case of isometric exercise [79,81].

The DBP response patter was very similar in both groups of soccer players, with no differences greater than 3 mmHg in the mean values. No influence of age or competitive level was noted in the observed response although some studies involving untrained healthy individuals reported a slight dependence of age on this response during isokinetic exercise [30,68]. This effect is decreased in highly trained individuals; thus, the DBP response is determined by the adaptations to training by soccer players.

However, certain variations in the DBP response according to field position were observed. In general, defenders had DBP throughout the protocol, with the forwards reporting lower values until the sixth measurement, after which they exceeded the mean DBP of the midfielders. These results differ from those of SBP; i.e., midfielders had higher SBP than forwards and defenders; at protocol completion, the differential BP of the midfielders (86 mmHg) was higher than that of the forwards (79.3 mmHg) and defenders (74 mmHg). These findings agree with those of previous studies that evaluated other types of exercises [82,83]; there is a linear relationship in which as the subject's training level, maximum TAS, and differential BP increase. Thus, due to the physical demands of their position, midfielders may have better BP adaptation to an intermittent protocol of isokinetic exercises at various velocities. However, this aspect is not recorded in continuous incremental aerobic exercises, as reflected in our ergospirometry results or those of Ramos [50], resulting in greater differences according to field position when faced with high-intensity intermittent efforts (isokinetic testing) than when performing a continuous incremental aerobic effort. This may all be influenced by an increasing interest in improving the aerobic capacity of field soccer players [84–87] regardless of their position, whereas adaptation to aerobic–anaerobic efforts are determined to a greater extent due to the demands of the footballer's position during competition.

Finally, MAP and RPP were determined because TAM has been previously used to assess BP response during isokinetic exercise [31,68,76,88], and RPP allows us to clinically objectify myocardial O_2 consumption during the test [89,90].

MAP progressively increased until the fourth measurement, with the cycling warm-up clearly resulting in a more marked increase in TAM (10.4 mmHg) and with values clearly lower than those recorded in other designs of isokinetic exercise both in young adults [68,76,88] and older, untrained subjects [31,68] No differences were observed in MAP according to the mean age of the participants in a previous study [68] similar to our results. There was no influence on the type of contraction selected because in general, a series of concentric contractions are considered more "hypertensive" than eccentric contractions at the same angular velocities [31,68,91] However, this influence on the MAP response according to the type of contraction selected appeared to be related only to samples from untrained and mainly older subjects, in which concentric-type isokinetic exercises trigger higher MAP, SBP, and DBP [31,68].

Regarding field positions, a slightly different MAP response was observed in the forwards, who had increased MAP in the final two measurements compared with those in the previous measurements, which, although not significant, showed increased BP near the end of the effort. This may be related to the type of physiological effort they usually perform, such as short and intense efforts but with longer recovery times; thus, an intermittent isokinetic testing protocol would reflect more differences in BP response according to the field position than commonly used treadmill tests.

However, this phenomenon was not reported for RPP, in which the behavior of the players was very similar in all groups. The clinical estimate of myocardial O_2 consumption that results from this parameter [89,92] would show a very homogeneous behavior among the groups of soccer players. The RPP values in our study are similar to those of other researchers who assessed this parameter in untrained participants [31,68,93] and with designs of isolated isokinetic exercises or with rest intervals greater than 90 s between each series, which results in higher BP and lower HR. Findings similar to the maximum RPP values in our participants during the isokinetic protocol were 15.000–17.000 units lower than those obtained by professional soccer players in an ergospirometry in previous studies [14,50].

This study shows at least one limitation. The between-groups and between-categories results are not strong. Some commonly utilized physiological parameters (e.g., HR or VO_2 max.) may not be sensitive enough to detect specific physiological adaptations occurring in response to fatigue/training [94–96]. One possible explanation for this may stem from the fact that these parameters provide little information on the specific nonlinear dynamic interactions between organic subsystems involved in exercise physiology [95]. Therefore, it would be interesting to evaluate the effects of isokinetic/treadmill protocols utilizing variables able to quantify how respiratory, cardiovascular systems, and neuromuscular systems coordinate during exercise in future studies.

5. Conclusions

The findings indicate that the performance of an intermittent isokinetic testing protocol of the knee triggers normal and safe BP and HR responses in healthy professional soccer players, with no values exceeding the recommended cardiovascular stability limits.

The angular velocity is not a determining element in the SBP and DBP response.

HR increased linearly during the isokinetic testing protocol until reaching submaximal values, and its increase depends to a great extent on the duration of the isokinetic effort than on its intensity.

The HR of the defenders was higher than those of the forwards and midfielders but was independent of the competitive level.

The SBP and HR values achieved at completion of the treadmill test were significantly higher than those during the isokinetic testing protocol. The final DBP in the isokinetic protocol was higher than that measured at completion of the treadmill test, but the results were not significantly different.

Author Contributions: Conceptualization, L.F.-R. and F.G.-M.S.J.; methodology, L.F.-R., O.C.-O. and F.G.-M.S.J.; formal analysis, A.P.-G. and T.P.-F.; investigation, A.P.-G. and F.G.-M.S.J.; writing—original draft preparation, A.P.-G. and O.C.-O.; writing—review and editing, F.G.-M.S.J. and T.P.-F.; supervision, L.F.-R. All authors have read and agreed to the published version of the manuscript.

Funding: This research received no external funding.

Institutional Review Board Statement: The study was conducted in accordance with the Declaration of Helsinki, and this study was approved by the Ethics Committee of the CEU San Pablo University in Madrid. No. 238/17/18; approval date: 30 July 2019. The study conforms with The Code of Ethics of the World Medical Association.

Informed Consent Statement: Informed consent was obtained from all subjects involved in the study.

Data Availability Statement: The data presented in this study are available on request from the corresponding author. The data are not publicly available due to ethical considerations.

Acknowledgments: We wish to acknowledge John Jairo Aguilera-Correa for his writing assistance.

Conflicts of Interest: The authors declare no conflict of interest.

References

1. Kunz, M. "265 Million Playing Football" Big Count Survey. *FIFA Magazine*, July 2007; pp. 10–15.
2. Ekblom, B. Applied physiology of soccer. *Sports Med.* **1986**, *3*, 50–60. [CrossRef]
3. Bangsbo, J.; Nørregaard, L.; Thorsø, F. Activity profile of competition soccer. *Can. J. Sport Sci.* **1991**, *16*, 110–116.
4. Bangsbo, J.; Iaia, F.M.; Krustrup, P. Metabolic Response and Fatigue in Soccer. *Int. J. Sports Physiol. Perform.* **2007**, *2*, 111–127. [CrossRef]
5. Clemente, F.M.; Couceiro, M.S.; Martins, F.M.L.; Ivanova, M.O.; Mendes, R. Activity profiles of soccer players during the 2010 world cup. *J. Hum. Kinet.* **2013**, *38*, 201–211. [CrossRef]
6. Stølen, T.; Chamari, K.; Castagna, C.; Wisløff, U. Physiology of Soccer. *Sport Med.* **2005**, *35*, 501–536. [CrossRef]
7. Shephard, R.J. Biology and medicine of soccer: An update. *J. Sports Sci.* **1999**, *17*, 757–786. [CrossRef]
8. Aslan, A.; Acikada, C.; Güvenç, A.; Gören, H.; Hazir, T.; Ozkara, A. Metabolic demands of match performance in young soccer players. *J. Sports Sci. Med.* **2012**, *11*, 170–179.
9. Reilly, T. Aspectos fisiológicos del futbol. *Actual Cienc. Deport.* **1996**, *4*, 1–14.
10. Baker, J.S.; McCormick, M.C.; Robergs, R.A. Interaction among Skeletal Muscle Metabolic Energy Systems during Intense Exercise. *J. Nutr. Metab.* **2010**, *2010*, 905612. [CrossRef]
11. Maron, B.J.; Doerer, J.J.; Haas, T.S.; Tierney, D.M.; Mueller, F.O. Sudden deaths in young competitive athletes: Analysis of 1866 deaths in the United States, 1980–2006. *Circulation* **2009**, *119*, 1085–1092. [CrossRef]
12. Suárez-Mier, M.P.; Aguilera, B.; Mosquera, R.M.; Sánchez-de-León, M.S. Pathology of sudden death during recreational sports in Spain. *Forensic Sci. Int.* **2013**, *226*, 188–196. [CrossRef]
13. Morentin, B.; Suárez-Mier, M.P.; Monzó, A.; Molina, P.; Lucena, J.S. Sports-related sudden cardiac death due to myocardial diseases on a population from 1–35 years: A multicentre forensic study in Spain. *Forensic Sci. Res.* **2019**, *4*, 257–266. [CrossRef]
14. Metaxas, T.I.; Koutlianos, N.A.; Kouidi, E.J.; Deligiannis, A.P. Comparative study of field and laboratory tests for the evaluation of aerobic capacity in soccer players. *J. Strength Cond. Res.* **2005**, *19*, 79–84.
15. Chamari, K.; Hachana, Y.; Ahmed, Y.; Galy, O.; Sghaïer, F.; Chatard, J.-C.; Hue, O.; Wisløff, U. Field and laboratory testing in young elite soccer players. *Br. J. Sports Med.* **2004**, *38*, 191–196. [CrossRef]
16. O'Reilly, J.; Wong, S.H. The development of aerobic and skill assessment in soccer. *Sports Med.* **2012**, *42*, 1029–1040. [CrossRef]
17. Ramos, J.; Segovia, J.; Lopez-Silvarrey Varela, F. Laboratory Test versus field test in football (soccer) players assessment. *Rev. Int. Med. Y Cienc. Act Física Y Deport.* **2009**, *9*, 312–321.
18. Bangsbo, J.; Mohr, M.; Krustrup, P. Physical and metabolic demands of training and match-play in the elite football player. *J. Sports Sci.* **2006**, *24*, 665–674. [CrossRef]
19. Fousekis, K.; Tsepis, E.; Poulmedis, P.; Athanasopoulos, S.; Vagenas, G. Intrinsic risk factors of non-contact quadriceps and hamstring strains in soccer: A prospective study of 100 professional players. *Br. J. Sports Med.* **2011**, *45*, 709–714. [CrossRef]

20. Della Villa, S.; Boldrini, L.; Ricci, M.; Danelon, F.; Snyder-Mackler, L.; Nanni, G.; Giulio Sergio, R. Clinical outcomes, and return-to-sports participation of 50 soccer players after anterior cruciate ligament reconstruction through a sport-specific rehabilitation protocol. *Sports Health* **2012**, *4*, 17–24. [CrossRef]
21. Pereira, M.T.; Della Villa, S.; Roi, G.S. Isokinetic rehabilitation after anterior cruciate ligament (ACL) reconstruction. *Arch. Med. Deport.* **2005**, *22*, 19–25.
22. Vidmar, M.F.; Baroni, B.M.; Michelin, A.F.; Mezzomo, M.; Lugokenski, R.; Pimentel, G.L.; Silva, M.F. Isokinetic eccentric training is more effective than constant load eccentric training on the quadriceps rehabilitation following anterior cruciate ligament reconstruction: A randomized controlled trial. *Braz. J. Phys. Ther.* **2020**, *24*, 424–432. [CrossRef]
23. Dauty, M.; Potiron-Josse, M.; Rochcongar, P. Consequences and prediction of hamstring muscle injury with concentric and eccentric isokinetic parameters in elite soccer players. *Ann. Readapt. Med. Phys.* **2003**, *46*, 601–606. [CrossRef]
24. Brito, J.; Figueiredo, P.; Fernandes, L.; Seabra, A.; Soares, J.M.; Krustrup, P.; Rebelo, A. Isokinetic strength effects of FIFA'a "The 11+" injury prevention training programme. *Isokinet. Exerc. Sci.* **2010**, *18*, 211–215. [CrossRef]
25. Dauty, M.; Menu, P.; Fouasson-Chailloux, A.; Ferréol, S.; Dubois, C. Prediction of hamstring injury in professional soccer players by isokinetic measurements. *Muscles Ligaments Tendons J.* **2016**, *6*, 116–123. [CrossRef]
26. Rahnama, N.; Lees, A.; Bambaecichi, E. A comparison of muscle strength and flexibility between the preferred and non-preferred leg in English soccer players. *Ergonomics* **2005**, *48*, 1568–1575. [CrossRef]
27. Bogdanis, G.; Kalapotharakos, V. Knee Extension Strength and Hamstrings-to-Quadriceps Imbalances in Elite Soccer Players. *Int. J. Sports Med.* **2015**, *37*, 119–124. [CrossRef]
28. Paul, D.J.; Nassis, G.P. Testing strength and power in soccer players: The application of conventional and traditional methods of assessment. *J. Strength Cond. Res.* **2015**, *29*, 1748–1758. [CrossRef]
29. Marcos, M.A.; Koulla, P.M.; Anthos, Z.I. Preseason maximal aerobic power in professional soccer players among different divisions. *J. Strength Cond. Res.* **2018**, *32*, 356–363. [CrossRef]
30. Horstmann, T.; Mayer, F.; Fischer, J.; Maschmann, J.; Röcker, K.; Dickhuth, H.H. The cardiocirculatory reaction to isokinetic exercises in dependence on the form of exercise and age. *Int. J. Sports Med.* **1994**, *15* (Suppl. S1), S50–S55. [CrossRef]
31. Thompson, E.; Versteegh, T.H.; Overend, T.J.; Birmingham, T.B.; Vandervoort, A.A. Cardiovascular responses to submaximal concentric and eccentric isokinetic exercise in older adults. *J. Aging Phys. Act.* **1999**, *7*, 20–31. [CrossRef]
32. Kleiner, D.M.; Blessing, D.L.; Mitchell, J.W.; Davis, W.R. A Description of the Acute Cardiovascular Responses to Isokinetic Resistance at Three Different Speeds. *J. Strength Cond. Res.* **1999**, *13*, 360–366.
33. Okamoto, T.; Masuhara, M.; Ikuta, K. Cardiovascular responses induced during high-intensity eccentric and concentric isokinetic muscle contraction in healthy young adults. *Clin. Physiol. Funct. Imaging* **2006**, *26*, 39–44. [CrossRef]
34. Lamotte, M.; Chevalier, A.; Jamon, A.; Brassine, E.; Van De Borne, P. Hemodynamic response of an isokinetic testing and training session. *Isokinet. Exerc. Sci.* **2009**, *17*, 135–143. [CrossRef]
35. Czamara, A.; Krzemińska, A.; Szuba, L. The influence of exercises under isokinetic conditions on heart rate in males aged between 40 and 51. *Acta Bioeng. Biomech.* **2011**, *13*, 95–104. [PubMed]
36. GRANMO. Sample Size and Power Calculator. 2012. Available online: https://www.imim.cat/ofertadeserveis/software-public/granmo/ (accessed on 15 June 2020).
37. UEFA. *UEFA Medical Regulations*; UEFA: Nyon, Switzerland, 2017; pp. 1–20.
38. American College of Sports Medicine. *ACSM's Resource Manual for Guidelines for Exercise Testing and Prescription*; 7a. Lippincot Williams and Wilkins; Wolters Kluwer Health: Philadelphia, PA, USA, 2013; 896p.
39. Myers, J.; Arena, R.; Franklin, B.; Pina, I.; Kraus, W.E.; McInnis, K.; Balady, G.J. Recommendations for clinical exercise laboratories: A scientific statement from the american heart association. *Circulation* **2009**, *119*, 3144–3161. [CrossRef]
40. AEMEF. *AEMEF Protocol: Medical Examination in the Transfer of Professional Football Players*; AEMEF: Bilbao, Spain, 2014; pp. 1–13.
41. Magnusson, S.P.; Geismar, R.A.; Gleim, G.W.; Nicholas, J.A. The effect of stabilization on isokinetic knee extension and flexion torque production. *J. Athl. Train.* **1993**, *28*, 221–225.
42. Johnson, J.; Siegel, D. Reliability of an isokinetic movement of the knee extensors. *Res. Q* **1978**, *49*, 88–90. [CrossRef]
43. Perrin, D.H. Reliability of isokinetic measures. *Athl. Train.* **1986**, *21*, 319–321.
44. Hackett, D.A.; Chow, C.-M. The Valsalva maneuver: Its effect on intra-abdominal pressure and safety issues during resistance exercise. *J. Strength Cond. Res.* **2013**, *27*, 2338–2345. [CrossRef]
45. Baltzopoulos, V.; Williams, J.G.; Brodie, D.A. Sources of error in isokinetic dynamometry: Effects of visual feedback on maximum torque. *J. Orthop. Sports Phys. Ther.* **1991**, *13*, 138–142. [CrossRef]
46. Kellis, E.; Baltzopoulos, V. Resistive eccentric exercise: Effects of visual feedback on maximum moment of knee extensors and flexors. *J. Orthop. Sports Phys. Ther.* **1996**, *23*, 120–124. [CrossRef]
47. Eniseler, N.; Sahan, C.; Vurgun, H.; Mavi, H.F. Isokinetic Strength Responses to Season-long Training and Competition in Turkish Elite Soccer Players. *J. Hum. Kinet.* **2012**, *31*, 159–168. [CrossRef]
48. Lehnert, M.; Xaverová, Z.; Croix, M.D.S. Changes in Muscle Strength in U19 Soccer Players during an Annual Training Cycle. *J. Hum. Kinet.* **2014**, *42*, 175–185. [CrossRef] [PubMed]
49. Segovia, J.; López-Silvarrey, F.; Ramos, J.; Legido Arce, J. Valoración funcional en el fútbol. In *El fútbol: Valoración Clínica y Funcional*; Segovia, J., Ramos, J., López-Silvarrey, F., Eds.; Fundación Instituto SEK: Madrid, Spain, 2013; pp. 191–238.

50. Ramos, J. *Valoración Ergoespirométrica en Futbolistas Profesionales: Estudio de la Recuperación Tras Prueba de Esfuerzo Máxima*; Universidad Complutense de Madrid: Madrid, Spain, 2007.
51. Bishop, D. Warm up II: Performance changes following active warm up and how to structure the warm up. *Sports Med.* **2003**, *33*, 483–498. [CrossRef]
52. Bishop, D. Warm up I: Potential mechanisms and the effects of passive warm up on exercise performance. *Sports Med.* **2003**, *33*, 439–454. [CrossRef] [PubMed]
53. Fletcher, G.F.; Ades, P.A.; Kligfield, P.; Arena, R.; Balady, G.J.; Bittner, V.A.; Coke, L.A.; Fleg, J.L.; Forman, D.E.; Gerber, T.C.; et al. Exercise standards for testing and training: A scientific statement from the American heart association. *Circulation* **2013**, *128*, 873–934. [CrossRef]
54. Gibbons, R.J.; Balady, G.J.; Bricker, J.T.; Chaitman, B.R.; Fletcher, G.F.; Froelicher, V.F.; Mark, D.B.; McCallister, B.D.; Mooss, A.N.; O'Reilly, M.G.; et al. ACC/AHA 2002 guideline update for exercise testing: Summary article. A report of the American College of Cardiology/American Heart Association Task Force on Practice Guidelines (Committee to Update the 1997 Exercise Testing Guidelines). *J. Am. Coll. Cardiol.* **2002**, *40*, 1531–1540. [CrossRef]
55. Sieira, M.C.; Ricart, A.O.; Estrany, R.S. Respuesta de la tensión arterial a la prueba de esfuerzo. *Apunt. Med. Esport.* **2010**, *45*, 191–200. [CrossRef]
56. Morris, S.N.; Phillips, J.F.; Jordan, J.W.; McHenry, P.L. Incidence and significance of decreases in systolic blood pressure during graded treadmill exercise testing. *Am. J. Cardiol.* **1978**, *41*, 221–226. [CrossRef]
57. Tanaka, H.; Bassett, D.R.; Turner, M.J. Exaggerated blood pressure response to maximal exercise in endurance-trained individuals. *Am. J. Hypertens.* **1996**, *9*, 1099–1103. [CrossRef]
58. Turmel, J.; Poirier, P.; Bougault, V.; Blouin, E.; Belzile, M.; Boulet, L.-P. Cardiorespiratory screening in elite endurance sports athletes: The Quebec study. *Phys. Sportsmed.* **2012**, *40*, 55–65. [CrossRef]
59. Holland, D.; Sacre, J.; McFarlane, S.; Coombes, J.; Sharman, J. Pulse wave analysis is a reproducible technique for measuring central blood pressure during hemodynamic perturbations induced by exercise. *Am. J. Hypertens.* **2008**, *21*, 1100–1106. [CrossRef]
60. Douris, P.C. Cardiovascular responses to velocity-specific isokinetic exercise. *J. Orthop. Sports Phys. Ther.* **1991**, *13*, 28–32. [CrossRef]
61. Kleiner, D.M. The effects of manipulating the speed of maximal isokinetic resistance training on heart rate. *Med. Sci. Sport Exerc.* **1990**, *22*, 45. [CrossRef]
62. Quitério, R.J.; Melo, R.C.; Takahashi, A.C.M.; Aniceto, I.a.V.; Silva, E.; Catai, A.M. Torque, myoeletric sygnal and heart rate responses during concentric and eccentric exercises in older men. *Rev. Bras. Fisioter.* **2011**, *15*, 8–14. [CrossRef] [PubMed]
63. Lamotte, M.; Fournier, F.; Vanissum, A.; van de Borne, P. Influence of rest period duration between successive muscular strength sets on acute modifications of blood pressure and heart rate in the healthy subject. *Isokinet. Exerc. Sci.* **2006**, *14*, 1–6. [CrossRef]
64. Kleiner, D.M.; Blessing, D.L.; Davis, W.R.; Mitchell, J.W. Acute Cardiovascular Responses to Various Forms of Resistance Exercise. *J. Strength Cond. Res.* **1996**, *10*, 56–61.
65. Gür, H.; Akova, B.; Pündük, Z.; Küçükoğlu, S. Effects of age on the reciprocal peak torque ratios during knee muscle contractions in elite soccer players. *Scand. J. Med. Sci. Sports* **1999**, *9*, 81–87. [CrossRef] [PubMed]
66. Śliwowski, R.; Grygorowicz, M.; Hojszyk, R.; Jadczak, Ł. The isokinetic strength profile of elite soccer players according to playing position. *PLoS ONE* **2017**, *12*, e0182177. [CrossRef]
67. Hayashi, N.; Koba, S.; Yoshida, T. The effect of muscle contraction velocity on cardiorespiratory responses to repetitive isokinetic exercise in humans. *Jpn. J. Physiol.* **2003**, *53*, 327–333. [CrossRef]
68. Overend, T.J.; Versteegh, T.H.; Thompson, E.; Birmingham, T.B.; Vandervoort, A.A. Cardiovascular stress associated with concentric and eccentric isokinetic exercise in young and older adults. *J. Gerontol. A Biol. Sci. Med. Sci.* **2000**, *55*, B177–B182. [CrossRef]
69. Haff, G.; Dumke, C. *Laboratory Manual for Exercise Physiology with Web Resource*; Human Kinetics: Champaign, IL, USA, 2012; p. 464.
70. Le, V.-V.; Mitiku, T.; Sungar, G.; Myers, J.; Froelicher, V. The blood pressure response to dynamic exercise testing: A systematic review. *Prog. Cardiovasc. Dis.* **2008**, *51*, 135–160. [CrossRef]
71. Freedson, P.; Chang, B.; Katch, F.; Kroll, W.; Rippe, J.; Alpert, J.S.; Byrnes, W. Intraarterial blood pressure during free weight and hydraulic resistive exercise. *Med. Sci. Sport Exerc.* **1984**, *16*, 131. [CrossRef]
72. Vincenzi da Silva, E.; Pila Hernández, H.; Estévez Perera, A. *Comportamiento de Parámetros Cardiovasculares Durante Evaluaciones Isocinética de Rodilla en Deportistas de Alto Rendimiento de Balonmano*; INDER: La Habana, Cuba, 2008.
73. Narloch, J.A.; Brandstater, M.E. Influence of breathing technique on arterial blood pressure during heavy weight lifting. *Arch. Phys. Med. Rehabil.* **1995**, *76*, 457–462. [CrossRef]
74. Palatini, P.; Mos, L.; Munari, L.; Valle, F.; Del Torre, M.; Rossi, A.; Varotto, L.; Macor, F.; Martina, S.; Pessina, A.C.; et al. Blood pressure changes during heavy-resistance exercise. *J. Hypertens Suppl.* **1989**, *7*, S72–S73. [CrossRef]
75. Sale, D.G.; Moroz, D.E.; McKelvie, R.S.; MacDougall, J.D.; McCartney, N. Comparison of blood pressure response to isokinetic and weight-lifting exercise. *Eur. J. Appl. Physiol. Occup. Physiol.* **1993**, *67*, 115–120. [CrossRef]
76. Iellamo, F.; Legramante, J.M.; Raimondi, G.; Castrucci, F.; Damiani, C.; Foti, C.; Peruzzi, G.; Caruso, I. Effects of isokinetic, isotonic and isometric submaximal exercise on heart rate and blood pressure. *Eur. J. Appl. Physiol. Occup. Physiol.* **1997**, *75*, 89–96. [CrossRef] [PubMed]

77. Huggett, D.L.; Elliott, I.D.; Overend, T.J.; Vandervoort, A.A. Comparison of heart-rate and blood-pressure increases during isokinetic eccentric versus isometric exercise in older adults. *J. Aging Phys. Act.* **2004**, *12*, 157–169. [CrossRef]
78. Chapman, J.H.; Elliott, P.W. Cardiovascular effects of static and dynamic exercise. *Eur. J. Appl. Physiol. Occup. Physiol.* **1988**, *58*, 152–157. [CrossRef]
79. Weippert, M.; Behrens, K.; Rieger, A.; Stoll, R.; Kreuzfeld, S. Heart rate variability and blood pressure during dynamic and static exercise at similar heart rate levels. *PLoS ONE* **2013**, *8*, e83690. [CrossRef]
80. Di Blasio, A.; Sablone, A.; Civino, P.; D'Angelo, E.; Gallina, S.; Ripari, P. Arm vs. Combined Leg and Arm Exercise: Blood Pressure Responses and Ratings of Perceived Exertion at the Same Indirectly Determined Heart Rate. *J. Sports Sci. Med.* **2009**, *8*, 401–409.
81. MacDougall, J.D.; Tuxen, D.; Sale, D.G.; Moroz, J.R.; Sutton, J.R. Arterial blood pressure response to heavy resistance exercise. *J. Appl. Physiol.* **1985**, *58*, 785–790. [CrossRef] [PubMed]
82. Kaşikçioğlu, E.; Oflaz, H.; Akhan, H.; Kayserilioğlu, A.; Umman, S. Peak pulse pressure during exercise and left ventricular hypertrophy in athletes. *Anadolu. Kardiyol. Derg.* **2005**, *5*, 64–65.
83. Rawlins, J.; Bhan, A.; Sharma, S. Left ventricular hypertrophy in athletes. *Eur. J. Echocardiogr.* **2009**, *10*, 350–356. [CrossRef] [PubMed]
84. Metaxas, T.; Sendelides, T.; Koutlianos, N.; Mandroukas, K. Seasonal variation of aerobic performance in soccer players according to positional role. *J. Sports Med. Phys. Fit.* **2006**, *46*, 520–525.
85. Lago-Peñas, C.; Casais, L.; Dellal, A.; Rey, E.; Domínguez, E. Anthropometric and physiological characteristics of young soccer players according to their playing positions: Relevance for competition success. *J. Strength Cond. Res.* **2011**, *25*, 3358–3367. [CrossRef]
86. Sales, M.M.; Brownec, R.A.V.; Asanod, R.Y.; Olher, R.; dos Reis, V.; Vila Novad, J.; Moraese; Simões, H.G. Physical fitness and anthropometric characteristics in professional soccer players of the United Arab Emirates. *Rev. Andal. Med. Deport.* **2014**, *7*, 106–110. [CrossRef]
87. Di Paco, A.; Catapano, G.a.; Vagheggini, G.; Mazzoleni, S.; Micheli, M.L.; Ambrosino, N. Ventilatory response to exercise of elite soccer players. *Multidiscip. Respir. Med.* **2014**, *9*, 20. [CrossRef] [PubMed]
88. Haennel, R.G.; Snydmiller, G.D.; Teo, K.K.; Greenwood, P.V.; Quinney, H.A.; Kappagoda, C.T. Change in blood pressure and cardiac output during maximal isokinetic exercise. *Arch. Phys. Med. Rehabil.* **1992**, *73*, 150–155. [PubMed]
89. Nelson, R.R.; Gobel, F.L.; Jorgensen, C.R.; Wang, K.; Wang, Y.; Taylor, H.L. Hemodynamic predictors of myocardial oxygen consumption during static and dynamic exercise. *Circulation* **1974**, *50*, 1179–1189. [CrossRef]
90. Moreu-Burgos, J.; Macaya-Miguel, C. Fisiopatología del miocardio isquémico. Importancia de la frecuencia cardiaca. *Rev Española Cardiol.* **2007**, *7* (Suppl. D), 19–25. [CrossRef]
91. Isner-Horobeti, M.-E.; Dufour, S.P.; Vautravers, P.; Geny, B.; Coudeyre, E.; Richard, R. Eccentric Exercise Training: Modalities, Applications and Perspectives. *Sport Med.* **2013**, *43*, 483–512. [CrossRef] [PubMed]
92. Kitamura, K.; Jorgensen, C.R.; Gobel, F.L.; Taylor, H.L.; Wang, Y. Hemodynamic correlates of myocardial oxygen consumption during upright exercise. *J. Appl. Physiol.* **1972**, *32*, 516–522. [CrossRef] [PubMed]
93. Solomon, K. Blood pressure and heart rate responses to a standard lower limb isokinetic test. *Aust. J. Physiother.* **1992**, *38*, 95–102. [CrossRef]
94. Garcia-Retortillo, S.; Gacto, M.; O'Leary, T.J.; Noon, M.; Hristovski, R.; Balagué, N.; Morris, M.G. Cardiorespiratory coordination reveals training-specific physiological adaptations. *Eur. J. Appl. Physiol.* **2019**, *119*, 1701–1709. [CrossRef] [PubMed]
95. Balagué, N.; Hristovski, R.; Almarcha, M.C.; Garcia-Retortillo, S.; Ivanov, P.C. Network Physiology of Exercise: Vision and Perspectives. *Front. Physiol.* **2020**, *11*, 611550. [CrossRef]
96. Ivanov, P.C. The New Field of Network Physiology: Building the Human Physiolome. *Front. Netw. Physiol.* **2021**, *1*, 711778. [CrossRef]

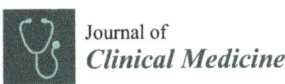

Article

Dynamic Ultrasound Assessment of the Anterior Tibial Translation for Anterior Cruciate Ligament Tears Diagnostic

Anca Gabriela Stoianov [1], Jenel Marian Pătrașcu [1], Bogdan Gheorghe Hogea [1], Bogdan Andor [1], Liviu Coriolan Mișcă [1], Sorin Florescu [1], Roxana Ramona Onofrei [2,*] and Jenel Marian Pătrașcu, Jr. [1,*]

[1] Department of Orthopedics and Trauma, "Victor Babes" University of Medicine and Pharmacy Timisoara, 300041 Timisoara, Romania; anca.stoianov@umft.ro (A.G.S.); patrascujenel@yahoo.com (J.M.P.); hogeabg@yahoo.com (B.G.H.); andormed@yahoo.com (B.A.); miscal.liviu@yahoo.com (L.C.M.); florescusorin@yahoo.com (S.F.)

[2] Department of Rehabilitation, Physical Medicine and Rheumatology, Research Center for Assessment of Human Motion, Functionality and Disability, "Victor Babes" University of Medicine and Pharmacy Timisoara, 300041 Timisoara, Romania

* Correspondence: onofrei.roxana@umft.ro (R.R.O.); jenel.patrascu@umft.ro (J.M.P.J.)

Citation: Stoianov, A.G.; Pătrașcu, J.M.; Hogea, B.G.; Andor, B.; Mișcă, L.C.; Florescu, S.; Onofrei, R.R.; Pătrașcu, J.M., Jr. Dynamic Ultrasound Assessment of the Anterior Tibial Translation for Anterior Cruciate Ligament Tears Diagnostic. *J. Clin. Med.* **2022**, *11*, 2152. https://doi.org/10.3390/jcm11082152

Academic Editors: Joel T. Cramer and Kevin L. Garvin

Received: 18 January 2022
Accepted: 7 April 2022
Published: 12 April 2022

Publisher's Note: MDPI stays neutral with regard to jurisdictional claims in published maps and institutional affiliations.

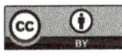

Copyright: © 2022 by the authors. Licensee MDPI, Basel, Switzerland. This article is an open access article distributed under the terms and conditions of the Creative Commons Attribution (CC BY) license (https://creativecommons.org/licenses/by/4.0/).

Abstract: The aim of our study was to investigate the accuracy of dynamic ultrasound assessment of the anterior tibial translation, in diagnosing anterior cruciate ligament tears, and to assess its test–retest reliability. Twenty-three patients (32 ± 8.42 years; 69.56% males) with a history of knee trauma and knee instability participated in the study. Knee ultrasound was performed by an experienced orthopedic surgeon. The anterior tibial translation was measured in both knees and differences between the injured and uninjured knee were calculated. Side-to-side differences > 1 mm were considered a positive diagnosis of an ACL tear. The anterior tibial translation values were 3.34 ± 1.48 mm in injured knees and 0.86 ± 0.78 mm in uninjured knees. Side-to-side differences > 1 mm were found in 22 cases (95.65%). The diagnosis accuracy was 91.30% (95%CI: 71.96–98.92%) and sensitivity 95.45% (95%CI: 77.15–99.88%). The intraclass correlation coefficient showed an excellent test–retest reliability (ICC$_{3,1}$ = 0.97 for the side-to-side difference in anterior tibial translation). The study highlights the accuracy and reliability of the dynamic ultrasound assessment of the anterior tibial translation in the diagnosis of unilateral anterior cruciate ligament tears. Ultrasound assessment is an accessible imaging tool that can provide valuable information and should be used together with physical examination in suspected cases of ACL injuries.

Keywords: dynamic ultrasound; ACL tears; anterior tibial translation; test–retest reliability

1. Introduction

Anterior cruciate ligament (ACL) tears are one of the most frequent ligament injuries of the knee, most of them needing surgical reconstruction [1,2]. In Romania, in 2015, there were 759 ACL/PCL reconstructions reported through the National ACL/PCL Reconstruction Register [3].

An accurate diagnosis of ACL injuries is essential for an appropriate treatment and a good prognosis. The American Academy of Orthopaedic Surgeons (AAOS) strongly recommends a detailed history and physical examination, as well as magnetic resonance imaging (MRI), for identifying ACL injuries [4]. However, the diagnostic accuracy of physical examination tests (anterior drawer test, Lachman test, pivot shift test) varies greatly in the literature [5]. Magnetic resonance imaging is considered highly accurate in diagnostic ACL tears [6]. However, performing MRI routinely for assessment of knee ligament injuries is not cost-effective and not always available [7]. Although arthroscopy is considered to be the gold standard for the diagnosis of ACL injuries, clinical diagnosis should be made with relevant imaging examinations [8]. In comparison with MRI, musculoskeletal ultrasound is more accessible, less expensive, with fewer impediments (e.g., metal implants, claustrophobia, pacemakers or other implants). Its reliability in assessing ligaments, tendons, muscles or joints has also been reported in several studies [9–16]. To date, there are several studies assessing the efficiency of ultrasound to identify ACL injuries. A systematic review performed by Wang et al. [17] showed that ultrasound can play a very important role in the diagnosis of ACL injury, although there are still some limitations, especially in identifying partial ACL tears (sensitivity of 15%).

In the literature, several ultrasound methods for ACL assessment are described that implies different patient positions (supine or prone, with the knee in different flexion degrees) and transducer placement (on the anterior or posterior aspect of the knee), static or dynamic evaluation, destabilizing strategies or different numbers of persons engaged in the examination [18]. One of the techniques used for the diagnosis of ACL injuries is the one described by Schwarz et al. [19], who used ultrasound to measure the anterior tibial translation to assess the ACL function.

The aim of our study was to investigate the accuracy of dynamic ultrasound assessment of the anterior tibial translation, in diagnosing anterior cruciate ligament tears, and to assess its test–retest reliability. The accuracy of this method has been addressed in previous studies on acute ACL tears. We have evaluated the accuracy on injuries older than 4 weeks. To the best of our knowledge, the test–retest reliability of this assessment method used for the diagnosis of chronic ACL tears has not been studied.

2. Materials and Methods

2.1. Participants and Study Design

In this prospective study, all patients presenting to the clinic between January 2020–May 2021 with complaints of knee instability were screened for inclusion in the study. The inclusion criteria were: (1) age over 18 years; (2) positive Lachman test; (3) positive anterior drawer test; (4) history of knee trauma within the last 6 months. After selecting patients based on the above-mentioned inclusion criteria, only patients who underwent either MRI or arthroscopy were further included in the study (to confirm or to infirm the ACL tear). Exclusion criteria were: (1) acute knee injury (<4 weeks since the traumatic event); (2) positive posterior drawer test; (3) multidirectional instability; (4) previous knee surgery (including ACL reconstruction); (5) open knee wounds. Informed consent was obtained from all subjects who met the inclusion criteria and agreed to participate in the study. The study was carried out in accordance with the Declaration of Helsinki and was approved by the Institutional Ethics Committee (14b/28.02.2020).

2.2. Assessments

All patients underwent an initial clinical evaluation, followed by knee ultrasound assessment and MRI and arthroscopic ACL reconstruction if a total ACL injury was diagnosed.

Knee ultrasound assessment was performed by an experienced orthopedic surgeon, using a Sonoscape S22 apparatus equipped with a 5–12 MHz linear-array transducer. The patient was lying prone with a roll under the lower legs in order to maintain the knee in 20° of flexion (Figure 1). Measurements were performed in both knees (injured and uninjured), at the postero-medial aspect of the knee. The distance between the tangent line to the medial femoral condyle and the tangent to the posterior aspect of the tibia was measured in static position (D1) and after applying manual pressure on the posterior proximal aspect of the calf (D2) [20] (Figure 2). For each knee, the difference between the two distances was calculated (D2 − D1). The translation differences between the injured and uninjured knee were calculated: $\Delta D = (D2_{injured} - D1_{injured}) - (D2_{uninjured} - D1_{uninjured})$ [20]. Schwarz et al. reported that a value greater than 1 mm for ΔD is a reliable threshold for the diagnosis of an ACL tear [19,20]. The measurements were repeated after 15 min, in order to assess the test–retest reliability.

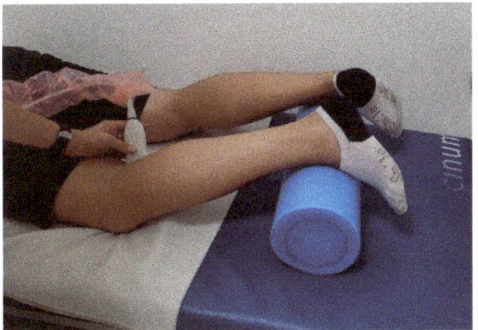

Figure 1. Patient position during ultrasound assessment.

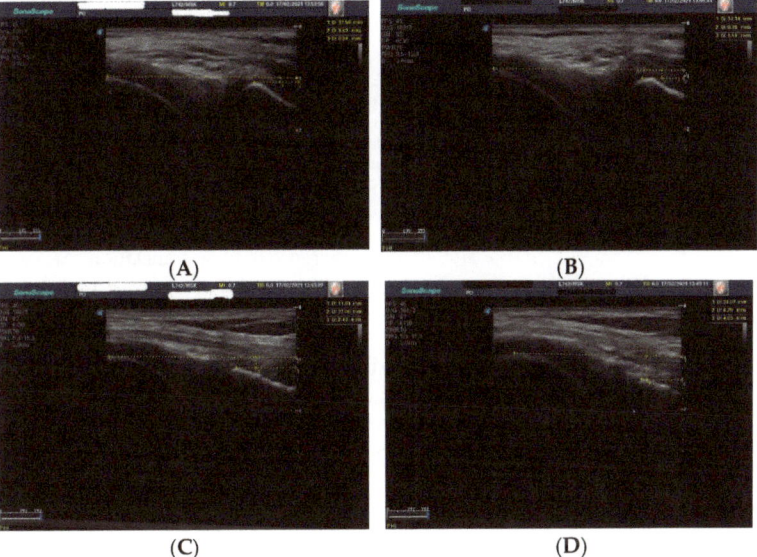

Figure 2. Anterior tibial translation measurements in uninjured and injured knee. (**A**) Static anterior tibial translation in uninjured knee (D1$_{uninjured}$ = 0.94 mm); (**B**) Dynamic anterior tibial translation (manual pressure was applied in the proximal posterior aspect of the calf) in uninjured knee (D2$_{uninjured}$ = 1.5 mm); (**C**) Static anterior tibial translation in injured knee (D1$_{injured}$ = 2.13 mm); (**D**) Dynamic anterior tibial translation (manual pressure was applied in the proximal posterior aspect of the calf) in injured knee (D2$_{injured}$ = 4.63 mm).

2.3. Statistical Analysis

Statistical analysis was performed with MedCalc Statistical Software version 20.014 (MedCalc Software Ltd., Ostend, Belgium). Data were tested for normality using Shapiro–Wilk test and descriptive statistics were performed. In order to assess the sensitivity and accuracy of the ultrasound-based diagnostic for complete ACL tear, a 2 × 2 contingency table was created, comparing the results from ultrasound with those obtained by arthroscopy. Intraclass correlation coefficient (ICC$_{3,1}$) was used to assess the test–retest reliability [21]. ICC values greater than 0.90 were considered as excellent, values between 0.75 and 0.90 as good and values less than 0.75 as moderate [21]. Standard error of measurement (SEM) was calculated according to the formula SEM = SDpooled × $\sqrt{1 - ICC}$ [22,23]. The measurements are considered more reliable if the SEM values are smaller [22]. The smallest detectable change at 95% confidence interval (SDC$_{95}$) assessed the magnitude of the real change between measurements necessary to exceed error. The lower the values for SDC_{95} are, the higher the reliability is [24]. SDC_{95} is calculated using the formula: $SDC_{95} = 1.96 \times \sqrt{2} \times SEM$ [23]. A paired sample t-test was performed in order to assess the systematic bias [22,23]. Statistical significance was set $p < 0.05$ for all tests.

3. Results

Twenty-three patients who met the inclusion criteria, agreed to participate in the study and were also evaluated by MRI and arthroscopy were included in the study. Mean age was 32 ± 8.42 years; 16 patients were males (69.56%). The traumatic event took place during amateur sporting activities (soccer—9 cases (39.13%); ski—10 cases (43.48%); basketball—2 cases (8.7%)) or professional sport activities (handball—1 case (4.34%); soccer—1 case (4.34%)).

The anterior tibial translations measured by ultrasound for the injured and non-injured knee, in both measurement sessions, are present in Table 1.

Table 1. Anterior tibial translation in injured and non-injured knee.

	Injured Knee	p *	Uninjured Knee	p **
Anterior tibial translation (D2 − D1), mm (mean ± SD)	3.34 ± 1.48	0.0002	0.86 ± 0.78	0.01
Anterior tibial translation (D2 − D1) − retest, mm (mean ± SD)	3.66 ± 1.64		0.95 ± 0.78	

p *—relates to the differences between test and retest for the injured knee; p **—relates to the differences between test and retest for the uninjured knee.

The side-to-side difference in tibial translation (ΔD) was greater than 1 mm in 22 cases (95.65%), with a mean of 2.47 ± 1.25 mm at the first measurement, and 2.71 ± 1.39 mm at retest (Figure 3). Complete ACL tears were confirmed in all 23 cases by MRI, and in 22 cases by arthroscopy (including the case non-confirmed by ultrasound). One case was diagnosed as partial ACL tear by arthroscopy and no ACL reconstruction was performed. Using the threshold of 1 mm for side-to-side differences of tibial translation, complete ACL tears have been correctly diagnosed in 22 cases, the sensitivity of the method being 95.45% (95%CI: 77.15–99.88%) and the accuracy 91.30% (95%CI: 71.96–98.92%).

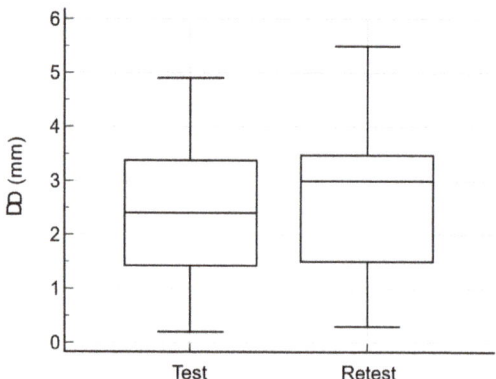

Figure 3. Side-to-side differences in tibial translation (ΔD).

Significant differences were found between test and retest values for the anterior tibial translation, for both injured (p = 0.0002) and uninjured knees (p = 0.01).

The $ICC_{3,1}$, SEM and SDC_{95} values for D1 and D2 measurement, for both injured and uninjured knee, as well as for ΔD, are presented in Table 2. Lower values for SEM and SDC_{95} were observed for both measurements (D1 and D2) in the uninjured knee.

Table 2. The $ICC_{3,1}$, SEM and SDC_{95} values for D1, D2 measurements and ΔD.

	$ICC_{3,1}$	95%CI	SEM	SDC_{95}
D1 injured knee	0.99	0.997–0.999	0.23	0.63
D2 injured knee	0.99	0.98–0.99	0.31	0.85
D1 uninjured knee	0.99	0.991–0.998	0.08	0.22
D2 uninjured knee	0.98	0.973–0.995	0.18	0.49
ΔD	0.97	0.945–0.99	0.22	0.6

$ICC_{3,1}$—intraclass correlation coefficient; 95%CI—95% confidence interval; SEM—standard error of measurement; SDC_{95}—smallest detectable change at 95% confidence interval; SEM and SDC_{95} are expressed in the same measurement units as the test.

4. Discussion

Although ultrasound is a frequently used method in the diagnosis of musculoskeletal injuries, in both orthopedics and rehabilitation medicine [25,26], ultrasound assessments for the diagnosis of ACL injuries showed varied results, mainly due to the different methodologies used (conventional ultrasound and functional/dynamic ultrasound) [7]. The aim of the present study was to investigate the accuracy of dynamic ultrasound assessment of the anterior tibial translation, in diagnosing anterior cruciate ligament tears, and to assess its test–retest reliability. We found a diagnostic accuracy of dynamic ultrasound measurement of anterior tibial translation of 91.30% and a sensitivity of 95.45% for the diagnosis of complete ACL tears.

The anterior tibial translation measurements showed a systematic bias between test–retest, for both injured and uninjured knees. Since these measurements were only taken 15 min apart, this is not surprising, given the viscoelastic properties of knee ligaments [27]. These findings suggest that the ligaments in the knee become stretched during the anterior tibial translation measurement, and the ligaments do not return to their original length within 15 min (the amount of time between test and retest). These findings also suggest that the manual pressure on the posterior proximal aspect of the calf applied by the tester is likely causing this systematic lengthening of the knee ligaments. Such pressure should be controlled to minimize variations among systematic lengthening of these ligaments during the test. Future studies should examine the reliability of this anterior tibial translation measurement with 2–3 days between the test and retest, rather than 15 min, to understand the full scope of reliability, systematic variability, and sensitivity of this assessment. Furthermore, future studies should also examine the time course of ligament lengthening to understand how long it takes for the affected ligaments to return to their original length between successive measurements. Such information would improve recommendations on how much time to wait between anterior tibial translation measurements when multiple tests are required.

In our study, we used the same method as Palm et al. [20], and found similar results in terms of sensitivity. In their study, Palm et al. [20] investigated if an examiner with basic expertise in ultrasonography and little or no experience in arthrosonography can use functional ultrasonography with the same high diagnostic accuracy as an experienced sonographer. They found a sensitivity of 97% for the method, the ACL tears being confirmed by arthroscopy in 32 of 33 cases.

Kumar et al. [28] also found a high sensitivity for this method (81.65%), after the assessment of 130 patients with a non-acute knee injury. They compared the efficacy of dynamic ultrasound in identifying ACL tears with MRI.

Gebhard et al. [29] used the ultrasound to quantify the anterior tibial translation in their study, the difference between the two methods being the way the tibial translation was induced. We used the same method as Palm et al. [20] in their study, applying manual pressure on the posterior proximal aspect of the calf. Gebhard et al. [29] manually lifted the lower leg under ultrasound control as far as possible, while the thigh remained in contact with the surface; after marking the tibial head, the lower leg was carefully released and drawn by gravity into anterior draw position. They opted for the gravity-induced anterior tibial translation as they noticed pain during dorsal force on most of the acute ACL lesions. For a minimum intra-individual difference of 5 mm, the authors reported a sensitivity of 96% [29].

We found excellent test–retest reliability in the dynamic ultrasound assessment of the anterior tibial translation, with patients lying prone and measurements being made in the postero-medial aspect of the knees ($ICC_{3,1}$ = 0.97 for the side-to-side difference in anterior tibial translation). A good intra-rater reliability of ultrasound assessment of the anterior tibial translation was reported by Teng et al. [30], but in participants with no ACL tears.

For the diagnosis of ACL injuries, direct and indirect signs, as well as signs of antero-posterior instability under ultrasound imaging were proposed, with different diagnosis accuracy and sensitivity [31]. As in physical examination, the anterior tibial translation is used as a sign of antero-posterior instability under ultrasound assessment, with greater values in the presence of ACL injuries compared to uninvolved knees [19,20,28,29]. In our study the anterior tibial translation of the affected knees was also greater than in uninjured knees (3.34 ± 1.48 mm vs. 0.86 ± 0.78 mm), similar to values found by Palm et al. [20] (3.8 ± 1.5 mm vs. 0.1 ± 0.7 mm). The values reported by Kumar et al. [28] for the anterior tibial translation for the injured and uninjured knee were slightly greater than our results (4.21 ± 2.93 mm and 2.16 ± 2.67 mm, respectively). Gebhard et al. [29] reported a mean anterior displacement of the medial tibial plateau of 14.1 ± 3.5 mm in ACL-injured knees and of 8.3 ± 3.4 mm in uninjured knees, values greater than those reported by us, Palm et al. [20] and Kumar et al. [28]. One explanation could be the different method of inducing anterior tibial translation. Using a different method (patient in a seated position, with the knee flexed to about 70–80°, the transducer placed onto the anterior aspect of the knee, above the level of tibial tuberosity, parallel with the patellar tendon; examiner in front of the patient; the patient's lower leg was pushed backwards with the examiner's foot), Grzelak et al. [32] reported absolute knee anterior translation values of 8.67 ± 2.65 mm in injured knees and 2.88 ± 1.26 mm in uninjured knees.

Schwarz et al. reported that a value greater than 1 mm for side-to-side differences in ultrasound-measured anterior tibial translation is a reliable threshold for the diagnosis of an ACL tear [19,20]. We found a side-to-side difference in tibial translation (ΔD) greater than 1 mm in 22 cases (95.65%), with a mean of 2.47 ± 1.25 mm. Palm et al. [20] and Kumar et al. [28] have also considered the threshold of 1 mm in side-to-side difference for anterior tibial translation for a diagnosis of ACL tear.

The examiner in our study was an orthopedic surgeon with significant prior experience with the use of ultrasound. However, the results from Palm et al. [20] showed that an examiner without specialist knowledge in ultrasonography can accurately diagnose acute ACL injuries using functional ultrasonography.

Ultrasound assessment of anterior tibial translation, as a side-to-side difference of more than 1 mm, proved to be accurate and reliable for the diagnosis of complete ACL tears. To the best of our knowledge, this is the first study that has assessed the test–retest reliability of the dynamic ultrasound assessment of anterior tibial translation for the diagnosis of chronic ACL tears. Our results showed an excellent test–retest reliability for this method. However, the method can be used only if the injury is unilateral, and this is a limitation. Further studies are needed to find a threshold value for the anterior tibial translation, to use it also in cases in which there is a laxity or instability in the contralateral knee and also to test the inter-rater reliability of this method. Some limitations of this study have to be considered. We have not evaluated acute ACL tears. Not examining the side-to-side differences with another device, such as an arthrometer, could also be a limitation of the study.

5. Conclusions

The study highlights the accuracy and reliability of the dynamic ultrasound assessment of the anterior tibial translation, in the diagnosis of unilateral anterior cruciate ligament tears. Ultrasound assessment is an accessible imaging tool that can provide valuable information and should be used together with the physical examination in suspected cases of ACL injuries.

Author Contributions: Conceptualization, A.G.S. and J.M.P.; methodology, A.G.S.; formal analysis, A.G.S.; investigation, A.G.S.; data curation, A.G.S. and R.R.O.; writing—original draft preparation, A.G.S., J.M.P, B.G.H., B.A., L.C.M., S.F., R.R.O. and J.M.P.J.; writing—review and editing, A.G.S., J.M.P., L.C.M., S.F., R.R.O. and J.M.P.J.; supervision, J.M.P. All authors have read and agreed to the published version of the manuscript.

Funding: This research received no external funding.

Institutional Review Board Statement: The study was conducted according to the guidelines of the Declaration of Helsinki, and approved by the Institutional Ethics Committee of "Victor Babes" University of Medicine and Pharmacy Timisoara, Romania (14b/28.02.2020).

Informed Consent Statement: Informed consent was obtained from all subjects involved in the study.

Conflicts of Interest: The authors declare no conflict of interest.

References

1. Abram, S.G.F.; Price, A.J.; Judge, A.; Beard, D.J. Anterior Cruciate Ligament (ACL) Reconstruction and Meniscal Repair Rates Have Both Increased in the Past 20 Years in England: Hospital Statistics from 1997 to 2017. *Br. J. Sports Med.* **2020**, *54*, 286–291. [CrossRef] [PubMed]
2. Sanders, T.L.; Maradit Kremers, H.; Bryan, A.J.; Larson, D.R.; Dahm, D.L.; Levy, B.A.; Stuart, M.J.; Krych, A.J. Incidence of Anterior Cruciate Ligament Tears and Reconstruction: A 21-Year Population-Based Study. *Am. J. Sports Med.* **2016**, *44*, 1502–1507. [CrossRef] [PubMed]
3. The Romanian Arthroplasty Register. Summary Findings on ACL/PCL Reconstruction Register. Available online: https://www.rne.ro/rnemedia/download/lia_lip1.pdf (accessed on 15 December 2021).
4. Shea, K.G.; Carey, J.L. Management of Anterior Cruciate Ligament Injuries: Evidence-Based Guideline. *JAAOS-J. Am. Acad. Orthop. Surg.* **2015**, *23*, e1–e5. [CrossRef] [PubMed]
5. Zhao, G.; Lyu, J.; Liu, C.; Wu, J.; Xia, J.; Huang, G. A Modified Anterior Drawer Test for Anterior Cruciate Ligament Ruptures. *J. Orthop. Surg. Res.* **2021**, *16*, 260. [CrossRef]
6. Crawford, R.; Walley, G.; Bridgman, S.; Maffulli, N. Magnetic Resonance Imaging versus Arthroscopy in the Diagnosis of Knee Pathology, Concentrating on Meniscal Lesions and ACL Tears: A Systematic Review. *Br. Med. Bull.* **2007**, *84*, 5–23. [CrossRef] [PubMed]
7. Lee, S.H.; Yun, S.J. Efficiency of Knee Ultrasound for Diagnosing Anterior Cruciate Ligament and Posterior Cruciate Ligament Injuries: A Systematic Review and Meta-Analysis. *Skelet. Radiol.* **2019**, *48*, 1599–1610. [CrossRef]
8. Ji, C.; Chen, Y.; Zhu, L.; Zhang, J. Arthroscopic Anterior Cruciate Ligament Injury in Clinical Treatment of Joint Complications and CT Observation. *J. Healthc. Eng.* **2021**, *2021*, 6667046. [CrossRef]
9. Grassi, W.; Filippucci, E.; Farina, A.; Cervini, C. Sonographic Imaging of Tendons. *Arthritis Rheum.* **2000**, *43*, 969–976. [CrossRef]
10. Ahmad, A.; Bandpei, M.A.M.; Gilani, S.A.; Munawar, A.; Ahmed, I.; Tanveer, F. Reliability of Musculoskeletal Ultrasound Imaging to Measure Supraspinatus Tendon Thickness in Healthy Subjects. *J. Phys. Ther. Sci.* **2017**, *29*, 1394–1398. [CrossRef]
11. Gellhorn, A.C.; Carlson, M.J. Inter-Rater, Intra-Rater, and Inter-Machine Reliability of Quantitative Ultrasound Measurements of the Patellar Tendon. *Ultrasound Med. Biol.* **2013**, *39*, 791–796. [CrossRef]
12. Gessl, I.; Balint, P.V.; Filippucci, E.; Keen, H.I.; Pineda, C.; Terslev, L.; Wildner, B.; D'Agostino, M.A.; Mandl, P. Structural Damage in Rheumatoid Arthritis Assessed by Musculoskeletal Ultrasound: A Systematic Literature Review by the Structural Joint Damage Task Force of the OMERACT Ultrasound Working Group. *Semin. Arthritis Rheum.* **2021**, *51*, 627–639. [CrossRef]
13. del Baño-Aledo, M.E.; Martínez-Payá, J.J.; Ríos-Díaz, J.; Mejías-Suárez, S.; Serrano-Carmona, S.; de Groot-Ferrando, A. Ultrasound Measures of Tendon Thickness: Intra-Rater, Inter-Rater and Inter-Machine Reliability. *Muscles Ligaments Tendons J.* **2017**, *7*, 192–199. [CrossRef]
14. Rossi, F.; Zaottini, F.; Picasso, R.; Martinoli, C.; Tagliafico, A.S. Ankle and Foot Ultrasound: Reliability of Side-to-Side Comparison of Small Anatomic Structures. *J. Ultrasound Med.* **2019**, *38*, 2143–2153. [CrossRef] [PubMed]
15. Stracciolini, A.; Boucher, L.; Jackson, S.; Brown, N.; Magrini, D.; McKee-Proctor, M.; d'Hemecourt, P.; Delzell, P. Feasibility and Reliability of Musculoskeletal Ultrasound Measurement of the Medial Patellofemoral Ligament. *Orthop. J. Sports Med.* **2020**, *8*, 2325967120S00185. [CrossRef]
16. Kandel, M.; Cattrysse, E.; de Maeseneer, M.; Lenchik, L.; Paantjens, M.; Leeuw, M. Inter-Rater Reliability of an Ultrasound Protocol to Evaluate the Anterolateral Ligament of the Knee. *J. Ultrason.* **2019**, *19*, 181–186. [CrossRef] [PubMed]
17. Wang, J.; Wu, H.; Dong, F.; Li, B.; Wei, Z.; Peng, Q.; Dong, D.; Li, M.; Xu, J. The Role of Ultrasonography in the Diagnosis of Anterior Cruciate Ligament Injury: A Systematic Review and Meta-Analysis. *Eur. J. Sport Sci.* **2018**, *18*, 579–586. [CrossRef]
18. Poboży, T.; Kielar, M. A Review of Ultrasonographic Methods for the Assessment of the Anterior Cruciate Ligament in Patients with Knee Instability—Diagnostics Using a Posterior Approach. *J. Ultrason.* **2016**, *16*, 288–295. [CrossRef]

19. Schwarz, W.; Hagelstein, J.; Minholz, R.; Schierlinger, M.; Danz, B.; Gerngroß, H. Manuelle Sonometrie Des KniegelenksEine Praxisnahe Methode Zur Diagnostik Der Frischen Ruptur Des Vorderen Kreuzbandes. *Der Unfallchirurg* **1997**, *100*, 280–285. [CrossRef]
20. Palm, H.-G.; Bergenthal, G.; Ehry, P.; Schwarz, W.; Schmidt, R.; Friemert, B. Functional Ultrasonography in the Diagnosis of Acute Anterior Cruciate Ligament Injuries: A Field Study. *Knee* **2009**, *16*, 441–446. [CrossRef]
21. Koo, T.K.; Li, M.Y. A Guideline of Selecting and Reporting Intraclass Correlation Coefficients for Reliability Research. *J. Chiropr. Med.* **2016**, *15*, 155–163. [CrossRef]
22. Atkinson, G.; Nevill, A. Statistical Methods for Asssing Measurement Error (Reliability) in Variables Relevant to Sports Medicine. *Sports Med.* **1998**, *26*, 217–238. [CrossRef] [PubMed]
23. Weir, J.P. Quantifying Test-Retest Reliability Using the Intraclass Correlation Coefficient and the SEM. *J. Strength Cond. Res.* **2005**, *19*, 231–240. [PubMed]
24. Hyong, I.H.; Kim, J.H. Test of Intrarater and Interrater Reliability for the Star Excursion Balance Test. *J. Phys. Ther. Sci.* **2014**, *26*, 1139–1141. [CrossRef] [PubMed]
25. Li, X.; Yi, P.H.; Curry, E.J.; Murakami, A.M. Ultrasonography as a Diagnostic, Therapeutic, and Research Tool in Orthopaedic Surgery. *JAAOS-J. Am. Acad. Orthop. Surg.* **2018**, *26*, 187–196. [CrossRef]
26. Özçakar, L.; Kara, M.; Chang, K.-V.; Lew, H.L.; Franchignoni, F. Musculoskeletal Ultrasound Liberating Physical and Rehabilitation Medicine: A Reinforcement for "Runners," a Reminder for "Walkers" and the Last Call for "Couch Potatoes". *Am. J. Phys. Med. Rehabil.* **2018**, *97*, e73–e74. [CrossRef]
27. Wojtys, E.M.; Wylie, B.B.; Huston, L.J. The Effects of Muscle Fatigue on Neuromuscular Function and Anterior Tibial Translation in Healthy Knees. *Am. J. Sports Med.* **1996**, *24*, 615–621. [CrossRef]
28. Kumar, S.; Kumar, A.; Kumar, S.; Kumar, P. Functional Ultrasonography in Diagnosing Anterior Cruciate Ligament Injury as Compared to Magnetic Resonance Imaging. *Indian J. Orthop.* **2018**, *52*, 638–644. [CrossRef]
29. Gebhard, F.; Authenrieth, M.; Strecker, W.; Kinzl, L.; Hehl, G. Ultrasound Evaluation of Gravity Induced Anterior Drawer Following Anterior Cruciate Ligament Lesion. *Knee Surg. Sports Traumatol. Arthrosc.* **1999**, *7*, 166–172. [CrossRef]
30. Teng, P.S.P.; Leong, K.F.; Yi Xian Phua, P.; Kong, P.W. An Exploratory Study of the Use of Ultrasound in the Measurement of Anterior Tibial Translation under Gastrocnemius Muscle Stimulation. *Res. Sports Med.* **2021**, *29*, 103–115. [CrossRef]
31. Wu, W.-T.; Lee, T.-M.; Mezian, K.; Naňka, O.; Chang, K.-V.; Özçakar, L. Ultrasound Imaging of the Anterior Cruciate Ligament: A Pictorial Essay and Narrative Review. *Ultrasound Med. Biol.* **2021**, *48*, 377–396. [CrossRef]
32. Grzelak, P.; Podgórski, M.T.; Stefańczyk, L.; Domżalski, M. Ultrasonographic Test for Complete Anterior Cruciate Ligament Injury. *Indian J. Orthop.* **2015**, *49*, 143–149. [CrossRef] [PubMed]

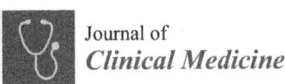

Article

Acute Effects of Sedentary Behavior on Ankle Torque Assessed with a Custom-Made Electronic Dynamometer

Iulia Iovanca Dragoi [1], Florina Georgeta Popescu [2,*], Teodor Petrita [3,*], Florin Alexa [3], Sorin Barac [1], Cosmina Ioana Bondor [4], Elena-Ana Pauncu [2], Frank L. Bowling [1,5], Neil D. Reeves [6] and Mihai Ionac [1]

1. Department of Vascular Surgery and Reconstructive Microsurgery, "Victor Babes" University of Medicine and Pharmacy, 2 Eftimie Murgu Square, 300041 Timisoara, Romania; contactfastfizioclinic@gmail.com (I.I.D.); sorin.barac@umft.ro (S.B.); frank.bowling@manchester.ac.uk (F.L.B.); mihai.ionac@umft.ro (M.I.)
2. Discipline of Occupational Health, "Victor Babes" University of Medicine and Pharmacy, 2 Eftimie Murgu Square, 300041 Timisoara, Romania; medicinamuncii@umft.ro
3. Department of Communications, Politehnica University Timisoara, 2 Vasile Parvan, 300223 Timisoara, Romania; florin.alexa@upt.ro
4. Department of Medical Informatics and Biostatistics, University of Medicine and Pharmacy "Iuliu Hatieganu", 8 Victor Babes, 400000 Cluj-Napoca, Romania; cbondor@umfcluj.ro
5. Department of Surgery & Translational Medicine, Faculty of Medical and Human Sciences, University of Manchester, Oxford Road, Manchester M13 9PL, UK
6. Research Centre for Musculoskeletal Science & Sports Medicine, Department of Life Sciences, Faculty of Science and Engineering, Manchester Metropolitan University, Oxford Road, Manchester M1 5GD, UK; n.reeves@mmu.ac.uk
* Correspondence: popescu.florina@umft.ro (F.G.P.); teodor.petrita@upt.ro (T.P.); Tel.: +40-745384732 (F.G.P.)

Abstract: Inactivity negatively influences general health, and sedentary behaviour is known to impact the musculoskeletal system. The aim of the study was to assess the impact of time spent in active and sedentary behaviour on foot muscle strength. In this observational study, we compared the acute effects of one day of prolonged sitting and one day of low-to-moderate level of activity on ankle torque in one group of eight healthy participants. Peak ankle torque was measured using a portable custom-made electronic dynamometer. Three consecutive maximal voluntary isometric contractions for bilateral plantar flexor and dorsiflexor muscles were captured at different moments in time. The average peak torque significant statistically decreased at 6 h ($p = 0.019$) in both static and active behaviours, with a higher average peak torque in the active behaviour ($p < 0.001$). Age, gender, body mass index and average steps did not have any significant influence on the average value of maximal voluntary isometric contraction. The more time participants maintained either static or active behaviour, the less force was observed during ankle torque testation. The static behaviour represented by the sitting position was associated with a higher reduction in the average peak ankle torque during a maximal voluntary isometric contraction when compared to the active behaviour.

Keywords: prolonged sitting; ankle torque; dynamometer; muscle strength; physical activity; sedentary behaviour

Citation: Dragoi, I.I.; Popescu, F.G.; Petrita, T.; Alexa, F.; Barac, S.; Bondor, C.I.; Pauncu, E.-A.; Bowling, F.L.; Reeves, N.D.; Ionac, M. Acute Effects of Sedentary Behavior on Ankle Torque Assessed with a Custom-Made Electronic Dynamometer. *J. Clin. Med.* **2022**, *11*, 2474. https://doi.org/10.3390/jcm11092474

Academic Editor: David Rodríguez-Sanz

Received: 5 April 2022
Accepted: 26 April 2022
Published: 28 April 2022

Publisher's Note: MDPI stays neutral with regard to jurisdictional claims in published maps and institutional affiliations.

Copyright: © 2022 by the authors. Licensee MDPI, Basel, Switzerland. This article is an open access article distributed under the terms and conditions of the Creative Commons Attribution (CC BY) license (https:// creativecommons.org/licenses/by/ 4.0/).

1. Introduction

Human physical activity and physiology of movement during daily activities, professional activities and sports in all age-related populations have gained increased scientist's interest. Physical activity level influences general health, and the expansion of sedentary behaviour and its chronic complications are of great concern lately. Studying how sedentary behaviour influences human health across a lifespan might help increase physical and psychological wellbeing among various populations.

Physical activity has been defined as movement produced by the action of the skeletal muscles and can be related to occupational, household, sports or any other activities. Physical fitness has been defined as planned, structured exercise and is different from physical activity. These two particular terms are often confounded. Physical fitness might be misused when defining physical activity [1].

When compared with the rest basal level, activity has been associated with higher energy expenditure, while the absence of activity has been defined as inactivity [1]. For a better thermology statement, the World Health Organization [2] and the National Institute of Health [3] have these definitions stated. Undertaking 7000–8000 steps/day is the border for physical activity to be categorised [4].

A sedentary lifestyle is considered when ≤5000 steps/day are undertaken, while ≈3500 steps/day is associated with an extremely low level of activity [5]. The same number of steps (just below 5000 steps/day) have been reported in the Framingham Heart Study [6].

Low-intensity physical activity (LIPA) and moderate to vigorous physical activity (MVPA) are the main two types of identified activity levels. A minimum of 150–300 min of weekly physical activity with moderate intensity, or 75–150 min of vigorous activity, or a combination of both types of activities is highly recommended [7]. By replacing the sedentary-spent time with light/moderate/heavy activities, a positive influence could be obtained on the human body's main functions [8]. Increasing heavy physical activity for only five minutes can resemble a reduction of one hour of sedentary time [9].

Despite the well-documented general health benefits of MVPA [10], the adult population still shows a high amount of daily sedentary behaviour time [11]. Sedentary behaviour has shown negative effects, with prolonged physical inactivity being considered a major risk factor for human health and a reduced life expectancy [12]. Sedentary behaviour has been characterised by reduced energy expenditure and was recognised even among individuals engaged in MVPA [13]. The World Health Organisation recommendations on the appropriate level of activity are only met in one of four adults [14]. Evidence from wearable devices monitoring the level of human physical activity reported a massive increment in sedentary-spent time [15,16], with increased exposure to risks in all demographics and age groups [17]. Individuals' sedentary behaviour can be identified by using self-reported questionnaires on daily time spent in any sedentary activities and mainly in a sitting position [18].

Increased sedentary time (ST) has been associated with an increased risk for type 2 diabetes mellitus, metabolic syndrome [19,20] and cardiovascular diseases (CVD) [19,21]. When comparing the acute effects of LIPA with inactivity in various populations, an impact on the cardiometabolic system [22], haemostasis [23], glucose and insulin responses have been observed in the case of inactivity [24]. When the time of sedentary behaviour, LIPA time and MVPA time were objectively analysed, exposure to risks was revealed in the case of sedentary behaviour in various age groups [25]. Physical inactivity and mainly prolonged sitting are involved in the mechanisms regulating proteins involved in disease susceptibility [26]. Due to daily reduced levels of muscle contractions, while maintaining a prolonged sitting position, modern society is experiencing the negative impact of inactivity [27]. Short-term studies demonstrated the unhealthy potential of one day of inactivity [28], with acute physiologically secondary effects of sitting being shown even in the active population [29]. Simulated microgravity has been shown to induce marked lower limb skeletal muscle atrophy when one limb was suspended for four weeks, and a similarity in the magnitude of muscle mass and strength reduction was obtained in the case of bed-rest [30].

Six weeks of unilateral suspension of the lower limb showed changes in the muscle morphology [31].

Few studies analysed the impact of sedentary behaviour on the muscles acting around the ankle joint, and even less data is available for healthy individuals.

In patients suffering from diabetes, prolonged sitting revealed a potential negative impact on the foot plantar skin health [32]. In subjects that underwent ankle immobilisation, no significant differences were seen at 48 h, but significant differences were seen at one week. This presumed that the accumulated effects of immobilisation are needed to explain the reduction in strength at one week [33]. When participants were placed under chronic unloading (90 days of simulated microgravitational situation), negative effects resulted on the mechanical properties of the human Achille's Tendon, while when participants were placed under resistive exercises, preventive effects were observed [34]. The effects of unloading on the tendon's mechanical properties when placed for six weeks on bed rest conditions were also reported [35].

Despite sitting being associated with physical inactivity and inactivity is further associated with risks, the amount of sitting time linked with risks for human health has not yet been defined [36,37]. Reeves et al. suggested that in the case of simulated microgravity, in order to completely prevent alterations in the Achille's Tendon mechanical properties, a certain level of muscle exercise is required [34].

Reducing sedentary behaviours was already strongly recommended and might be considered a preventive strategy [7].

One of the multiple proposed strategies for reducing sedentary behaviour was increasing the number of daily steps; thereafter, foot abilities to generate strength and endurance are requested for an effective gait. Walking is efficient if supported by the lower limb's performance. Sitting, mainly prolonged sitting, as well as the association of sitting with sedentary behaviour, places one's feet in an inactivity situation. Assessing foot muscles performance, despite being a difficult procedure that implies both technologies and testators' skills, is essential. Determining the relationship between muscle action dose–response in particular functional activities could explain the side-effects of muscle inactivity and, in particular, during being in sitting positions.

No agreement has been stated on the most appropriate method for measuring the strength of the foot intrinsic muscles [38]. From electromyographic studies [39] to toe flexor muscles (TFM) custom-made dynamometry [40], diverse methods for measuring foot intrinsic muscle's function have been described [34].

By capturing ankle torque through the evaluation of maximal voluntary isometric contraction (MVIC), foot and ankle muscles that generated strength during a particular time interval and at the selected range of ankle joint motion can be precisely measured. Custom-made electronic dynamometry showed to be a reliable method for the measurement of ankle torque in humans [41] and a reproducible dynamic method when foot muscle strength was assessed in two moments in time [42].

Acute and accumulated effects of sitting on the intrinsic foot muscles and all muscles acting around the ankle joint need in-depth research, and the capturing of ankle torque by dynamometric means could be of relevance in both clinical and experimental fields.

This study is, to the best of our knowledge, the first to examine the impact of active and sedentary behaviour on ankle torque when assessed with a custom-made electronic dynamometer.

The aims of this study were: to analyse the impact and compare the effects of two different types of activities (short-time sedentary versus a short-time active behaviour) on the evolution of peak ankle torque in time; to assess the two types of routine lifestyles (sedentary and active) on ankle torque when participants were subjected to a short-time active and a short-time sedentary behaviour.

Despite the impact of sedentary behaviour on ankle torque as the main focus of this paper, describing the measurement system (custom-made electronic dynamometer) as an innovative way to assess muscle strength in relation to inactivity is of great importance. In order to better profit from the measurement device's practical use, we considered that an extensive outline of the measurement principles and measurement system description is required to ensure that any further replication of our study would be conducted with ease when a custom-made device is being used.

The more time either short-time static or short-time active behaviour was maintained, the less force was observed during ankle torque testation. Peak torque during maximal isometric contraction was higher during a short time spent in active behaviour.

2. Materials and Methods

2.1. Participants

Eight healthy adult consenting participants were selected for the study, and written signed consent was obtained before the enrolment. Ethical approval from the University of Medicine and Pharmacy "Victor Babes" Timisoara Ethics Committee was released and registered under Nr. 50/21.09-14.10.2020. The included participants had their measurements of peak ankle torque captured at maximum 2-weeks intervals in October 2021. All measurements were performed in the same physiotherapy unit placed in Timisoara, Romania. Based on their daily average number of steps recovered from the wearable devices, four of the participants were considered routinely active ($\geq$6000 steps/day), and the other four participants were considered routinely sedentary (<6000 steps/day), further named routinely active and sedentary group, respectively. Only the average number of daily steps of the last month were recovered from the participant's smartwatches. The data extracted from the devices did not represent the exact type of activity the participants underwent during their last month. Thereafter, neither physical activity or physical fitness had been recognised or identified from the recovered data. Nor a systematical control of the data derived from smartwatches, nor was a correlation between the data and participant reports applied for a possible correlation with a specific type of activity during the last month. Routinely active participants self-declared an active lifestyle during their occupational work, including light to moderate physical activity level and a regularly active lifestyle during off-work hours, respectively. Three of the four routinely active participants were engaged in recreational sports during the week, declaring a history of participation in performance sports. One participant practised soccer for eight years, one participant was a performant swimmer for five years and one participant practised acrobatic dancing for six years. All four routinely sedentary participants declared a sedentary lifestyle during their occupational work, including mainly sitting posture-spent time and no specific light to moderate intensity of physical activity during off-work hours. Only one participant from the four routinely sedentary group declared a history of 12 years of professional gymnastics.

We considered for exclusion any systemic diseases affecting the foot and ankle, past/present foot or lower limb trauma or surgery interventions that might have altered the foot mobility or function, or physical congenital foot and ankle deformities or malformations. Any cognitive/neurological conditions altering lower limb functionality, as well as psychiatric issues affecting the participant's ability to participate, were also considered exclusion criteria.

2.2. Data Collection

Anthropometric data, including age, gender, height, weight and foot length, were registered/measured at the first visit.

The average number of daily steps during the last month prior to measurements (independent of being considered physical activity or physical fitness) were registered after being recovered from the participant's wearable devices (smartwatches), and a general physical activity level was established for each enrolled participant [43].

For a better framing of the off-work hours type of activity level, questions on daily activities were asked, targeting overall sedentary time spent in a sitting position, screen and tv time [18].

2.3. Description of the Measurement System and Measurement Procedure

2.3.1. Measurement System Description

Bilaterally ankle torque measurements were performed for all participants using a reliable [41], reproducible [42], portable custom-made electronic dynamometer [44]. A simple diagram with the measurement system components is represented in Figure 1.

The dynamometers pedal construction permitted the measurement of ankle torque at different joint angles by setting the desired pedal angle using an electronic inclinometer. Torque was converted into force, permitting that the applied force on the load cell was to be further converted into voltage. By the connected load cell amplifier, the load cell imbalance was converted into voltage, further evaluated with an oscilloscope (PicoScope Model 2204A) [45] connected to the personal computer (PC). The PicoScope®6 software used (manufactured by Pico Technology, PC Oscilloscope software version: 6.14.54.6108Copyright © 1995–2021, Pico Technology Ltd., St Neots, UK) [46] permitted the data acquisition and the recording of the whole measurement period. The apparatus construction, calibration and the full disclosure of the measurement system and protocol intervention have been described elsewhere [41]. A representation of the measurement system components and the participant's general position on the chair is captured in Figure 2. Figure 2 demonstrates the minimum required amount of space (~3 m²) needed for the whole measurement system components and the participants' chair to be positioned in order to proceed to measurements.

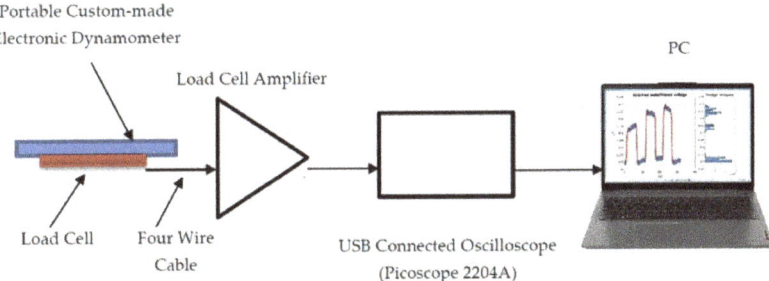

Figure 1. Diagram of graphic representation of the measurement system components comprising the portable custom-made electronic dynamometer, dynamometer load cell, a load cell amplifier connected to the dynamometer's load cell through a four-wire cable, the USB connected oscilloscope (PicoScope 2204A) and the personal computer (PC).

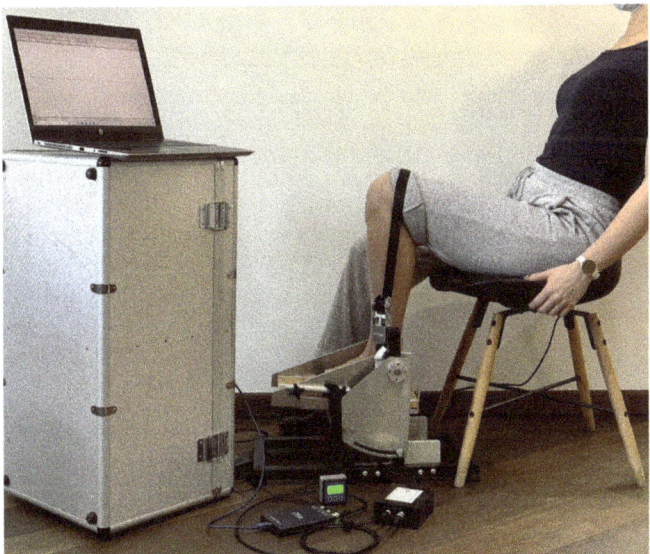

Figure 2. The system components used for ankle torque measurement and participant position on the chair; the measurement system components include: portable custom-made electronic dynamometer with an incorporated load cell, electronic inclinometer, a load cell amplifier, oscilloscope, connection wires and a PC.

The PicoScope®6 software graphic user interface allowed for the particular parameter configuration seen in Figure 3.

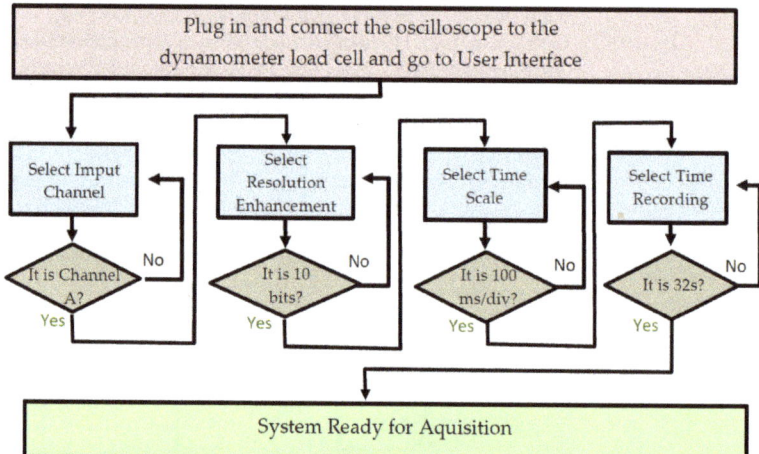

Figure 3. Flow chart representing the steps needed for the selection of the oscilloscope software graphic user interface configuration parameters: Channel A on, direct current (DC) coupling, input = 2 V/div, time base = 100 ms/div (32 s length record) and 10 bits resolution enhancement.

During active ankle plantar flexion, a positive voltage value variation was obtained, as seen in Figure 4—trace A, while during dorsiflexion, a negative voltage value variation was obtained, as seen in Figure 4—trace B. The voltage values were transformed into torque in Nm. The actual voltage value, represented in V, corresponds to the voltage signal seen on the PC screen. Two sources of displacement of the voltage off-set are present in the set-up: the pedal remanent off-set (own pedal weight and permanent mechanical tension), as seen in Figure 4—trace E, and the participant-generated off-set, as seen in Figure 4—traces C and D (comprised of the lower limb weight in the absence of any ankle motion without tension generated by the fixation belt, and the lower limb weight in the absence of any ankle motion with the tension generated by the fixation belt, respectively).

After each measurement, the data recordings were saved as a folder from the PicoScope interface, containing 32 text files of voltage values. For the validation of each measurement, a MATLAB [47] application was developed. The application allowed for the inspection of the saved text files by loading the multi-file contents of each measurement and concatenating them in a single time graph. By inspection of the resulted time graphs the operator appreciated the quality of each measurement and concluded for validation. Time graphs not passing the validation procedure were followed by another measurement trial. Measurements considered valid received a numerical code for each participant. The saved valid measurements were later sent for data processing. For accurate time graphs, low-pass filtering and scaling with the pedal constant were applied [41]. Voltage offset and peak torque during MVIC were processor-estimated and summarised into an Excel spreadsheet [48]. The summarised Excel data of voltage were converted into torque data [41]. Both time graphs of the voltage data, as well as time graphs of torque data, were visualised as graphic representations in time of the voltage variations in V, as seen in Figure 5a, or torque variations in Nm, as seen in Figure 5b–d. Automatically computed peak torque values (highlighted with a red circle, as seen in Figure 5c,d) and offset means (indicated by the red line in the time graphs, as seen in Figure 5c,d) were included in the torque time graphs.

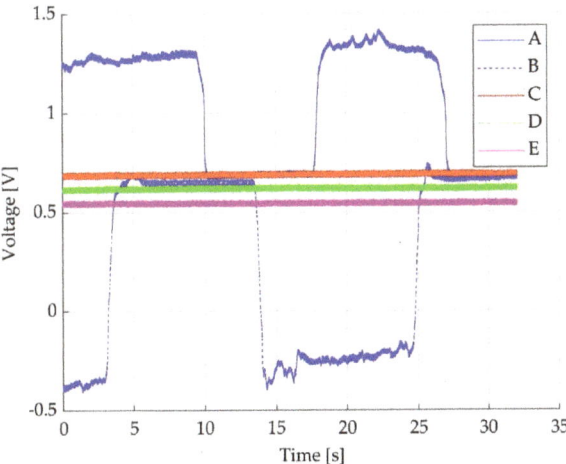

Figure 4. Time graph representing five different situations. Trace A represents a positive transition of voltage from the off-set level during two MVICs while the participant actively plantarflexes the foot; Trace B represents a negative transition of voltage from the off-set level during two MVICs while the participant actively dorsiflexes the foot; Trace C represents the off-set voltage level while the participant's foot is relaxed on the pedal with fixation strap not tightened; Trace D represents the off-set voltage level while the participant's foot is relaxed on the pedal with the fixation strap being tightened on the thigh just above the knee level; Trace E represents the pedal off-set in the absence of the participant's foot on the dynamometer pedal.

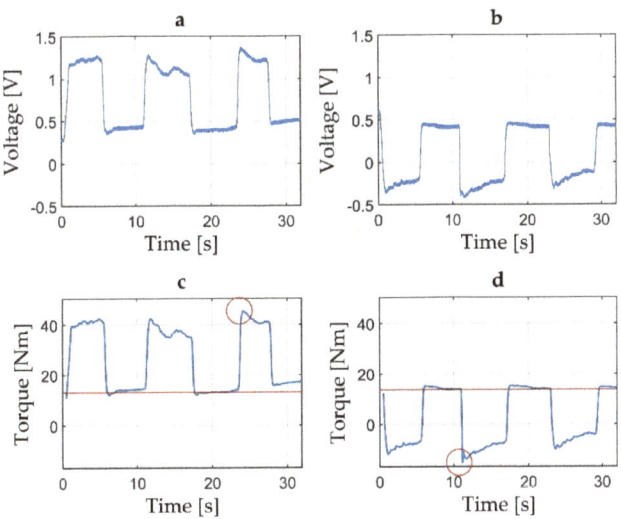

Figure 5. Three time graphs representing a succession of three MVIC of 5 s each followed by 5 s of relaxation between contractions: (**a**) time graph of voltage during ankle plantar flexion with the period being represented in seconds (s) on the Ox axis and voltage represented in V on the Oy axis; (**b**) an example of the same time graph for ankle dorsiflexion with the period being represented in seconds (s) on the Ox axis and torque represented in Nm on the Oy axis; (**c**) torque represented in Nm during ankle plantar flexion, where the peak torque is highlighted with a red circle and the mean off-set level is marked with a red line; (**d**) torque represented in Nm during ankle dorsiflexion, where the peak torque is highlighted with a red circle and the mean off-set level is marked with a red line.

2.3.2. Methods of Participant Preparation for Measurement Procedure

Each measurement session consisted of measuring ankle torque during plantar flexion and dorsiflexion using a custom-made electronic dynamometer. All measurements were performed in the same testing laboratory with a constant room temperature (22 °C), allowing for an acclimatisation period of one hour before measurements. All possible adverse effects and the complete measurement protocol [41] were fully detailed to the participants. Possible adverse reactions, such as muscle cramps/fatigue/pain, or any other physical/emotional discomfort, were written and verbally presented to the participants and followed by cessation of the session in case such reactions might appear during the measurements. The participants were encouraged to fully relax while maintaining a sitting position with their trunk resting on the chair back-rest. Knee and hip joints were kept flexed, and the examined foot was resting in a plantigrade position on the dynamometer plate. Using nonelastic fibre belts, the fixation of the foot and thigh were ensured. For accurate measurements, the thigh strap was fixed just above the knee joint using one rigid fixation belt, and the foot was fixed in place using a second rigid fixation belt placed just above the dorsal aspect of the metatarsal-phalangeal joints (MPJ). This specific fixation allowed for the foot and ankle to remain stable and the heel to remain fixed in place during all measurements, as shown in Figure 6a,b. The foot positioning considered the ankle joint axis of rotation (defined as the line passing through the ankle malleoli) being aligned with the dynamometer's pivotal point. The dynamometer's pivotal point is marked with a blue horizontal line, as represented in Figure 6b.

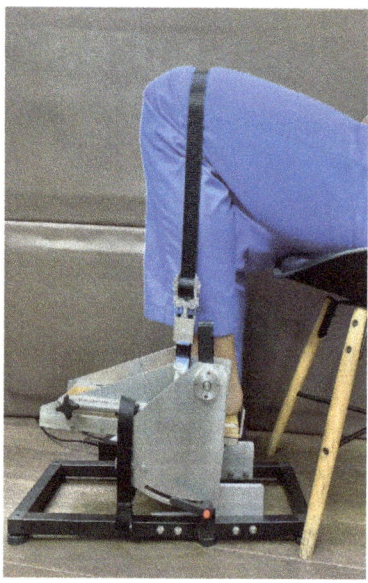 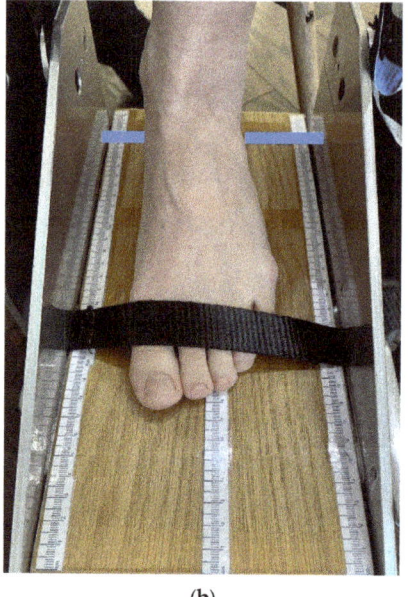

(a)   (b)

Figure 6. The participant's sitting position: (**a**) fixation of the lower limb using a rigid fixation belt over the thigh right above the knee joint and the knee joint angle settled between 90° and 110°; (**b**) foot positioned on the dynamometer plate, with the ankle joint axis of rotation above the apparatus's pivotal line marked on the device pedal with a blue line, with fixation of the rigid belt on the dorsum of the foot just above the MPJs level.

A more flexed knee position [49] allowed for the better isolation of the foot's small muscles (flexor digitorum longus, flexor hallucis longus and the long toe flexor muscles) also involved in plantar flexing of the ankle. The strap fixation just above the MPJs level allowed for the attenuation of the anterior tibialis muscle impact as an ankle dorsiflexor.

After all of the participants understood the type of requested muscle efforts, a succession of contractions followed as an experimental trial for better participant acclimatisation. Voltage acquisitions started while the clinician vocally commanded the direction of the ankle movements. After the acclimatisation test, a trial of three consecutive MVICs were registered for each ankle while the participants actively plantarflexed and dorsiflexed the foot. The acquisition period for the three consecutive MVICs was settled for 32 s. To better prevent muscle fatigue, a two-minute recovery break was permitted between the measurements for all pedal inclinations and all muscle groups. We measured the passive moment at rest and ankle torque at $0°$, $+5°$, $-5°$ of pedal inclination during three consecutive MVIC of 5 s, each separated by 5 s relaxation time for both plantar and dorsiflexor muscle groups, resulting in 12 measurements for each participant. The selected pedal inclinations ($0°$, $+5°$, $-5°$) corresponded to the same range of the participant's ankle joint. When the tibia's long axis was perpendicular to the ground, having the foot resting on the dynamometer at $0°$ of pedal inclination, we defined the ankle as being in a neutral position ($90°$ of ankle dorsiflexion). From the neutral ankle position, we considered $95°$ of ankle dorsiflexion when $+5°$ of pedal inclination and $5°$ of ankle plantar flexion when $-5°$ of pedal inclination.

All participants were measured during two separate six-hour sessions. One session comprised six hours of sedentary behaviour (further named static behaviour) while maintaining a prolonged sitting position. The other session comprised of six hours of active behaviour (further named active behaviour) defined by low and moderate levels of physical activity.

A two-week interval was allowed between the two separate sessions.

The static behaviour was represented by six hours of prolonged sitting posture, with only small breaks allowed for participant's urgent personal needs. The active behaviour consisted of six hours of mixed activities (short or long-distance walking, ascending/descending stairs, orthostatic postures) without exceeding the moderate level of physical activity.

Three ankle torque measurements were performed at three different moments during each individual session: at two, four and six hours. The first measurement on each session was performed after two hours of the initiation of static/active behaviour.

The ankle torque measurement recordings from both the first and second sessions were later used for data processing.

2.3.3. Methods for Validation of Acquired Data

One validation procedure during the measurements and two validation procedures during the interpretation of the results were performed for all of the acquired data. Participant-related errors (due to indiscipline or improper clinician commands) appeared and were considered errors during the measurements. When such errors were encountered, new measurements were requested.

All recorded voltage time graphs resulting from the oscilloscope were inspected by the main researcher immediately after each performed measurement, and only valid measurements were selected. Errors were kept for statistical analysis without being considered valid measurements.

Participant errors derived from off-set instability, improper contraction/break time (s), muscle efforts not corresponding with the clinician's vocal commands, insufficient number of MVIC, fatigue, insufficiently sustained MVIC, pain or participant's errors derived from testator command are possibly seen during measurements, and some of the most commonly encountered errors are represented in Figure 7a–d.

By a simple analysis of the time graphs obtained with the developed application, the human or apparatus errors were easily recognised. Improperly recorded data derived from both participant and/or operator errors or apparatus errors were eliminated.

The obtained results from the three consecutive MVIC, the difference between the maximum obtained level of torque and the minimum obtained level of torque (defined as peak torque in Nm), were registered and statistically analysed.

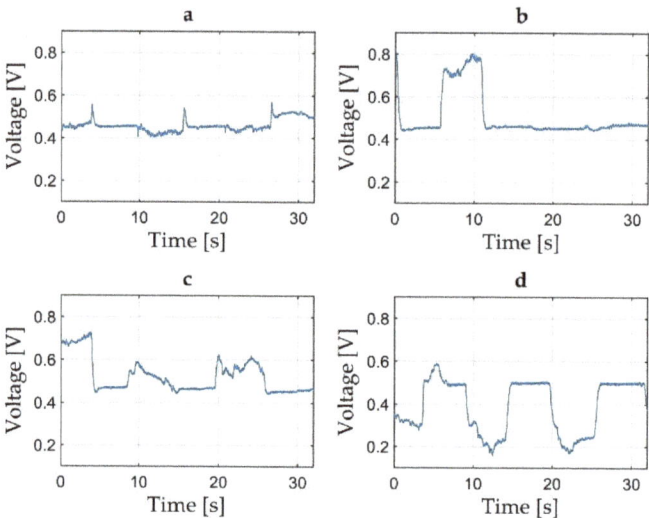

Figure 7. Time graphs representing invalid measurements due to errors derived from: (**a**) probable momentary fraction without participant's proper sustain of MVIC; (**b**) insufficient number of MVIC probable due to the testator's command error; (**c**) two insufficient and inconsistent MVIC following a good MVIC due to subject's inability to focus on the testator command; (**d**) erroneous plantarflexion during dorsiflexion requests.

2.4. Other Clinical and Functional Performed Tests

A hand grip strength (HGS) test [50,51] for both right and left hands was performed using a factory-calibrated Hand Grip Dynamometer KERN MAP 80 K1 [52]. The testation was in accordance with the manufacturer's instructions. The participants were asked to stand in an upright position having their testing arm resting close to their trunk and the elbow flexed at 90°. Three consecutive maximal volitional hand grip contractions were requested using the dynamometer's 80 kg spring, and the maximal value of strength in kg was registered for the right and left hands. Right/left arm dominance was asked and registered.

Bilateral calf circumference (CC) in cm at the calf's greatest girth was registered after being measured using a flexible nonelastic ruler. To measure CC, the participants were asked to stand in an upright position having their feet apart at shoulder width with their body weight equally distributed on both legs [53].

The number of repetitions during the Calf Raise Senior Test (CRST) [54,55] was registered for all participants. The participants were asked, while barefoot with their knees in maximum extension, to raise their heels simultaneously as high as possible, maintaining the same range of movement for all repetitions. To ensure stability, keeping their fingers on a vertical wall was permitted. While CRST was performed, muscle fatigue and muscle pain appeared during testation, and the onset moment of both fatigue and pain were registered.

The Calf Raise Test (CRT) [56] was performed starting from a unilateral weight bearing stance, and the number of repetitions for both legs was registered. Participants were asked to unilaterally raise their heel as high as possible, maintaining the same range of movement for all repetitions. To ensure stability, keeping fingers on a vertical wall was permitted. Muscle pain and muscle fatigue that appeared during CRT and the onset moment of both fatigue and pain were registered.

The chair raise test [57] was performed, and the total number of repetitions of chair raises in one minute was registered. Participants were asked to repetitively fully stand up in an upright position having their legs apart with their body weight symmetrically distributed on both legs, and then to sit down on a chair and perform as many repetitions as possible.

2.5. Statistical Analysis

For the study group, demographic data were reported as the arithmetic mean ± standard deviation or with absolute and relative frequencies. The normal distribution was tested with Shapiro–Wilk's test.

The collected time graphs during measurements were analysed for errors. The peak torque was considered missing in case errors were found. Other missing data were due to fatigue, muscle pain or discomfort of the participant.

Clinical measurements were compared between the moments of measurements (at 2, 4 and 6 h) and between the active versus static behaviour with one-way ANOVA for repeated measures, separately for each flexion, foot and degree. The *p*-value for the comparisons between the moments (different measurements in time) and the *p*-value for the comparisons between active and static behaviour was reported. The number of data entered in the one-way ANOVA with repeated measures was 8 for each moment (one measurement for each participant).

When all the data were analysed (576 measurements), multivariate analysis was performed with linear mixed models for repeated data because the data were not independent between the participants (each participant had 12 measurements in each moment). Independent factors were considered, and they were entered into the analysis as fixed factors: the active/static behaviour, the moments, the flexion, the foot and the degree. The data were analysed and reported to the first considered moment at 2 h. The data at 0 h were not available due to the protocol design.

Arithmetic means of the clinical measurements were computed. These arithmetic means were compared between the moments of the measurements with *t*-test for paired samples for normally distributed data and with Wilcoxon signed-rank test for non-normally distributed data. Post-hoc analysis was performed using Bonferroni correction.

Correlations between two parameters were analysed by computing the Pearson and Spearman coefficients of correlation.

The *p*-value was considered statistically significant for values smaller than 0.05. Analysis was performed using SPSS application (manufactured by IBM Corp., Armonk, NY, USA, 2017) [58].

3. Results

3.1. Participant's Characteristics

Our participant's characteristics are described in Table 1. The average participants' age was 35.88 years old, with a minimum age of 23 and a maximum age of 58 years; three participants (37.5%) were male; four participants (50%) reported an average daily number of steps higher than 6000; five participants (62.5%) had a normal body mass index (BMI). For the studied sample, the HGS, CC, CRST, CRT, chair raise test and muscle pain and fatigue moment of onset during CRST, CRT and chair raise test for all participants and results are reported in Table 1.

Table 1. Demographic and anthropometric data of the sample.

Parameters	Arithmetic Mean ± Standard Deviation (n = 8) [1]
Age (years)	35.88 ± 12.65
Male, no. [7] (%)	3 (37.5)
Foot length (cm)	25.36 ± 2.56
BMI [2] (kg/m²)	25.02 ± 4.43
Average no. [7] of daily steps (steps/day)	6125 ± 2279.57
AHGS [3] (kg)	28.01 ± 10.62
ACC [4] (cm)	37.25 ± 3.17
CRST [5] (no. [7] of repetitions)	57.25 ± 17.69
Muscle pain during CRST [5] (no. [7] of repetitions)	42.75 ± 21.37
Muscle fatigue during CRST [5] (no. [7] of repetitions)	40.5 ± 10.57
ACRT [6] (no. [7] of repetitions)	30.44 ± 4.92
Chair raise test bilateral	41.88 ± 13.44
Muscle pain ACRT [6] (no. [7] of repetitions)	23.38 ± 5.71
Muscle fatigue ACRT [6] (no. [7] of repetitions)	25.31 ± 3.95

[1] Total sample (n = 8); [2] BMI—Body Mass Index; [3] AHGS—Average Hand Grip Strength; [4] ACC—Average Calf Circumference; [5] CRST—Calf Raise Senior Test; [6] ACRT—Average Calf Raise Test; [7] no.—number.

3.2. Clinical Measurements Results

In Table 2, the descriptive statistic parameters for peak ankle torque during MVIC (dMVIC) in the case of active and static behaviour for each moment in time were presented and analysed with an ANOVA repeated measure for each foot, flexion and degree. The number of data entered in the ANOVA repeated measure analysis was $n = 8$ (one measurement of dMVIC for each participant).

When we analysed all the data with linear mixed models without taking into consideration the foot, the flexion or the degree, we found that the active versus static behaviour ($p = 0.005$) and the moments (2 h vs. 6 h $p = 0.040$, 2 h vs. 4 h $p = 0.128$) had a significant effect on the dMVIC. The number of data entered in the linear mixed models' analysis was $n = 288$ (for each subject 36 measurements of dMVIC).

The averages of dMVIC measured on different flexion, foot and degree on different moments per static/active behaviour are presented in Figure 8. There were significant differences between dMVIC after two hours compared with dMVIC after six hours ($p = 0.019$). There were no significant differences between dMVIC after two hours compared with dMVIC after four hours ($p = 0.224$) and also between dMVIC after four hours compared with dMVIC after six hours ($p = 0.815$). The average dMVIC in the case of active behaviour was significant statistically greater than the average dMVIC during static behaviour.

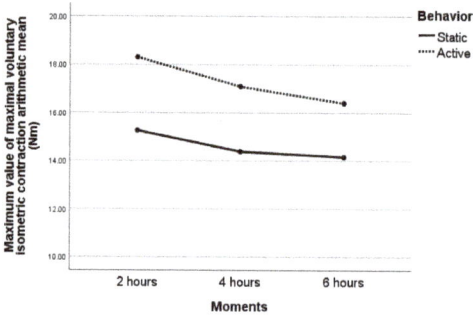

Figure 8. Impact of the moments of testing and the behaviour on dMVIC.

Table 2. Descriptive statistics (arithmetic mean +/− standard deviation; median (25th; 75th percentile)) for dMVIC in the cases of active and static behaviours.

Flexion	Foot	Degree	Time Moment	dMVIC * (Nm) Static (n = 8)	dMVIC * (Nm) Active (n = 8)	p ** between Moments	p ** between Active and Static
Dorsi	Left	−5	2	17.78 ± 12.21	21.97 ± 14.05	0.087	0.560
			4	18.01 ± 10.1	21.35 ± 10.99		
			6	16.89 ± 11.08	19.01 ± 10.39		
		0	2	19.10 ± 12.40	26.11 ± 14.10	0.172	0.459
			4	18.01 ± 9.83	19.7 ± 10.82		
			6	18.02 ± 13.15	18.91 ± 11.96		
		5	2	20.2 ± 8.44	21.57 ± 11.03	0.150	0.632
			4	17.67 ± 8.22	19.73 ± 9.88		
			6	18.30 ± 12.15	17.24 ± 11.47		
	Right	−5	2	17.72 ± 12.33	23.99 ± 13.29	0.469	0.269
			4	18.46 ± 10.71	21.16 ± 11.66		
			6	17.60 ± 11.63	22.27 ± 12.01		
		0	2	15.76 ± 10.17	21.43 ± 12.85	0.098	0.783
			4	14.49 ± 8.19	21.32 ± 12.37		
			6	13.53 ± 9.56	18.44 ± 10.41		
		5	2	18.53 ± 10.5	21.58 ± 13	0.324	0.381
			4	16.26 ± 11.22	21.48 ± 12.03		
			6	15.29 ± 10.43	21.45 ± 14.04		
Plantar	Left	−5	2	14.7 ± 7.5	19.41 ± 11.31	0.922	0.267
			4	15.1 ± 7.88	18.50 ± 9.82		
			6	16.17 ± 8.50	17.10 ± 11		
		0	2	2.63 ± 5.10	5.95 ± 7.91	0.535	0.227
			4	3.17 ± 5.72	3.26 ± 6.99		
			6	3.83 ± 7.06	3.55 ± 7.66		
		5	2	17.84 ± 4.93	21.19 ± 17.43	0.340	0.313
			4	15.51 ± 4.72	20.48 ± 13.28		
			6	20.32 ± 13.75	19.50 ± 12.81		
	Right	−5	2	18.15 ± 9.38	20.50 ± 13.48	0.821	0.682
			4	18.10 ± 8.26	18.59 ± 11.04		
			6	16.59 ± 9.91	19.33 ± 14.99		
		0	2	3.49 ± 5.61	2.05 ± 1.21	0.752	0.188
			4	3.52 ± 5.87	1.71 ± 2.53		
			6	2.43 ± 4.78	2.31 ± 2.76		
		5	2	21.17 ± 8.10	20.69 ± 13.70	0.308	0.356
			4	17.9 ± 6.37	20.57 ± 12.59		
			6	16.87 ± 6.47	20.36 ± 14.47		

* dMVIC—peak torque (maximum value of maximal voluntary isometric contraction with pedal off-set correction),
** p-value from ANOVA with repeated measure.

When we tested the other factors: age, gender, BMI, average steps, AHGS, ACC, CRST, CRT, chair raise test, muscle pain during CRST, muscle pain during CRT, muscle fatigue during CRST and muscle fatigue during CRT in a repeated-measure ANOVA model, we did not find any significant influence on average dMVIC.

We analysed the impact of the daily activity as the average number of steps (Table 3) or as the difference between the group of routinely active and routinely sedentary, but we did not find any significant statistical correlation (r = −0.313, p = 0.450) or association (p = 0.882) with dMVIC.

Table 3. Correlation between average dMVIC and the other parameters.

Parameters	Pearson/Spearman Coefficient of Correlation	p
Age (years)	0.229	0.586
BMI [1] (kg/m^2)	0.580	0.132
Foot length (cm)	0.483	0.226
Average no. [6] of daily steps (steps/day)	−0.313 *	0.450
AHGS [2] (kg)	0.573	0.137
ACC [3] (cm)	0.359 *	0.382
CRST [4] (no. [6] of repetitions)	0.535	0.171
Muscle pain during CRST [4] (no. [6] of repetitions)	0.569	0.141
Muscle fatigue during CRST [4] (no. [6] of repetitions)	0.365	0.373
ACRT [5] (no. [6] of repetitions)	0.411	0.360
Chair raise test bilateral	0.048	0.911
Muscle pain ACRT [5] (no. [6] of repetitions)	−0.252 *	0.585
Muscle fatigue ACRT [5] (no. [6] of repetitions)	−0.131	0.779

[1] BMI—Body Mass Index; [2] AHGS—Average Hand Grip Strength; [3] ACC—Average Calf Circumference; [4] CRST—Calf Raise Senior Test; [5] CRT—Calf Raise Test; [6] no.—number. * Spearman coefficient of correlation.

When we tested the correlation with The Pearson and Spearman coefficients of correlation, the same not-significant statistical relationship between average dMVIC and the other factors was found (Table 3).

4. Discussion

Based on previous studies, we hypothesised that a sitting posture could negatively influence foot and ankle muscle strength.

One day of inactivity was associated with an unhealthy potential on human health [28], and sitting showed secondary negative effects even in the active population [29].

In our study, both routinely active and routinely sedentary participants showed a significant statistically decrement in average peak ankle torque when subjected to six hours of prolonged sitting. In our group, foot and ankle muscle strength suffered a reduction over time even when participants were subjected to six hours of low to moderate physical activity.

Chronic unloading of negative effects on the Achilles' tendon was demonstrated, but when resistive exercises were added, some preventive effects were observed [34].

Considering the results demonstrated by Reeves et al. [34], we could estimate that when some type of exercise is associated, preventive effects of inactivity might be installed.

In our study, we demonstrated that all eight participants, when subjected to low to moderate physical activity, showed higher values for average peak ankle torque when compared to the values obtained when subjected to sedentary behaviour.

In the case of traumatic events, immobilisation effects have been reported. A decrease in ankle plantar flexor muscle strength has been observed after one week of immobilisation, but no significant differences were seen after two days of ankle immobilisation. The accumulated effects of immobilisation in time could explain the differences [33].

In our study, we evaluated the acute effects of six hours of inactivity on the plantar flexors' muscles through the measurement of ankle torque in nontraumatic events. There were significant differences between dMVIC after two hours compared with dMVIC after six hours ($p = 0.019$). We should further consider that the same study could be replicated related to traumatic events.

In our study, only after six hours of prolonged sitting a significant decrement in average peak torque was observed, with no significant differences between measurements at two hours and at four hours. We can state that in our group of participants placed under static behaviour, ankle torque decreased after the accumulated effects of prolonged sitting.

In patients suffering from diabetes, some electrophysiological reports analysed the soleus muscle activity in different sedentary postures, comparing chair-sitting with squat-like sitting [32].

In our group of participants, when sitting activity (static behaviour) was compared with a low to moderate physical activity (active behaviour), we found that even in healthy individuals', inactivity has negative potential on foot and ankle muscles strength.

Optimisation of the effects of muscle activity for promoting health in the general population and reducing sedentary behaviour strategies, daily contraction duration of skeletal muscle and the role of contractile duration were studied [7].

Our study reports the effects on ankle torque when individuals were placed in a short-time sedentary behaviour. Due to the insignificant reduction in torque at four hours but the significant decrement in torque after six hours, new considerations should be evaluated for proper preventive strategies to reduce the negative effects of prolonged sitting on foot and ankle muscle strength.

Based on our findings on the acute effects of six hours of sedentary behaviour on ankle torque, we might consider that while individuals adopt a prolonged sitting position, interposing activity-based breaks after at least four hours of inactivity might positively influence lower limb muscle performance. We only found a significant statistically decrement in ankle torque after six hours of inactivity, but no significant statistically decrement was found after two hours and four hours. These findings could help in establishing more rigorous prevention strategies for reducing sedentary behaviour effects of prolonged sitting in individuals. Such prevention strategies could address modifications of break time and break frequencies, time of work in sitting postures and routine behaviour modifications, as other previous studies showed [59].

In sports medicine and rehabilitation medicine, foot and ankle muscle strength assessments are essential, and one indicator of muscle performance tested in clinical practice is measuring ankle torque by assessing MVIC [60].

As no agreement has been stated on the most appropriate method for measuring the strength of the foot's intrinsic muscles [38], our study analysed peak ankle torque by measuring MVIC using a reliable [41] and reproducible [42] custom-made electronic dynamometer.

As per our knowledge, no particular study has assessed the impact of sedentary behaviour on ankle torque using a custom-made electronic dynamometer; therefore, describing the measurement system in detail as an innovative way to measure muscle strength in relation to inactivity was of great importance.

The hand grip strength cut-off values and CC have been stated in relation to muscle strength reduction in sarcopenia [50,53], and some correlations with lower limb muscle strength have been reported [51].

We found no significant statistically relationship between average dMVIC and the average values of HGS and CC, probably due to the small sample (8 participants).

The number of repetitions during the Calf Raise Senior Test (CRST) [54,55] has previously been used to assess plantar flexor muscle strength.

We applied CRST to our group of participants, and muscle pain/muscle fatigue appearance and the onset moment of both fatigue and pain were registered. We found no significant statistical relationship between average dMVIC and the average values of CRST fatigue and pain during CRST.

The Calf Raise Test (CRT) for evaluating calf muscle properties is a well-known clinical method [56], and based on a systematic review, the standards have been reported.

When we tested CRT in our group, muscle pain and muscle fatigue appeared, and the onset moment of both fatigue and pain were registered. We found no significant statistical relationship between average dMVIC and the average values of CRT, fatigue and pain during CRT.

The chair raise test, another commonly used method for assessing lower limb muscle parameters [57], was performed on our group of participants, and the total number of repetitions of chair raises in one minute was registered, with no significant statistical relationship between average dMVIC and the average values of the number of repetitions during the chair raise test.

Although a massive increment in sedentary-spent time was reported [16], with increased exposure to risks in all demographics and age groups [17], no particular study has analysed the impact of short-time sedentary time on ankle torque.

We found no significant statistical relationship between average dMVIC and the other factors, such as age, BMI, foot length and average no. of daily steps.

We analysed the impact of the type of daily activity (defined by the average number of steps, which differentiates the two groups of routinely active and routinely sedentary participants), but we did not find any significant statistical correlation ($r = -0.313$, $p = 0.450$) association ($p = 0.882$) with dMVIC.

Despite sitting being associated with physical inactivity and further health risks, the amount of sitting time linked with risks for human health has not yet been defined [36,37].

Understanding the acute effects of prolonged sitting on ankle torque could better frame the long-term effects of sedentary behaviour on both routinely active and routinely sedentary individuals.

Correlations between physical inactivity and diseases need a better understanding.

In this study, we took into consideration only the measurements at two hours from the initiation of the behaviour, but not measurements at the baseline. The authors think that they ensured that after maintaining two hours of static/active behaviour, all participants had the same level of physical activity before the initiation of measurements. However, a better approach can be considered. Ideally, the study should have implemented a baseline measure in the protocol with a levelled physical activity for each participant. We considered our study limitations to have not established a levelled baseline of physical activity for the participants before being subjected to the measurement in both types of behaviour. To consider the baseline measurements when reporting the impact of the testing moments and the impact of two types of behaviour on ankle torque would have been desirable.

We took into consideration only the measurements at two hours from the initiation of the behaviour. This further ensured that after maintaining two hours of static/active behaviour, all participants had the same level state of physical activity before the measurements.

This particular limitation is also due to the inconsistency of the participant's data recovered from their wearable devices (smartwatches). We could only recover an average of daily steps from the participant's last month of activity. Unfortunately, the data extracted from such devices does not represent the exact type of undertaken activity, with physical activity nor physical fitness being identifiable from the recovered data. To better identify the exact type of activity through the data derived from smartwatches, a more systematic control should be considered and eventually correlated with participants' reports of activity questionnaires/scales [61].

Another limitation of our study is due to the small sample. Because of that, the comparison between samples with eight data (Table 2) was not found to be statistically significantly different, but the same data, when compared with multivariate techniques, were statistically significant.

Further studies should implement the baseline measurement in the protocol when a levelled physical activity before the measurements are ensured and identify the exact type of physical activity through modern technology or by using validated questionnaires.

5. Conclusions

The more time participants maintained either short-term static or short-term active behaviour, the lower the average peak ankle torque resulted in both situations. Both routinely active and routinely sedentary participants showed a decrement of force in time when maintaining both types of behaviours, with the sitting position being associated with a lower value of average peak ankle torque during maximal voluntary isometric contraction.

Future studies should target the establishment of a threshold for the time spent in a sitting position, sedentary behaviour, in relation to foot muscle strength and establish whether breaking the routine during a specific activity might positively change the muscle force results.

Our force measurement results could complete ergonomic improvements for the achievement of healthy foot status in individuals spending prolonged time in a sitting position and especially when sitting while working.

Future studies should consider repeating the experiment in other types of groups of participants and possibly in groups affected by different conditions.

Author Contributions: Conceptualisation, I.I.D. and F.G.P.; methodology, T.P. and F.A.; software, T.P.; validation, S.B. and F.A.; formal analysis, C.I.B. and T.P.; investigation, I.I.D.; resources, E.-A.P.; data curation, T.P. and F.G.P.; writing—original draft preparation, I.I.D.; writing—review and editing, F.G.P.; visualisation, I.I.D., F.G.P., T.P. and F.A.; supervision, M.I., F.L.B. and N.D.R.; project administration, I.I.D. All authors have read and agreed to the published version of the manuscript.

Funding: This research received no external funding.

Institutional Review Board Statement: The study was conducted in accordance with the Declaration of Helsinki, and approved by Ethics Committee of University of Medicine and Pharmacy "Victor Babes" Timisoara, released and registered under Nr. 50/21.09-14.10.2020.

Informed Consent Statement: Informed consent was obtained from all subjects involved in the study. Written informed consent has been obtained from the patient(s) to publish this paper.

Acknowledgments: We thank all participants that voluntarily enrolled in the study.

Conflicts of Interest: The authors declare no conflict of interest.

References

1. Caspersen, C.J.; Powell, K.E.; Christenson, G.M. Physical activity, exercise, and physical fitness: Definitions and distinctions for health-related research. *Public Health Rep.* **1985**, *100*, 126–131. [PubMed]
2. Physical Inactivity. Available online: https://www.who.int/data/gho/indicator-metadata-registry/imr-details/3416 (accessed on 4 March 2022).
3. Adult Physical Inactivity Prevalence Maps by Race/Ethnicity. Available online: https://www.cdc.gov/physicalactivity/data/inactivity-prevalence-maps/index.html (accessed on 4 March 2022).
4. Tudor-Locke, C.; Craig, C.L.; Brown, W.J.; Clemes, S.A.; De Cocker, K.; Giles-Corti, B.; Hatano, Y.; Inoue, S.; Matsudo, S.M.; Mutrie, N.; et al. How many steps/day are enough? For adults. *Int. J. Behav. Nutr. Phys. Act.* **2011**, *8*, 79. [CrossRef] [PubMed]
5. Tudor-Locke, C.; Hatano, Y.; Pangrazi, R.P.; Kang, M. Revisiting "how many steps are enough?". *Med. Sci. Sports Exerc.* **2008**, *40*, 537–543. [CrossRef]
6. Nayor, M.; Chernofsky, A.; Spartano, N.L.; Tanguay, M.; Blodgett, J.B.; Murthy, V.L.; Malhotra, R.; Houstis, N.E.; Velagaleti, R.S.; Murabito, J.M.; et al. Physical activity and fitness in the community: The Framingham Heart Study. *Eur. Heart J.* **2021**, *42*, 4565–4575. [CrossRef] [PubMed]

7. Bull, F.C.; Al-Ansari, S.S.; Biddle, S.; Borodulin, K.; Buman, M.P.; Cardon, G.; Carty, C.; Chaput, J.P.; Chastin, S.; Chou, R.; et al. World Health Organization 2020 guidelines on physical activity and sedentary behaviour. *Br. J. Sports Med.* **2020**, *54*, 1451–1462. [CrossRef] [PubMed]
8. World Health Organization. *Global Action Plan on Physical Activity 2018–2030: More Active People for a Healthier World*; World Health Organization: Geneva, Switzerland, 2018. Available online: https://apps.who.int/iris/handle/10665/272722 (accessed on 6 March 2022).
9. Van der Velde, J.H.P.M.; Koster, A.; Van der Berg, J.D.; Sep, S.J.S.; Van der Kallen, C.J.H.; Dagnelie, P.C.; Schram, M.T.; Henry, R.M.A.; Eussen, S.J.P.M.; Van Dongen, M.C.J.M.; et al. Sedentary Behavior, Physi-cal Activity, and Fitness-The Maastricht Study. *Med. Sci. Sports Exerc.* **2017**, *49*, 1583–1591. [CrossRef]
10. Tucker, J.M.; Welk, G.J.; Beyler, N.K. Physical activity in U.S.: Adults' compliance with the physical activity guidelines for Americans. *Am. J. Prev. Med.* **2011**, *40*, 454–461. [CrossRef]
11. Owen, N.; Healy, G.N.; Matthews, C.E.; Dunstan, D.W. Too much sitting: The population health science of sedentary behavior. *Exerc. Sport Sci. Rev.* **2010**, *38*, 105–113. [CrossRef]
12. Lee, I.M.; Shiroma, E.J.; Lobelo, F.; Puska, P.; Blair, S.N.; Katzmarzyk, P.T. Lancet Physical Activity Series Working Group. Effect of physical inactivity on major non-communicable diseases worldwide: An analysis of burden of disease and life expectancy. *Lancet* **2012**, *380*, 219–229. [CrossRef]
13. Sedentary Behaviour Research Network. Letter to the editor: Standardized use of the terms "sedentary" and "sedentary behaviours". *Appl. Physiol. Nutr. Metab.* **2012**, *37*, 540–542. [CrossRef]
14. Guthold, R.; Stevens, G.A.; Riley, L.M.; Bull, F.C. Worldwide trends in insufficient physical activity from 2001 to 2016: A pooled analysis of 358 population-based surveys with 1·9 million participants. *Lancet Glob. Health* **2018**, *6*, e1077–e1086. [CrossRef]
15. Loprinzi, P.D.; Herod, S.M.; Cardinal, B.J.; Noakes, T.D. Physical activity and the brain: A review of this dynamic, bi-directional relationship. *Brain Res.* **2013**, *20*, 95–104. [CrossRef] [PubMed]
16. Schuna, J.M., Jr.; Johnson, W.D.; Tudor-Locke, C. Adult self-reported and objectively monitored physical activity and sedentary behavior: NHANES 2005-2006. *Int. J. Behav. Nutr. Phys. Act.* **2013**, *10*, 126. [CrossRef] [PubMed]
17. Hamilton, M.T.; Healy, G.N.; Dunstan, D.W.; Zderic, T.W.; Owen, N. Too Little Exercise and Too Much Sitting: Inactivity Physiology and the Need for New Recommendations on Sedentary Behavior. *Curr. Cardiovasc. Risk Rep.* **2008**, *2*, 292–298. [CrossRef] [PubMed]
18. Healy, G.N.; Clark, B.K.; Winkler, E.A.; Gardiner, P.A.; Brown, W.J.; Matthews, C.E. Measurement of adults' sedentary time in population-based studies. *Am. J. Prev. Med.* **2011**, *41*, 216–227. [CrossRef]
19. Wilmot, E.G.; Edwardson, C.L.; Achana, F.A.; Davies, M.J.; Gorely, T.; Gray, L.J.; Khunti, K.; Yates, T.; Biddle, S.J. Sedentary time in adults and the association with diabetes, cardiovascular disease and death: Systematic review and meta-analysis. *Diabetologia* **2012**, *55*, 2895–2905. [CrossRef]
20. Hamilton, M.T.; Hamilton, D.G.; Zderic, T.W. Sedentary behavior as a mediator of type 2 diabetes. *Med. Sport Sci.* **2014**, *60*, 11–26.
21. Brocklebank, L.A.; Falconer, C.L.; Page, A.S.; Perry, R.; Cooper, A.R. Accelerometer-measured sedentary time and cardiometabolic biomarkers: A systematic review. *Prev. Med.* **2015**, *76*, 92–102. [CrossRef]
22. Saunders, T.J.; Larouche, R.; Colley, R.C.; Tremblay, M.S. Acute sedentary behaviour and markers of cardiometabolic risk: A systematic review of intervention studies. *J. Nutr. Metab.* **2012**, *2012*, 712435. [CrossRef]
23. Howard, B.J.; Fraser, S.F.; Sethi, P.; Cerin, E.; Hamilton, M.T.; Owen, N.; Dunstan, D.W.; Kingwell, B.A. Impact on hemostatic parameters of interrupting sitting with intermittent activity. *Med. Sci. Sports Exerc.* **2013**, *45*, 1285–1291. [CrossRef]
24. Dunstan, D.W.; Kingwell, B.A.; Larsen, R.; Healy, G.N.; Cerin, E.; Hamilton, M.T.; Shaw, J.E.; Bertovic, D.A.; Zimmet, P.Z.; Salmon, J.; et al. Breaking up prolonged sitting reduces postprandial glucose and insulin responses. *Diabetes Care* **2012**, *35*, 976–983. [CrossRef]
25. Spittaels, H.; Van Cauwenberghe, E.; Verbestel, V.; De Meester, F.; Van Dyck, D.; Verloigne, M.; Haerens, L.; Deforche, B.; Cardon, G.; De Bourdeaudhuij, I. Objectively measured sedentary time and physical activity time across the lifespan: A cross-sectional study in four age groups. *Int. J. Behav. Nutr. Phys. Act.* **2012**, *9*, 149. [CrossRef]
26. Hamilton, M.T. The role of skeletal muscle contractile duration throughout the whole day: Reducing sedentary time and promoting universal physical activity in all people. *J. Physiol.* **2018**, *596*, 1331–1340. [CrossRef] [PubMed]
27. Raichlen, D.A.; Pontzer, H.; Zderic, T.W.; Harris, J.A.; Mabulla, A.Z.P.; Hamilton, M.T.; Wood, B.M. Sitting, squatting, and the evolutionary biology of human inactivity. *Proc. Natl. Acad. Sci. USA* **2020**, *117*, 7115–7121. [CrossRef]
28. Duvivier, B.M.; Schaper, N.C.; Hesselink, M.K.; van Kan, L.; Stienen, N.; Winkens, B.; Koster, A.; Savelberg, H.H. Breaking sitting with light activities vs structured exercise: A randomised crossover study demonstrating benefits for glycaemic control and insulin sensitivity in type 2 diabetes. *Diabetologia* **2017**, *60*, 490–498. [CrossRef] [PubMed]
29. Stephens, B.R.; Granados, K.; Zderic, T.W.; Hamilton, M.T.; Braun, B. Effects of 1 day of inac-tivity on insulin action in healthy men and women: Interaction with energy intake. *Metabolism* **2011**, *60*, 941–949. [CrossRef]
30. Berg, H.E.; Dudley, G.A.; Haggmark, T.; Ohlsen, H.; Tesch, P.A. Effects of lower limb unloading on skeletal muscle mass and function in humans. *J. Appl. Physiol.* **1991**, *70*, 1882–1885. [CrossRef] [PubMed]
31. Hather, B.M.; Adams, G.R.; Tesch, P.A.; Dudley, G.A. Skeletal muscle responses to lower limb suspension in humans. *J. Appl. Physiol.* **1992**, *72*, 1493–1498. [CrossRef]

32. Henshaw, F.R.; Bostan, L.E.; Worsley, P.R.; Bader, D.L. Evaluating the effects of sedentary behaviour on plantar skin health in people with diabetes. *J. Tissue Viability* **2020**, *9*, 277–283. [CrossRef]
33. Caplan, N.; Forbes, A.; Radha, S.; Stewart, S.; Ewen, A.; St Clair Gibson, A.; Kader, D. Effects of 1 week of unilateral ankle immobilization on plantar-flexor strength, balance, and walking speed: A pilot study in asymptomatic volunteers. *J. Sport Rehabil.* **2015**, *24*, 156–162. [CrossRef]
34. Reeves, N.D.; Maganaris, C.N.; Ferretti, G.; Narici, M.V. Influence of 90-day simulated microgravity on human tendon mechanical properties and the effect of resistive countermeasures. *J. Appl. Physiol.* **2005**, *98*, 2278–2286. [CrossRef] [PubMed]
35. Berg, H.E.; Larsson, L.; Tesch, P.A. Lower limb skeletal muscle function after 6 wk of bed rest. *J. Appl. Physiol.* **1997**, *82*, 182–188. [CrossRef] [PubMed]
36. Hamilton, M.T.; Hamilton, D.G.; Zderic, T.W. Exercise physiology versus inactivity physiology: An essential concept for understanding lipoprotein lipase regulation. *Exerc. Sport Sci. Rev.* **2004**, *32*, 161–166. [CrossRef]
37. Hamilton, M.T.; Hamilton, D.G.; Zderic, T.W. Role of low energy expenditure and sitting in obesity, metabolic syndrome, type 2 diabetes, and cardiovascular disease. *Diabetes* **2007**, *56*, 2655–2667. [CrossRef] [PubMed]
38. Soysa, A.; Hiller, C.; Refshauge, K.; Burns, J. Importance and challenges of measuring intrinsic foot muscle strength. *J. Foot Ankle Res.* **2012**, *5*, 29. [CrossRef]
39. Arinci Incel, N.; Genc, H.; Erdem, H.R.; Yorgancioglu, Z.R. Muscle imbalance in hallux valgus: An electromyographic study. *Am. J. Phys. Med. Rehabil.* **2003**, *82*, 345–349. [CrossRef]
40. Goldmann, J.-P.; Brüggemann, G.-P. The potential of human toe flexor muscles to produce force. *J. Anat.* **2012**, *221*, 187–194. [CrossRef]
41. Drăgoi, I.I.; Popescu, F.G.; Petrița, T.; Tatu, R.F.; Bondor, C.I.; Tatu, C.; Bowling, F.L.; Reeves, N.D.; Ionac, M. A Custom-Made Lower Limb Dynamometer for Assessing Ankle Joint Torque in Humans: Calibration and Measurement Procedures. *Sensors* **2022**, *22*, 135. [CrossRef]
42. Dragoi, I.I.; Popescu, F.G.; Petrita, T.; Alexa, F.; Tatu, R.F.; Bondor, C.I.; Tatu, C.; Bowling, F.L.; Reeves, N.D.; Ionac, M. A Custom-Made Electronic Dynamometer for Evaluation of Peak Ankle Torque after COVID-19. *Sensors* **2022**, *22*, 2073. [CrossRef] [PubMed]
43. Tudor-Locke, C.; Bassett, D.R., Jr. How many steps/day are enough? Preliminary pedometer indices for public health. *Sports Med.* **2004**, *34*, 1–8. [CrossRef]
44. Research Solutions (Alsager) LTD Overview—Find and Update Company Information—GOV.UK. Available online: https://find-and-update.company-information.service.gov.uk/company/07746832 (accessed on 16 October 2021).
45. PicoScope Model 2204A, Manufactured by Pico Technology, St Neots, UK. Available online: https://www.picotech.com/ (accessed on 16 October 2021).
46. PC Oscilloscope, Data Logger & RF Products | Pico Technology. Available online: https://www.picotech.com/ (accessed on 10 January 2022).
47. MATLAB, Version 9.9.0.1570001 (R2020b); Update 4. 2020. Available online: https://www.mathworks.com/products/matlab.html (accessed on 18 February 2022).
48. Microsoft Corporation. Microsoft Excel. Available online: https://www.microsoft.com/en-us/microsoft-365/excel (accessed on 26 October 2021).
49. Landin, D.; Thompson, M.; Reid, M. Knee and Ankle Joint Angles Influence the Plantarflexion Torque of the Gastrocnemius. *J. Clin. Med. Res.* **2015**, *7*, 602–606. [CrossRef] [PubMed]
50. Cruz-Jentoft, A.J.; Bahat, G.; Bauer, J.; Boirie, Y.; Bruyère, O.; Cederholm, T.; Cooper, C.; Landi, F.; Rolland, Y.; Sayer, A.A.; et al. Writing Group for the European Working Group on Sarcopenia in Older People 2 (EWGSOP2), and the Extended Group for EWGSOP2. Sarcopenia: Revised European consensus on definition and diagnosis. *Age Ageing* **2019**, *48*, 16–31. [CrossRef] [PubMed]
51. Bohannon, R.W.; Magasi, S.R.; Bubela, D.J.; Wang, Y.-C.; Gershon, R.C. Grip and knee extension muscle strength reflect a common construct among adults. *Muscle Nerve* **2012**, *46*, 555–558. [CrossRef] [PubMed]
52. Hand Grip Dynamometer MAP-KERN & SOHN GmbH (kern-sohn.com). Available online: https://www.kern-sohn.com/shop/en/medical-scales/hand-grip-dynamometers/MAP/ (accessed on 10 February 2022).
53. Kim, S.; Kim, M.; Lee, Y.; Kim, B.; Yoon, T.Y.; Won, C.W. Calf Circumference as a Simple Screening Marker for Diagnosing Sarcopenia in Older Korean Adults: The Korean Frailty and Aging Cohort Study (KFACS). *J. Korean Med. Sci.* **2018**, *33*, e151. [CrossRef] [PubMed]
54. Andre, H.I.; Carnide, F.; Borja, E.; Ramalho, F.; Santos-Rocha, R.; Veloso, A.P. Calf-raise senior: A new test for assessment of plantar flexor muscle strength in older adults: Protocol, validity, and reliability. *Clin. Interv. Aging* **2016**, *11*, 1661–1674. [CrossRef]
55. Andre, H.I.; Moniz-Pereira, V.; Ramalho, F.; Santos-Rocha, R.; Veloso, A.; Carnide, F. Respon-siveness of the Calf-Raise Senior test in community-dwelling older adults undergoing an exercise intervention program. *PLoS ONE* **2020**, *15*, e0231556. [CrossRef]
56. Hébert-Losier, K.; Newsham-West, R.J.; Schneiders, A.G.; Sullivan, S.J. Raising the standards of the calf-raise test: A systematic review. *J. Sci. Med. Sport* **2009**, *12*, 594–602. [CrossRef]
57. Johansson, J.; Strand, B.H.; Morseth, B.; Hopstock, L.A.; Grimsgaard, S. Differences in sarcopenia prevalence between upper-body and lower-body based EWGSOP2 muscle strength criteria: The Tromsø study 2015–2016. *BMC Geriatr.* **2020**, *20*, 461. [CrossRef]
58. IBM Corp. *Released 2017. IBM SPSS Statistics for Windows, Version 25.0*; IBM Corp.: Armonk, NY, USA, 2017.

59. Ding, Y.; Cao, Y.; Duffy, V.G.; Zhang, X. It is Time to Have Rest: How do Break Types Affect Muscular Activity and Perceived Discomfort During Prolonged Sitting Work. *Saf. Health Work.* **2020**, *11*, 207–214. [CrossRef]
60. Hou, Z.C.; Miao, X.; Ao, Y.F.; Hu, Y.L.; Jiao, C.; Guo, Q.W.; Xie, X.; Zhao, F.; Pi, Y.B.; Li, N.; et al. Characteristics and predictors of muscle strength deficit in mechanical ankle instability. *BMC Musculoskelet. Disord.* **2020**, *21*, 730. [CrossRef]
61. Strath, S.J.; Kaminsky, L.A.; Ainsworth, B.E.; Ekelund, U.; Freedson, P.S.; Gary, R.A.; Richardson, C.R.; Smith, D.T.; Swartz, A.M. American Heart Association Physical Activity Committee of the Council on Lifestyle and Cardiometabolic Health and Cardiovascular, Exercise, Cardiac Rehabilitation and Prevention Committee of the Council on Clinical Cardiology, and Council. Guide to the assessment of physical activity: Clinical and research applications: A scientific statement from the American Heart Association. *Circulation* **2013**, *128*, 2259–2279. [PubMed]

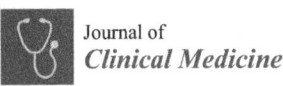

Article

Cardiopulmonary Exercise Testing and Cardiac Biomarker Measurements in Young Football Players: A Pilot Study

Alexandru-Dan Costache [1,2,†], Mihai Roca [1,2,*], Cezar Honceriu [3,†], Irina-Iuliana Costache [1,4,†], Maria-Magdalena Leon-Constantin [1,2], Ovidiu Mitu [1,4,†], Radu-Ștefan Miftode [1,4,†], Alexandra Maștaleru [1,2,†], Dan Iliescu-Halițchi [1,5], Codruța-Olimpiada Halițchi-Iliescu [6,7], Adriana Ion [1,4], Ștefania-Teodora Duca [1,4], Delia-Melania Popa [1], Beatrice Abălasei [3], Veronica Mocanu [8] and Florin Mitu [1,2]

1 Department of Internal Medicine I, Faculty of Medicine, University of Medicine and Pharmacy "Grigore T. Popa", 700115 Iasi, Romania; adcostache@yahoo.com (A.-D.C.); irina.costache@umfiasi.ro (I.-I.C.); leon_mariamagdalena@yahoo.com (M.-M.L.-C.); mituovidiu@yahoo.co.uk (O.M.); radu.miftode@yahoo.com (R.-Ș.M.); alexandra.mastaleru@gmail.com (A.M.); iliescud@gmail.com (D.I.-H.); adriana.ion@hotmail.com (A.I.); stefaniateodoraduca@gmail.com (Ș.-T.D.); deliamelaniapopa@gmail.com (D.-M.P.); mitu.florin@yahoo.com (F.M.)
2 Department of Cardiovascular Rehabilitation, Clinical Rehabilitation Hospital, 700661 Iasi, Romania
3 Faculty of Physical Education and Sports, "Alexandru Ioan Cuza" University, 700115 Iasi, Romania; chonceri@yahoo.fr (C.H.); beatrice.abalasei@uaic.ro (B.A.)
4 Department of Cardiology, "St. Spiridon" Emergency County Hospital, 700111 Iasi, Romania
5 Department of Cardiology, Arcadia Hospital, 700620 Iasi, Romania
6 Department of Mother and Child Medicine-Pediatrics, University of Medicine and Pharmacy "Grigore T. Popa", 700115 Iasi, Romania; codrutzache@yahoo.co.uk
7 Department of Pediatrics, Arcadia Hospital, 700620 Iasi, Romania
8 Department of Morphofunctional Sciences II, Faculty of Medicine, University of Medicine and Pharmacy "Grigore T. Popa", 700115 Iasi, Romania; veronica.mocanu@gmail.com
* Correspondence: roca2m@yahoo.com; Tel.: +40-721661446
† These authors contributed equally to this work.

Abstract: Constant and intense physical activity causes physiological adaptive changes in the human body, but it can also become a trigger for adverse events, such as sudden cardiac arrest or sudden cardiac death. Our main objective was to assess the use of combined cardiopulmonary exercise testing (CPET) and cardiac biomarker determinants in young professional athletes. We conducted a study which involved the full examination of 19 football players, all male, aged between 18 and 20 years old. They underwent standard clinical and paraclinical evaluation, a 12-lead electrocardiogram (ECG), and transthoracic echocardiography (TTE). Afterwards, a tailored CPET was performed and peripheral venous blood samples were taken before and 3 h after the test in order to determine five biomarker levels at rest and post-effort. The measured biomarkers were cardiac troponin I (cTnI), myoglobin (Myo), the MB isoenzyme of creatine-kinase (CK-MB), the N-terminal prohormone of brain natriuretic peptide (NT-proBNP) and D-dimers. While cTnI and NT-proBNP levels were undetectable both at rest and post-effort in all subjects, the variations in Myo, CK-MB and D-dimers showed significant correlations with CPET parameters. This highlights the potential use of combined CPET and biomarker determinants to evaluate professional athletes, and encourages further research on larger study groups.

Keywords: athletes; cardiopulmonary exercise testing; cardiac biomarkers

1. Introduction

Regular physical activity has many beneficial effects with regard to the cardiovascular system: it induces a physiological remodeling of the heart and results in molecular and cellular adaptive changes, which themselves have a cardioprotective effect. The long-term and moderate practice of sports, especially aerobic–isotonic ones, are even encouraged in those with chronic cardiac diseases [1]. Even in the older population, regular physical activity has been shown to slow degenerative cardiac changes and significantly improve quality of life [2].

Concerning young athletes, there are both morphological and functional adaptations of the heart in relation to sustained and intense physical activity. Morphologically, the myocardium suffers a process of hypertrophy and the chambers become dilated, as to adapt to the increased hemodynamic stress. The main difference between these physiological adaptative changes and the pathological ones, which are encountered in chronic cardiac diseases, lies in the fact that hemodynamic stress is intermittent in physical activity, whereas in chronic cardiac disease it is continuous. These structural modifications, especially the enlargement of the chambers, together with the increased vagal tonus, are the ones that, in turn, lead to electrophysiological modifications [3].

Most of the electrophysiological changes, in the context of constant physical activity, which have an electrocardiographic (ECG) expression, can be interpreted as within the normal limits without warranting further investigation. However, they are not to be confused with pathological ECG patterns, which have an underlying cardiac pathology and which can act as triggers for adverse events, such as sudden cardiac death [4,5] (see Table 1).

Table 1. Electrocardiographic patterns in athletes and their interpretation (RBBB—right bundle branch block; AV—atrio-ventricular; PCV—premature ventricular contraction) (adapted from Sharma et al. [5]).

ECG Patterns in Athletes			References
Normal	*Borderline*	*Abnormal*	
<ul><li>Increased QRS voltage</li><li>Incomplete RBBB</li><li>Early repolarization</li><li>Black athlete repolarization variant</li><li>Juvenile T wave pattern</li><li>Sinus bradycardia</li><li>Sinus arrhythmia</li><li>Ectopic atrial rhythm</li><li>Junctional escape rhythm</li><li>1st-degree atrioventricular block</li><li>Mobitz Type I 2nd-degree atrioventricular block</li></ul>	<ul><li>Left axis deviation</li><li>Left atrial enlargement</li><li>Right axis deviation</li><li>Right atrial enlargement</li><li>Complete RBBB</li></ul>	<ul><li>T wave inversion</li><li>ST-segment depression</li><li>Pathologic Q waves</li><li>Complete left bundle branch block</li><li>Profound nonspecific intra-ventricular conduction delay</li><li>Epsilon wave</li><li>Ventricular pre-excitation</li><li>Prolonged QT interval</li><li>Brugada Type 1 pattern</li><li>Profound sinus bradycardia</li><li>Profound 1st-degree AV block</li><li>Mobitz Type II 2nd-degree AV block</li><li>3rd-degree AV block</li><li>Atrial tachyarrhythmias</li><li>PVC</li><li>Ventricular arrhythmias</li></ul>	[5]

The 2020 European Society of Cardiology (ESC) guidelines on sports cardiology and exercise in patients with cardiovascular disease are a milestone in both the field of cardiology and sports medicine. As the first edition, they introduce numerous up-to-date information and recommendations for the practice of physical exercise in both healthy individuals and persons with known cardiovascular pathologies. Among the potential adverse cardiovascular events, the two most dangerous are sudden cardiac arrest (SCA) and sudden cardiac death (SCD). As tragic as they may be, especially if occurring in young healthy individuals, SCA and SCD are not reported in all countries; therefore, their incidences cannot be accurately estimated. However, according to most recent statistics, SCA is diagnosed in 1 out of 80,000 high-school-aged athletes and in 1 out of 50,000 college-aged athletes. Based on gender, ethnicity, and type of sports practiced, the most at-risk group is represented by male, black, basketball athletes in the United States, or football athletes in Europe [6–11] (see Table 2).

Table 2. Exercise-related major adverse cardiovascular events (MACE) [6].

Exercise-Related MACE	References
• Sudden cardiac arrest (SCA) • Sudden cardiac death (SCD) • Acute coronary syndromes (ACS) • Transient ischemic attacks (TIA) • Cerebrovascular accidents (CVA) • Supraventricular tachyarrhythmias	[6]

The most important etiology of SCD in young athletes is congenital cardiac structural disorders; yet, a significant number of autopsies (44%) cannot identify a cause, these being the autopsy-negative sudden unexplained deaths (AN-SUD) [6,7,12–15].

The current guidelines recommend, for the routine screening for cardiovascular disease in young athletes, the patient's history, a physical examination, and a 12-lead standard ECG, which actually outweighs the first two. Although the cardiac ultrasound could offer significantly more information, especially regarding the congenital anomalies, a lack of evidence restricts its implementation in the standard screening protocols [6,16–22].

There are a few methods that allow the assessment of cardiorespiratory fitness (CRF) in youths which are currently used, such as the 20-m shuttle run test (20mSRT). It is a feasible, reliable, and easy to put in practice method of evaluation, and is currently being discussed to be included in the standardized evaluation protocols [23].

Given the wide spectrum of parameters evaluated (pulmonary, cardiovascular, muscular and oxidative) and the multitude of data and correlations it provides, the cardiopulmonary exercise testing (CPET) is an essential tool in current practice [24]. It is also useful in healthy individuals and in the athletic performance assessment, as maximal oxygen uptake (VO_2 max) is directly linked to the exercise capacity [25,26]. Of course, normal parameters vary, as elite aerobic athletes can reach VO_2 max values over 80 mL/kg/min, compared to untrained individuals who are in the 30–45 mL/kg/min range [27]. The test can be performed on a treadmill (mostly in the United States) or on the cycle ergometer (mostly in Europe). The cycle ergometer testing has a low associated cardiovascular risk in evaluating young healthy athletes [28,29] (see Table 3).

A particular role of CPET in evaluating athletes is to differentiate between their physiological left-ventricular hypertrophy (LVH) and hypertrophic cardiomyopathy (HCM) [30,31].

Table 3. CPET indications (adapted from Löllgen et al. [31]).

CPET Indications			References
Asymptomatic individuals	Patients	Follow-up assessment during training	
• Latent disease diagnosis • Risk factor identifications • Physical performance ability assessment • Guidance/monitorization of training	• Cardiac/respiratory disease diagnosis • Symptom evaluation	• Training regimen recommendations	[31]

Cardiac troponins (cTn) are regulatory components of the cardiac muscle contraction. Cardiac troponin I (cTnI) is of interest due to its phosphorylation sites, which regulate different contractile responses [32,33]. It has been shown that physiological left ventricular hypertrophy, which is specific to trained persons, causes a reversible increase in Ca^{2+}-dependent force production and in Ca^{2+}-sensitivity in left ventricular (LV) cardiomyocytes. Together with a reduction in cTnI phosphorylation, it is suggestive for an adaptive measure and for the preserved or even increased contractile function, despite the morphology changes [34]. In contrast, untrained persons who are subjected to a sudden physical effort do register increases in cTnI levels, although they are not pathological [35]. Additionally, of interest is the fact that peak levels of hs-cTn are registered between 3 and 4 h after peak physical stress [36].

Myoglobin is a biomarker produced by both the myocardial and skeletal muscle cells. Therefore, its levels rise in cardiac diseases (myocarditis, acute coronary syndromes) as well as muscular stress or strenuous physical effort. It can aid the differential diagnosis of cardiac or muscular damage, whether its levels rise independently or in conjunction with other cardiac biomarkers. Its use in establishing the diagnosis of acute coronary syndrome is low in the absence of other biomarkers' elevation (CK-MB, cTn); however, it is the one whose levels rise earliest in the serum [37–39].

The MB isoenzyme of creatine-kinase (CK-MB) is specific to the cardiac muscle. On its own it cannot predict the cardiovascular risk accurately, unless it is associated with the rise of cTn; thus, its use is still being debated. Its practical utility resides in situations where the estimated glomerular filtration rate (eGFR) is below 15 mL/min/m^2, or in recent-onset acute coronary syndromes [40,41].

The N-terminal prohormone of brain natriuretic peptide (NT-proBNP) levels do increase during intense physical exercise, especially in non-trained, amateur athletes. Yet, when not correlated with ECG changes, they are not significant for a cardiovascular pathology [35]. Its release in the blood is more associated with aging and with the effort-generated hypertensive stress on the ventricular and atrial walls [42–44]. Of course, it is essential in diagnosing potential ischemic changes in the myocardium, especially in conjunction with cTn, and with proven benefit in risk stratification in athletes [45–47].

While not being specific markers of myocardial cytolysis, D-dimers levels reflect intravascular fibrinolysis and show higher concentrations in patients with severe atherosclerosis or other causes of coronary stenosis [48]. They have more use in confirming or infirming venous thromboembolism, acute aortic dissection, cardioembolic stroke, or left atrium thrombosis in patients with atrial fibrillation [49]. Additionally, an independent rise in their levels can be specific in persons with implantable cardiac devices [50].

The aim of our study was to assess the relationship between effort-induced cardiac biomarker variations and CPET parameters, and their usefulness in the evaluation of young athletes.

2. Materials and Methods

2.1. Experimental Approach

We conducted a complete cardiovascular evaluation of professional football players, with an emphasis on cardiopulmonary exercise testing (CPET) and blood biomarkers (cTnI, myoglobin, CK-MB, NT-proBNP and D-dimers) in order to evaluate and assess the cardiovascular risk. The study was designed following the recommendations for clinical research contained in the Helsinki Declaration of the World Medical Association, and the protocol was approved by both the Ethics Committee of the Clinical Rehabilitation Hospital in Iași, Romania, approved on 24 March 2021, and the Ethics Research Committee of the "Grigore T. Popa" University of Medicine and Pharmacy in Iași, Romania, nr. 72, approved on 25 April 2021.

2.2. Participants and Protocol

We evaluated professional football players (n = 19). Football club trainers from the region of Moldova in the counties of Iași and Vaslui were informed of the ongoing study and were given our contact data. They themselves informed the registered football players aged between 18 and 20 years, and the first 30 to voluntarily contact us were automatically selected to be evaluated. In order for them to be included, they had to participate actively in regular training during the season of the last year, or at least the last months. Those who had missed part of the last months of training or playing due to injury, or who were in the recovery period after an injury of any sort, were excluded, as well as those with cardio-pulmonary pathological findings during the initial evaluation.

The participants were all male, aged between 18 and 20 years old (mean 18.47 ± 0.841), and fully informed about the procedures, research, and protocols used. They were asked to halt any strenuous training sessions or games a minimum of 24 h before the evaluation, and not to consume any foods or beverages other than water before the initial blood sampling, so as not to interfere with the blood sugar values. Afterwards, they could have a small snack or light meal at least an hour before the CPET. They were admitted through day hospitalization in August and September 2021. Upon admission, they filled out the informed consent forms regarding all the procedures and their inclusion in the study, and underwent rapid COVID-19 antigen testing, which, if negative, would allow them to further proceed with the investigations. They underwent a clinical and paraclinical evaluation with an emphasis on the cardiovascular system, followed by a 12-lead resting ECG, TTE, and CPET. Blood samples for the measurements of cardiac biomarkers values were taken at rest before the procedures and 3 h after finishing the CPET.

2.3. Initial Evaluation

After the initial blood samples were taken, a complete clinical evaluation was conducted with an emphasis on the cardiovascular system with its four major components (inspection, palpation, percussion and auscultation). The resting blood pressure (BP) and heart rate (HR) values were measured comparatively on the both upper limbs and in the orthostatism using a Rossmax X3 BT automatic blood pressure monitor with a brachial cuff. Height and weight were measured on a SECA digital measuring station.

2.4. Resting ECG

A standard 12-lead resting ECG was performed on a BTL-08 LC device, both in post-expiratory apnea and in deep post-inspiratory apnea, and every morphological change was analyzed to be considered as either normal for an athlete or pathological (see Table 1), and possibly contraindicate further procedures.

2.5. Cardiac Ultrasound

The standard transthoracic echocardiographic evaluation was performed on a Toshiba Aplio device, prior to the CPET, to assess the cardiac function and to exclude any possible contraindications, using the M-mode, pulse wave Doppler (PWD), continuous wave Doppler (CWD), and color Doppler methods, according to the European Society of Cardiology (ESC) and European Association of Cardiovascular Imaging (EACVI) protocols.

2.6. Cardiopulmonary Exercise Testing

Functional capacity was assessed by cardiopulmonary exercise testing (CPET) on the BTL CardioPoint software (version 2.32 manufactured by BTL Industries Ltd., Herfordshire, UK) and the BTL-compatible device. We used a progressive maximal symptom-limited CPET protocol on the cycle ergometer, specifically tailored for the athletes: they started on a workload of 15 Watts which was set to increase every 30 s with 12.5 Watts. The duration of the testing was between 10 and 12 min and the recovery period was 10 min.

The most important CPET parameters were: maximal work rate (absolute value, WR (Watt) and percentage of the predicted value, WR% (%)); oxygen uptake with maximal aerobic capacity (absolute value, VO_2 max (mL per min) and percentage of the predicted value, VO_2 max%); carbon dioxide output (VCO_2 (mL per min)); oxygen uptake at the anaerobic threshold (AT) (mL per min); peak value of the respiratory exchange ratio (RER) defined as the ratio between VCO_2 and VO_2; maximal heart rate (HR (bpm)); O_2 pulse as the ratio of VO_2 to heart rate, reflecting the amount of O_2 extracted per heartbeat; ventilatory efficiency expressing the rise in minute ventilation (VE) relative to VCO_2 (VE/VCO_2 slope); and heart rate reserve (difference between maximal HR and resting HR, HRR (bpm)). VO_2, VCO_2, and AT were also expressed as values normalized by body weight (mL per min per km).

Metabolic efficiency was assessed by measuring the increase in VO_2 over the rate of increase in work rate ($\Delta VO_2/\Delta WR$). The slope of this relationship expresses the ability of the muscle to extract O_2 during exercise.

Blood pressure was monitored every 2 min using the auscultatory method, while a real-time 12-lead ECG was recorded.

To clinically determine the intensity of the exercise, a subjective rating of the intensity of perceived fatigue was determined by a 6 to 20 Borg scale of perceived exertion.

The test was halted, according to current recommendations, when the subject requested it, upon symptoms or fatigue occurrence, when the blood pressure (BP) measurement exceeded 220 mmHg for the systolic value, or 120 mmHg for the diastolic value, or when suggestive ischemic ECG patterns appeared.

2.7. Cardiac Biomarker Determination

Peripheral venous blood was collected at rest for the basic laboratory parameters and also to determine the mentioned biomarker values at rest. Three hours after finalizing the CPET, another sample was taken to measure the variations of the biomarker values after the stress test, so as to allow them time to appear and reach certain levels in the blood. All blood sampling was taken from the antecubital veins and in kept dedicated vacutainers (with sodium citrate for D-dimers and lithium heparin for CK-MB, Myo, cTnI, and NT-proBNP). Their measurements were performed immediately after, using whole blood on the FIA 8000 device from Getein Biotechnology Co. Ltd. on its dedicated panels: triple tests for CK-MB, myoglobin, and cTnI (CK-MB: measuring range 2.5–80 ng/mL, lower detection limit $\leq$ 2.5 ng/mL, recovery 96%; myoglobin: measuring range 30–1000 ng/mL, lower detection limit $\leq$ 30 ng/mL, recovery 95%; cTnI: measuring range 0.5–50 ng/mL, lower detection limit $\leq$ 0.5 ng/mL, recovery rate 95%, measuring time 15 min), double tests for cTnI and NT-proBNP (cTnI: measuring range 0.5-50 ng/mL, lower detection limit $\leq$ 0.5 ng/mL, recovery rate 95%; NT-proBNP: measuring range 10–12,000 pg/mL, lower detection limit $\leq$ 100 ng/mL, recovery 99%, measuring time 18 min) and a single test for D-dimers (D-dimers: measuring range 0.1–10 mg/L, lower detection limit $\leq$ 0.1 mg/L, recovery rate 99%, measuring time 7 min) were completed. All the assays were stored, according to manufacturer specifications, at a temperature between 4 and 30 degrees Celsius and used before the expiration date was reached and within 1 h since each foil was opened.

2.8. Data analysis and Statistics

Data analysis was performed using SPSS 20.0 (Statistical Package for the Social Sciences, Chicago, IL, USA). Data were presented as mean $\pm$ standard deviation (SD), or as median with an interquartile range for continuous variables. These variables were compared by the non-parametric Mann–Whitney U test, considering that their distribution did not satisfy the assumption of normality, due to the small number of subjects included in the study. For the same reason, correlations between continuous variables were assessed by calculating the Spearman correlation coefficients. A two-sided p-value < 0.05 was considered significant for all analyses.

3. Results

3.1. Anthropometric Data and Initial Clinical and Paraclinical Evaluation

During the clinical evaluation, no significant pathological findings were encountered. The resting systolic blood pressure (SBP), diastolic blood pressure (DBP), and heart rate (HR) were within the normal range and no significant BP differences were noticed between the upper limbs or in the orthostatic position. Using the measured height and weight values, the body mass index (BMI) was calculated using the formula weight/(height)^2.

Most of them had a normal BMI (18.55–24.99 kg/m^2), while four of them had a BMI of 25 kg/m^2 or above. Therefore, we measured the abdominal circumference and none of them had a value above 102 cm (see Table 4.).

Table 4. Anthropometric and baseline BP and HR values.

Parameter	Mean	Standard Deviation
Age (years)	18.47	0.84
SBP baseline (mmHg)	120.47	6.97
DBP baseline (mmHg)	75.74	6.35
HR baseline (bpm)	63.68	13.55
Height (m)	1.77	0.06
Weight (kg)	72.89	7.26
BMI (kg/m^2)	23.13	1.84

3.2. 12-Lead Resting ECG

All subjects were in sinus rhythm and 14 had sinus bradycardia (HR < 60 bpm), while the other 5 had normal baseline HR. Two athletes had a right-heart axis deviation, and one had a 90-degree axis. Four of them had normal morphology, while in fourteen a high QRS-complex voltage was encountered, three showed a complete RBBB (RSR' pattern in the V1 and V2 leads and a QRS duration >0.12 s), and three displayed an incomplete RBBB (RSR' pattern only in the V1 lead and a QRS duration <0.12 s). By analyzing these patterns, the increased QRS complex voltage, the incomplete RBBB and the sinus bradycardia were considered to be normal for an athlete, while the complete RBBB and the right-axis deviation were considered borderline changes (see Table 1). However, they were not considered to be a reason to contraindicate further investigations.

3.3. Transthoracic Cardiac Ultrasound

The TTE parameters were within the normal limits and no significant pathological encounters were made: two subjects had a mild tricuspid valve regurgitation, two had an anterior mitral valve prolapse, and two had a mild mitral valve regurgitation. However, these findings were considered benign and not a reason to contraindicate further investigations (see Table 5).

3.4. CPET

In 12 out of 19 subjects, the CPET had to be halted due to the recorded systolic BP values of 220 mmHg or higher, while in the remaining 7, the test was stopped due to muscle fatigue. No ECG ischemic patterns were identified, nor any symptoms such as angina were declared. Eleven of them did not reach the 85% heart rate threshold, yet only two had a peak VO$_2$ value below 85% of the predicted. The respiratory exchange ratio (RER) was, in all cases, over 1.00 and only in three cases below 1.0 (see Table 6).

3.5. Cardiac Biomarkers

cTnI and NT-proBNP levels were below the lower detection limit of the assays in the blood samples in all participants, both at rest and 3 h after the CPET, while seven of the athletes had values below the lower detection limit of the assays for all biomarkers. In four subjects, myoglobin levels increased after 3 h compared to the at-rest values, while in three subjects they decreased. In two participants, CK-MB levels increased post-CPET, while in one athlete they decreased. The D-dimer levels decreased after CPET in five subjects, while in three the values increased. For the statistical analysis, all participants were considered and for those with undetectable values, the lower detection limit value for each biomarker was assigned (see Table 7).

Table 5. TTE parameters.

Parameter	Mean	Standard Deviation
EDV (Teich, mL)	115.24	23.53
ESV (Teich, mL)	33.84	8.40
SV (Teich, mL)	81.50	19.42
EF (Teich, %)	70.42	5.99
FS (%)	40.19	4.85
SI (Teich, mL/m^2)	42.90	9.96
IVSTd (mm)	10.17	1.49
LVIDd (mm)	49.22	4.33
LVPWTd (mm)	10.56	1.49
IVSTs (mm)	13.63	1.90
LVIDs (mm)	43.27	60.55
LVPWTs (mm)	16.54	2.27
LV MASSd (ASE, g)	234.63	50.18
LV MASSd Index (ASE, g/m^2)	123.66	25.17
LV MASSs (ASE, g)	191.16	54.05
LV MASSs Index (ASE, g/m^2)	103.95	25.46
E Vel (cm/s)	76.96	13.63
A Vel (cm/s)	44.15	8.08
E/A	1.78	0.38
A/E	0.58	0.13
DcT (s)	0.25	0.05
MVArea PHT (cm^2)	4.51	6.45
PHT (s)	0.07	0.01
LVOT Diam (mm)	25.53	1.51
Ao Diam (mm)	30.44	2.30
LA Diam (mm)	27.88	3.82
LA/Ao	0.91	0.12

Abbreviations: EDV—end-diastolic volume; ESV—end-systolic volume; SV—stroke volume; EF—ejection fraction; FS—fractional shortening; SI—stroke-volume index; IVSTd—interventricular septum thickness at end-diastole; LVIDd—left ventricular internal dimension at end-diastole; LVPWTd—left ventricular posterior wall thickness at end-diastole; IVSTs—interventricular septum thickness at end-systole; LVIDs—left ventricular internal dimension at end-systole; LVPWTs—left ventricular posterior wall thickness at end-systole; LV MASSd—left ventricular mass at end-diastole; LV MASSd Index—left ventricular mass at end-diastole adjusted to body surface index; LV MASSs—left ventricular mass at end-systole; LV MASSs Index—left ventricular mass at end-systole adjusted to body surface index; E Vel—peak velocity of early diastolic mitral annular motion as determined by pulsed wave Doppler; A Vel—peak velocity of diastolic mitral annular motion as determined by pulsed wave Doppler; E/a—ratio of E to A; A/E—ratio of A to E; DcT—deceleration time MV area; PHT—mitral valve area at pressure half time; PHT—pressure half time; LVOT Diam—left ventricular outflow tract diameter; Ao Diam—aortic annulus diameter; LA Diam—left atrium diameter; LA/Ao—ratio of the left atrial dimension to the aortic annulus dimension.

Table 6. CPET parameters.

Parameter	Mean	Standard Deviation
VO_2 max (mL/min)	3565.58	599.96
VO_2 max body weight (mL/min/kg)	49.20	8.29
%VO_2 max	106.89	17.13
VO_2@AT (mL/min)	2558.84	703.16
VO_2@AT body weight (mL/min/kg)	35.43	9.97
RER	1.12	0.08
VE/VCO_2	23.54	3.37
$\Delta VO_2/\Delta WR$ (mL/min/Watt)	13.24	1.54
WR max (Watt)	249.68	25.36
%WR max	85.37	9.47
O_2_pulse (mL/beat)	21.28	3.55
%O_2_pulse	128.66	20.57
HR max (bpm)	170.89	11.28
%HR max	84.79	5.63
HR_rez (bpm)	107.21	13.75
SBP max (mmHg)	215.53	16.57
DBP max (mmHg)	83.42	4.42

Abbreviations: VO_2 max—maximum oxygen uptake; VO_2 max body weight—ratio of maximum oxygen uptake to body weight; %VO_2 max—percentage of maximum oxygen uptake from the predicted value; VO_2@AT—oxygen uptake at the anaerobic threshold; VO_2@AT body weight—ratio of oxygen uptake at the anaerobic threshold to body weight; RER—respiratory exchange ratio; VE/VCO_2—ventilatory equivalent for carbon dioxide; $\Delta VO_2/\Delta WR$—slope of the relation VO_2–power in W; WR max—maximum load; %WR max—percentage of maximum load from the predicted value; O_2_pulse—oxygen pulse; HR max—maximum heart rate; %HR max—percentage of maximum heart rate from the predicted value; HR_rez—heart rate reserve; SBP max—maximum systolic blood pressure; DBP max—maximum diastolic blood pressure.

Table 7. Biomarker variation analysis.

Parameter	Mean	Standard Deviation	Number of Subjects with Values above the Lower Detection Limit
Myoglobin baseline (ng/mL)	37.71	19.74	5
Myoglobin 3 h (ng/mL)	53.70	93.94	5
CK-MB baseline (ng/mL)	2.76	1.17	1
CK-MB 3 h (ng/mL)	2.86	1.40	3
D-dimer baseline (mg/L)	0.16	0.14	7
D-dimer 3 h (mg/L)	0.14	0.10	8

3.6. Interrelations between Cardiac Biomarkers and Functional Parameters

Statistically, in the Mann–Whitney nonparametric tests, CK-MB changes showed significant differences in the heart rate (HR) on the resting ECG ($p = 0.047$), the VO_2 max at the CPET ($p = 0.008$), and with the peak load (WR max) on the CPET ($p = 0.014$) between those with and those without changes in CK-MB levels (see Table 8 and Figure 1).

Table 8. Significant differences between the groups without changes (No) and with changes (Yes) in CK-MB values.

Parameter	CK-MB Change (No)	CK-MB Change (Yes)	p-Value
HR ECG (bpm)	54.50 (50.00–57.50)	67.00 (61.50–72.50)	0.047
VO$_2$ max (mL/min)	3391.50 (2908.75–3907.50)	4148.00 (4116.00–4463.50)	0.008
Watt max (Watt)	241.50 (223.00–260.00)	285.00 (285.00–285.00)	0.014
Number of subjects	16	3	

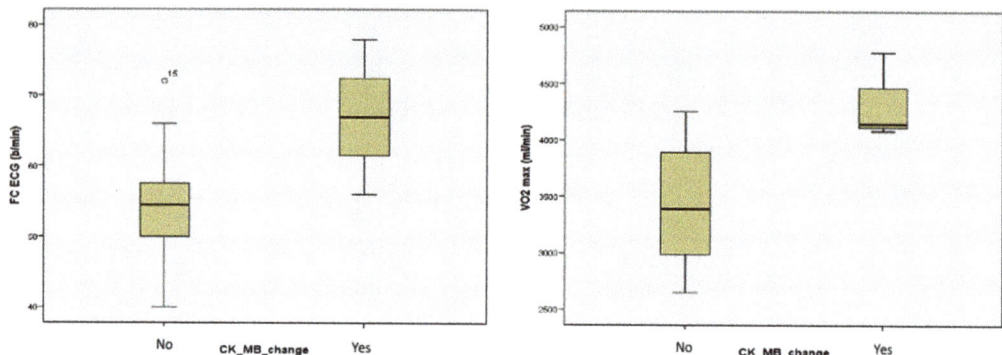

Figure 1. Significant differences between the groups without changes (No) and with changes (Yes) in CK-MB values on resting ECG heart rate (**left**) and on CPET VO$_2$ max (**right**), respectively.

D-dimers showed significant differences within the %WR max on the CPET ($p = 0.035$), between those with and those without changes in D-dimers levels (see Table 9 and Figure 2).

Table 9. Significant differences between the groups without changes (No) and with changes (Yes) in D-dimers values.

Parameter	D-Dimers Change (No)	D-Dimers Change (Yes)	p-Value
%Watt max	87.50 (85.00–93.25)	84.00 (79.50–85.50)	0.035
Number of subjects	10	9	

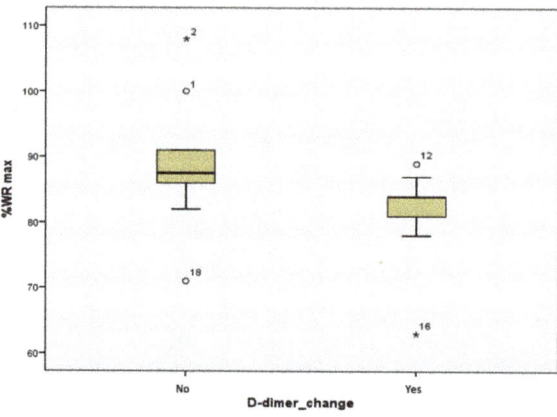

Figure 2. Significant differences between the groups without changes (No) and with changes (Yes) in D-dimers values on CPET %WR max.

Myoglobin showed significant differences between those with and those without changes in myoglobin levels for E/A and A/E ultrasound parameters ($p = 0.036$), VO$_2$ at the anaerobic threshold (VO$_2$ @ AT) on CPET ($p = 0.045$), and with VO$_2$ @ AT/body weight on CPET ($p = 0.017$). Additionally, significant differences were observed with % Watt max on CPET ($p = 0.045$), with % O$_2$ pulse on CPET ($p=0.028$) and with HR max ($p = 0.013$) and % HR max ($p = 0.017$) on CPET (see Table 10 and Figure 3).

Table 10. Significant differences between the groups without changes (No) and with changes (Yes) in myoglobin values.

Parameter	Myoglobin Change (No)	Myoglobin Change (Yes)	p-Value
E/A	1.90 (1.70–2.09)	1.57 (1.23–1.64)	0.036
A/E	0.53 (0.47–0.58)	0.640 (0.61–0.81)	0.036
VO$_2$ @ AT (mL/min)	2688.00 (2211.25–3401.25)	2215.00 (1995.00–2431.00)	0.045
VO$_2$ @ AT/body weight (mL/min/kg)	40.34 (31.91–46.16)	27.94 (23.47–35.15)	0.017
% WR max	87.00 (84.50–89.75)	82.00 (71.00-84.00)	0.045
% O$_2$ Pulse	136.57 (123.38–150.21)	114.11 (96.70–137.10)	0.028
HR max (bpm)	165.00 (161.25–167.75)	183.00 (175.00–190.00)	0.013
% HR max	81.50 (80.00–83.75)	91.00 (87.00–94.00)	0.017
Number of subjects	12	7	

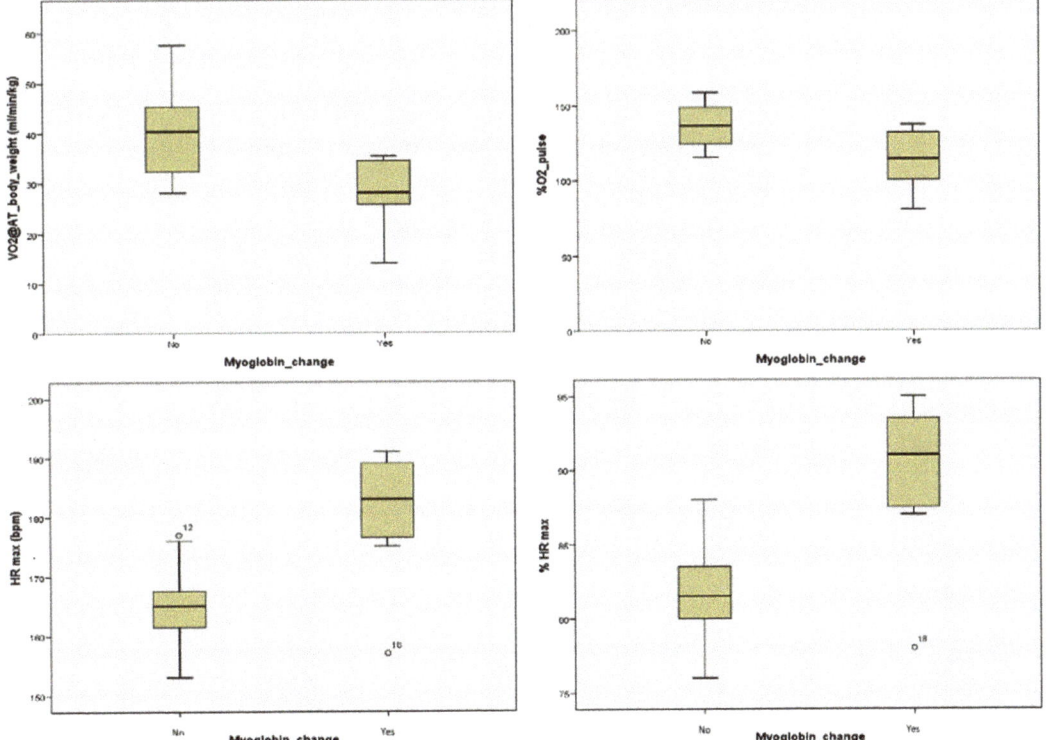

Figure 3. Significant differences between the groups without changes (No) and with changes (Yes) in myoglobin values.

4. Discussion

Laboratory explorations are gaining more and more ground and sports cardiology represents the new trend in medicine. Therefore, as confirmed by previous studies, their combination is an opportunity for future research [51].

The initial evaluation showed findings consistent with athletes with a normal BMI. In the few cases where BMI was over 25 kg/m^2, this was due to the higher muscle mass, as the abdominal circumference was normal. ECG interpretation also showed heart rate and morphology patterns which are considered normal in an athletic population as part of the effort adaptation process (sinus bradycardia, right bundle branch block). The cardiac ultrasound highlighted parameters of increased cardiovascular performance, such as a higher ejection fraction and a mild left ventricular hypertrophy, which, once again, is part of the adaptation to effort process in athletes.

In addition, cardiorespiratory functional evaluations are becoming more used in current practice and screening. As obesity and the sedentary lifestyle are becoming more prevalent, especially among the young population, cardiorespiratory functional evaluations are useful tools for assessing the fitness level. In recent studies, CRF has been proven to correlate negatively with parameters such as BMI and the sedentary lifestyle at younger ages [52].

A study published by Olekšák et al. involved the evaluation of CPET on young Slovenian footballers. They compared the CPET parameters on children and adolescents and concluded that some of them were physiologically higher in athletes and with growing age (VO$_2$ max, Watt max) [53].

The CPET parameters evaluated on the 19 subjects were comparable with those in other studied athlete cohorts. It is interesting to note that some of the registered values, such as a lower VO$_2$ max than predicted, were consistent with the tests which were halted for high BP values. This once again proves the utility of this particular evaluation and shows how physical performance CRF can be limited by an abrupt rise in BP.

Other investigations whose utility has been confirmed in recent studies include biomarker measurements. In a paper published by Mahanty et al., cTn, BNP and hypoxanthine were proven as means of assessing the cardiovascular impact of intense physical activity. Therefore, they are being considered to be implemented in the future as part of screening protocols [54].

A metanalysis published in 2015 concluded that cTnT, hs-cTnT, BNP, NT-proBNP, and D-dimers do suffer serum level changes when a person is performing a high-intensity physical effort, which may interfere with their interpretation in an emergency unit when an acute coronary syndrome, heart failure or pulmonary embolism can be suspected [55].

When investigating young football players, after a full-time football match, cTnI and NT-proBNP levels rose above the baseline and remained elevated even 24 h after the game, yet they never reached pathologically significant values. This rise, compared to our study can be attributed to the higher intensity and duration of the football match (90 min, on average) compared to a CPET [56]. Similarly, blood samples taken from participants in the 2016 Barcelona marathon showed an increase in NT-proBNP levels; however, the intensity of the physical stress and its duration were considerably higher than during a CPET [44].

Another study published in 2021 included individuals that participated in 2018 in the North Sea Race, a 91 km leisure sport mountain bike race. Prior to the race, they performed a CPET. Their cTnI levels were measured before, 3 h, and 24 h after both the race and CPET. The peak values were reached at the 3-h mark, though it should be once again mentioned that, in both cases, the duration and intensity of the physical exercise were higher than in the CPET which we conducted. However, a noticeable inter-individual variation was also observed [57].

There are several mechanisms incriminated for this pattern of variation in biomarker blood levels, such as microvascular ischemia, deficiencies in cardiac metabolism, a systemic inflammatory surge, or even an impaired renal function during intense exercise [58]. This particular dynamic of cTnI concentrations, with an early peak followed by a rapid normalization within hours (maximum 48–72 h), renders an active myocyte necrosis highly improbable, and rather suggests the above-mentioned secondary mechanisms. In our study, including highly trained athletes, we did not observe any variation of cTnI or NT-proBNP, compared to baseline. These somehow atypical kinetics can be explained by the rather short duration of the CPET, performed by apparently healthy, well-trained individuals, without the deleterious effects of prolonged and exhausting sports that can presumably represent important triggers for the release of cardiac biomarkers. This finding is consistent with the results of Marshall et al., who recently highlighted a similar pattern of troponin fluctuation, with significant variations compared to baseline occurring only in subjects who performed a moderate or intense training regimen. Very interestingly, the same authors noted that a shorter duration of high-intensity exercise induced a more important increase in troponin compared to prolonged, but less intensive, training [59]. Basically, these heterogeneous patterns outline the importance of the duration, intensity, and type of training when assessing cardiac biomarkers. A promising future scenario also assumes the use of novel cardiac biomarkers, such as the soluble suppression of tumorigenesis-2 (sST2) for the early detection of subclinical myocardial injury during sports. Being a marker of increased myocardial strain, fibrosis, and neurohormonal activation, sST2 exhibits a superior prognosis value compared to NT-proBNP or cTnI in patients presenting acute myocardial injury [60,61].

Recent studies have shown that cardiac biomarkers have an important negative predictive value. Thus, low or undetectable hs-cTnI levels can help exclude an inducible myocardial ischemia, in both patients with known coronary artery disease (CAD) and patients without [62–64].

Comparing male and female football players who had CK-MB values measured before, immediately after, and 15 min after a running training session, researchers described a slight increase in CK-MB values immediately post-exercise, most notably in the women's group, yet these values returned to baseline at the 15 min timepoint. The groups comprised both genders and the measurements were performed at different timepoints (immediately after and 15 min after). This study was comparable to ours with regard to the type of sports practiced and the number of participants [65].

Another study measured myoglobin and CK levels immediately after, at the 24 h, 48 h and 72 h timepoints after a high-intensity intermittent running protocol. The results showed a higher increase in myoglobin levels and a more modest one in CK levels, with a return to the baseline values within 24 h for both parameters [66].

On a longer time span, CK and myoglobin levels were measured during a 12-day training period, with blood samples taken prior, at the 6-day mark, and on the 12th day at the end of the training period. CK values peaked on the 6th day, with a drop afterward, while myoglobin peaked on the 12th day [67].

By combining the results of both the cardiac biomarker measurements and of the CPET we can observe how biomarkers are also useful in the assessment of CRF, as they are released into the bloodstream when the cardiovascular stress is at higher values.

The main limitation of our study is represented by the small number of participants, which was not sufficient for more complex statistical analysis tests and could not offer sufficient data for further correlations (see Appendix A).

However, given the low number of publications and existing studies of this design, which combines the complete cardiovascular evaluation of athletes starting from the history, physical examination, 12-lead ECG and cardiac ultrasound and focusing on the combination of the CPET and cardiac biomarker measurements, it is definitely a starting point for further research and future studies. This is also supported by the significant statistical results which were obtained.

Our study offers a more complete approach than other studies, with the combination of CPET and biomarker measurements, and the established correlations so far encourage future research on larger groups, even though the biomarkers which suffered blood level changes (CK-MB, myoglobin, D-dimers) were not specific on their own for coronary diseases [37–41,48]. This association of CPET and biomarkers is also useful to be implemented in cardiac and respiratory rehabilitation evaluations, as shown by a 2021 study conducted by Wang et al., where the improvement of CHF patients' parameters was monitored using these dynamics [68]. Apart from a higher number of subjects, serial measurements of cardiac biomarkers at more timepoints, especially at 12 and 24 h, would offer more indication of their full dynamics in relation to induced physical stress.

5. Conclusions

The current study showed that when subjected to an induced physical effort, biomarkers such as CK-MB, myoglobin, and D-dimers suffer changes in their blood levels. Additionally, between these biomarkers which suffered changes in relation to induced physical stress and the parameters which evaluated the functional capacity in the CPET, significant correlations were observed. This highlights the potential of the combined CPET and biomarker determinations for the functional evaluation of young professional athletes and the assessment of cardiovascular risk, alongside the 12-lead ECG and the cardiac ultrasound. However, additional research on a larger study group is needed to further ascertain these findings.

Author Contributions: Conceptualization, A.-D.C., I.-I.C. and F.M.; methodology, C.H., M.R. and V.M.; software, O.M.; validation, R.-Ș.M.; formal analysis, M.-M.L.-C. and A.M.; investigation, A.-D.C.; resources, D.I.-H. and C.-O.H.-I.; data curation, M.R. and B.A.; writing—original draft preparation, A.-D.C.; writing—review and editing A.I., Ș.-T.D. and D.-M.P.; visualization, I.-I.C.; supervision, F.M. All authors have read and agreed to the published version of the manuscript.

Funding: This research received no external funding.

Institutional Review Board Statement: The study was designed following the recommendations for clinical research contained in the Helsinki Declaration of the World Medical Association, and the protocol was approved by both the Ethics Committee of the Clinical Rehabilitation Hospital in Iași, Romania, approved on 24 March 2021 and the Ethics Research Committee of the "Grigore T. Popa" University of Medicine and Pharmacy in Iași, Romania, nr. 72 approved on 25 April 2021.

Informed Consent Statement: Informed consent was obtained from all subjects involved in the study. Written informed consent has been obtained from the patient(s) to publish this paper.

Data Availability Statement: Not applicable.

Conflicts of Interest: The authors declare no conflict of interest.

Appendix A

This is a pilot study from a much larger research project in a doctoral study conducted within the "Grigore T. Popa" University of Medicine and Pharmacy in Iași, Romania, entitled "The evaluation of the correlations between the cardiac biomarkers and the risk of cardiovascular events during sustained physical effort", under the direct coordination and supervision of Professor Habil. Florin Mitu, MD, PhD.

References

1. Makar, O.; Siabrenko, G. Influence of Physical Activity on Cardiovascular System and Prevention of Cardiovascular Diseases (Review). *Georgian Med. News* **2018**, *285*, 69–74.
2. Jakovljevic, D.G. Physical activity and cardiovascular aging: Physiological and molecular insights. *Exp. Gerontol.* **2018**, *109*, 67–74. [CrossRef] [PubMed]
3. Franklin, B.A.; Thompson, P.D.; Al-Zaiti, S.S.; Albert, C.M.; Hivert, M.F.; Levine, B.D.; Lobelo, F.; Madan, K.; Sharrief, A.Z.; Eijsvogels, T.M.H. Exercise-related acute cardiovascular events and potential deleterious adaptations following long-term exercise training: Placing the risks into perspective-an update: A scientific statement from the American Heart Association. *Circulation* **2020**, *141*, e705–e736. [CrossRef] [PubMed]
4. Poddębska, I.; Kosielski, P.; Gałczyński, S.; Wranicz, K.; Cygankiewicz, I.; Kaczmarek, K. ECG abnormalities in athletes as compare to healthy subjects. *Pol. Merkur. Lek. Organ Pol. Tow. Lek.* **2020**, *48*, 387–390.

5. Sharma, S.; Drezner, J.A.; Baggish, A.; Papadakis, M.; Wilson, M.G.; Prutkin, J.M.; La Gerche, A.; Ackerman, M.J.; Borjesson, M.; Salerno, J.C.; et al. International recommendations for electrocardiographic interpretation in athletes. *Eur. Heart J.* **2018**, *39*, 1466–1480. [CrossRef]
6. Pelliccia, A.; Sharma, S.; Gati, S.; Bäck, M.; Börjesson, M.; Caselli, S.; Collet, J.P.; Corrado, D.; Drezner, J.A.; Halle, M.; et al. 2020 ESC Guidelines on sports cardiology and exercise in patients with cardiovascular disease. *Eur. Heart J.* **2021**, *42*, 17–96. [CrossRef]
7. Harmon, K.G.; Asif, I.M.; Maleszewski, J.J.; Owens, D.S.; Prutkin, J.M.; Salerno, J.C.; Zigman, M.L.; Ellenbogen, R.; Rao, A.L.; Ackerman, M.J.; et al. Incidence, Cause, and Comparative Frequency of Sudden Cardiac Death in National Collegiate Athletic Association Athletes: A Decade in Review. *Circulation* **2015**, *132*, 10–19. [CrossRef]
8. Drezner, J.A.; Harmon, K.G.; Marek, J.C. Incidence of sudden cardiac arrest in Minnesota high school student athletes: The limitations of catastrophic insurance claims. *J. Am. Coll. Cardiol.* **2014**, *63*, 1455–1456. [CrossRef]
9. Maron, B.J.; Haas, T.S.; Ahluwalia, A.; Rutten-Ramos, S.C. Incidence of cardiovascular sudden deaths in Minnesota high school athletes. *Heart Rhythm* **2013**, *10*, 374–377. [CrossRef]
10. Harmon, K.G.; Asif, I.M.; Maleszewski, J.J.; Owens, D.S.; Prutkin, J.M.; Salerno, J.C.; Zigman, M.L.; Ellenbogen, R.; Rao, A.L.; Ackerman, M.J.; et al. Incidence and Etiology of Sudden Cardiac Arrest and Death in High School Athletes in the United States. *Mayo Clin. Proc.* **2016**, *91*, 1493–1502. [CrossRef]
11. Toresdahl, B.G.; Rao, A.L.; Harmon, K.G.; Drezner, J.A. Incidence of sudden cardiac arrest in high school student athletes on school campus. *Heart Rhythm* **2014**, *11*, 1190–1194. [CrossRef] [PubMed]
12. Suárez-Mier, M.P.; Aguilera, B.; Mosquera, R.M.; Sánchez-de-León, M.S. Pathology of sudden death during recreational sports in Spain. *Forensic Sci. Int.* **2013**, *226*, 188–196. [CrossRef] [PubMed]
13. Finocchiaro, G.; Papadakis, M.; Robertus, J.L.; Dhutia, H.; Steriotis, A.K.; Tome, M.; Mellor, G.; Merghani, A.; Malhotra, A.; Behr, E.; et al. Etiology of Sudden Death in Sports: Insights from a United Kingdom Regional Registry. *J. Am. Coll. Cardiol.* **2016**, *67*, 2108–2115. [CrossRef] [PubMed]
14. Ullal, A.J.; Abdelfattah, R.S.; Ashley, E.A.; Froelicher, V.F. Hypertrophic Cardiomyopathy as a Cause of Sudden Cardiac Death in the Young: A Meta-Analysis. *Am. J. Med.* **2016**, *129*, 486–496.e2. [CrossRef]
15. Thiene, G.; Rizzo, S.; Schiavon, M.; Maron, M.S.; Zorzi, A.; Corrado, D.; Maron, B.J.; Basso, C. Structurally Normal Hearts Are Uncommonly Associated with Sudden Deaths in Athletes and Young People. *J. Am. Coll. Cardiol.* **2019**, *73*, 3031–3032. [CrossRef]
16. Malhotra, A.; Sharma, S. Outcomes of Cardiac Screening in Adolescent Soccer Players. *N. Engl. J. Med.* **2018**, *379*, 524–534. [CrossRef]
17. Hevia, A.C.; Fernández, M.M.; Palacio, J.M.; Martín, E.H.; Castro, M.G.; Reguero, J.J. ECG as a part of the preparticipation screening programme: An old and still present international dilemma. *Br. J. Sports Med.* **2011**, *45*, 776–779. [CrossRef]
18. Fudge, J.; Harmon, K.G.; Owens, D.S.; Prutkin, J.M.; Salerno, J.C.; Asif, I.M.; Haruta, A.; Pelto, H.; Rao, A.L.; Toresdahl, B.G.; et al. Cardiovascular screening in adolescents and young adults: A prospective study comparing the Pre-participation Physical Evaluation Monograph 4th Edition and ECG. *Br. J. Sports Med.* **2014**, *48*, 1172–1178. [CrossRef]
19. Drezner, J.A.; Prutkin, J.M.; Harmon, K.G.; O'Kane, J.W.; Pelto, H.F.; Rao, A.L.; Hassebrock, J.D.; Petek, B.J.; Teteak, C.; Timonen, M.; et al. Cardiovascular screening in college athletes. *J. Am. Coll. Cardiol.* **2015**, *65*, 2353–2355. [CrossRef]
20. Drezner, J.A.; Owens, D.S.; Prutkin, J.M.; Salerno, J.C.; Harmon, K.G.; Prosise, S.; Clark, A.; Asif, I.M. Electrocardiographic Screening in National Collegiate Athletic Association Athletes. *Am. J. Cardiol.* **2016**, *118*, 754–759. [CrossRef]
21. Price, D.E.; McWilliams, A.; Asif, I.M.; Martin, A.; Elliott, S.D.; Dulin, M.; Drezner, J.A. Electrocardiography-inclusive screening strategies for detection of cardiovascular abnormalities in high school athletes. *Heart Rhythm* **2014**, *11*, 442–449. [CrossRef] [PubMed]
22. Rizzo, M.; Spataro, A.; Cecchetelli, C.; Quaranta, F.; Livrieri, S.; Sperandii, F.; Cifra, B.; Borrione, P.; Pigozzi, F. Structural cardiac disease diagnosed by echocardiography in asymptomatic young male soccer players: Implications for pre-participation screening. *Br. J. Sports Med.* **2012**, *46*, 371–373. [CrossRef] [PubMed]
23. Tomkinson, G.R.; Lang, J.J.; Blanchard, J.; Léger, L.A.; Tremblay, M.S. The 20-m Shuttle Run: Assessment and Interpretation of Data in Relation to Youth Aerobic Fitness and Health. *Pediatr. Exerc. Sci.* **2019**, *31*, 152–163. [CrossRef] [PubMed]
24. Guazzi, M.; Bandera, F.; Ozemek, C.; Systrom, D.; Arena, R. Cardiopulmonary Exercise Testing: What Is its Value. *J. Am. Coll. Cardiol.* **2017**, *70*, 1618–1636. [CrossRef]
25. Tran, D. Cardiopulmonary Exercise Testing. *Methods Mol. Biol.* **2018**, *1735*, 285–295.
26. Arena, R.; Canada, J.M.; Popovic, D.; Trankle, C.R.; Del Buono, M.G.; Lucas, A.; Abbate, A. Cardiopulmonary exercise testing—Refining the clinical perspective by combining assessments. *Expert Rev. Cardiovasc. Ther.* **2020**, *18*, 563–576. [CrossRef]
27. Gibson, M.E.; Gray, K. Exercise Testing. *Curr. Sports Med. Rep.* **2019**, *18*, 349–350. [CrossRef]
28. Mezzani, A. Cardiopulmonary Exercise Testing: Basics of Methodology and Measurements. *Ann. Am. Thorac. Soc.* **2017**, *14*, S3–S11. [CrossRef]
29. Foster, C. Is There Risk in Exercise Testing of Athletes. *Int. J. Sports Physiol. Perform.* **2017**, *12*, 849–850. [CrossRef]
30. Guazzi, M.; Adams, V.; Conraads, V.; Halle, M.; Mezzani, A.; Vanhees, L.; Arena, R.; Fletcher, G.F.; Forman, D.E.; Kitzman, D.W.; et al. EACPR/AHA Scientific Statement. Clinical recommendations for cardiopulmonary exercise testing data assessment in specific patient populations. *Circulation* **2012**, *126*, 2261–2274. [CrossRef]
31. Löllgen, H.; Leyk, D. Exercise Testing in Sports Medicine. *Dtsch. Arztebl. Int.* **2018**, *115*, 409–416. [CrossRef] [PubMed]
32. Katrukha, I.A. Human cardiac troponin complex. Structure and functions. *Biochemistry* **2013**, *78*, 1447–1465. [CrossRef] [PubMed]

33. Van der Velden, J.; Stienen, G.J.M. Cardiac Disorders and Pathophysiology of Sarcomeric Proteins. *Physiol. Rev.* **2019**, *99*, 381–426. [CrossRef] [PubMed]
34. Bódi, B.; Oláh, A.; Mártha, L.; Tóth, A.; Radovits, T.; Merkely, B.; Papp, Z. Exercise-induced alterations of myocardial sarcomere dynamics are associated with hypophosphorylation of cardiac troponin I. *Rev. Cardiovasc. Med.* **2021**, *22*, 1079–1085. [CrossRef] [PubMed]
35. Kosowski, M.; Młynarska, K.; Chmura, J.; Kustrzycka-Kratochwil, D.; Sukiennik-Kujawa, M.; Todd, J.A.; Jankowska, E.A.; Banasiak, W.; Reczuch, K.; Ponikowski, P. Cardiovascular stress biomarker assessment of middle-aged non-athlete marathon runners. *Eur. J. Prev. Cardiol.* **2019**, *26*, 318–327. [CrossRef]
36. Samaha, E.; Avila, A.; Helwani, M.A.; Ben Abdallah, A.; Jaffe, A.S.; Scott, M.G.; Nagele, P. High-Sensitivity Cardiac Troponin After Cardiac Stress Test: A Systematic Review and Meta-Analysis. *J. Am. Heart Assoc.* **2019**, *8*, e008626. [CrossRef]
37. Fan, J.; Ma, J.; Xia, N.; Sun, L.; Li, B.; Liu, H. Clinical Value of Combined Detection of CK-MB, MYO, cTnI and Plasma NT-proBNP in Diagnosis of Acute Myocardial Infarction. *Clin. Lab.* **2017**, *63*, 427–433. [CrossRef]
38. Tota, Ł.; Piotrowska, A.; Pałka, T.; Morawska, M.; Mikuľáková, W.; Mucha, D.; Żmuda-Pałka, M.; Pilch, W. Muscle and intestinal damage in triathletes. *PLoS ONE* **2019**, *14*, e0210651. [CrossRef]
39. Bjørnsen, T.; Wernbom, M.; Paulsen, G.; Berntsen, S.; Brankovic, R.; Stålesen, H.; Sundnes, J.; Raastad, T. Frequent blood flow restricted training not to failure and to failure induces similar gains in myonuclei and muscle mass. *Scand. J. Med. Sci. Sports* **2021**, *31*, 1420–1439. [CrossRef]
40. Safdar, B.; Bezek, S.K.; Sinusas, A.J.; Russell, R.R.; Klein, M.R.; Dziura, J.D.; D'Onofrio, G. Elevated CK-MB with a normal troponin does not predict 30-day adverse cardiac events in emergency department chest pain observation unit patients. *Crit. Pathw. Cardiol.* **2014**, *13*, 14–19. [CrossRef]
41. Sahadeo, P.A.; Dym, A.A.; Berry, L.B.; Bahar, P.; Singla, A.; Cheta, M.; Bhansali, R.; LaVine, S.; Laser, J.; Richman, M. The Best of Both Worlds: Eliminating Creatine Kinase-Muscle/Brain (CK-MB) Testing in the Emergency Department Leads to Lower Costs Without Missed Clinical Diagnoses. *Cureus* **2021**, *13*, e15150. [CrossRef] [PubMed]
42. Zhang, Z.L.; Li, R.; Yang, F.Y.; Xi, L. Natriuretic peptide family as diagnostic/prognostic biomarker and treatment modality in management of adult and geriatric patients with heart failure: Remaining issues and challenges. *J. Geriatr. Cardiol.* **2018**, *15*, 540–546.
43. Vassalle, C.; Masotti, S.; Lubrano, V.; Basta, G.; Prontera, C.; Di Cecco, P.; Del Turco, S.; Sabatino, L.; Pingitore, A. Traditional and new candidate cardiac biomarkers assessed before, early, and late after half marathon in trained subjects. *Eur. J. Appl. Physiol.* **2018**, *118*, 411–417. [CrossRef] [PubMed]
44. Roca, E.; Nescolarde, L.; Lupon, J.; Barallat, J.; Januzzi, J.L.; Liu, P.; Cruz Pastor, M.; BayesGenis, A. The dynamics of cardiovascular biomarkers in non-elite marathon runners. *J. Cardiovasc. Transl. Res.* **2017**, *10*, 206–208. [CrossRef]
45. Cocking, S.; Landman, T.; Benson, M.; Lord, R.; Jones, H.; Gaze, D.; Thijssen, D.H.J.; George, K. The impact of remote ischemic preconditioning on cardiac biomarker and functional response to endurance exercise. *Scand. J. Med. Sci. Sports* **2017**, *27*, 1061–1069. [CrossRef] [PubMed]
46. Pearson, M.J.; King, N.; Smart, N.A. Effect of exercise therapy on established and emerging circulating biomarkers in patients with heart failure: A systematic review and meta-analysis. *Open Heart* **2018**, *5*, e000819. [CrossRef]
47. Limkakeng, A.T.; Leahy, J.C.; Griffin, S.M.; Lokhnygina, Y.; Jaffa, E.; Christenson, R.H.; Newby, L.K. Provocative biomarker stress test: Stress-delta N-terminal pro-B type natriuretic peptide. *Open Heart* **2018**, *5*, e000847. [CrossRef]
48. Koch, V.; Biener, M.; Müller-Hennessen, M.; Vafaie, M.; Staudacher, I.; Katus, H.A.; Giannitsis, E. Diagnostic performance of D-dimer in predicting venous thromboembolism and acute aortic dissection. *Eur. Heart J. Acute Cardiovasc. Care* **2020**, *online ahead of print*. [CrossRef]
49. Almorad, A.; Ohanyan, A.; Pintea Bentea, G.; Wielandts, J.Y.; El Haddad, M.; Lycke, M.; O'Neill, L.; Morissens, M.; De Keyzer, E.; Nguyen, T.; et al. D-dimer blood concentrations to exclude left atrial thrombus in patients with atrial fibrillation. *Heart* **2021**, *107*, 195–200. [CrossRef]
50. Miller, M.J.; Maier, C.L.; Duncan, A.; Guarner, J. Assessment of Coagulation and Hemostasis Biomarkers in a Subset of Patients with Chronic Cardiovascular Disease. *Clin. Appl. Thromb. Hemost.* **2021**, *27*, 10760296211032292. [CrossRef]
51. Lombardo, B.; Izzo, V.; Terracciano, D.; Ranieri, A.; Mazzaccara, C.; Fimiani, F.; Cesaro, A.; Gentile, L.; Leggiero, E.; Pero, R.; et al. Laboratory medicine: Health evaluation in elite athletes. *Clin. Chem. Lab. Med.* **2019**, *57*, 1450–1473. [CrossRef] [PubMed]
52. Pepera, G.; Hadjiandrea, S.; Iliadis, I.; Sandercock, G.R.H.; Batalik, L. Associations between cardiorespiratory fitness, fatness, hemodynamic characteristics, and sedentary behaviour in primary school-aged children. *BMC Sports Sci. Med. Rehabil.* **2022**, *14*, 16. [CrossRef] [PubMed]
53. Olekšák, F.; Dvoran, P.; Jakušová, Ľ.; Ďurdík, P.; Igaz, M.; Bánovčin, P. Reference Values for Cardiopulmonary Exercise Testing in Young Male Slovak Athletes. *Acta Med.* **2021**, *64*, 119–124. [CrossRef] [PubMed]
54. Mahanty, A.; Xi, L. Utility of cardiac biomarkers in sports medicine: Focusing on troponin, natriuretic peptides, and hypoxanthine. *Sports Med. Health Sci.* **2020**, *2*, 65–71. [CrossRef]
55. Sedaghat-Hamedani, F.; Kayvanpour, E.; Frankenstein, L.; Mereles, D.; Amr, A.; Buss, S.; Keller, A.; Giannitsis, E.; Jensen, K.; Katus, H.A.; et al. Biomarker changes after strenuous exercise can mimic pulmonary embolism and cardiac injury—A metaanalysis of 45 studies. *Clin. Chem.* **2015**, *61*, 1246–1255. [CrossRef]

56. Hosseini, S.M.; Azizi, M.; Samadi, A.; Talebi, N.; Gatterer, H.; Burtscher, M. Impact of a Soccer Game on Cardiac Biomarkers in Adolescent Players. *Pediatr. Exerc. Sci* **2018**, *30*, 90–95. [CrossRef]
57. Bjørkavoll-Bergseth, M.; Erevik, C.B.; Kleiven, Ø.; Eijsvogels, T.M.H.; Skadberg, Ø.; Frøysa, V.; Wiktorski, T.; Auestad, B.; Edvardsen, T.; Moberg Aakre, K.; et al. Determinants of Interindividual Variation in Exercise-Induced Cardiac Troponin I Levels. *J. Am. Heart Assoc.* **2021**, *10*, e021710. [CrossRef]
58. Scherr, J.; Braun, S.; Schuster, T.; Hartmann, C.; Moehlenkamp, S.; Wolfarth, B.; Pressler, A.; Halle, M. 72-h kinetics of high-sensitive troponin T and inflammatory markers after marathon. *Med. Sci. Sports Exerc.* **2011**, *43*, 1819–1827. [CrossRef]
59. Marshall, L.; Lee, K.K.; Stewart, S.D.; Wild, A.; Fujisawa, T.; Ferry, A.V.; Stables, C.L.; Lithgow, H.; Chapman, A.R.; Anand, A.; et al. Effect of Exercise Intensity and Duration on Cardiac Troponin Release. *Circulation* **2020**, *141*, 83–85. [CrossRef]
60. Costache, A.-D.; Costache, I.-I.; Miftode, R.-Ș.; Stafie, C.-S.; Leon-Constantin, M.-M.; Roca, M.; Drugescu, A.; Popa, D.-M.; Mitu, O.; Mitu, I.; et al. Beyond the Finish Line: The Impact and Dynamics of Biomarkers in Physical Exercise—A Narrative Review. *J. Clin. Med.* **2021**, *10*, 4978. [CrossRef]
61. Miftode, R.-S.; Constantinescu, D.; Cianga, C.M.; Petris, A.O.; Timpau, A.-S.; Crisan, A.; Costache, I.-I.; Mitu, O.; Anton-Paduraru, D.-T.; Miftode, I.-L.; et al. A Novel Paradigm Based on ST2 and Its Contribution towards a Multimarker Approach in the Diagnosis and Prognosis of Heart Failure: A Prospective Study during the Pandemic Storm. *Life* **2021**, *11*, 1080. [CrossRef] [PubMed]
62. Hammadah, M.; Kim, J.H.; Tahhan, A.S.; Kindya, B.; Liu, C.; Ko, Y.A.; Al Mheid, I.; Wilmot, K.; Ramadan, R.; Alkhoder, A.; et al. Use of High-Sensitivity Cardiac Troponin for the Exclusion of Inducible Myocardial Ischemia: A Cohort Study. *Ann. Intern. Med.* **2018**, *169*, 751–760. [CrossRef] [PubMed]
63. Walter, J.E.; Honegger, U.; Puelacher, C.; Mueller, D.; Wagener, M.; Schaerli, N.; Strebel, I.; Twerenbold, R.; Boeddinghaus, J.; Nestelberger, T.; et al. Prospective Validation of a Biomarker-Based Rule Out Strategy for Functionally Relevant Coronary Artery Disease. *Clin. Chem.* **2018**, *64*, 386–395. [CrossRef] [PubMed]
64. Lima, B.B.; Hammadah, M.; Kim, J.H.; Uphoff, I.; Shah, A.; Levantsevych, O.; Almuwaqqat, Z.; Moazzami, K.; Sullivan, S.; Ward, L.; et al. Relation of High-sensitivity Cardiac Troponin I Elevation with Exercise to Major Adverse Cardiovascular Events in Patients with Coronary Artery Disease. *Am. J. Cardiol.* **2020**, *136*, 1–8. [CrossRef] [PubMed]
65. Chamera, T.; Spieszny, M.; Klocek, T.; Kostrzewa-Nowak, D.; Nowak, R.; Lachowicz, M.; Buryta, R.; Ficek, K.; Eider, J.; Moska, W.; et al. Post-Effort Changes in Activity of Traditional Diagnostic Enzymatic Markers in Football Players' Blood. *J. Med. Biochem.* **2015**, *34*, 179–190. [CrossRef] [PubMed]
66. Joo, C.H. Development of a non-damaging high-intensity intermittent running protocol. *J. Exerc. Rehabil.* **2015**, *11*, 112–118. [CrossRef] [PubMed]
67. Radzimiński, Ł.; Jastrzębski, Z.; López-Sánchez, G.F.; Szwarc, A.; Duda, H.; Stuła, A.; Paszulewicz, J.; Dragos, P. Relationships between Training Loads and Selected Blood Parameters in Professional Soccer Players during a 12-Day Sports Camp. *Int. J. Environ. Res. Public Health* **2020**, *17*, 8580. [CrossRef]
68. Wang, Y.; Cao, J.; Kong, X.; Wang, S.; Meng, L.; Wang, Y. The effects of CPET-guided cardiac rehabilitation on the cardiopulmonary function, the exercise endurance, and the NT-proBNP and hscTnT levels in CHF patients. *Am. J. Transl. Res.* **2021**, *13*, 7104–7114.

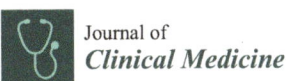

Article

An Intervention of 12 Weeks of Nordic Walking and Recreational Walking to Improve Cardiorespiratory Capacity and Fitness in Older Adult Women

Nebojsa Cokorilo [1], Pedro Jesús Ruiz-Montero [2,*], Francisco Tomás González-Fernández [2] and Ricardo Martín-Moya [2]

1. Faculty of Sport, University UNION Nikola Tesla, 11158 Belgrade, Serbia; cokorilon@gmail.com
2. Physical Education and Sport Department, Faculty of Education and Sport Sciences, Campus of Melilla, University of Granada, 52005 Melilla, Spain; ftgonzalez@ugr.es (F.T.G.-F.); rmartinm@ugr.es (R.M.-M.)
* Correspondence: pedrorumo@ugr.es

Abstract: (1) Background: The main aim of this study was to examine the effect of an intervention of 12 weeks in three groups on anthropometric measurement and heart rate (HR) variables, fitness index, and maximal oxygen consumption (VO_2max) in older women. (2) Methods: In total, 166 Serbian adult women, aged 50 to 69 years old, participated in this study, comprising a control group (60 participants, μ_{age} = 57.8 + 6.6), Nordic-walking (NW) group (53 participants, μ_{age} = 57.5 + 6.8), and recreational-walking (RW) group (53 participants, μ_{age} = 57.8 + 6.6) in a physical fitness programme for 12 weeks. (3) Results: Anthropometric measurement variables were measured using a stadiometer and an electronic scale. The data showed differences in walking heart rate (bt/min) ($p < 0.001$; $\eta^2 = 0.088$) between control, NW, and RW groups in the pretest analysis. Moreover, there were significant differences in walking heart rate (bt/min) ($\eta^2 = 0.155$), heart rate at the end of the test (bt/min) ($\eta^2 = 0.093$), total time of fitness index test (min) ($\eta^2 = 0.097$), fitness index ($\eta^2 = 0.130$), and VO_2max ($\eta^2 = 0.111$) (all, $p < 0.001$) between control, NW, and RW groups in the posttest analysis. (4) Conclusions: NW group training resulted in slightly greater benefits than RW group training. The present study demonstrated that both groups could act as modalities to improve the functionality and quality of life of people during the ageing process, reflected mainly in HR variables; UKK test measurements, and VO_2max. It also contributes to the extant research on older women during exercise and opens interesting avenues for future research.

Keywords: ageing; physical fitness; walkers; well-being; physical exercise programme

1. Introduction

In recent decades, growing evidence from various experimental approaches has shown that the ageing process with a sedentary lifestyle (e.g., sitting and engaging with television and other electronic devices) leads to a greater likelihood of suffering health problems [1]. The majority of this research shows that more sedentary time is linked with increased risk for cardiovascular disease [2] and adverse metabolic effects such as obesity and insulin resistance in women, among other effects [3]. In fact, global health organisations such as the World Health Organisation (WHO) and the American College of Sports Medicine (ACSM) report that sedentary life in adult and older adult women is apparently related to inactivity behaviour during occupational and domestic activities and little participation in physical exercise (PE) during leisure and free-time activities [4].

Previous studies indicate that ageing and a low level of PE are directly related to cardiovascular and pulmonary changes that lead to a reduction in functional capacities [5–7]. In this sense, different physiologic mechanisms that affect health are caused by sedentary time. For example, sedentary time decreases the metabolic activity of muscle and decreases energy utilisation, causing insulin resistance and metabolic disorders [8]. Therefore, chronic

Citation: Cokorilo, N.; Ruiz-Montero, P.J.; González-Fernández, F.T.; Martín-Moya, R. An Intervention of 12 Weeks of Nordic Walking and Recreational Walking to Improve Cardiorespiratory Capacity and Fitness in Older Adult Women. *J. Clin. Med.* **2022**, *11*, 2900. https://doi.org/10.3390/jcm11102900

Academic Editor: David Rodríguez-Sanz

Received: 25 March 2022
Accepted: 19 May 2022
Published: 20 May 2022

Publisher's Note: MDPI stays neutral with regard to jurisdictional claims in published maps and institutional affiliations.

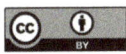

Copyright: © 2022 by the authors. Licensee MDPI, Basel, Switzerland. This article is an open access article distributed under the terms and conditions of the Creative Commons Attribution (CC BY) license (https://creativecommons.org/licenses/by/4.0/).

PE could help to combat a sedentary lifestyle. In fact, numerous studies have shown the beneficial effects of PE on overall health, specifically in physical fitness and anthropometric measurement [9–11]. Recent systematic reviews and meta-analyses have concluded that physical exercise helps to reduce the risk of various conditions associated with ageing, such as frailty [12], cognitive decline [13], low muscle power, or poor functional capacity [14]. There is also evidence that exercise intervention programmes can prevent falls in older people with mild comorbidities [15]. However, the literature shows that, in addition to preventing functional capacities, PE also prevents mental diseases and supports health benefits across the older adult lifespan [16]. In addition, it is well-documented that changes in body composition and anthropometric measurement are strongly related to ageing; the main effects are lean body mass and fat mass [17,18]. In this respect, variations in body composition and anthropometric measurement in older people have also been associated with loss of muscle mass and, therefore, with muscle strength, physical capacity, and quality of life and well-being [19,20].

Other important physiologic mechanisms that influence ageing are the heart rate (HR) and maximal oxygen consumption (VO_2max). One study showed that age-related declines in VO_2max were approximately 0.35, 0.44, and 0.62 mL/kg/min per year for sedentary, physically fit, and physically trained females, respectively [21]. In this sense, an intervention of 16 weeks of combined aerobic exercise training and resistance exercise training produced a significant improvement in muscular strength, cardiovascular fitness, and functional tasks in older women [22]. Overall, the majority of effects of ageing on the heart can be decreased by chronic exercise; therefore, PE can help people maintain cardiovascular fitness as well as muscular fitness as they age [23].

Healthy ageing is the key to maintaining an adequate level of physical performance, which is needed to be able to successfully perform everyday activities [24]. Currently, there is a large number of tests whose objective is to assess the physical condition of different population groups. From the point of view of health care and biomedical fields, tests have the main objective of prescribing a PE programme according to individual characteristics. In this sense, obtaining correct values could help to assess the initial fitness level of each subject. Urho Kaleva Kekkonen (UKK) test has a very simple application, reliability, health-related validity, and physical-activity-related safety and feasibility [25], especially for adults aged 18–69. In addition, the UKK test has a large correlation with VO_2max [25]. Due to having all these properties, the UKK test may show the variability of physical performance over time and provide evidence for maintaining good physical fitness and promoting healthy ageing in different age groups [26].

As mentioned above, a low level of PE among older adults, caused by a sedentary lifestyle, leads to reduced functional capacities and, therefore, damage to health over time. To overcome this issue, the literature suggests that individuals practice regular PE of low-to-moderate intensity, such as recreational walking (RW) or Nordic walking (NW), which may encourage older people to practice regular PE [27,28]. RW may be a simple and efficient means of PE for older people due to the low risk of injury, and irrespective of individual level [29], it is an effective way to improve the level of PE, requires no equipment, and can be performed almost anywhere at any time. Thus, RW involves moderate intensity that can provoke positive changes to health and minimise the risk of premature death [30]. With regard to NW, a systematic review reveals its enormous positive benefit on health [31]. NW has grown in popularity recently and is considered a good PE for older people due to its safety and low cost. Originally derived from RW, NW is highly popular and accepted by the population [32]. The literature has shown that NW reduces the load of the lumbar spine and lower limb joints and increases energy expenditure in comparison with RW [33]. Finally, the beneficial effects of NW on different health parameters such as resting HR, blood pressure, exercise capacity, and VO_2max have been established in different populations [34,35]. In addition, recent studies have shown the effectiveness of programmes of regular PE based on NW [36]. Taking into account the current literature, there is strong scientific evidence that regular physical activity has extensive health benefits for adults aged 65 and above, but there is little evidence to suggest which are the most suitable practices if we talk about Nordic-walking or recreational-walking modalities [34], and how they can serve to improve the physical condition and quality of life of older adults. In fact, older adults perceive them as easy and enjoyable types of exercise, and they provide effective ways to promote an active lifestyle for improved health. Thus, the aim of the present study was to examine the effect of a 12-week intervention in three groups (control, RW, and NW groups) on anthropometric measurement variables (body mass and body mass index (BMI)), HR variables (walking HR and HR at the end of the test), UKK test measurement (total time and fitness index), and VO_2max in older women.

2. Materials and Methods

A total of 166 older women (50–69 years; μ_{age} = 57.6 ± 5.6) from the north of Serbia (city of Novi Sad) were recruited through social groups from Novi Sad University (Serbia), leaflets, local newspapers, and social media. Specifically, there were 60 participants in the control group (μ_{age} = 57.75 ± 3.51), 53 participants in the RW group (μ_{age} = 57.85 ± 6.64) and 53 in the NW group (μ_{age} = 57.53 ± 6.85) (see Figure 1). As initial contact with potential recruits yielded only seven men, researchers decided to recruit only female participants in the study to avoid problems of statistical power with a low male sample.

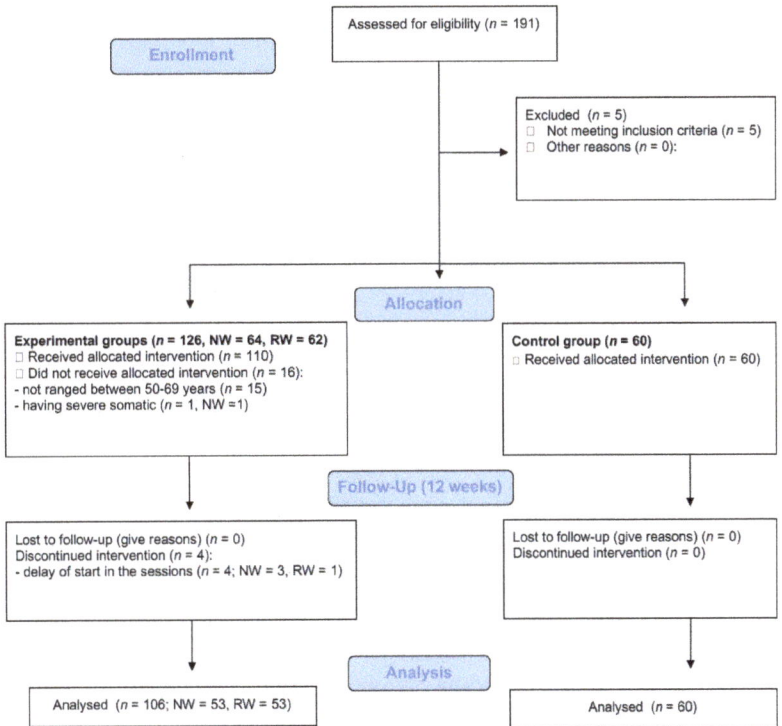

Figure 1. Participant's flow diagram based on CONSORT reporting guidelines.

Based on a statistical power of 80% (z), a type 1 margin of error or alpha of 0.05, a response distribution of 50% (r), and a sample population of older women (50–69 years) ($N_{recommended}$ = 164) in the city, the sample size of the present study was in the recommended range. The following formulas were used [37]:

$$x = Z(c/100)\, 2r\, (100 - r)$$

$$n = N x/((N - 1) E2 + x)$$
$$E = \text{Sqrt} [(N - n) x/n(N - 1)]$$

Anthropometric measurement variables (body mass and BMI), HR variables (walking HR and HR at the end of the test), UKK test measurements (total time and fitness index), and VO$_2$max were gathered.

All participants were provided with a written document that specified the research objective. They were recruited via telephone or direct contact from an association of women that used to gather together in the Faculty of Sport Science of Novi Sad to engage in several leisure activities (not involving physical activity or sport). We informed all participants not to modify their daily behavioural patterns and not to engage in other extra physical exercises, to avoid conflation of results. A sampling strategy was determined for convenience.

The inclusion criteria for all women who participated in this study were (1) 50–69 years of age, (2) no severe somatic or psychiatric disorders, (3) ability to complete the walking test of two kilometres without assistance, and (4) oral and written communications ability. Exclusion criteria for this study were (1) not to be diagnosed with an acute or terminal illness; (2) to have suffered a major cardiovascular event (i.e., myocardial infarction, angina, or stroke) in the past 6 months; (3) presence of neuromuscular disease or drugs affecting neuromuscular function, (4) unwillingness to complete the study requirements, and (5) presence of neuromuscular disease or drugs affecting neuromuscular function.

This study was conducted in accordance with the ethical principles of the Declaration of Helsinki, and it was approved by the Ethical Committee (no. 46-06-03/2020-1), with the purpose of ensuring a responsible investigation. Moreover, this study was registered as a controlled and non-randomised design in ISRCT (ISRCTN44310625).

2.1. Measures

2.1.1. Anthropometric Measurement Variables

Age and gender were determined by two ad hoc questions. Body height was measured to ± 0.1 mm using a stadiometer (SECA 213, Hamburg, Germany), and body mass (kg) was measured with an electronic scale (SECA 799, Hamburg, Germany), with participants wearing light indoor clothing and no shoes. BMI was calculated as weight (kg)/height^2 (m). Prior to measurement, participants were asked to have fasted for 4 h, to not have consumed alcohol for 8 h, and to not have performed physical exercise for the previous 8 h. All tests were repeated in the same space and at the same time after 12 weeks under the same humidity condition (30–40%), as recommended by Morente-Oria et al. [24]. BMI was calculated as kg/m^2.

2.1.2. Cardiorespiratory Fitness

To measure the cardiorespiratory capacity, achieved by brisk walking and prediction of VO$_2$max, the UKK walking test for adults aged 18–69 [25], developed by the Urho Kaleva Kekkonen Institute for Health Promotion Research (the UKK Institute), was used. The UKK walking test involves walking two kilometres on a flat surface at as brisk a pace as possible. The results of this test indicate a fitness index, taking into consideration the age, gender, body mass, duration of the walk, and HR at the end of the test. Furthermore, we measured the walking HR average over the two kilometres. The fitness index by cardiorespiratory capacity fitness index uses five levels, where the lowest level is <70 (considerably below average) and the highest is >130 (considerably above average). The equation to calculate UKK fitness index by the cardiorespiratory capacity of women was as follows [38]:

1° step: (walking time-min * 8.5) + (walking time-seconds * 0.14) + (HR at the end of the test-beats/minutes * 0.32) + (BMI-kg/m^2 * 1.1) = X; 2° step: X − (age * 0.4) = Y; 3° step: 304 − Y = UKK fitness index.

To calculate the VO₂max, an equation predicting maximal aerobic power on the basis of the results obtained in the UKK walking test was used for women in this study as follows [38]:

116.2 − 2.98 * time(minutes/seconds) − 0.11 * HR (at the end of the test) − 0.14 * age − 0.30 * BMI (kg/m^2).

2.1.3. Heart Rate (HR)

The HR at the end of the UKK walking test and the walking HR during the UKK walking test were measured by a pulse watch and chest belt (Polar FT2, Kempele, Finland). The measured values were obtained immediately after finishing the pretest and posttest intervention evaluations of the UKK walking test.

2.1.4. Patient and Public Involvement

Data were collected twice: a test performed during the month of August 2021 (pretest) and after 12 weeks (posttest), performed in October 2021.

The participants visited the measuring area at the University of Novi Sad (Serbia), and their anthropometric measurements were measured 48 h before starting the interventional programme and 48 h after the programme. They were evaluated in the morning, and environmental conditions were controlled.

Both training programmes (RW and NW) were performed three times a week for 12 weeks (3 months) in the morning, with a duration from 35 to 45 min, in line with the requirements laid out by the ACSM [4]. During this intervention, participants took part in no other physical activity.

The participants from the experimental NW group used specific telescope aluminium poles (100–135 cm) for 3 months. Participants from the experimental RW group used no poles.

The programme was carried out on a trim track (park "Sremska Kamenica", Novi Sad, Serbia), which offered good conditions for this activity. The training programme was supervised by physical exercise specialists and adapted individually for each of the participants, depending on participant age and in compliance with sports training principles. In addition, each specialist controlled a different studied variable (anthropometric measurement, HR, UKK test measurements, and VO₂max variables. Thus, any bias related to assessors and researchers was minimum. Participants' individual physical limitations were considered in controlling for the range and intensity of exercise.

Prior to each activity, participants were made aware of the necessary HR during the training, and the programme was conceptualised in such a way that participants were always in the aerobic zone of performance. During the walking exercise, HR was monitored by a pulse meter and was used to determine load intensity. Both programmes were divided into three parts, different by volume (frequency of sessions per week and length) and intensity (percentage of maximum heart rate (%HRmax) according to the age and physical activity level of participants). Participants performed three weekly training sessions of 35 min of continuous aerobic work during the first 4 weeks (first month of the training programme), and the intensity was 60–65% of the total. From the fifth to eighth training week (second month of the training programme), the duration of training sessions was 40 min of continuous aerobic work three times per week at 65–70% %HRmax. Finally, in the last 4 weeks (third month), the sessions were 45 min in length three times per week, with an %HRmax of 75–80%. The differences in burdening (training intensity) according to age were calculated by using the percentage of maximum heart rate and optimal intensity of burdening within the limits of 50–90% [39] (Table 1).

Table 1. Timeline of the study.

									2021					
	Pretest Intervention				Intervention								Posttest Intervention
Months	July	August			September					October			December
Week		1	2	3	4	5	6	7	8	9	10	11	12	
Control group	Pretest				35 min of continuous aerobic (60–65% %HRmax)									Posttest
Nordic-walking group	Pretest				40 min of continuous aerobic (65–70% %HRmax)									Posttest
Recreational-walking group	Pretest				45 min of continuous aerobic (75–80% %HRmax)									Posttest

For the RW and NW groups, participants had to do a 10 min warm-up in a dedicated area of the trim track. Specifically, the participants performed movement exercises with different specific gestures such as lateral steps, knee elevation, tiptoe walk, and fast arms movement. After the warm-up, the main block of the session was followed by 20 min (weeks 1–4), 25 min (weeks 5–8), and 30 min (weeks 9–12) of continuous RW or NW depending on the experimental group. This was followed by a 5 min cool-down period, featuring mainly stretching exercises. Participants of the control group did not undergo supervised training and were asked not to modify daily activities. However, as physical exercise and active life are beneficial to health, participants in the control group attended three workshops (one per month) addressing the benefits of being physically active. The attendance at these workshops aimed to maintain participation in the control group and their commitment to completing the entire 12 weeks of intervention.

Finally, participants received a report of the results and conclusions obtained in the study after the elaboration and discussion of the data, thanking them for their participation.

2.1.5. Statistical Analysis

The Kolmogorov–Smirnov test with mean values was used to test the normality of distribution. The mean (μ) and standard deviation (DT) of the anthropometric measurement variables (body mass and BMI), HR variables (walking HR and HR at the end of the test), UKK test measurements (total time and fitness index), and VO_2max of the participants were determined. In addition, test reliability was determined by calculating the coefficient of variation of VO_2max between pretest and posttest in the RW and NW groups.

A mixed-design ANOVA for participants was used between groups (control, Nordic walking, and recreational walking) and moment intervention (pretest–posttest). To establish the differences in outcomes, we used a one-way analysis of variance (ANOVA) in the pre- and posttest. Pairwise comparisons were performed with Bonferroni's adjustment. Effect size is indicated with partial eta squared (η^2) for Fs [40]. The Greenhouse–Geisser correction was applied when sphericity was violated [41]. In such a case, corrected probability values were reported. Differences in participant groups were found in the five categories of UKK fitness index. Regarding the pretest and posttest differences among all groups, a repeated-measures ANOVA test was used for two dependent samples. This process was carried out with regard to anthropometric measurement variables, HR variables, UKK test measurements, and VO_2max in all groups.

All statistical analyses were performed using the Statistical Package for Social Science (IBM SPSS Statistics for Windows 21.0. Armonk, NY, USA).

3. Results

3.1. Comparison of the Participant Groups (Control, RW, and NW) Relative to Anthropometric Measurement Variables, HR Variables, UKK Test Measurements, and VO_2max

Table 2 shows only one significant difference among the three participant groups in the pretest. The walking HR was lower in the RW group than that in the control and NW groups (79.17 ± 9.45 bt/min vs. 82.13 ± 9.36 bt/min and 87.12 ± 12.36 bt/min, respectively, $p < 0.001$).

Table 2. ANOVA for anthropometric measurement variables, heart rate, UKK walking test time and fitness index, and VO2max for pretest, with mean values (SD).

Variables Involved in UKK Walking Test	Pretest			F	p	η^2
	Control Group (n = 60)	Nordic-Walking Group (n = 53)	Recreational-Walking Group (n = 53)			
Body mass (kg)	69.35 ± 9.26	70.27 ± 9.61	69.40 ± 8.38	0.177	0.838	0.002
BMI (kg/m^2)	25.52 ± 3.58	26.20 ± 3.88	25.83 ± 4.13	0.436	0.648	0.005
Walking heart rate (bt/min)	82.13 ± 9.36 [b]	87.12 ± 12.36 [ab]	79.17 ± 9.45 [a]	7.847	0.001	0.088
Heart rate at the end of the test (bt/min)	114.35 ± 12.48	112.68 ± 15.75	117.26 ± 15.07	1.374	0.256	0.017
UKK total time (min)	23.32 ± 1.65	23.98 ± 1.48	23.80 ± 2.12	2.123	0.123	0.025
UKK fitness index	72.75 ± 15.76	65.42 ± 20.61	69.28 ± 19.01	2.211	0.113	0.026
VO$_2$max (mL·min^{-1}·kg^{-1})	19.61 ± 5.52	16.85 ± 5.42	18.39 ± 7.31	2.839	0.061	0.034

Note. UKK: Urho Kaleva Kekkonen; BMI: body mass index; VO$_2$max: maximal oxygen consumption; m: metre; kg: kilogram; bt: beat; min: minute; mL: millilitre; η^2: effect size by eta square; SD: standard deviation; df: degrees of freedom (2, 163 for pretest); [a,b] superscripts with the same letter show a degree of significant difference between both groups ($p < 0.05$). Pairwise comparisons were performed with Bonferroni's adjustment.

However, Table 3 reveals several significant differences among the control, NW, and RW groups, such as the walking HR (82.35 ± 9.09 bt/min vs. 79.45 ± 9.36 bt/min and 73.54 ± 7.32 bt/min, respectively, $p < 0.001$) and HR at the end of the test (114.13 ± 11.56 bt/min vs. 105.09 ± 11.61 bt/min and 106.51 ± 14.81 bt/min, respectively, $p < 0.001$). The results of measurements of the UKK test in terms of the UKK total time spent to walk two kilometres and the fitness index were significantly worse in the control group than those for the NW and RW groups, as detailed below. Participants in the RW group spent the shortest time to walk two kilometres (RW group = 22.06 ± 1.91 min; NW group = 22.11 ± 1.76 min; control group = 23.32 ± 1.84 min; $p < 0.001$) and obtained the best UKK fitness index (RW group = 88.92 ± 19.42; NW group = 84.72 ± 15.94; control group = 72.95 ± 18.13; $p < 0.001$). Finally, the RW group showed higher VO$_2$max than the NW and control groups (24.51 ± 6.41 mL·min^{-1}·kg^{-1} vs. 23.58 ± 6.05 mL·min^{-1}·kg^{-1} and 19.59 ± 6.14 mL·min^{-1}·kg^{-1}, respectively, $p < 0.001$). According to the coefficient of variation of VO$_2$max, it is possible to observe an increase of 23.59% in the difference between pretest and posttest results in RW and 30.20% in NW.

Table 3. ANOVA posttest results in terms of anthropometric measurement variables, heart rate, UKK walking test time and fitness index, and VO$_2$max, with mean values (SD).

Variables Involved in UKK Walking Test	Posttest			F	p	η^2
	Control Group (n = 60)	Nordic-Walking Group (n = 53)	Recreational-Walking Group (n = 53)			
Body mass (kg)	69.37 ± 9.25	68.44 ± 9.64	67.18 ± 8.25	0.823	0.441	0.010
BMI (kg/m^2)	25.53 ± 3.55	25.52 ± 3.85	25.01 ± 4.05	0.332	0.718	0.004
Walking heart rate (bt/min)	82.35 ± 9.09 [b,c]	79.45 ± 9.36 [a,b]	73.54 ± 7.32 [a,c]	14.919	0.001	0.155
Heart rate at the end of the test (bt/min)	114.13 ± 11.56 [a,b]	105.09 ± 11.61 [a]	106.51 ± 14.81 [b]	8.402	0.001	0.093
UKK total time (min)	23.32 ± 1.84 [a,b]	22.11 ± 1.76 [a]	22.06 ± 1.91 [b]	8.748	0.001	0.097
UKK fitness index	72.95 ± 18.13 [a,b]	84.72 ± 15.94 [a]	88.92 ± 19.42 [b]	12.230	0.001	0.130
VO$_2$max (mL·min^{-1}·kg^{-1})	19.59 ± 6.14 [a,b]	23.58 ± 6.05 [a]	24.51 ± 6.41 [b]	10.168	0.001	0.111

Note. UKK: Urho Kaleva Kekkonen; BMI: body mass index; VO$_2$max: maximal oxygen consumption; m: metre; kg: kilogram; bt: beat; min: minute; mL: millilitre; η^2: Effect size by eta square; SD: standard deviation; df: degrees of freedom (2, 163 for posttest intervention); [a,b,c] superscripts with the same letter show a degree of significant difference between both groups ($p < 0.05$). Pairwise comparisons were performed with Bonferroni's adjustment.

3.2. Differences in Body Composition Variables, HR Variables, UKK Test Measuring, and VO$_2$max between Pretest and Posttest by Participant Group (Control, RW, and NW)

A mixed-design ANOVA with mean data of body mass (F = 410.13, $p < 0.001$, $\eta^2 <= 0.72$) and BMI (F = 412.63, $p < 0.001$, $\eta^2 = 0.71$) revealed a significant main effect of participant groups (control, RW and NW). The interaction between group and pretest–posttest intervention showed a significant effect in body mass (F = 113.33, $p < 0.001$, $\eta^2 = 0.58$) and BMI (F = 111.73, $p < 0.001$, $\eta^2 = 0.57$). Moreover, a repeated-measures ANOVA test between pretest and posttest in the RW and NW groups demonstrated differences in body mass (RW group, $t = 14.49$, $p < 0.001$; NW group, $t = 15.09$, $p < 0.001$), BMI (RW group, $t = 14.37$, $p < 0.001$; NW group, $t = 15.16$, $p < 0.001$), and walking HR (RW group, $t = -14.36$, $p < 0.001$; NW group, $t = -9.41$, $p < 0.001$). This is shown in Figure 2.

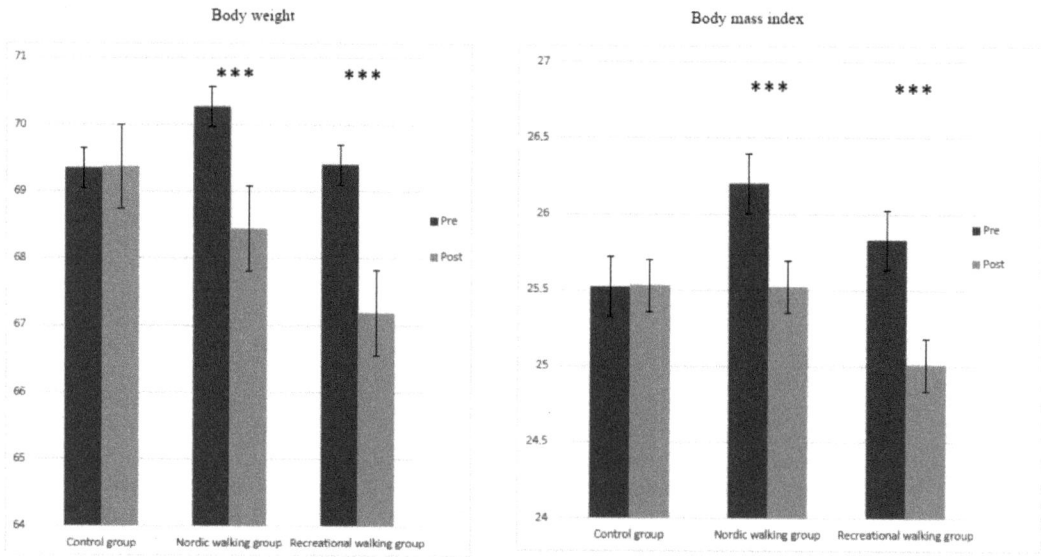

Figure 2. Differences in body weight and body mass index at pretest and posttest interventions in the three studied groups. *** $p < 0.001$.

The mean data of walking HR (F = 62.94, $p < 0.001$, $\eta^2 = 0.28$) and the HR at the end of the UKK walking test (F = 82.59, $p < 0.001$, $\eta^2 = 0.31$) determined by a mixed-design ANOVA revealed a significant main effect of participant groups (control, RW and NW). The interaction between group and pretest–posttest intervention showed a significant effect in walking HR (F = 19.25, $p < 0.001$, $\eta^2 = 0.19$) and the HR at the end of the test (F = 21.77, $p < 0.001$, $\eta^2 = 0.21$). The HR at the end of the test showed differences between the pretest and posttest (RW group, $t = 8.99$, $p < 0.001$; NW group, $t = 4.45$, $p < 0.001$), while the walking HR during the test also showed significant differences (RW group, $t = 5.90$, $p < 0.001$; NW group, $t = 5.60$, $p < 0.001$) (Figure 3).

The mean data of UKK total time (F = 183.01, $p < 0.001$, $\eta^2 <= 0.53$) and UKK fitness index (F = 132.81, $p < 0.001$, $\eta^2 <= 0.45$) determined by a mixed-design ANOVA revealed a significant main effect of participant groups (control, RW and NW). The interaction between group and pretest–posttest intervention showed a significant effect in UKK total time (F = 47.55, $p < 0.001$, $\eta^2 <= 0.36$) and UKK fitness index (F = 33.55, $p < 0.001$, $\eta^2 <= 0.29$). The significant differences between before and after 12 weeks of intervention in terms of UKK test measurements are shown in Figure 4—namely, UKK total time (RW group, $t = 13.03$, $p < 0.001$; NW group, $t = 8.29$, $p < 0.001$) and UKK fitness index (RW group, $t = -6.79$, $p < 0.001$; NW group, $t = -6.41$, $p < 0.001$).

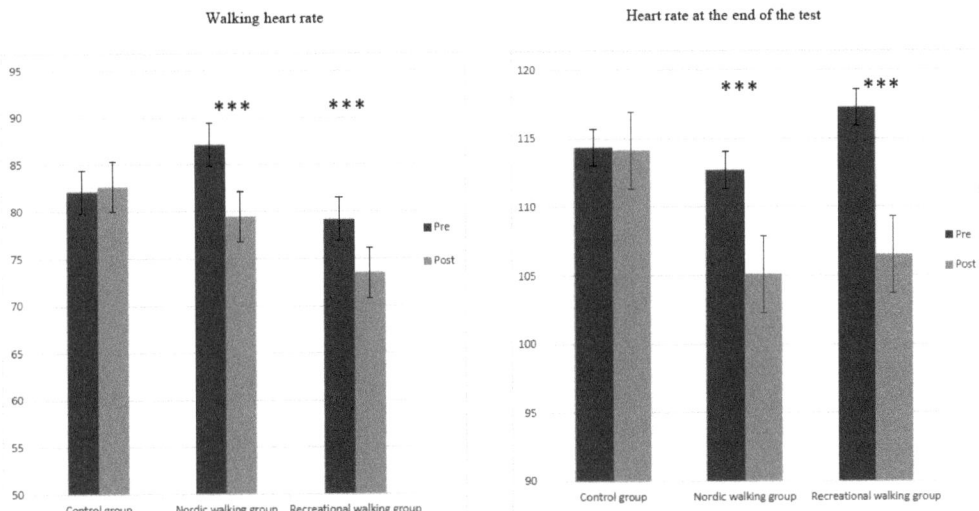

Figure 3. Differences in walking heart rate and heart rate at the end of the test in pretest and posttest interventions in the three studied groups. *** $p < 0.001$.

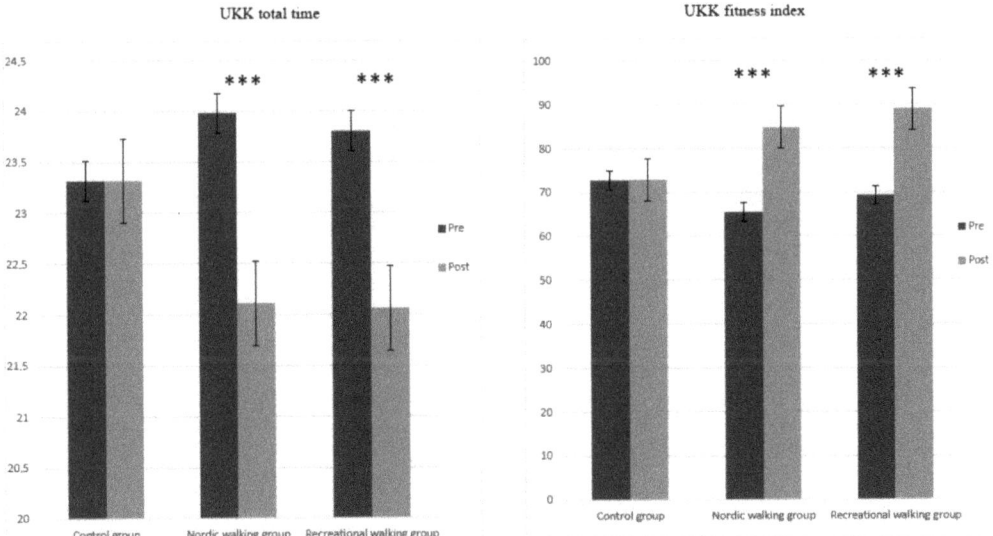

Figure 4. Differences in UKK total time and UKK fitness index in pretest and posttest interventions in the three studied groups. *** $p < 0.001$.

Finally, the results of the mixed-design ANOVA for VO$_2$max (F = 230.89, $p < 0.001$, $\eta^2 <= 0.58$) showed the significant main effect of participant groups (control, RW, and NW). The interaction between groups and pretest–posttest intervention also showed a significant effect in VO$_2$max (F = 60.91, $p < 0.001$, $\eta^2 <= 0.43$). Figure 5 shows significant differences in VO$_2$max between pretest and posttest in the RW group ($t = -14.36$, $p < 0.001$) and the NW group ($t = -9.40$, $p < 0.001$). The control group showed no significant differences between pretest and posttest interventions in any variable studied.

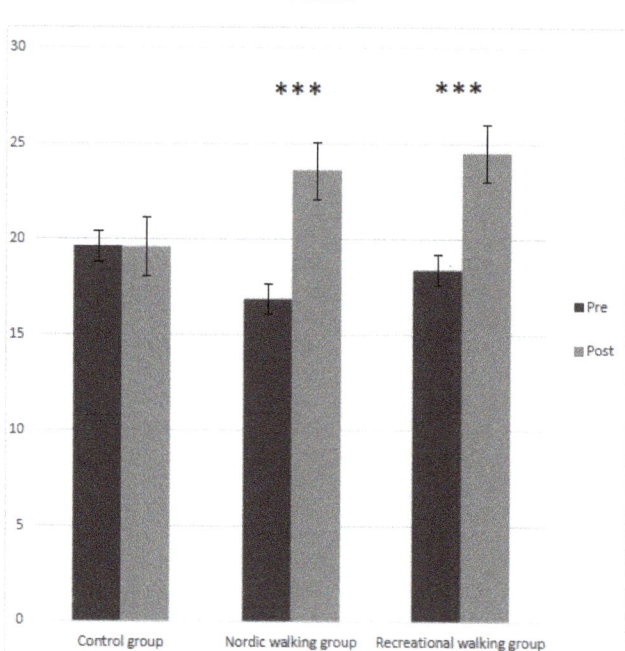

Figure 5. Differences in VO$_2$max in pretest and posttest interventions in the three studied groups. *** $p < 0.001$.

4. Discussion

The objective of the present study was to examine the effects of a 12-week intervention in three groups (control, RW, and NW groups) on anthropometric measurement variables (body mass and BMI), HR variables (walking HR and HR at the end of the test), UKK test measurements (total time and fitness index), and VO$_2$max in older adult women. Given the specific nature of exercise adaptations and the need to maintain muscle mass, muscle strength, and flexibility throughout life, and even more in the ageing process, a comprehensive training programme consisting of resistance, aerobic, and flexibility exercises is recommended [4]. NW can improve muscle strength and flexibility, as well as aerobic endurance capability [35]. Likewise, RW, together with a muscular strength programme, can produce the same improvements as the NW discipline, because the disciplines do not differ considerably [29]. The main finding of this study showed that NW group training resulted in slightly greater benefits than RW group training; nevertheless, both were shown to be valid modalities to improve the functionality and quality of life of people during the ageing process.

In regard to the variable of walking HR, we found that the lowest mean was presented by the RW group, followed by NW. In accordance with a recent systematic review and meta-analysis carried out by Bullo et al. [34], these data contradict the majority of studies. These results could be due to the fact that it has been shown that healthy older adults can maintain their gait speed with or without poles, thus matching the physical demands required [36]. The same results were found in a study by Takeshima et al. [33]. Both disciplines showed improvements after the training programme. These data are in line with those found for participants of the same age range in the literature [28] or for those registered in control groups of physical training programmes [37], which confirms favourable results in the experimental groups of this study. We observed that, after the intervention, RW produced better values than NW in terms of walking HR and HR at the end of the test; NW values were also significant and showed improvements very similar to those of the RW modality. These data are in accordance with those found by Gomeñuka et al. [35], in which the NW discipline did not result in greater benefits than RW related to participants' quality of life.

As expected, the improvements in the average walking HR were greater in the NW group than in the RW group at the end of the program. These data could be explained by the fact that NW increases the activity (muscular) of the upper part of the body during practice and, with it, the energy expenditure with higher oxygen consumption [38]. If we compare our results with the findings of Pellegrini et al. [28], it can be deduced that NW group participants of the present study showed lower bt/min during the 2 km test. However, in a study by Sugiyama et al. [42], participants were evaluated for 5 km, whereas we studied only 2 km. Therefore, increases in both strength and aerobic capacity contribute to the reduction in submaximal HR when NW and RW are performed at the same walking speed [39]. In the present study, UKK total time was similar for both disciplines. Regarding the variable HR at the end of the test, the NW group presented the best average. In a similar way, we found comparable results for RW, elucidating how both modalities generated improvements in the reduction in mean beats per minute at the end of the programme [35]. Similar improvements were shown for the rest of the variables described above and below (HR, fitness index, and VO_2max).

NW and RW are two aerobic activities capable of improving anthropometric measurement through the ageing process, and a 12-week programme using these two modalities, such as that used in the present study, results in significant changes in terms of body mass loss and BMI [41,43]. Although both exercise disciplines showed comparable results, we found that RW produced slightly better results than NW in body mass and BMI after 12 weeks of intervention. According to a study by Figard-Fabre et al. [44], even with a correct NW technique, the difference in energy expenditure is not greater than that in RW. This minimal difference in energy expenditure could explain how RW obtained slightly better results in the current study, underlining that NW has also shown improvements in this regard. These results are not in line with the fact that energy expenditure is higher in the NW pattern, and this would mean a greater body mass loss [28,45].

Given the nature of the NW modality, gait speed is greater with the use of poles versus walking without any help [46]. Although the time to complete the activity was similar, the RW group presented a slightly shorter time. This is consonant with data found by Gomeñuka et al. [35] and contrary to what is found in other studies [31,33,46]. This could be explained by the fact that if the poles do not push the ground in the correct way for the propulsion of the movement, the dynamic stability is impaired; thus, the movement is not as efficient and fast, requiring more time to complete a given distance [47].

In the final measurement, UKK fitness level and VO_2max showed slightly higher values in the RW group compared with the NW group, which points to a greater improvement in functional capacities in the former group, compared with the control group. This increase was manifested as an improved UKK fitness level, increased general cardiorespiratory capacity, and higher percentages of VO_2max, which were considered the best indicators of lung capacity and air intake. A study by Pellegrini et al. [46] reported NW and RW as acceptable forms of exercise for the ageing population regardless of their VO_2max. The results found in this study would contradict those shown in the literature, since, as previously described, NW generally showed higher energy expenditure and, with it, the expectation that UKK fitness level and VO_2max values should also be higher in this group [46]. These data could be explained by the fact that if participants' NW technique was incorrect, resulting in a weak NW style instead of the suggested technique, this could decrease the effectiveness of the training programme [28]. Hansen and Smith [48] found that when participants are taught to perform a particularly energetic NW technique, characterised by long strides and pole pushes, oxygen consumption exceeds that measured during walking, by up to 67%. In contrast, in line with the findings of the present study, NW and RW showed similar results, which can be explained by the fact that both modalities share muscle synergies that mainly involve the activation of the muscles of the lower extremities and the trunk.

Therefore, walking with the use of poles does not produce considerable changes in the muscular demands of the lower body [31].

If each modality and variable is analysed separately, NW produced greater improvements with respect to RW. In a study carried out by Mikalački et al. [49], in which they evaluated the effects of a 12-week NW programme on functional capacities using the UKK test, results showed improvements in UKK fitness values, which is consistent with our findings. Other studies on NW have shown that VO_2max increases at the end of the intervention [34,50], which is also consistent with our study, showing significant results for NW training in the variables mentioned above.

The outcomes of this study support NW as a secure, viable, and helpful form of physical training that can improve several components of fitness in older adults. RW also has a multitude of other documented benefits, and it is often used as a primary and secondary preventive alternative to PE [4]. Both RW and NW can be performed by individuals or in groups, which may provide social well-being benefits. Additionally, although NW is often performed outdoors, it can also be practised indoors with the use of rubber-tipped poles, turning it into an activity that can be accomplished all year round, even during adverse weather conditions [33]. NW appears to be more effective in providing more cardiorespiratory fitness benefits, compared with RW. Consequently, NW may be more effective than RW in improving and maintaining the overall health and function of adults in the ageing process [51]. Therefore, it is important to know the benefits of both modalities, and it would be convenient to carry out future research in different segments of the older adult population and during longer intervention periods.

In terms of limitations, the present study shows its potential due to the lack of related studies that have compared NW and RW in this population group. On the one hand, the intervention time of 12 weeks should be extended in future research to obtain more significant results, especially in physiological variables and time spent covering the distance of the UKK test. On the other hand, far from being a constraint, the Nordic-walking technique of participants was controlled during the study and supervised by physical exercise specialists. In fact, participants' individual physical limitations were considered in controlling for the range and intensity of the exercise.

Another variable that could have completed the study would have been to evaluate muscular grip strength and, thus, be able to explain the possible adaptations in terms of upper body strength and physiological changes. Regarding the different groups and the modalities used, it is worth highlighting the need to expand the given consideration to the technique when using poles in NW. Additionally, in the context of control, it would be advisable to control the dietary intake of study participants; if the decrease in body mass is to be taken into account, diet is one of the variables most affected. Likewise, evaluating the improvements in the anthropometric measurement of the participants should include changes in the different variables through electrical bioimpedance.

5. Conclusions

The novelty of this study lies in its comparative results between NW and RW interventions for older adults and, with it, guiding healthy alternatives to improve the quality of life and health in the ageing process. The main findings revealed that, after 12 weeks, NW training resulted in slightly greater benefits than RW training; nevertheless, both were shown to be valid modalities to improve the functionality and quality of life of people during the ageing process.

Moreover, our study suggested that the NW technique is a beneficial training method for improving the physical condition of healthy older adults. The practice of the NW and RW modalities represents an optimal continuity of kinesiological activity, particularly in older adults, to maintain and improve their functional capabilities. The present study showed that 12 weeks of Nordic walking and recreational walking improved HR variables, UKK test measurements, and VO_2max. In fact, this research highlighted the clinical importance of chronic exercise and its considerably positive benefits on health and quality of everyday life. However, caution is required concerning participants' extensive use without the presence of specialists to control the individual training in older people.

Author Contributions: Conceptualisation, P.J.R.-M. and F.T.G.-F.; methodology, P.J.R.-M.; formal analysis, P.J.R.-M. and F.T.G.-F.; investigation, N.C. and P.J.R.-M.; resources, N.C.; data curation, P.J.R.-M.; writing—original draft preparation, P.J.R.-M.; writing—review and editing, P.J.R.-M., F.T.G.-F. and R.M.-M.; visualisation, P.J.R.-M., F.T.G.-F. and R.M.-M.; supervision, N.C. and R.M.-M.; project administration, N.C. All authors have read and agreed to the published version of the manuscript.

Funding: This research received no external funding.

Institutional Review Board Statement: This study was conducted in accordance with the Declaration of Helsinki and approved by the Ethics Committee of the University of Novi Sad (Serbia) (protocol code 46-06-03/2020-1 at 6 October 2020).

Informed Consent Statement: Informed consent was obtained from all subjects involved in the study. Written informed consent has been obtained from the patients to publish this paper.

Data Availability Statement: Not applicable.

Acknowledgments: The authors would like to thank the people who participated in the study for the extra time they spent with the test and questionnaires. All of them consented to the acknowledgement.

Conflicts of Interest: The authors declare no conflict of interest.

References

1. Seguin, R.; Lamonte, M.; Tinker, L.; Liu, J.; Woods, N.; Michael, Y.L.; Bushnell, C.; Lacroix, A.Z. Sedentary Behavior and Physical Function Decline in Older Women: Findings from the Women's Health Initiative. *J. Aging Res.* **2012**, *2012*, 271589. [CrossRef] [PubMed]
2. Manson, J.E.; Greenland, P.; LaCroix, A.Z.; Stefanick, M.L.; Mouton, C.P.; Oberman, A.; Perri, M.G.; Sheps, D.S.; Pettinger, M.B.; Siscovick, D.S. Walking Compared with Vigorous Exercise for the Prevention of Cardiovascular Events in Women. *N. Engl. J. Med.* **2002**, *347*, 716–725. [CrossRef] [PubMed]
3. Rader, D.J. Effect of Insulin Resistance, Dyslipidemia, and Intra-Abdominal Adiposity on the Development of Cardiovascular Disease and Diabetes Mellitus. *Am. J. Med.* **2007**, *120*, S12–S18. [CrossRef] [PubMed]
4. American College of Sports Medicine. *American College of Sports Medicine ACSM's Guidelines for Exercise Testing and Prescription*, 10th ed.; Wolters Kluwer Health: Philadelphia, PA, USA, 2018.
5. dos Santos, V.R.; Gobbo, L.A. Physical Activity Is Associated with Functional Capacity of Older Women with Osteosarcopenic Obesity: 24-Month Prospective Study. *Eur. J. Clin. Nutr.* **2020**, *74*, 912–919. [CrossRef]
6. Nelson, M.E.; Rejeski, W.J.; Blair, S.N.; Duncan, P.W.; Judge, J.O.; King, A.C.; Macera, C.A.; Castaneda-Sceppa, C. Physical Activity and Public Health in Older Adults: Recommendation from the American College of Sports Medicine and the American Heart Association. *Med. Sci. Sports Exerc.* **2007**, *39*, 1435–1445. [CrossRef]
7. Pepera, G.; Christina, M.; Katerina, K.; Argirios, P.; Varsamo, A. Effects of Multicomponent Exercise Training Intervention on Hemodynamic and Physical Function in Older Residents of Long-Term Care Facilities: A Multicenter Randomized Clinical Controlled Trial. *J. Bodyw. Mov. Ther.* **2021**, *28*, 231–237. [CrossRef]
8. Bey, L.; Hamilton, M.T. Suppression of Skeletal Muscle Lipoprotein Lipase Activity during Physical Inactivity: A Molecular Reason to Maintain Daily Low-Intensity Activity. *J. Physiol.* **2003**, *551*, 673–682. [CrossRef]
9. Bergamin, M.; Ermolao, A.; Tolomio, S.; Berton, L.; Sergi, G.; Zaccaria, M. Water- versus Land-Based Exercise in Elderly Subjects: Effects on Physical Performance and Body Composition. *Clin. Interv. Aging* **2013**, *8*, 1109–1117. [CrossRef]
10. Crombie, I.K.; Irvine, L.; Williams, B.; McGinnis, A.R.; Slane, P.W.; Alder, E.M.; McMurdo, M.E.T. Why Older People Do Not Participate in Leisure Time Physical Activity: A Survey of Activity Levels, Beliefs and Deterrents. *Age Ageing* **2004**, *33*, 287–292. [CrossRef]
11. Ruiz-Montero, P.J.; Castillo-Rodriguez, A.; Mikalački, M.; Nebojsa, Č.; Korovljev, D. 24-Weeks Pilates-Aerobic and Educative Training To Improve Body Fat Mass in Elderly Serbian Women. *Clin. Interv. Aging* **2014**, *9*, 243–248. [CrossRef]
12. García-Hermoso, A.; Ramirez-Vélez, R.; Sáez de Asteasu, M.L.; Martínez-Velilla, N.; Zambom-Ferraresi, F.; Valenzuela, P.L.; Lucia, A.; Izquierdo, M. Safety and Effectiveness of Long-Term Exercise Interventions in Older Adults: A Systematic Review and Meta-Analysis of Randomized Controlled Trials. *Sports Med.* **2020**, *50*, 1095–1106. [CrossRef] [PubMed]
13. Zheng, G.; Xia, R.; Zhou, W.; Tao, J.; Chen, L. Aerobic Exercise Ameliorates Cognitive Function in Older Adults with Mild Cognitive Impairment: A Systematic Review and Meta-Analysis of Randomised Controlled Trials. *Br. J. Sports Med.* **2016**, *50*, 1443–1450. [CrossRef]
14. Chase, J.A.D.; Phillips, L.J.; Brown, M. Physical Activity Intervention Effects on Physical Function among Community-Dwelling Older Adults: A Systematic Review and Meta-Analysis. *J. Aging Phys. Act.* **2017**, *25*, 149–170. [CrossRef] [PubMed]

15. Sherrington, C.; Michaleff, Z.A.; Fairhall, N.; Paul, S.S.; Tiedemann, A.; Whitney, J.; Cumming, R.G.; Herbert, R.D.; Close, J.C.T.; Lord, S.R. Exercise to Prevent Falls in Older Adults: An Updated Systematic Review and Meta-Analysis. *Br. J. Sports Med.* **2017**, *51*, 1750–1758. [CrossRef] [PubMed]
16. Paterson, D.H.; Warburton, D.E.R. Physical Activity and Functional Limitations in Older Adults: A Systematic Review Related to Canada's Physical Activity Guidelines. *Int. J. Behav. Nutr. Phys. Act.* **2010**, *7*, 1–22. [CrossRef]
17. He, Q.; Heo, M.; Heshka, S.; Wang, J.; Pierson, R.N.; Albu, J.; Wang, Z.; Heymsfield, S.B.; Gallagher, D. Total Body Potassium Differs by Sex and Race across the Adult Age Span. *Am. J. Clin. Nutr.* **2003**, *78*, 72–77. [CrossRef]
18. Poehlman, E.T.; Toth, M.J.; Fishman, P.S.; Vaitkevicius, P.; Gottlieb, S.S.; Fisher, M.L.; Fonong, T. Sarcopenia in Aging Humans: The Impact of Menopause and Disease. *J. Gerontology Ser. A Biol. Sci. Med. Sci.* **1995**, *50*, 73–77.
19. Katula, J.A.; Sipe, M.; Rejeski, W.J.; Focht, B.C. Strength Training in Older Adults: An Empowering Intervention. *Med. Sci. Sports Exerc.* **2006**, *38*, 106–111. [CrossRef]
20. Mankowski, R.T.; Anton, S.D.; Axtell, R.; Chen, S.H.; Fielding, R.A.; Glynn, N.W.; Hsu, F.C.; King, A.C.; Layne, A.S.; Leeuwenburgh, C.; et al. Device-Measured Physical Activity As a Predictor of Disability in Mobility-Limited Older Adults. *J. Am. Geriatr. Soc.* **2017**, *65*, 2251–2256. [CrossRef]
21. Kim, C.H.; Wheatley, C.M.; Behnia, M.; Johnson, B.D. The Effect of Aging on Relationships between Lean Body Mass and VO2max in Rowers. *PLoS ONE* **2016**, *11*, e0160275. [CrossRef]
22. Fisher, G.; McCarthy, J.P.; Zuckerman, P.A.; Bryan, D.R.; Bickel, C.S.; Hunter, G.R. Frequency of Combined Resistance and Aerobic Training in Older Women. *J. Strength Cond. Res.* **2013**, *27*, 1868–1876. [CrossRef]
23. Campbell, E.; Petermann-Rocha, F.; Welsh, P.; Celis-Morales, C.; Pell, J.P.; Ho, F.K.; Gray, S.R. The Effect of Exercise on Quality of Life and Activities of Daily Life in Frail Older Adults: A Systematic Review of Randomised Control Trials. *Exp. Gerontol.* **2021**, *147*, 111287. [CrossRef] [PubMed]
24. Morente-Oria, H.; Jesus Ruiz-Montero, P.; Chiva-Bartoll, O.; Tomas Gonzalez-Fernandez, F. Effects of 8-Weeks Concurrent Strength and Aerobic Training on Body Composition, Physiological and Cognitive Performance in Older Adult Women. *Sustainability* **2020**, *12*, 1944. [CrossRef]
25. Suni, J.; Husu, P.; Rinne, M. *Fitness for Health: The ALPHA-FIT Test. Battery for Adults Aged 18–69. Tester's Manual*; European Union DS: Tampere, Finland; UKK Institute for Health Promotion Research: Tampere, Finland, 2009.
26. Jantunen, H.; Wasenius, N.; Salonen, M.K.; Perälä, M.M.; Osmond, C.; Kautiainen, H.; Simonen, M.; Pohjolainen, P.; Kajantie, E.; Rantanen, T.; et al. Objectively Measured Physical Activity and Physical Performance in Old Age. *Age Ageing* **2017**, *46*, 232–237. [CrossRef] [PubMed]
27. Gobbo, S.; Bullo, V.; Roma, E.; Duregon, F.; Bocalini, D.S.; Rica, R.L.; Di Blasio, A.; Cugusi, L.; Vendramin, B.; Bergamo, M.; et al. Nordic Walking Promoted Weight Lost in Overweight and Obese People: A Systematic Review for Future Exercise Prescription. *J. Funct. Morphol. Kinesiol.* **2019**, *4*, 36. [CrossRef]
28. Pellegrini, B.; Boccia, G.; Zoppirolli, C.; Rosa, R.; Stella, F.; Bortolan, L.; Rainoldi, A.; Schena, F. Muscular and Metabolic Responses to Different Nordic Walking Techniques, When Style Matters. *PLoS ONE* **2018**, *13*, e0195438. [CrossRef]
29. Notthoff, N.; Carstensen, L.L. Positive Messaging Promotes Walking in Older Adults. *Psychol. Aging* **2014**, *29*, 329–341. [CrossRef]
30. Ogawa, K.; Oka, J.; Yamakawa, J.; Higuchi, M. A Single Bout of Exercise Influences Natural Killer Cells in Elderly Women, Especially Those Who Are Habitually Active. *J. Strength Cond. Res.* **2005**, *19*, 45–50. [CrossRef]
31. Tschentscher, M.; Niederseer, D.; Niebauer, J. Health Benefits of Nordic Walking: A Systematic Review. *Am. J. Prev. Med.* **2013**, *44*, 76–84. [CrossRef]
32. Boccia, G.; Zoppirolli, C.; Bortolan, L.; Schena, F.; Pellegrini, B. Shared and Task-Specific Muscle Synergies of Nordic Walking and Conventional Walking. *Scand. J. Med. Sci. Sports* **2018**, *28*, 905–918. [CrossRef]
33. Takeshima, N.; Islam, M.M.; Rogers, M.E.; Rogers, N.L.; Sengoku, N.; Koizumi, D.; Kitabayashi, Y.; Imai, A.; Naruse, A. Effects of Nordic Walking Compared to Conventional Walking and Band-Based Resistance Exercise on Fitness in Older Adults. *J. Sports Sci. Med.* **2013**, *12*, 422–430. [PubMed]
34. Bullo, V.; Gobbo, S.; Vendramin, B.; Duregon, F.; Cugusi, L.; di Blasio, A.; Bocalini, D.S.; Zaccaria, M.; Bergamin, M.; Ermolao, A. Nordic Walking Can Be Incorporated in the Exercise Prescription to Increase Aerobic Capacity, Strength, and Quality of Life for Elderly: A Systematic Review and Meta-Analysis. *Rejuvenation Res.* **2018**, *21*, 141–161. [CrossRef] [PubMed]
35. Gomeñuka, N.A.; Oliveira, H.B.; Silva, E.S.; Costa, R.R.; Kanitz, A.C.; Liedtke, G.V.; Schuch, F.B.; Peyré-Tartaruga, L.A. Effects of Nordic Walking Training on Quality of Life, Balance and Functional Mobility in Elderly: A Randomized Clinical Trial. *PLoS ONE* **2019**, *14*, e0211472. [CrossRef] [PubMed]
36. Cugusi, L.; Manca, A.; Yeo, T.J.; Bassareo, P.P.; Mercuro, G.; Kaski, J.C. Nordic Walking for Individuals with Cardiovascular Disease: A Systematic Review and Meta-Analysis of Randomized Controlled Trials. *Eur. J. Prev. Cardiol.* **2017**, *24*, 1938–1955. [CrossRef]
37. Vardeman, S.; Hamburg, M.; Zuwaylif, F.H. Basic Statistics, A Modern Approach. *J. Am. Stat. Assoc.* **1980**, *75*, 2287210. [CrossRef]
38. Ojala, K. *UKK Walk Test. Tester's Guide*, 4th ed.; UKK Institute for Health Promotion Research: Tampere, Finland, 2013.
39. Beam, W.C.; Adams, G.M. *Exercise Physiology. Laboratory Manual*, 7th ed.; McGraw-Hill: New York, NY, USA, 2014.
40. Sawilowsky, S.S. New Effect Size Rules of Thumb. *J. Mod. Appl. Stat. Methods* **2009**, *8*, 26. [CrossRef]
41. Panou, H.; Giovanis, V.; Tsougos, E.; Angelidis, G. Influence of the Nordic Walking Intervention Program on the Improvement of Functional Parameters in Older Women. *Top. Geriatr. Rehabil.* **2019**, *35*, 129–133. [CrossRef]

42. Sugiyama, K.; Kawamura, M.; Tomita, H.; Katamoto, S. Oxygen Uptake, Heart Rate, Perceived Exertion, and Integrated Electromyogram of the Lower and Upper Extremities during Level and Nordic Walking on a Treadmill. *J. Physiol. Anthropol.* **2013**, *32*, 2. [CrossRef]
43. Beauchet, O.; Annweiler, C.; Lecordroch, Y.; Allali, G.; Dubost, V.; Herrmann, F.R.; Kressig, R.W. Walking Speed-Related Changes in Stride Time Variability: Effects of Decreased Speed. *J. NeuroEngineering Rehabil.* **2009**, *6*, 32. [CrossRef]
44. Figard-Fabre, H.; Fabre, N.; Leonardi, A.; Schena, F. Physiological and Perceptual Responses to Nordic Walking in Obese Middle-Aged Women in Comparison with the Normal Walk. *Eur. J. Appl. Physiol.* **2010**, *108*, 1141–1151. [CrossRef]
45. Sanchez-Lastra, M.A.; Miller, K.J.; Martinez-Lemos, R.I.; Giraldez, A.; Ayan, C. Nordic Walking for Overweight and Obese People: A Systematic Review and Meta-Analysis. *J. Phys. Act. Health* **2020**, *17*, 762–772. [CrossRef] [PubMed]
46. Pellegrini, B.; Peyré-Tartaruga, L.A.; Zoppirolli, C.; Bortolan, L.; Bacchi, E.; Figard-Fabre, H.; Schena, F. Exploring Muscle Activation during Nordic Walking: A Comparison between Conventional and Uphill Walking. *PLoS ONE* **2015**, *10*, e0138906. [CrossRef] [PubMed]
47. Schiffer, T.; Knicker, A.; Montanarella, M.; Strüder, H.K. Mechanical and Physiological Effects of Varying Pole Weights during Nordic Walking Compared to Walking. *Eur. J. Appl. Physiol.* **2011**, *111*, 1121–1126. [CrossRef] [PubMed]
48. Hansen, E.A.; Smith, G. Energy Expenditure and Comfort During Nordic Walking With Different Pole Lengths. *J. Strength Cond. Res.* **2009**, *23*, 1187–1194. [CrossRef]
49. Mikalacki, M.; Cokorilo, N.; Katić, R. Effect of Nordic Walking on Functional Ability and Blood Pressure in Elderly Women. *Coll. Antropol.* **2011**, *35*, 889–894.
50. Kukkonen-Harjula, K.; Hiilloskorpi, H.; Mänttäri, A.; Pasanen, M.; Parkkari, J.; Suni, J.; Fogelholm, M.; Laukkanen, R. Self-Guided Brisk Walking Training with or without Poles: A Randomized-Controlled Trial in Middle-Aged Women. *Scandinavian J. Med. Sci. Sports* **2007**, *17*, 316–323. [CrossRef]
51. Pérez-Soriano, P.; Encarnación-Martínez, A.; Aparicio-Aparicio, I.; Giménez, J.; Llana-Belloch, S. Nordic Walking: A Systematic Review. *Eur. J. Hum. Mov.* **2014**, *33*, 26–45.

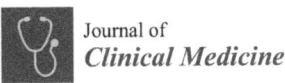

Article

Measurement of Lipid Peroxidation Products and Creatine Kinase in Blood Plasma and Saliva of Athletes at Rest and following Exercise

Aleksandr N. Ovchinnikov [1,2,*], Antonio Paoli [2,3], Vladislav V. Seleznev [4] and Anna V. Deryugina [2,5]

1. Department of Sports Medicine and Psychology, Lobachevsky University, 603022 Nizhny Novgorod, Russia
2. Laboratory of Integral Human Health, Lobachevsky University, 603022 Nizhny Novgorod, Russia; antonio.paoli@unipd.it (A.P.); derugina69@yandex.ru (A.V.D.)
3. Department of Biomedical Sciences, University of Padova, 35122 Padova, Italy
4. Department of Theory and Methodology of Sport Training, Lobachevsky University, 603022 Nizhny Novgorod, Russia; vseleznev92@mail.ru
5. Department of Physiology and Anatomy, Lobachevsky University, 603022 Nizhny Novgorod, Russia
* Correspondence: alexander_ovchinnikov91@mail.ru

Abstract: This study aimed to assess the agreement between quantitative measurements of plasmatic and salivary biomarkers capable of identifying oxidative stress and muscle damage in athletes at rest and following exercise. Thirty-nine high-level athletes participating in track and field (running), swimming or rowing were recruited and assigned to one of three groups depending on the sport. Each athlete group underwent its specific exercise. Blood and saliva samples were collected before and immediately after the exercise. Diene conjugates (DC), triene conjugates (TC), Schiff bases (SB), and creatine kinase (CK) were measured. Comparisons were made using Wilcoxon signed-rank test. Correlation analysis and Bland–Altman method were applied. DC levels were elevated in plasma ($p < 0.01$) and saliva ($p < 0.01$) in response to exercise in all three groups, as were the plasmatic ($p < 0.01$) and salivary ($p < 0.01$) TC and SB concentrations. CK activity was also significantly higher at postexercise compared to pre-exercise in both plasma ($p < 0.01$) and saliva ($p < 0.01$) in all groups. Strong positive correlation between salivary and plasmatic DC ($p < 0.001$), TC ($p < 0.001$), SB ($p < 0.01$), and CK ($p < 0.001$) was observed at rest and following exercise in each athlete group. The bias calculated for DC, TC, SB, and CK using the Bland–Altman statistics was not significant at both pre-exercise and postexercise in all three groups. The line of equality was within the confidence interval of the mean difference. All of the data points lay within the respective agreement limits. Salivary concentrations of DC, TC, SB, and CK are able to reliably reflect their plasma levels.

Keywords: saliva; blood plasma; oxidative stress; lipid peroxidation products; muscle damage; creatine kinase; exercise; athletes

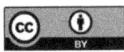

1. Introduction

Accurate monitoring of oxidative stress and muscle damage caused by exercise is essential in sports and exercise medicine [1]. Recently, the use of saliva has been carefully considered and examined as an attractive option for the assessment of oxidative stress and muscle damage in exercise science due to its non-invasive nature and analyte availability compared to blood analysis [2–15]. Saliva availability allows for the collection of multiple specimens, including continuous supply during each training session, which is not possible with blood sampling [1]. These beneficial aspects of saliva make possible the early recognition of excessive adverse effects induced by exercise.

Additional advantage of saliva over blood collection can be attributed to the simplicity of collection device. Blood sampling requires sample tubes containing clot-activating factors, anti-coagulating and ligand-binding compounds to safely collect and stabilize blood components, while saliva collection simply involves a sterilized tube [4]. Importantly, saliva sampling allows for reduced risk of cross-contamination and personalized timing of sample collection, which does not require a phlebotomist for obtaining a sample [1,14]. Furthermore, blood collection is associated with pain, which may affect secretion of stress hormones. This becomes especially important in studies quantifying oxidative stress following exercise that may lead to false-positive results and overestimation of exercise-induced disruption in redox control.

Concentrations of salivary biomarkers such as cortisol, testosterone, alpha-amylase, glucose, lactate, uric acid, and secretory immunoglobulins have been reported to reliably reflect serum levels [2,4,16–22]. Despite these advances, salivary biomarkers that are capable of providing accurate information regarding exercise-induced oxidant stress and muscle damage remain to be established. Containing a variety of enzymes, hormones, proteins and lipids, saliva is a potentially ideal medium for the assessment of oxidative stress and muscle damage imposed by the exercise. The most commonly used salivary biomarkers that relate to oxidant stress are thiobarbituric acid reactive substances (TBARS), in particular malondialdehyde (MDA) [1,11,12]. MDA, which is well known, is an intermediate product of lipid peroxidation, and its level cannot give an accurate estimation of the lipid peroxidation process. In addition, only certain lipid peroxidation products generate MDA, and MDA is neither the sole end product of fatty peroxide formation and decomposition, nor a substance generated exclusively through lipid peroxidation. Therefore, the use of MDA analysis and/or the TBA test, as well as interpretation of sample MDA content and TBA test response in studies of lipid peroxidation, require caution, discretion, and correlative data from other indices of fatty peroxide formation and decomposition, especially in biological systems [23]. However, the above-mentioned limitations to use MDA do not apply to some other products of lipid peroxidation such as diene conjugates (DC), triene conjugates (TC) and Schiff bases (SB), which together may provide a reliable indication of oxidative stress. DC are one of the main primary products of lipid peroxidation that refer to two double bonds separated by a single bond [24,25]. TC, in turn, are also alkenes but with three double bonds separated by a single bond in a molecule that can be formed as secondary products during lipid peroxidation [25]. Despite their relative stability compared with free radicals, the chemical structure of DC and TC makes these electrophilic molecules highly reactive [26]. Thus, to better understand the lipid peroxidation rates, it is necessary to also measure the end products of lipid peroxidation with a relatively high stability. The major end product that is derived from the oxidation of arachidonic acid and larger polyunsaturated fatty acids through enzymatic or nonenzymatic processes is α, β-unsaturated aldehyde 4-hydroxynonenal (4-HNE) [26,27]. However, 4-HNE has an extraordinary reactivity that relies upon both the Michael addition of thiol or amino compounds on the C3 of the C2=C3 double bond and the SB formation between the C1 carbonyl group and primary amines [27]. Despite slow and reversible kinetics of SB formation, SB are relatively more stable products than their direct precursor. The advantage over Michael-adducts, and the biggest, is that SB as well as DC and TC are able to be detected by means of simple UV spectrophotometry in both blood plasma and saliva, including under exercise conditions [28]. Collectively, it could make DC, TC and SB predominant to quantify exercise-induced lipid peroxidation and thus oxidative stress.

There is growing evidence that excessive accumulation of toxic lipid peroxidation products during exercise can lead to damage of cellular components in damaged muscle after exercise, what is reflected by increased plasma and saliva levels of soluble muscle enzymes such as creatine kinase (CK) [28–31]. Consequently, elevated CK activity in saliva following exercise may also be considered as a sign of exercise-induced muscle damage.

There is no study that has evaluated the agreement between quantitative measurements of plasmatic and salivary biomarkers capable of identifying oxidant stress and muscle damage in athletes under exercise conditions. Our aim was to assess the agreement between quantitative measurements of plasmatic and salivary DC, TC, SB, and CK at rest and following exercise. Since exercise has been reported to induce similar pattern of antioxidant response in both blood plasma and saliva [13], as well as the corresponding changes in plasmatic and salivary CK activities [32,33], we hypothesize that salivary DC, TC, SB, and CK could accurately represent plasma concentrations in athletes participating in different sports under special exercise conditions.

2. Materials and Methods

2.1. Subjects

Thirty nine high-level athletes (sex: Male; age: 19.6 ± 1.1 years; height: 173.3 ± 2.5 cm; body mass: 63.7 ± 2.1 kg; body mass index: 21.2 ± 0.6 kg/m^2), i.e., athletes who bear qualification in accordance with the Unified Russian Sports Classification System: winners and/or prize-winners of national sports events and international sports events, were recruited from the Olympic Reserve Center (Nizhny Novgorod, Russia) through advertising directly to coaches. Exclusion criteria for all subjects were chronic use of any medication, ingestion of antioxidant supplements, periodontal disease, respiratory infection, and orthopedic injury (sprain, contusion, or fracture within 14 days of enrollment). Each subject participated in one of the three kinds of sports (track and field (running), swimming, rowing) for at least 5 years and thus was assigned to one of three groups depending on the sport. Anthropometric baseline characteristics of subjects are shown in Table 1.

Table 1. Baseline characteristics of athletes.

	Runners	Swimmers	Rowers
Age (years)	19.7 ± 1.2	19.4 ± 1.0	19.6 ± 1.0
Height (cm)	173.2 ± 3.1	173.7 ± 1.3	173.0 ± 3.0
Body mass (kg)	63.4 ± 1.7	64.6 ± 2.4	63.0 ± 2.3
BMI (kg/m^2)	21.2 ± 0.5	21.4 ± 0.6	21.0 ± 0.6

Values are mean ± SD.

Before any procedures, informed written consent was obtained from each of the participants. The study was conducted in accordance with the Declaration of Helsinki and was approved by the Bioethics Committee of Lobachevsky University (approval number: 43) [34].

2.2. Study Design

After signing the informed consent and two weeks before exercise testing, the participants were invited to refer to the Integral Human Health Laboratory of the Faculty of Physical Education and Sport of Lobachevsky University. During the visit, the athletes underwent medical screening and food interview to ensure eligibility for the study and to gather information on the subjects' dietary habits. Participants were instructed to maintain their usual diet two weeks before the exercise testing. Subjects were also instructed to have breakfast one hour before the training session and refrain from consuming alcohol and caffeinated beverages for at least 24 h before exercise testing. Adherence to study medications was assessed by a qualified dietician with a face-to-face interview.

Each athlete group kept a typical training routine, which was the same for all participants depending on the sport. The group of swimmers comprised short-distance athletes (100 m). Swimmers underwent high-intensity interval exercise (HIIE), which consisted of 4 sets of 50 m distance in their preferred swimming style at the top-most speed interspersed with 45 s of recovery periods in a 25 m swimming pool. The group of runners included only sprinters (100–200 m). Runners underwent their specific HIIE on a 400 m outdoor track of stadium. HIIE protocol applied to the runners consisted of 3 repetitions of 100 m distance at the top-most speed interspersed with 45 s of recovery time. The group of rowers comprised middle-distance rowers specialized in 2000 m. High-intensity continuous exercise (HICE), consisting of 2000 m distance, was performed by rowers at the top-most speed using a rowing ergometer (Concept2, Morristown, VT, USA). Each exercise protocol was selected due to its widespread use in the training process among categories of athletes participated in the study. Exercise testing was performed in the morning. Subjects were examined before and immediately after exercise for blood and saliva sample collection, followed by measurements of oxidative stress and muscle damage biomarkers.

2.3. Measurement of Exercise Performance

Runners underwent HIIE consisting of 3 sets of 100 m distance with 45 s rest between the sets. The aim of the test was to complete each set in the shortest possible time. Results were determined by the time taken to complete each set with the subsequent calculation of mean. Timing was recorded using a stopwatch from the start signal until the runner crossed the finish line.

Swimmers underwent HIIE consisting of 4 sets of 50 m distance with 45 s rest between the sets. The aim of the test was to complete each set in the shortest possible time. Results were determined by the time taken to complete each set with the subsequent calculation of mean. Timing was recorded using a stopwatch from the start signal until the swimmer touched the wall to finish. Due to the lack of uniformity requirement for swimming style, in order to unify the results of swimmers, average time to overcome a distance of 50 m by the preferred stroke was converted into the corresponding number of points according to a single assessment system developed and approved by the International Swimming Federation (FINA points).

Rowers underwent HICE consisting of 2000 m distance. The aim of the test was to cover the distance in the shortest possible time. Results were determined by the time taken to overcome the distance. Timing was recorded using a stopwatch from the start signal until the rower overcame the 2000 m.

2.4. Sample Collection

Blood from the median cubital vein (approximately 4 mL per collection) was collected and placed in EDTA-coated tubes by a qualified phlebotomist using standardized venipuncture techniques. Saliva samples were collected into the plastic conical centrifuge tubes by a spitting method without stimulation for 3 min. Athletes rinsed their mouth with water before saliva sampling. Subjects were also instructed to swallow the remaining water in the oral cavity and to wait a minute before saliva collection. Blood and saliva samples were taken no more than 5 min before exercise (at rest) and immediately after the exercise. All collection procedures were performed in the morning. Blood and saliva samples were centrifuged at 3000 rpm for 15 min, and supernatant was aliquoted. All samples were stored at $-40\,°C$ until analysis.

2.5. Measurement of Lipid Peroxidation Products

DC, TC and SB were photometrically determined using spectrophotometer (SF 2000, Saint-Petersburg, Russian Federation). To obtain lipid extract, 0.5 mL of sample (plasma or saliva) was added to 8 mL of heptane–isopropanol mixture in a 1:1 ratio. Then, the sample and heptane–isopropanol mixture were stirred for 15 min and centrifuged at 3000 rpm for 15 min. Subsequently, 5 mL of heptane–isopropanol mixture was added to the lipid extract in a 3:7 ratio. To separate phases and remove non-lipid impurities, 2 mL of aqueous solution of HCl (0.01 N) was added. After phase separation, an upper (heptane) phase was transferred into a clean test tube. To dehydrate the isopropanol extract, 1 g of NaCl was added to a lower phase. Thereafter, the lower phase was transferred to a clean tube. Optical densities (E) were measured at the following wavelengths: 220 nm (absorption of isolated double bonds), 232 nm (absorption of DC), 278 nm (absorption of TC), and 400 nm (absorption of SB). Each phase was assessed against the corresponding control sample, which was prepared in the same way as the test, but distilled water was added instead of plasma or saliva. Sample concentrations of DC, TC and SB are presented as continuous variables and were calculated using standard equations (E232/E220 for calculating DC, E278/E220 for calculating TC, and E400/E220 for calculating SB, respectively) [3,25,28,31,35].

2.6. Measurement of Creatine Kinase Activity

CK activity was measured by enzymatic kinetic assay in the range of 1–1100 U/L on biochemical analyzer (Clima MC-15, RAL, Barcelona, Spain) using a CK-NAC DiaS reagent set (Hannover, Germany). When preparing a monoreagent, preheated (37 °C) reagent 1 and reagent 2 were mixed in a 4:1 ratio, respectively. Subsequently, 50 µL of sample (plasma or saliva) was added into a cuvette intended for the sample. Then, 500 µL of monoreagent was added into a cuvette intended for the reagent. Control cuvette was left blank, without reagents and sample. Preheated (37 °C) monoreagent and sample (plasma or saliva) were mixed in a 10:1 ratio. Enzyme activity was measured at 340 nm [3,28,31,33,35].

2.7. Statistical Analysis

Descriptive statistical analysis was carried out for all study variables. Data are presented as median and interquartile range (Me, 25th percentile and 75th percentile). Assumption of normality was verified using the Shapiro–Wilk test. Since not all data were normally distributed, comparisons were made using Wilcoxon signed-rank test for all study variables. Statistical relationships between plasmatic and salivary biomarkers at pre-exercise and postexercise were evaluated using Spearman's correlation coefficient (r_s). After ensuring that the differences between paired measurements of plasmatic and salivary biomarkers are normally distributed, Bland–Altman plot analysis was applied to assess the agreement between quantitative measurements of the same biomarkers in blood plasma and saliva. For all analyses, a p value < 0.05 was considered statistically significant. All statistical analyses were performed using RStudio, version 1.3.1093 for macOS (RStudio, PBC).

3. Results

All the recruited subjects successfully completed the study. Exercise performance of subjects is shown in Table 2.

Table 2. Exercise performance of athletes.

	HIIE (Runners)	HIIE (Swimmers)	HICE (Rowers)
Time to completion (s)	11.15 ± 0.14	-	-
FINA points (a.u.)	-	621.00 ± 34.23	-
Time to completion (min)	-	-	6.36 ± 0.04

Values are mean ± SD. HIIE: high-intensity interval exercise; HICE: high-intensity continuous exercise.

Measurements of DC, TC, SB, and CK concentrations in both blood plasma and saliva of athletes at rest and following exercise are presented in Figure 1.

The content of plasmatic and salivary DC, TC and SB significantly increased at postexercise compared to pre-exercise in all three groups. Plasmatic and salivary CK activities were also significantly elevated in response to exercise in each group of athletes.

Correlation between plasmatic and salivary concentrations of DC, TC, SB, and CK was evaluated at both pre-exercise and postexercise (Figure 2).

A strong positive correlation between salivary and plasmatic DC, TC and SB levels was observed at rest and following exercise in all groups. It was also verified to have a high positive correlation between plasmatic and salivary CK activities at both pre-exercise and postexercise in each athlete group.

Bland and Altman plots allowed us to demonstrate the difference between quantitative measurements of DC, TC, SB, and CK in blood plasma and saliva against the average of the measurements in two biological fluids. In relation to plasmatic and salivary DC concentrations at rest and following exercise, the bias was not significant in all groups because the line of equality was within the confidence interval of the mean difference. At the same time, all of the data points lay within ± 1.96 SD of the mean difference (Figure 3).

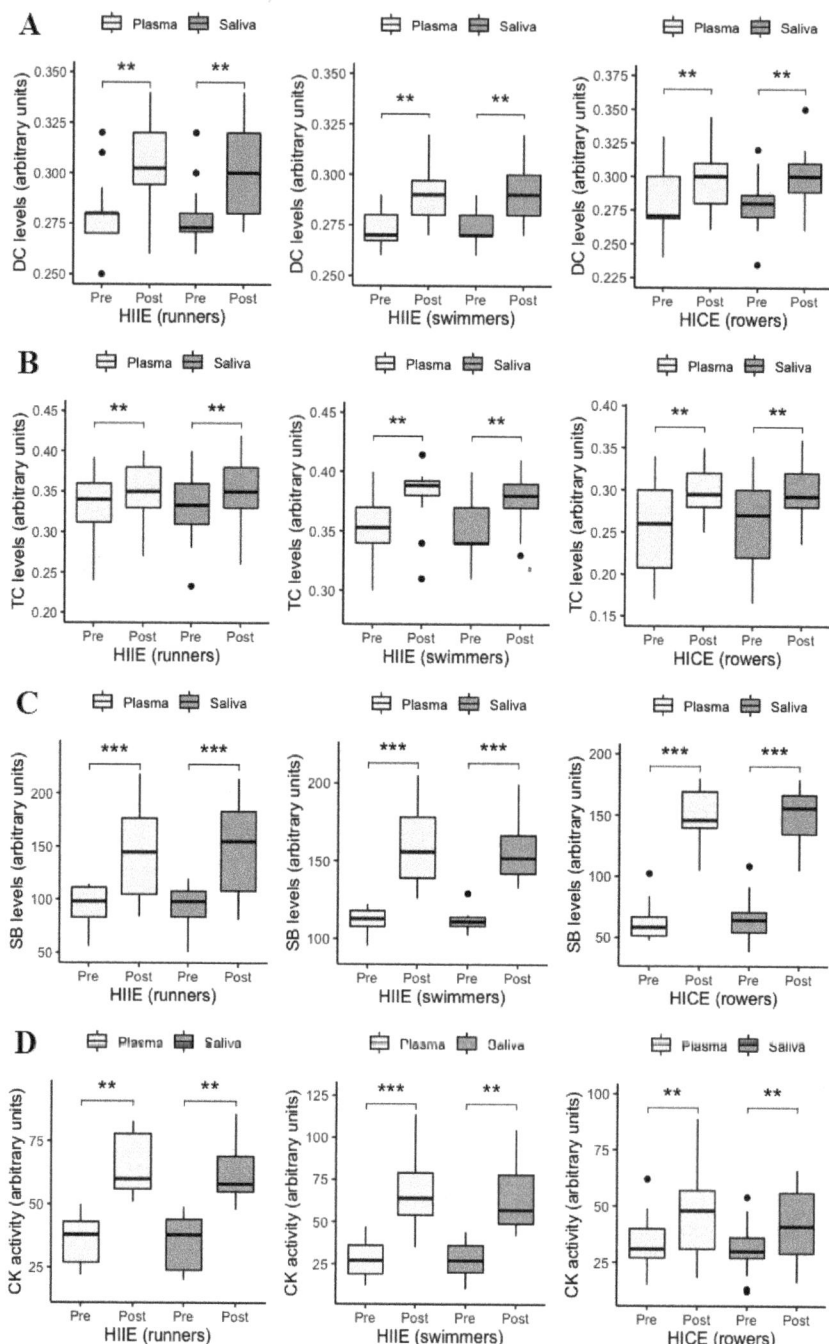

Figure 1. Plasmatic and salivary levels of DC (**A**), TC (**B**), SB (**C**), and CK (**D**) at pre-exercise and postexercise. Data are given as median and interquartile range and compared by Wilcoxon signed-rank test. $n = 13$ per group. ** $p < 0.01$. *** $p < 0.001$. DC: diene conjugates; TC: triene conjugates; SB: Schiff bases; CK: creatine kinase; HIIE: high-intensity interval exercise; HICE: high-intensity continuous exercise.

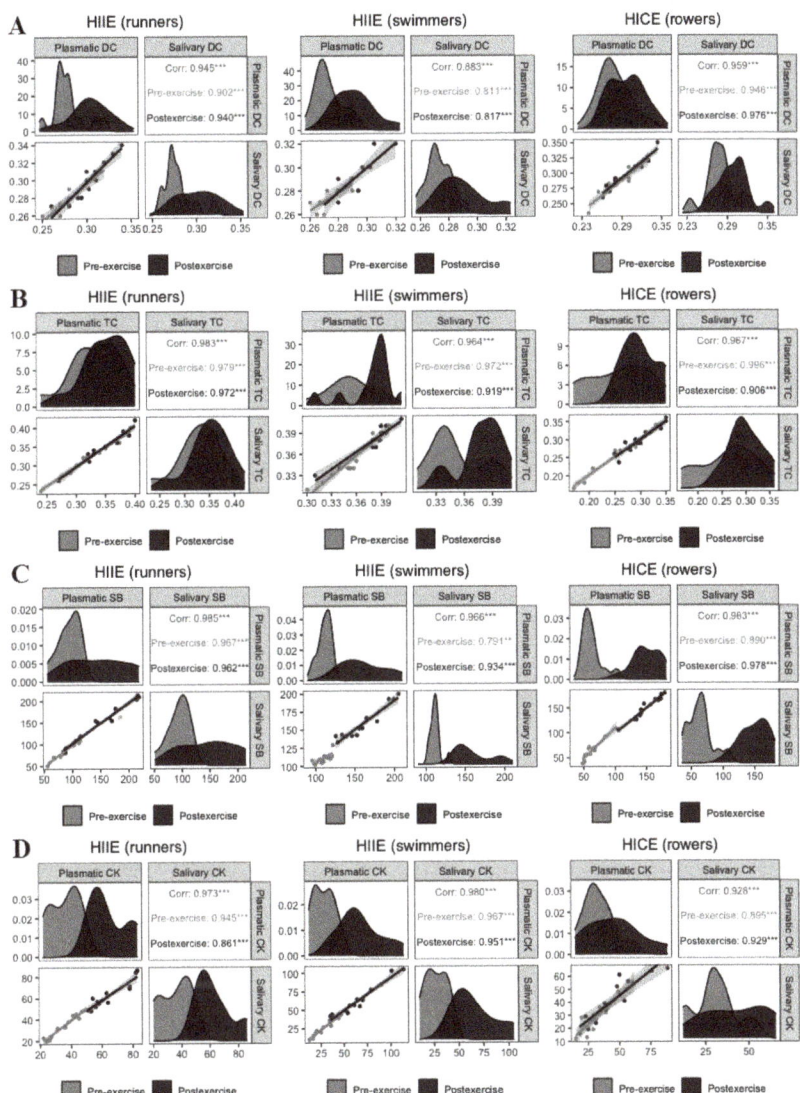

Figure 2. Generalized pairs plots, including density plot, scatter plot and correlation matrix, for displaying distribution and relationship between plasmatic and salivary concentrations of DC (**A**), TC (**B**), SB (**C**), and CK (**D**). $n = 13$ per group. ** $p < 0.01$. *** $p < 0.001$. Corr: Spearman's correlation coefficient for both pre-exercise and postexercise; Pre-exercise: Spearman's correlation coefficient at pre-exercise; Postexercise: Spearman's correlation coefficient at postexercise; DC: diene conjugates; TC: triene conjugates; SB: Schiff bases; CK: creatine kinase; HIIE: high-intensity interval exercise; HICE: high-intensity continuous exercise.

The average difference between plasmatic and salivary TC content both at pre-exercise and at postexercise was also not significant in each group of athletes (Figure 4).

Regarding SB levels in plasma and saliva, they were also shown to have a line of equality within the confidence interval of the mean difference both before and immediately after exercise in all three groups (Figure 5).

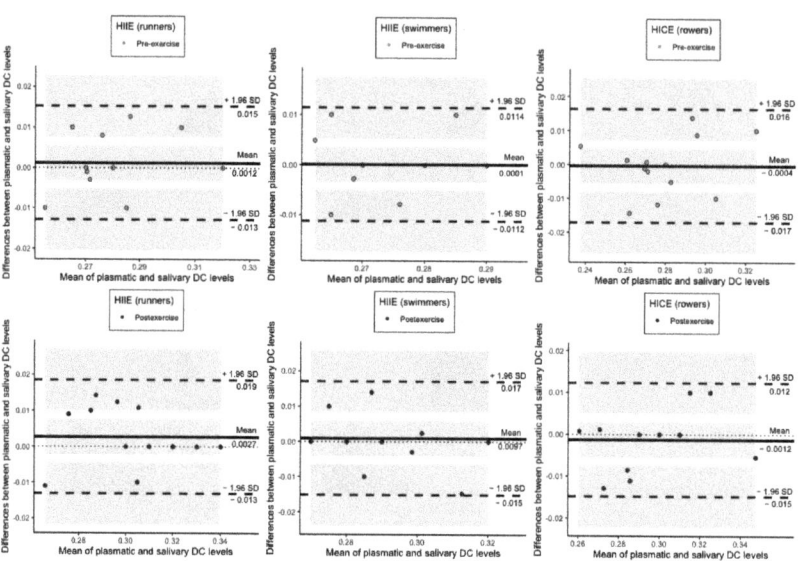

Figure 3. Plots of difference between the measurements of DC levels in plasma and saliva vs. the mean of the measurement. The bias (mean difference) is represented by a solid line parallel to the X axis. The limits of agreement are represented by the dashed lines parallel to the X axis at −1.96 and +1.96 SD. Shaded areas present confidence interval limits for mean and agreement limits. DC: diene conjugates; HIIE: high-intensity interval exercise; HICE: high-intensity continuous exercise; SD: standard deviation.

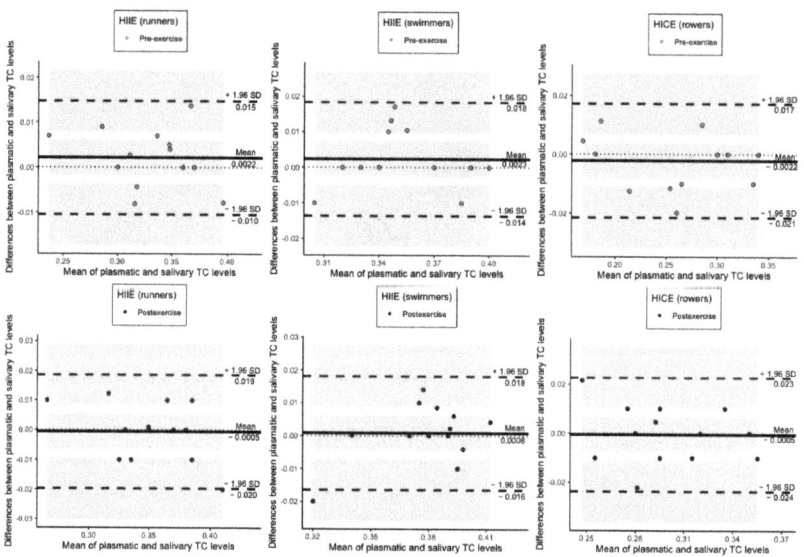

Figure 4. Plots of difference between the measurements of TC levels in plasma and saliva vs. the mean of the measurement. The bias (mean difference) is represented by a solid line parallel to the X axis. The limits of agreement are represented by the dashed lines parallel to the X axis at −1.96 and +1.96 SD. Shaded areas present confidence interval limits for mean and agreement limits. TC: triene conjugates; HIIE: high-intensity interval exercise; HICE: high-intensity continuous exercise; SD: standard deviation.

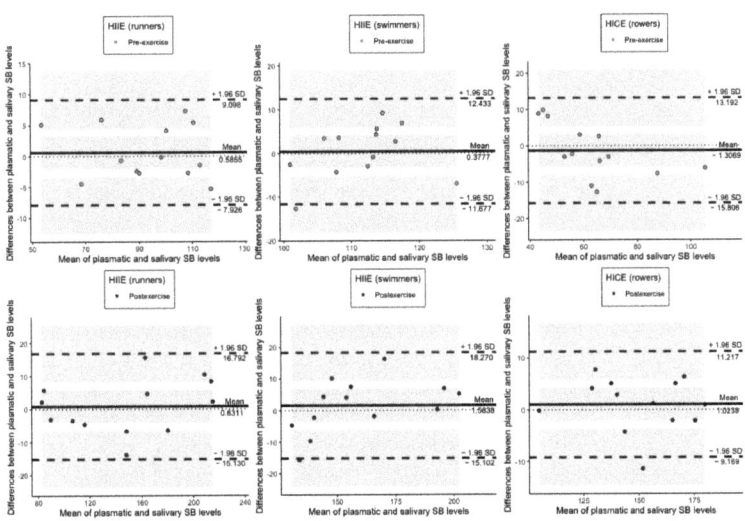

Figure 5. Plots of difference between the measurements of SB levels in plasma and saliva vs. the mean of the measurement. The bias (mean difference) is represented by a solid line parallel to the X axis. The limits of agreement are represented by the dashed lines parallel to the X axis at -1.96 and $+1.96$ SD. Shaded areas present confidence interval limits for mean and agreement limits. SB: Schiff bases; HIIE: high-intensity interval exercise; HICE: high-intensity continuous exercise; SD: standard deviation.

As for the measurement of plasmatic and salivary CK activities at rest and following exercise, the bias was not significant in each group of athletes since the line of equality was in the confidence interval (Figure 6).

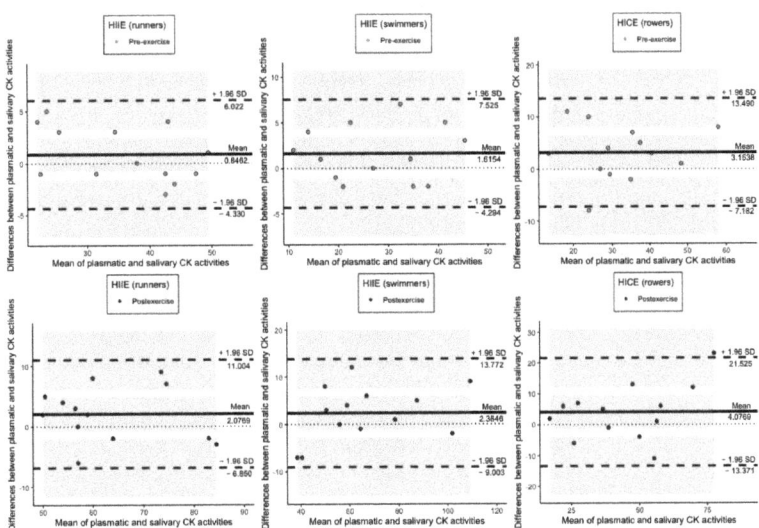

Figure 6. Plots of difference between the measurements of CK activity in plasma and saliva vs. the mean of the measurement. The bias (mean difference) is represented by a solid line parallel to the X axis. The limits of agreement are represented by the dashed lines parallel to the X axis at -1.96 and $+1.96$ SD. Shaded areas present confidence interval limits for mean and agreement limits. CK: creatine kinase; HIIE: high-intensity interval exercise; HICE: high-intensity continuous exercise; SD: standard deviation.

Simultaneously, all of the data points lay within the agreement limits.

4. Discussion

To the best of our knowledge, this is the first study to evaluate the agreement between quantitative measurements of plasmatic and salivary DC, TC, SB, and CK in athletes under exercise conditions. Our results demonstrated that HIIEs associated with running and swimming and HICE related to rowing induce an increase in the content of lipid peroxidation products in both blood plasma and saliva. Although HIIE generally implies less oxygen consumption (due to shorter efforts) than HICE, it could be responsible for significant production of reactive oxygen species (ROS) capable of initiating lipid peroxidation in the active skeletal muscles [36]. Recent data reveal that the rate of electron leakage in the electron transport chain during contractile activity is low enough, enabling only 0.15% of total oxygen consumption to be converted to superoxide radical [30,37,38]. Concurrently, other metabolic pathways such as activation of nicotinamide adenine dinucleotide phosphate oxidase, xanthine oxidase, monoamine oxidase, lipoxygenases are mainly implicated in ROS generation in contracting muscle [38,39]. Exercise-induced changes in salivary DC, TC and SB were shown to be similar to those found in plasma in each athlete group. Moreover, DC, TC and SB levels in saliva reliably reflected the concentrations of these compounds in blood plasma at both pre-exercise and postexercise in all three groups. Similar levels of plasmatic and salivary DC, TC and SB at rest and following exercise may be associated with the fact that these compounds are able to diffuse from serum through capillaries, accumulating in saliva according to the concentration gradient [40]. Our previous work partially confirms these findings where specific HIIEs performed by swimmers and runners induced lipid peroxidation propagation in saliva, which was identified by the measurements of salivary DC, TC and SB levels [3]. However, unlike the present study, there was no blood sampling together with saliva collection (i.e., simultaneously) before and immediately after the exercise, which did not allow us to assess the agreement between quantitative measurements of DC, TC and SB in plasma and saliva.

In addition, it was found that HIIEs for runners and swimmers and HICE for rowers cause increased levels of plasmatic and salivary CK. Importantly, salivary CK activity was consistent with plasmatic CK activity at both pre-exercise and postexercise in each athlete group. These results correspond with our preliminary findings and suggest that salivary CK activity may represent plasma levels of this enzyme at rest and in response to exercise [33]. In a recent study from Barranco et al. [32], the authors also found an increase in CK levels in both plasma and saliva following exercise consisting of a futsal match. More recently, Fernández et al. [41] observed the elevated CK activity in saliva after serial matches of rugby seven.

Increased CK levels found in blood indicate surface membrane damage and disruption of the sarcomere architecture, which may be mediated in part by oxidative stress [29,42]. As is well known, muscle contraction requires a transient increase in intracellular calcium, which is released from the sarcoplasmic reticulum into the cytosol through the excitation–contraction coupling system [29]. An overload of intracellular calcium activates calcium-dependent protease such as calpain-1, which destroys sarcomeric proteins [43]. Although there is no evidence for direct activation of calpain-1 by oxidative stress, the calcium-dependent protease activity is thought to be induced by ischemia/reperfusion damage during exercise due to calcium overload [29,44]. Another mechanism by which oxidant stress-mediated increases in protease activity can occur is activation/sensitization of the ryanodine receptor Ca^{2+}-release channels [45]. Current evidence suggests that calpain-1-induced proteolysis of sarcomere proteins is an early process in myocyte injury, and that excess levels of ROS may play a meaningful role in the initiation of signaling events related to muscle damage [29]. Cell membrane modifications triggered by lipid peroxidation propagation often precede irreversible biomolecular damage, being an early cause of cell death [30,46,47]. High concentrations of plasmatic and salivary SB (also known as 4-HNO-protein adducts) were observed in the present study, suggesting that large amounts of 4-HNE were produced during exercise. Lipid peroxidation end-products are able to affect membrane proteins, causing function impairment, increased nonspecific permeability to ions, fluidity changes and inactivation of membrane-bound receptors and enzymes [48–50]. Therefore, increased CK levels after exercise may be directly related to lipid peroxidation propagation during exercise [30]. In turn, elevated activity of salivary CK following exercise may be associated with diffusion of this enzyme from the bloodstream via transcellular/paracellular pathways [40,51].

This study has some limitations that should be noted. The first limitation derives from the origin of the sample. The fact that all athletes participated in sprinting, short-distance swimming or middle-distance rowing prompts us to be cautious in generalizing the results to athletes who represent other events and sports. In addition, the results of the present study cannot be extrapolated to the general population, taking into account that the subjects were only athletes. We consider that our research can serve as a basis for further studies enrolling a wider range of participants in order to confirm these findings. Second, it has been stated that CK activity is influenced by gender. Therefore, our results may be conditioned by the lack of women in the sample. However, since CK levels in men are usually higher than in women [52–54], we preferred to study a more homogeneous and representative sample. Nevertheless, our study had an important strength because there are no studies that have analyzed the agreement between quantitative measurements of plasmatic and salivary DC, TC, SB, and CK as biomarkers capable of providing a reliable indication of exercise-induced oxidative stress and muscle damage in athletes. Further studies examining whether the levels of salivary DC, TC, SB, and CK can reliably reflect plasma concentrations in male and female athletes who represent different sports will be important.

5. Conclusions

This study demonstrates that specific HICE for rowers and HIIEs for runners and swimmers induce lipid peroxidation chain reactions and muscle damage, which can be identified by the measurements of DC, TC, SB, and CK in both blood plasma and saliva. An important finding in that original study was that the concentrations of salivary DC, TC, SB, and CK are able to represent plasma levels in athletes under exercise conditions. Visual examination of the Bland–Altman plots allowed us to detect the high agreement between quantitative measurements of plasmatic and salivary DC, TC, SB, and CK both at rest and following exercise in each athlete group. The established relationship between plasmatic and salivary DC, TC, SB, and CK makes it possible to consider the use of saliva as a similarly reliable alternative to blood analysis in athletes for monitoring oxidative stress and muscle damage imposed by the exercise.

Author Contributions: Conceptualization, A.N.O.; methodology, A.N.O.; formal analysis, A.N.O.; investigation, A.N.O., V.V.S. and A.V.D.; resources, A.N.O., V.V.S. and A.V.D.; data curation, A.N.O. and A.V.D.; writing—original draft preparation, A.N.O. and A.P.; writing—review and editing, A.N.O. and A.P.; visualization, A.N.O.; supervision, A.P. All authors have read and agreed to the published version of the manuscript.

Funding: This research was funded by Lobachevsky University, grant number H-439-99_2020-2021. The study was approved by the Bioethics Committee of Lobachevsky University (approval number: 43) and complies with the Declaration of Helsinki. All participants signed informed consent forms prior to enrolment.

Institutional Review Board Statement: The study was conducted in accordance with the Declaration of Helsinki, and approved by the Bioethics Committee of Lobachevsky University (approval number: 43).

Informed Consent Statement: Informed consent was obtained from all subjects involved in the study.

Data Availability Statement: All relevant data analyzed during the current trial are included in the article. Access to raw datasets may be provided upon reasonable request to the corresponding author.

Acknowledgments: Authors thank the athletes for their participation and their coaches for help in conducting this research.

Conflicts of Interest: The authors declare no conflict of interest.

References

1. Lindsay, A.; Costello, J.T. Realising the Potential of Urine and Saliva as Diagnostic Tools in Sport and Exercise Medicine. *Sports Med.* **2017**, *47*, 11–31. [CrossRef] [PubMed]
2. Seshadri, D.R.; Li, R.T.; Voos, J.E.; Rowbottom, J.R.; Alfes, C.M.; Zorman, C.A.; Drummond, C.K. Wearable sensors for monitoring the physiological and biochemical profile of the athlete. *NPJ Digit. Med.* **2019**, *2*, 72. [CrossRef] [PubMed]
3. Ovchinnikov, A.N.; Deryugina, A.V. Saliva as highly informative substrate for non-invasive analysis of lipoperoxide processes and muscle damage in highly skilled athletes. *Klin. Lab. Diagn.* **2019**, *64*, 405–408. [CrossRef] [PubMed]
4. Lindsay, A.; Lewis, J.; Scarrott, C.; Gill, N.; Gieseg, S.P.; Draper, N. Assessing the effectiveness of selected biomarkers in the acute and cumulative physiological stress response in professional rugby union through non-invasive assessment. *Int. J. Sports Med.* **2015**, *36*, 446–454. [CrossRef] [PubMed]
5. Mortatti, A.L.; Moreira, A.; Aoki, M.S.; Crewther, B.T.; Castagna, C.; de Arruda, A.F.S.; Filho, J.M. Effect of competition on salivary cortisol, immunoglobulin A, and upper respiratory tract infections in elite young soccer players. *J. Strength Cond. Res.* **2012**, *26*, 1396–1401. [CrossRef]
6. Elloumi, M.; Maso, F.; Michaux, O.; Robert, A.; Lac, G. Behaviour of saliva cortisol [C], testosterone [T] and the T/C ratio during a rugby match and during the post-competition recovery days. *Eur. J. Appl. Physiol.* **2003**, *90*, 23–28. [CrossRef]
7. Beaven, C.M.; Gill, N.D.; Cook, C.J. Salivary testosterone and cortisol responses in professional rugby players after four resistance exercise protocols. *J. Strength Cond. Res.* **2008**, *22*, 426–432. [CrossRef]
8. Ghigiarelli, J.J.; Sell, K.M.; Raddock, J.M.; Taveras, K. Effects of strongman training on salivary testosterone levels in a sample of trained men. *J. Strength Cond. Res.* **2013**, *27*, 738–747. [CrossRef]
9. Neville, V.; Gleeson, M.; Folland, J.P. Salivary IgA as a risk factor for upper respiratory infections in elite professional athletes. *Med. Sci. Sports Exerc.* **2008**, *40*, 1228–1236. [CrossRef]
10. Gonzalez, D.; Marquina, R.; Rondon, N.; Rodriguez-Malaver, A.J.; Reyes, R. Effects of aerobic exercise on uric acid, total antioxidant activity, oxidative stress, and nitric oxide in human saliva. *Res. Sports Med.* **2008**, *16*, 128–137. [CrossRef]
11. Deminice, R.; Sicchieri, T.; Payao, P.O.; Jordao, A.A. Blood and salivary oxidative stress biomarkers following an acute session of resistance exercise in humans. *Int. J. Sports Med.* **2010**, *31*, 599–603. [CrossRef]
12. Sant'Anna, M.; Casimiro-Lopes, G.; Boaventura, G.; Marques, S.T.; Sorenson, M.M.; Simão, R.; Pinto, V.S. Anaerobic exercise affects the saliva antioxidant/oxidant balance in high performance pentathlon athletes. *Hum. Mov.* **2016**, *17*, 50–55. [CrossRef]
13. Souza, A.V.; Giolo, J.S.; Teixeira, R.R.; Vilela, D.D.; Peixoto, L.G.; Justino, A.B.; Caixeta, D.C.; Puga, G.M.; Espindola, F.S. Salivary and Plasmatic Antioxidant Profile following Continuous, Resistance, and High-Intensity Interval Exercise: Preliminary Study. *Oxid. Med. Cell. Longev.* **2019**, *2019*, 5425021. [CrossRef] [PubMed]
14. Hofman, L.F. Human saliva as a diagnostic specimen. *J. Nutr.* **2001**, *131*, 1621S–1625S. [CrossRef]
15. Chiappin, S.; Antonelli, G.; Gatti, R.; De Palo, E.F. Saliva specimen: A new laboratory tool for diagnostic and basic investigation. *Clin. Chim. Acta* **2007**, *383*, 30–40. [CrossRef]
16. McLellan, C.P.; Lovell, D.I.; Gass, G.C. Creatine kinase and endocrine responses of elite players pre, during, and post rugby league match play. *J. Strength Cond. Res.* **2010**, *24*, 2908–2919. [CrossRef] [PubMed]
17. Cadore, E.; Lhullier, F.; Brentano, M.; Silva, E.; Ambrosini, M.; Spinelli, R.; Silva, R.; Kruel, L. Correlations between serum and salivary hormonal concentrations in response to resistance exercise. *J. Sports Sci.* **2008**, *26*, 1067–1072. [CrossRef]
18. Hough, J.; Robertson, C.; Gleeson, M. Blunting of exercise-induced salivary testosterone in elite-level triathletes with a 10-day training camp. *Int. J. Sports Physiol. Perform.* **2015**, *10*, 935–938. [CrossRef]
19. De Oliveira, V.; Bessa, A.; Lamounier, R.; de Santana, M.G.; de Mello, M.T.; Espindola, F.S. Changes in the salivary biomarkers induced by an effort test. *Int. J. Sports Med.* **2010**, *31*, 377–381. [CrossRef]
20. Kivlighan, K.T.; Granger, D.A. Salivary a-amylase response to competition: Relation to gender, previous experience, and attitudes. *Psychoneuroendocrinology* **2006**, *31*, 703–714. [CrossRef]
21. MacKinnon, L.T.; Jenkins, D.G. Decreased salivary immunoglobulins after intense interval exercise before and after training. *Med. Sci. Sports Exerc.* **1993**, *25*, 678–683. [CrossRef] [PubMed]
22. Mackinnon, L.T.; Chick, T.W.; Van As, A.; Tomasi, T.B. Decreased secretory immunoglobulins following intense endurance exercise. *Res. Sports Med.* **1989**, *1*, 209–218. [CrossRef]
23. Janero, D.R. Malondialdehyde and thiobarbituric acid-reactivity as diagnostic indices of lipid peroxidation and peroxidative tissue injury. *Free Radic. Biol. Med.* **1990**, *9*, 515–540. [CrossRef]
24. Corongiu, F.P.; Banni, S. Detection of conjugated dienes by second derivative ultraviolet spectrophotometry. *Methods Enzymol.* **1994**, *233*, 303–310. [PubMed]
25. Bel'skaya, L.V.; Kosenok, V.K.; Massard, G. Endogenous Intoxication and Saliva Lipid Peroxidation in Patients with Lung Cancer. *Diagnostics* **2016**, *6*, 39. [CrossRef]

26. Ayala, A.; Muñoz, M.F.; Argüelles, S. Lipid peroxidation: Production, metabolism, and signaling mechanisms of malondialdehyde and 4-hydroxy-2-nonenal. *Oxid. Med. Cell. Longev.* **2014**, *2014*, 360438. [CrossRef]
27. Dalleau, S.; Baradat, M.; Guéraud, F.; Huc, L. Cell death and diseases related to oxidative stress: 4-hydroxynonenal (HNE) in the balance. *Cell Death Differ.* **2013**, *20*, 1615–1630. [CrossRef]
28. Ovchinnikov, A.N. The Effect of the Combination of Royal Jelly and Exogenous Coenzyme Q10 on the Indicators of Functional Status among Athletes under Exercise. PhD Thesis, Lobachevsky University, Nizhny Novgorod, Russia, 2019.
29. Aoi, W.; Naito, Y.; Yoshikawa, T. Role of oxidative stress in impaired insulin signaling associated with exercise-induced muscle damage. *Free Radic. Biol. Med.* **2013**, *65*, 1265–1272. [CrossRef]
30. Kozakowska, M.; Pietraszek-Gremplewicz, K.; Jozkowicz, A.; Dulak, J. The role of oxidative stress in skeletal muscle injury and regeneration: Focus on antioxidant enzymes. *J. Muscle Res. Cell Motil.* **2015**, *36*, 377–393. [CrossRef]
31. Kontorshchikova, K.N.; Tikhomirova, Y.R.; Ovchinnikov, A.N.; Kolegova, T.I.; Churkina, N.N.; Kuznetsova, S.Y.; Krylov, V.N. Indices of Free Radical Oxidation in the Oral Fluid as Markers of Athletes' Functional State. *Sovrem. Tehnol. V Med.* **2017**, *9*, 82–86. [CrossRef]
32. Barranco, T.; Tvarijonaviciute, A.; Tecles, F.; Carrillo, J.M.; Sánchez-Resalt, C.; Jimenez-Reyes, P.; Rubio, M.; García-Balletbó, M.; Cerón, J.J.; Cugat, R. Changes in creatine kinase, lactate dehydrogenase and aspartate aminotransferase in saliva samples after an intense exercise: A pilot study. *J. Sports Med. Phys. Fit.* **2017**, *58*, 910–916. [CrossRef] [PubMed]
33. Ovchinnikov, A.N.; Paoli, A.; Deryugina, A.V.; Yarygina, D.A. Salivary and Plasmatic Creatine Kinase and Lactate Dehydrogenase Responses Following High-intensity Continuous Exercise. *Med. Sci. Sports Exerc.* **2021**, *53*, 377. [CrossRef]
34. World Medical Association Declaration of Helsinki. Recommendations guiding physicians in biomedical research involving human subjects. *JAMA* **1997**, *277*, 925–926. [CrossRef]
35. Kontorschikova, K.; Tikhomirova, J.; Ovchinnikov, A.; Okrut, I.; Krylov, V.; Kolegova, T. The evaluation of highly qualified sportsmen's biochemical homeostasis. *Clin. Chem. Lab. Med.* **2017**, *55*, S811.
36. Powers, S.K.; Deminice, R.; Ozdemir, M.; Yoshihara, T.; Bomkamp, M.P.; Hyatta, H. Exercise-induced oxidative stress: Friend or foe? *J. Sport Health Sci.* **2020**, *9*, 415–425. [CrossRef]
37. Vasilaki, A.; Jackson, M.J. Role of reactive oxygen species in the defective regeneration seen in aging muscle. *Free Radic. Biol. Med.* **2013**, *65*, 317–323. [CrossRef]
38. Sakellariou, G.K.; Jackson, M.J.; Vasilaki, A. Redefining the major contributors to superoxide production in contracting skeletal muscle. The role of NAD(P)H oxidases. *Free Radic. Res.* **2014**, *48*, 12–29. [CrossRef]
39. Beckendorf, L.; Linke, W.A. Emerging importance of oxidative stress in regulating striated muscle elasticity. *J. Muscle Res. Cell Motil.* **2015**, *36*, 25–36. [CrossRef]
40. Wang, J.; Schipper, H.M.; Velly, A.M.; Mohit, S.; Gornitsky, M. Salivary biomarkers of oxidative stress: A critical review. *Free Radic. Biol. Med.* **2015**, *85*, 95–104. [CrossRef]
41. Fernández, A.G.; de la Rubia Ortí, J.E.; Franco-Martinez, L.; Ceron, J.J.; Mariscal, G.; Barrios, C. Changes in Salivary Levels of Creatine Kinase, Lactate Dehydrogenase, and Aspartate Aminotransferase after Playing Rugby Sevens: The Influence of Gender. *Int. J. Environ. Res. Public Health* **2020**, *17*, 8165. [CrossRef]
42. Gissel, H.; Clausen, T. Excitation-induced Ca^{2+} influx and skeletal muscle cell damage. *Acta Physiol. Scand.* **2001**, *171*, 327–334. [CrossRef] [PubMed]
43. Gissel, H. The role of Ca^{2+} in muscle cell damage. *Ann. N. Y. Acad. Sci.* **2005**, *1066*, 166–180. [CrossRef] [PubMed]
44. Inserte, J.; Hernando, V.; Garcia-Dorado, D. Contribution of calpains to myocardial ischaemia/reperfusion injury. *Cardiovasc. Res.* **2012**, *96*, 23–31. [CrossRef]
45. Allen, D.G.; Lamb, G.D.; Westerblad, H. Skeletal muscle fatigue: Cellular mechanisms. *Physiol. Rev.* **2008**, *88*, 287–332. [CrossRef] [PubMed]
46. Khanum, R.; Thevanayagam, H. Lipid peroxidation: Its effects on the formulation and use of pharmaceutical emulsions. *Asian J. Pharm. Sci.* **2017**, *12*, 401–411. [CrossRef] [PubMed]
47. Barbieri, E.; Sestili, P. Reactive oxygen species in skeletal muscle signaling. *J. Signal Transduct.* **2012**, *2012*, 982794. [CrossRef] [PubMed]
48. Schaur, R.J. Basic aspects of the biochemical reactivity of 4-hydroxynonenal. *Mol. Asp. Med.* **2003**, *24*, 149–159. [CrossRef]
49. Halliwell, B.; Chirico, S. Lipid peroxidation: Its mechanism, measurement, and significance. *Am. J. Clin. Nutr.* **1993**, *57*, 715S–724S. [CrossRef]
50. Roche, L.D. Oxidative stress: The dark side of soybean-oil-based emulsions used in parenteral nutrition. *Oxid. Antioxid. Med. Sci.* **2012**, *1*, 11–14. [CrossRef]
51. Sharma, A.; Badea, M.; Tiwari, S.; Marty, J.L. Wearable Biosensors: An Alternative and Practical Approach in Healthcare and Disease Monitoring. *Molecules* **2021**, *26*, 748. [CrossRef]
52. Mougios, V. Reference intervals for serum creatine kinase in athletes. *Br. J. Sports Med.* **2007**, *41*, 674–678. [CrossRef] [PubMed]
53. Yen, C.H.; Wang, K.T.; Lee, P.Y.; Liu, C.C.; Hsieh, Y.C.; Kuo, J.Y.; Bulwer, B.E.; Hung, C.L.; Chang, S.C.; Shih, S.C.; et al. Gender-differences in the associations between circulating creatine kinase, blood pressure, body mass and non-alcoholic fatty liver disease in asymptomatic asians. *PLoS ONE* **2017**, *12*, e0179898. [CrossRef] [PubMed]
54. Oosthuyse, T.; Bosch, A.N. The Effect of Gender and Menstrual Phase on Serum Creatine Kinase Activity and Muscle Soreness Following Downhill Running. *Antioxidants* **2017**, *6*, 16. [CrossRef] [PubMed]

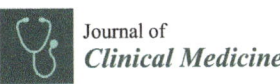

Article

Efficacy of Core Training in Swimming Performance and Neuromuscular Parameters of Young Swimmers: A Randomised Control Trial

Ahmad Khiyami [1], Shibili Nuhmani [1,*], Royes Joseph [2], Turki Saeed Abualait [1] and Qassim Muaidi [1]

[1] Department of Physical Therapy, College of Applied Medical Sciences, Imam Abdulrahman Bin Faisal University, Dammam 31451, Saudi Arabia; 2190500137@iau.edu.sa (A.K.); tsabualait@iau.edu.sa (T.S.A.); qmuaidi@iau.edu.sa (Q.M.)

[2] Department of Pharmacy Practice, College of Clinical Pharmacy, Imam Abdulrahman Bin Faisal University, Dammam 31451, Saudi Arabia; rjchacko@iau.edu.sa

* Correspondence: snuhmani@iau.edu.sa; Tel.: +966-554270531

Abstract: Background: This study aimed to investigate the efficacy of core training in the swimming performance and neuromuscular properties of young swimmers. Methods: Eighteen healthy male swimmers (age: 13 ± 2 years, height: 159.6 ± 14.5 cm, weight: 48.7 ± 12.4 kg) were recruited from the Public Authority for Sports swimming pool in Dammam and randomly assigned to the experimental and control groups. The experimental group performed a six-week core-training program consisting of seven exercises (three times/week) with regular swimming training. The control group maintained its regular training. Swimming performance and neuromuscular parameters were measured pre- and post-interventions. Results: The experimental group benefitted from the intervention in terms of the 50 m swim time (−1.4 s; 95% confidence interval −2.4 to −0.5) compared with the control group. The experimental group also showed improved swimming velocity (+0.1 m.s^{-1}), stroke rate (−2.8 cycle.min^{-1}), stroke length (+0.2 m.cycle^{-1}), stroke index (+0.4 m^2·s^{-1}), total strokes (−2.9 strokes), and contraction time for erector spinae (ES; −1.5 ms), latissimus dorsi (LD; −7 ms), and external obliques (EO; −1.9 ms). Maximal displacement ES (DM-ES) (+3.3 mm), LD (0.5 mm), and EO (+2.2 mm) were compared with the baseline values for the experimental group, and TC-ES (5.8 ms), LD (3.7 ms), EO (2.5 ms), DM-ES (0.2 mm), LD (−4.1 mm), and EO (−1.0 mm) were compared with the baseline values for the control group. The intergroup comparison was statistically significant ($p < 0.05$; DM-ES $p > 0.05$). Conclusion: The results indicate that a six-week core-training program with regular swimming training improved the neuromuscular properties and the 50 m freestyle swim performance of the experimental group compared with the control group.

Keywords: core muscles; swimming performance; tensiomyography; sports training

Citation: Khiyami, A.; Nuhmani, S.; Joseph, R.; Abualait, T.S.; Muaidi, Q. Efficacy of Core Training in Swimming Performance and Neuromuscular Parameters of Young Swimmers: A Randomised Control Trial. *J. Clin. Med.* **2022**, *11*, 3198. https://doi.org/10.3390/jcm11113198

Academic Editor: David Rodríguez-Sanz

Received: 14 April 2022
Accepted: 2 June 2022
Published: 3 June 2022

Publisher's Note: MDPI stays neutral with regard to jurisdictional claims in published maps and institutional affiliations.

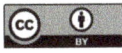

Copyright: © 2022 by the authors. Licensee MDPI, Basel, Switzerland. This article is an open access article distributed under the terms and conditions of the Creative Commons Attribution (CC BY) license (https://creativecommons.org/licenses/by/4.0/).

1. Introduction

The main goal of competitive swimming is to cover a certain distance in the least possible time. Performance in swimming depends on producing propelling forces and reducing resistance to movement in the water [1]. Maintaining streamlined balance and body position is crucial in enhancing the proficiency of swimmers' performance, which depends on the strength of the core muscles [2]. Several studies recommended adding core strength training to be an integral part of swimming training to improve performance [2–4]. Exercises to train core muscles can be exceptionally beneficial for sprint swimmers, allowing the effective transmission of force between the trunk and the upper and lower extremities to propel the body through the water, which leads to increased athletic performance and improved functional skills [5].

The enhancement of force production resulting from core training is achieved by improving neural adaptation, leading to faster nervous system activation, improved synchronisation of motor units, increased neural recruitment patterns, and lowered neural inhibitory reflexes [3,4]. These elements can be particularly beneficial for sprint swimmers [3]. Moreover, they reduce training costs and effort and help coaches choose the most appropriate training program to assess which swimmers could improve their performance effectively. Furthermore, they can reduce the rate of injuries by improving the efficacy of core muscles [3]. A strong core enables athletes to perform more effectively and conduct swift body movements, enhancing force distribution throughout the body [6]. A weak core leads to energy leakage, resulting in less powerful kicks and a decreased overall amount of power produced [7].

Previous studies focused on the effects of land-based limb power and strength interventions, with inconsistent findings with regard to swimming [8]. Furthermore, there is limited evidence regarding applying core-training programs to swimmers in terms of swimming performance. Weston et al. [9] reported an improvement in front crawl swimming time and core muscle functions following a 12-week isolated core-training program among young swimmers. A recent study by Karpiński et al. [10] also reported an improvement in swimming performance following a six-week core-training program among national-level Polish swimmers. Patil et al. [2] also reported an improvement in sprint time following six weeks of a core-training program in competitive swimmers. At the same time, Martens et al. [11] did not show a direct relationship between improvement in core muscle strength and swimming performance. There is also a lack of accurate performance measurements in core muscle training among swimmers [9,12]. Even though few studies are available that have assessed swimming speed, most of these studies did not assess accurate swimming parameters such as stroke rate, stroke length, sprint time, stroke index, etc., following the core-training program. It is also important to assess the performance parameters of the key core muscles that maintain the body position during swimming, such as the external oblique, erector spinae, and latissimus dorsi.

Tensiomyography (TMG) is a novel and non-invasive neuromuscular measurement used to quantify the contractile properties of the muscles and provide information about how the muscles respond to the exercises and the load [13,14]. It has also been used to assess muscle stiffness and composition [15]. The assessment of the contractile properties of the muscles can provide valuable information about the adaptations of the muscles in response to the training. Several researchers used TMG to measure the effect of various training loads in soccer [16–18], volleyball [19,20], and basketball players [21] and monitor the effects of physical training in soccer and basketball players throughout the season [21,22]. TMG has also been used to establish the relationship between neuromuscular parameters and sports performance indicators in cyclists [23] soccer [24] and rugby players [25]. To the best of the authors' knowledge, TMG has never been used to quantify the effect of core training among swimmers. Therefore, this study aimed to investigate the efficacy of a six-week core-training program in the swimming performance and neuromuscular properties of young swimmers. We hypothesised that an additional core-training program, along with a regular swimming training program, would lead to positive changes in the performance of young swimmers. This is the first study to use TMG to measure the effect of core-training exercises on swimmers.

2. Materials and Methods

2.1. Participants

Twenty-six healthy male young swimmers were approached for possible participation. Two subjects were excluded because they did not meet the inclusion criteria. Six subjects were dropped during the study because they did not attend the post-test and were absent from three training sessions (one participant). Nine male swimmers (age: 13 ± 2 years, height: 158.8 ± 17.3 cm, weight: 48.3 ± 14.2 kg, swimming experience 2.8 ± 0.4 years) were assigned to the experimental group and another nine male swimmers (age: 13.11 ± 2.6 years, height: 160.4 ± 11.9 cm, weight: 49.1 ± 11.3 kg, swimming experience 2.9 ± 0.7 years) to the control group (Figure 1). The inclusion criteria were as follows: (1) healthy subjects aged 10–16 years, (2) normal body mass index, and (3) swimming experience of more than one year. The exclusion criteria were as follows: (1) any previous injury of the shoulder or back muscles that could affect the training or measurement as reported by the participant, (2) any neurological or systemic disease as reported by the participant, (3) biomechanical abnormality of the participant that could affect the training and measurements, and (4) any medication that could affect performance. At baseline, the swimmers in both groups were performing a similar regular training program as they were enrolled under the same coach. The regular training consisted of seven sessions of pool-based training and two sessions of a land-based training program. The participants were covering an equal swimming distance per week with an average of 28 km. The major component of the regular training was endurance training. All the participants were familiar with core training, but not actively engaged in any core-training program. The idea of the research (including benefits, risks, and time needed) and the procedures were explained to the swimmers and their legal guardians, and written informed consent was taken from them. The participants were randomly assigned to two groups equally using the envelope drawing method, in which the envelope contained a number pertaining to the groups. Randomisation was conducted by a researcher who was unrelated to the study. Ethical approval was obtained from the Institutional Review Board of Imam Abdulrahman Bin Faisal University (IRB-PGS-2019-03-241).

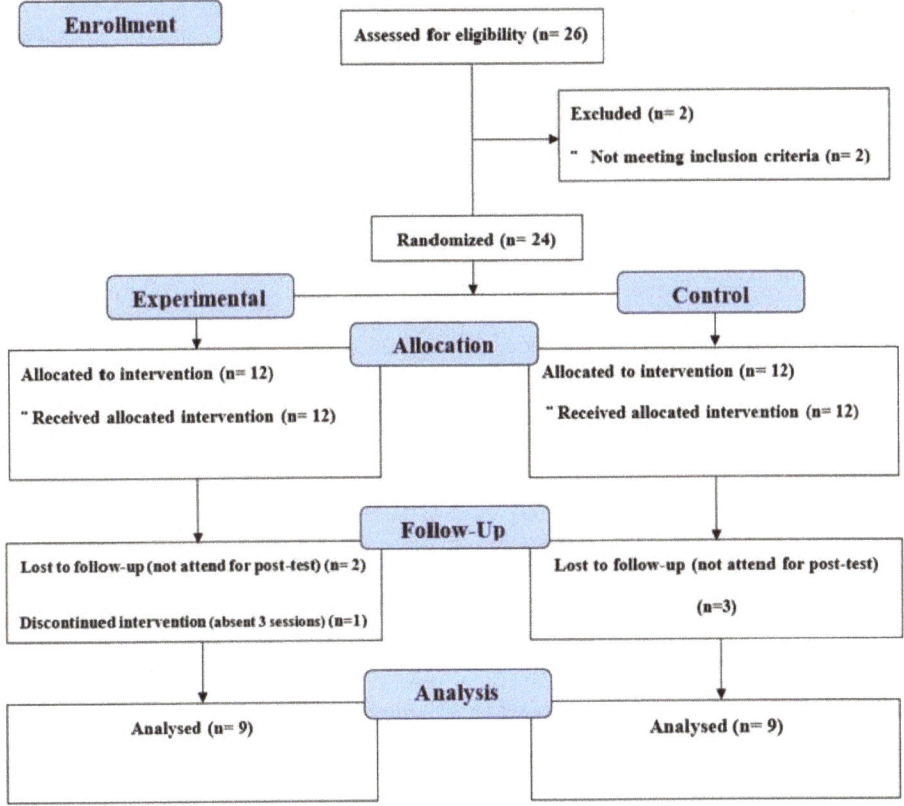

Figure 1. Consort diagram of participants' flow.

2.2. Design

This study followed a randomised control trial with a pre-test–post-test control group (parallel design). The experiment was performed in the swimming pool of the Public Authority for Sports in Dammam. The calculation of the sample size was based on a previous randomised control trial by S. Girold et al. [26], who examined the effect of speed training exercises on a 50 m swim time (ST) by calculating the mean and standard deviation (SD) of the two groups, with 80% power and 0.05 type 1 error. Group 1 (experimental $n = 11$) had a mean of 29.69 and SD of (2.45), and Group 2 (control $n = 11$) had a mean of 32.85 and SD of (2.77). The ratio between the two groups was 1:1, with a 0.05 significance level (alpha) and 80% power. The results showed that 18 subjects were required, with nine subjects in each group.

2.3. Procedure

The experimental group performed a six-week core-training program in addition to regular training, and the control group continued their regular training. The participants were asked not to participate in any research or training other than their regular swimming training during the study. The swimmer's dominant side was chosen for measurement. The dominant side is the same as the hand used in writing. TMG and swimming parameter measurements for the control group were performed twice: before the research began and after six weeks. For the experimental group, these were performed before and after the intervention. The reporting of this study followed the Consolidated Standards of Reporting Trials guidelines [27].

2.4. Intervention

The exercise program was based on existing literature and continued for 18 sessions for six weeks (three sessions per week, one hour per session, lasting no more than one hour in total) [9,28]. The progression of the exercise was performed by gradually increasing the number of repetitions and sets and the level of resistance/hold time (Table 1). All exercises were performed under the researchers' supervision. All standard safety procedures were followed, including warm-up and cool-down exercises, rest time between exercises, and the use of correct techniques. The participants had to perform 10 min of warm-up exercises (i.e., bent over twist, criss-cross crunches, forward shoulder rotation, and backward shoulder rotation) followed by 30 min of seven core exercises. A 1 min rest was given between the exercises and a 10 min rest after the core exercises. One hour of regular training then followed. Finally, the swimmers performed cool-down exercises. Table 1 presents the details of the training program.

2.5. Outcome Measures

2.5.1. Neuromuscular Properties

TMG was used to determine the neuromuscular properties of the external oblique (EO), erector spinae (ES), and latissimus dorsi (LD) muscles. These muscles were chosen for the measurement because they are the key muscles to maintain position during swimming and affect core stability and strength [9]. Moreover, our training program targeted these muscles. The LD is an extrinsic back muscle that contributes to arm adduction, extension movement, and stabilising the trunk during movement. The EO contributes to stabilising trunk movement and maintaining abdominal pressure and anatomical position. The ES muscle acts as a stabiliser for the entire vertebral column and the cranio-cervical region [29]. The participants were asked to remain in a relaxed supine position during measurement of the EO muscle, whereas a relaxed prone position was used to measure the ES and LD muscles [30]. The TMG sensor was positioned with regard to the muscle being measured, with a spring constant of 0.17 N mm^{-1}. Two self-adhesive stimulating electrodes were positioned at proximal and distal distances of 1.5 cm from the sensor. An initial stimulation current of 10 mA was used with a single square wave monophasic 1 ms-long pulse, and the stimulation was gradually increased by 10 mA until no more increase in the response amplitude or when the maximal stimulator output was reached. To prevent the effects of muscular fatigue and potentiation, an interval of ≥ 10 s was preferred between consecutive measurements. TMG software instantaneously showed muscle displacement in the form of a graph and recorded it. The total test time was 30 min. The validity and reliability of TMG has been established by measuring neuromuscular properties [28]. TMG has five outcome measures: TC, TS, TD, DM, and $\frac{1}{2}$ TR. In this study, we used TC and DM as the key parameters because they have high reliability in representing the effect of training on muscles. Contraction time is the period between the moment when muscular contraction is 10% and the moment when contraction reaches 90% of the maximum (ms), with the value of the TC depending on the percentage of slow or fast muscle fibres. The amplitude of DM (mm) is also linked to the TC values and depends on muscular flexibility [16].

Table 1. Core training program for the swimmers.

Exercises	Progression	Week 1 Repetitions	Week 1 Sets	Week 1 Weight	Week 2 Repetitions	Week 2 Sets	Week 2 Weight	Week 3 Repetitions	Week 3 Sets	Week 3 Weight
Prone Bridge *	Volume	30 s Hold	Two	-	60 s Hold	Two	-	90 s Hold	Two	-
Side Bridge *	Volume	30 s Hold	Two	-	60 s Hold	Two	-	90 s Hold	Two	-
Bird Dog *	Volume	10 Repetitions	Three	-	15 Repetitions	Three	-	20 Repetitions	Three	-
Leg Raising *	Volume	10 Repetitions	Three	-	15 Repetitions	Three	-	20 Repetitions	Three	-
Overhead Squat **	Resistance	10 Repetitions	Three	3 kg	10 Repetitions	Three	4 kg	15 Repetitions	Three	5 kg
Sit Twist **	Resistance	15 Repetitions	Three	3 kg	15 Repetitions	Three	4 kg	15 Repetitions	Three	5 kg
Shoulder Press ***	Volume	10 Repetitions	Three	3 kg	10 Repetitions	Four	3 kg	15 Repetitions	Three	3 kg
		Week Four			Week Five			Week Six		
Prone Bridge *	Volume	90 s Hold	Three	-	120 s Hold	Two	-	120 s Hold	Three	-
Side Bridge *	Volume	90 s Hold	Three	-	120 s Hold	Two	-	120 s Hold	Three	-
Bird Dog *	Volume	25 Repetitions	Three	-	25 Repetitions	Four	-	30 Repetitions	Three	-
Leg Raising *	Volume	25 Repetitions	Three	-	25 Repetitions	Four	-	30 Repetitions	Three	-
Overhead Squat **	Resistance	20 Repetitions	Three	6 kg	20 Repetitions	Four	7 kg	25 Repetitions	Three	7 kg
Sit Twist **	Resistance	20 Repetitions	Three	6 kg	20 Repetitions	Four	7 kg	25 Repetitions	Three	7 kg
Shoulder Press ***	Volume	20 Repetitions	Three	3 kg	20 Repetitions	Four	3 kg	25 Repetitions	Three	3 kg

* The exercises were performed by body weight. ** The exercises were performed with a medicine ball. *** The exercises were performed with a dumbbell. Core-training exercise details: Prone bridge (plank): hold a straight body position and use elbow and toes to support and pull abdomen and back in a natural position. Side bridge (side plank): start by lying on one side and push the body line straight through the feet and hips. Bird dog: stand on one knee and opposite hand, back in normal position, slowly extend one leg backwards, and raise opposite arm horizontally to the back level. The pelvis should not tilt and back arm should go to start position, and repeat on the other side. Leg raise: Lie supine on the floor with extended knees and lift one leg straight till 75-degree hip, then return to start position and swap the other side. Overhead squat: stand on both legs and hold medicine ball overhead using both hands; back should be vertical and straight. Squat as low as possible while maintaining balance. Sit twist: sit on the floor with knees bent 45 degrees and keep in natural position. While holding a medicine ball with both hands, twist the waist and shoulder to one side. The ball should be held out and front. Return to the neutral position, and repeat the other side. Shoulder press: lie prone with extended arms, hold a dumbbell in both hands, raise one arm, return, and repeat the other arm.

2.5.2. Swimming Parameters

All swimming performance measurements were taken in the same indoor swimming pool (50 m) at a temperature of 30 °C. Safety procedures were followed to ensure minimal risk, and this included a rescue team being available in the swimming pool. Furthermore, safety equipment, such as safety ropes and safety rings, was available in the swimming pool to prevent the risk of drowning. Special preparations were followed to determine the stroke parameters, including setting up a straight-line sector in the swimming pool [31]. Divider markers in the form of spiral float line lane ropes of 50 m were placed in the swimming pool. Three high-speed waterproof video cameras (GoPro HERO7, GoPro Inc, San Mateo, CA, USA) were used. One camera was placed on a wall 10 m away from the swimming pool to detect the total ST from the start point to the end point. The second camera was placed 0.15 m underwater in the centre of the lane to detect the stroke parameters [31]. The third camera was movable by the researcher to keep track of the entire trial (Figure 2). A chronometer was used by the coach to detect the ST to avoid possible time error. This measure is widely used to identify the stroke parameters [31,32]. To calculate the stroke parameters, the swimmers were asked to perform 15 min of warm-up exercises before the trial. Each swimmer was asked to take up a starting position in the swimming pool, followed by a 50 m front crawl swim with a maximum performance from a push-off start from the wall at the surface level (to isolate the effect of a dive) to the 50 m end point. The swimmers were asked to swim in a straight line at the whistle signal. Data were saved on the investigator's laptop with password protection, which means that only the researchers had access to the information. The trial measurement time took a total of 1.5 h. After taking the measurements, we used Pinnacle 22 software (https://www.pinnaclesys.com, accessed on 23 January 2021) to analyse the stroke parameters by viewing the trials and calculating the strokes. This program is valid and reliable [33].

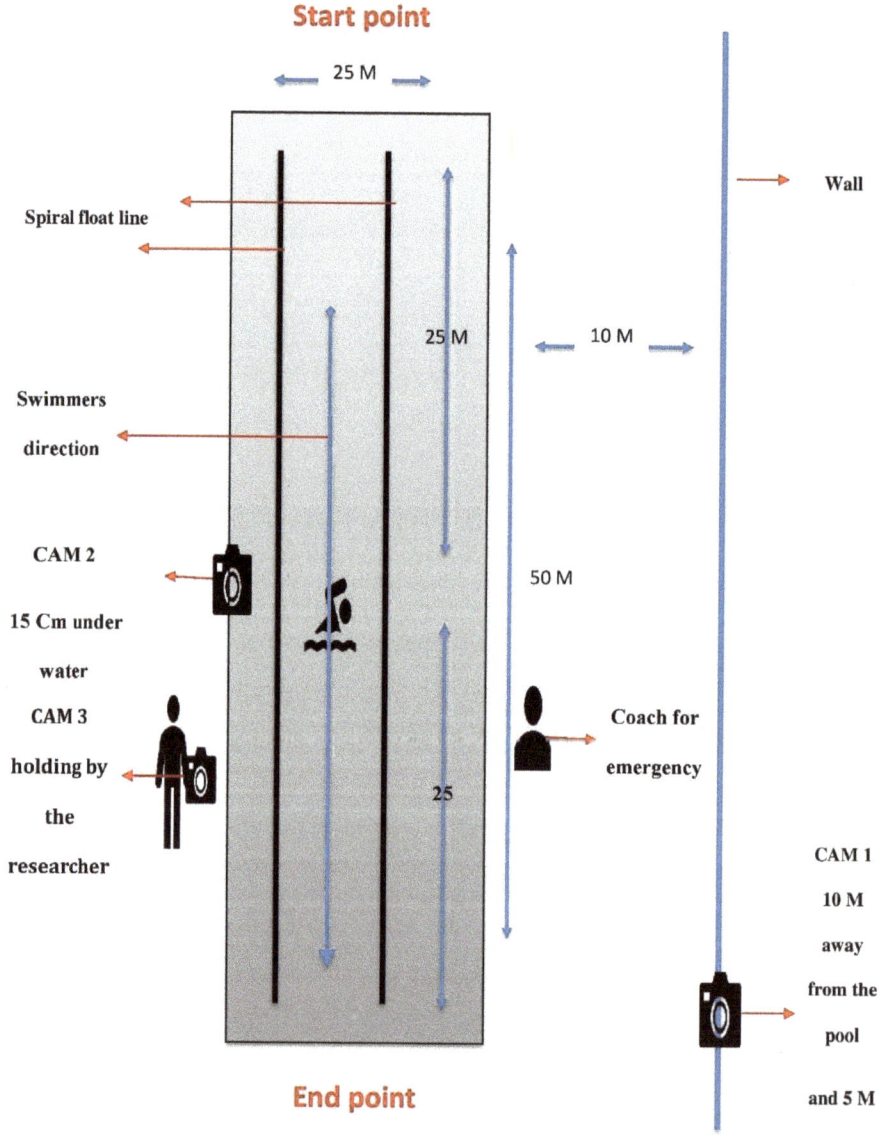

Figure 2. Swimming performance measurements.

The following parameters were measured:

1. Swimming velocity or swimming speed (SV; m.s^{-1}): Total distance covered (50 m) divided by the time required to cover that distance (s) [31,34,35] $\left(SV = \frac{D}{T}\right)$;
2. Stroke rate (SR; cycle.min^{-1}): The average time to perform a complete arm stroke $SR = (T_{stroke}^{-1}) \times 60$. SR was measured by taking the average of three complete cycles divided by three, and we used the equal sign in the equation [31,34,35]. SR = (3/3 CYCLE TIME) × 60;
3. Stroke length (SL; m. cycle^{-1}): SV (m.s^{-1}) divided by SR (cycle.min^{-1}) yields the cycle length in meters [31,34,35]. $SL = \left(\frac{V}{SR}\right) \times 60$;
4. Total strokes (NX): The total of the arm stroke cycles performed during the maximal test divided by the total test time [31,34,35]. N = (SR × T) / 60;
5. Sprint time (ST): The total time (s) covered in a 50 m distance from start to end [9];
6. Stroke index (SI; m^2·s^{-1}): SL (in m) and SV [36]. SI = (SL × V).

2.6. Program Compliance

Program compliance was assessed according to the swimmers' rate of participation using an attendance log. We considered compliance in training and decided to exclude subjects who would miss 15% of the required exercise sessions (three sessions). The researchers and team coaches monitored the exercise program in both the experimental and control groups to encourage the swimmers and prevent the risk of any injury.

2.7. Statistical Analysis

Data are presented as the mean ± SD. The difference was obtained between the post-test and pre-test to quantify the changes in athletic performance with an estimated 95% confidence interval (CI). SPSS version 20.0 was used to analyse the effect of the core-training intervention on all the outcome measures. Analysis of covariance was used to compare the two groups, with body mass, age, and pre-test score as the covariates to manage any imbalances in the measures between the intervention and the control group at baseline [9,37]. The change in the baseline method was used to represent the absolute change in the mean within-group [38]. Probabilistic magnitude-based inferences were made about the true value of the outcomes based on the likelihood that the true population difference was considerably positive or substantially negative [9,39]. The magnitude thresholds that were used as thresholds were 0.1, 0.3, and 0.5 for small, moderate, and large correlation coefficients, respectively, as suggested by Cohen [40] (1988). The standardised thresholds of 0.20, 0.60, and 1.20 [9,37] for the standardised differences in the means (the mean difference divided by the between-subjects SD) were derived from the between-subjects standard deviations of the baseline value to assess the magnitude of the effects. Effect size = mean difference ($X_1 - X_2$)/pooled SD. Statistical analysis was set to a significance level of $p \leq 0.05$. The normal distribution for the data was tested using the Shapiro–Wilks test, observation of histograms, and Q-Q plots.

3. Results

Table 2 presents the characteristics of the subjects. No statistically significant difference was found between the groups. Table 3 shows the core-training intervention, which had a positive effect on the swimming performance outcomes and neuromuscular outcomes. TC-ES, TC-LD, and SL showed a large beneficial effect after the training with the effect size d = 1.47, 1.01, and 0.7, respectively. TC-EO (effect size d = 0.5), DM-ES (effect size d = 0.33), DM-LD (effect size d = 0.45), DM-OE (effect size d = 0.5), SI (effect size d = 0.5), and NX (effect size d = 0.4) showed a moderate beneficial effect, while SR (effect size d = 0.3) and SV (effect size d = 0.28) showed a small effect. The group comparison was statistically significant ($p \leq 0.01$) in all the swimming performance outcomes. Moreover, the core-training intervention had a beneficial effect on ES, LD, and EO, with TC reduced and DM increased. The control group showed an increase in TC-ES, TC-LD, TC-EO, and DM-ES and a decrease in DM-LD and DM-EO. The group comparison after the core training was statistically significant ($p \leq 0.05$) for TC-ES, TC-LD, TC-EO, DM-LD, and DM-EO.

Table 2. Characteristics of the subjects. No statistically significant difference was found between the group. Values are presented as mean ± standard deviation.

Variable	Core Training Group (n = 9)	Control Group (n = 9)
Age (year)	13 ± 2	13.11 ± 2.6
Body Weight (kg)	48.3 ± 14.2	49.1 ± 11.3
Height (cm)	158.8 ± 17.3	160.4 ± 11.9

Table 3. The outcome measures between- and within-group comparison.

Performance Parameters	Core Training Group			Control Group			Group Comparison		
	Baseline Value	Post-Test Value	Adjusted Changed Score Lower—Upper 95% CI	Baseline Value	Post-Test Value	Adjusted Changed Score Lower—Upper 95% CI	Differences between Groups 95% CI	QI	p
TC ES (ms)	17.4 ± 3.4	15.8 ± 2.7	−1.5; −6.5 to 3.4	20.8 ± 4.3	26.5 ± 9.7	5.8; 0.92 to 10.8	−7.3; −14.7 to −0.007	Large +	0.05
TC LD (ms)	26.7 ± 6.8	24.4 ± 4.7	−7; −11.3 to −2.7	39.7 ± 9.6	38.6 ± 5.7	3.7; −0.6 to 8	−10.7; −17.6 to −3.8	Large +	0.01
TC OE (ms)	22.3 ± 5.8	20.8 ± 5.8	−1.9; −5 to 1.1	24 ± 6.8	26.1 ± 3.1	2.5; −0.5 to 5.6	−4.5; −8.9 to −0.1	Moderate +	0.05
DM ES (mm)	14.3 ± 7.3	17.3 ± 8.8	3.3; 0.4 to 6.2	13.4 ± 7.6	13.8 ± 6.4	0.2; −2.7 to 3.1	3.1; −1 to 7.3	Moderate +	0.12
DM LD (mm)	14.8 ± 8.7	15.6 ± 9.5	0.5; −2.7 to 3.8	17.4 ± 7.6	13 ± 4.1	−4.1; −7.4 to −0.9	4.7; 0.01 to 9.3	Moderate +	0.05
DM OE (mm)	9.3 ± 6.7	11.6 ± 8.5	2.2; 0.1 to 4.4	7.7 ± 2.5	6.5 ± 2.3	−1.0; −3.2 to 1.1	3.3; 0.3 to 6.3	Moderate +	0.04
ST (seconds)	39.2 ± 8.4	37.6 ± 8.3	−1.6; −2.2 to −0.9	37.6 ± 4.0	37.5 ± 4.1	−0.1; −0.8 to 0.5	−1.4; −2.4 to −0.5	small +	0.01
SV (m.s^{-1})	1.3 + 0.3	1.3 ± 0.2	0.06; 0.03 to 0.1	1.3 ± 0.2	1.3 ± 0.1	0.004; −0.02 to 0.03	0.1; 0.02 to 0.1	Small +	<0.01
SR (cycle.min^{-1})	49.6 ± 8.0	46 ± 8.1	−3.5; −4.8 to −2.2	46.1 ± 4.3	45.4 ± 4.3	−0.7; −2 to 0.6	−2.8; −4.7 to −1	Small +	0.01
SL (m.cycle^{-1})	1.6 ± 0.3	2.5 ± 0.8	0.2; 0.2 to 0.3	1.8 ± 0.2	2.4 ± 0.5	0.02; −0.04 to 0.1	0.2; 0.1 to 0.3	Large +	<0.01
SI (m^2·s^{-1})	2.2 + 0.7	1.8 ± 0.3	0.4; 0.3 to 0.5	2.4 + 0.5	1.8 ± 0.2	0.03; −0.1 to 0.2	0.4; 0.2 to 0.5	Moderate +	<0.01
NX	31.7 + 5.5	28.3 ± 5.5	−3.4; −4.2 to −2.6	28.8 ± 4.3	28.4 ± 4.2	−0.5; −1.4 to 0.3	−2.9; −4.1 to −1.6	Moderate +	<0.01

QI, qualitative inference; CI, confidence interval; +, positive effect on core-training group compared with controls; TC, time contraction; DM, muscle displacement; ES, erector spinae; LD, latissimus dorsi; OE, obliques external; ST, sprint time; SV, swimming velocity; SL, stroke length; SR, stroke rate; SI, stroke index; NX, total strokes.

4. Discussion

This study investigated the efficacy of a six-week core-training program in the swimming performance and TMG neuromuscular properties of young swimmers. To the best of our knowledge, previous studies have focused mostly on the effects of land-based limb power and strength interventions, with inconsistent findings with regard to swimming [8]. Moreover, there is limited evidence regarding the application of a core-training program to swimmers in terms of functional performance. Moreover, no study has used TMG to measure the effect of core-training exercises on swimmers. In our study, the core-training program had a beneficial effect on swimming performance and neuromuscular outcomes compared with the control group. Therefore, our finding rejected the null hypothesis and agreed with the alternate hypothesis that a six-week core-training program significantly affects the swimming performance parameters and TMG neuromuscular parameters of young swimmers ($p < 0.05$).

4.1. Swimming Performance and Core Training

The change in the swimming performance time required to improve swimmers' performance was 0.5% [9,39]. The beneficial effect was (−1.4 s) ≅ 3.47% on sprint swimming performance time after the core-training program, as calculated by $\frac{\text{post}-\text{pre}}{\text{pre}} \times 100$, which represents the estimated percentage differences [9,39]. Furthermore, SV (+0.1 m·s^{-1}), SR (−2.8 cycle·min^{-1}), SL (+0.2 m·cycle^{-1}), SI (+0.4 m^2·s^{-1}), and NX (−2.9 total strokes) represented a positive performance improvement [41]. These results showed that the beneficial effect was moderate on SL, SI, and NX and small on ST, SR, and SV after the training. The group comparison (95%) CI was statistically significant ($p \leq 0.01$) for ST, SV, SR, SL, SI, and NX. These findings are consistent with those of previous studies [2,9,32].

Weston et al. [9] studied the effect of 12 weeks of core training on swimming performance, which included ST and the physiological change in core muscles assessed by electromyography. The findings showed a significant improvement in ST and core muscle function starting from the sixth week. Moreover, the beneficial effect of ST was positively large. In the present study, the effect was positively small. Nevertheless, the variation in effect size depended on the mean difference between the groups and the mean difference method. Additionally, it was not associated with the p-value, as it could be beneficial, but not significant [42]. D. Patil et al. [2] reported that a six-week core-training program could significantly enhance swimming performance, including ST, SV, and SI, among young competitive swimmers in the 50 m freestyle. S. Iizuka et al. [32] reported that trunk muscle training could significantly improve swimming performance by reducing the starting time. The current study results are not consistent with those of H. Tanaka et al. [43], who reported that land-based training did not improve swimming performance and that improved power and strength did not affect swimming performance. This variation in the results may be due to the methodological issues in Tanaka et al.'s study, as they did not use a control group to measure the effect of the intervention on the group. A possible explanation for our result is that core training can enhance the production and transmutation of forces in the lower and upper extremities [3–5]. The enhancement of force production in core training is achieved by improving neural adaptation, leading to faster nervous system activation, improved synchronisation of motor units, increased neural recruitment patterns, and decreased neural inhibitory reflexes [3]. These can help sustain the efficient posture needed while swimming, thus generating powerful movement effectively. They can also help to stabilise the pelvis and the lumbar spine during kicks, enabling powerful strokes and assisting swimmers to move faster in water. They can also help the abdominal muscles maintain balance in the water and stabilise the trunk to prevent sagging down, which leads to decreased drag force [2]. If these aspects are ignored, resistive forces at the extremities increase, and the stroke technique breaks down, leading to inefficient strokes [44]. In our study, the core power of the swimmers increased, which enhanced their capability to sustain an efficient technique throughout the entire race.

4.2. Swimming Parameters

The swimming parameters such as ST, SV, SR, SL, SI, and NX are connected. For example, SV and SI increase when SL increases and SR decreases; NX increases SV; SI increases when SL increases, with no change in SR, in freestyle swimmers [45]. SR, SL, and SV are the main swimming parameters in the 50 m freestyle that demonstrate improvement in swimming performance [33,46]. As previously mentioned, our results showed that the SR value for the experimental group decreased by 3.5 and that SL, SV, and SI increased by 0.2 m·cycle^{-1}, 0.06 m·s^{-1}, and 0.4 m^2·s^{-1}, respectively. The control group showed a decrease of 0.7 cycle·min^{-1} in SR and an increase of 0.02 m·cycle^{-1}, 0.004 m·s^{-1}, and 0.03 m^2·s^{-1} in SL, SV, and SI, respectively. The group comparison was SR (−2.8) $p < 0.01$; SL (0.2) $p < 0.00$; SV (0.1) $p < 0.00$; and SI (0.4) $p < 0.00$. Our findings are similar to those in previous studies [43,45–48].

Hay et al. [47] showed that an increase in SL was associated with improved SV, which led to performance enhancement. Thus, a decrease in SL is linked to a decrease in SV [45]. Girold et al. [48], Aspenes et al. [49], and Roberts et al. [50] also found that the improvement in performance after training was associated with increased SL and decreased SR. The results of the current study are not consistent with those of some previous studies [26,43].

Tanaka et al. [43] found that an increase in performance did not result in an increase in SL. Girold et al. [26] found a significant decrease in SL with a significant increase in SR. This variation in results may be due to the training program, as previous studies used static sprint training and resistance training focused on the arms and shoulders. The authors suggested that low repetitions with a high SV are needed for improving SL. Increasing the strength level could lead to an increased SL [46]. Furthermore, as swimming distance increases to >400 m, SR becomes less of a determining factor [51], but increases because of a decrease in SL at volitional exhaustion [45]. Moreover, SL tends to be shorter for butterfly and longer for backstroke and freestyle, while SR is less in backstroke and freestyle and increases in butterfly and breaststroke. These may depend on neuromotor control and muscular endurance [44]. Our findings support the idea that an increase in SL and a decrease in SR represent an improvement in ST and swimmers' speed, leading to improvement in SI.

4.3. Neuromuscular Properties

Our intervention improved core muscle functionality, which was assessed by the TMG parameters. TC decreased (−1.5 ms) for ES, (−7 ms) LD, and (−1.9 ms) EO, and DM increased (+3.3 mm) for ES, (+0.5 mm) LD, and (+2.2 mm) EO compared with the baseline value. The control group was (5.8 ms) TC-ES, (3.7 ms) LD, (2.5 ms) EO, (0.2 mm) DM-ES, (−4.1 mm) LD, and (−1.0 mm) EO compared with the baseline value. The beneficial effect was large for TC-ES and TC-LD and moderate for TC-EO, DM-ES, DM-LD, and DM-EO. The group comparison (95% CI) was statistically significant $p \leq 0.05$ for TC-ES, TC-LD, TC-EO, DM-LD, and DM-EO and $p \leq 0.12$ for DM-ES. We assumed that the increase in TC and the decrease in DM for the control group were due to the slow process of recruiting motor units [16]. Our findings are consistent with some previous studies [16,22,52].

Rusu et al. [16] showed that a six-week isometric–concentric training could improve muscle functionality associated with a decrease in TC and an increase in DM values, leading to a high rate of Type II muscle fibres and a faster process of motor unit recruiting for the experimental group. Conversely, the control group showed an increase in TC and a decrease in DM values, indicating a slow motor unit recruiting process. Valverde et al. [22] found that a decrease in TC and increased DM values indicated a good response following muscle training. Monteiro and Massuca [52] showed that a decrease in muscle TC and an increase in DM had a beneficial effect on the muscle following training. Rusu et al. [16] suggested that concentric training could lead to an increased TC and a reduced DM, which is the opposite effect of isometric–concentric training and could occur due to the enlargement of the muscle as a result of concentric training. Muscle fatigue could change the TMG parameters, as it could increase TC and decrease DM as a result of high-intensity resistance, interval training, or endurance training over short periods [53]. However, our findings support that a decrease in TC and an increase in DM following isometric–concentric training could improve muscle functionality.

4.4. Practical Application

The results showed that a core-training intervention can enhance swimmers' performance and improve muscular functionality. The findings from this study can be generalised to any swimmer in the age group studied. Therefore, our findings can be helpful as evidence to assist coaches, trainers, and therapists in applying a core-training program along with regular training to improve the swimming performance of young swimmers. Nevertheless, this study has several limitations. First, puberty, maturation, and testosterone hormones could have influenced the results. They vary from child to child, cannot be controlled, and may mask training effects [54]. Further research should include or control for the effect of growth and maturation, which is a major hurdle when studying young athletes. Second, only male swimmers were recruited for the study, and thus, our findings cannot be generalised to female swimmers. Third, we investigated only the effect of a core-training intervention on the 50 m freestyle. We recommend that other swimming styles and long-distance swimming be included. Further studies are needed to investigate larger groups and athletes at different levels and those from different places or clubs. Fourth, some of the exercises used in the core-training program (e.g., shoulder press) might have caused an improvement in the upper and lower limb strength, which may influence the swimming performance. Fifth, we were unable to demonstrate the effect of the core-training intervention on stroke depth. Further research is needed to demonstrate the effect of core training on stroke depth. Nevertheless, we found a significant improvement in our performance measures after considering the effects of body mass and age.

5. Conclusions

A six-week core-training program along with regular swimming training significantly improved the freestyle swimming performance and core muscle properties, such as contractility (contraction time), excitability, extensibility, and elasticity, of the experimental group compared with the group that did not undergo the core-training program. These results can serve as evidence to assist coaches, trainers, and therapists in improving the swimming performance of young swimmers.

Author Contributions: A.K. and S.N. made substantial contributions to the concept, design, and study preparation. R.J., T.S.A. and Q.M. reviewed and edited the manuscript. All authors have read and agreed to the published version of the manuscript.

Funding: This research received no external funding.

Institutional Review Board Statement: The study was conducted according to the guidelines of the Declaration of Helsinki and approved by the Institutional Review Board of Imam Abdulrahman Bin Faisal University (IRB-PGS-2019-03-241).

Informed Consent Statement: Informed consent was obtained from all subjects involved in the study.

Data Availability Statement: The data that support the findings of this study are available from the corresponding author upon request.

Acknowledgments: Special thanks to the staff of the public authority for the sport swimming pool in Dammam for helping us throughout the data collection and giving us all the resources that we needed. The funding for this article was supported by each author from their own sources, to design the study and apply the training program. We also thank the Saudi Ministry of Health and Imam Abdulrahman Bin Faisal University, which allowed us to use their equipment for research and supported us throughout the research.

Conflicts of Interest: The authors declare no conflict of interest.

References

1. Toussaint, H.M.; Beek, P.J. Biomechanics of competitive front crawl swimming. *Sports Med.* **1992**, *13*, 8–24. [CrossRef] [PubMed]
2. Patil, D.; Salian, S.; Yardi, S. The effect of core strengthening on performance of young competitive swimmers. *Int. J. Sci. Res.* **2014**, *3*, 2470–2477.
3. Hibbs, A.E.; Thompson, K.G.; French, D.; Wrigley, A.; Spears, I. Optimizing performance by improving core stability and core strength. *Sports Med.* **2008**, *38*, 995–1008. [CrossRef] [PubMed]
4. Reed, C.A.; Ford, K.R.; Myer, G.D.; Hewett, T.E. The effects of isolated and integrated 'core stability' training on athletic performance measures: A systematic review. *Sports Med.* **2012**, *42*, 697–706. [CrossRef]
5. Dingley, A.A.; Pyne, D.B.; Youngson, J.; Burkett, B. Effectiveness of a dry-land resistance training program on strength, power, and swimming performance in paralympic swimmers. *J. Strength Cond. Res.* **2015**, *29*, 619–626. [CrossRef]
6. Kibler, W.B.; Press, J.; Sciascia, A. The role of core stability in athletic function. *Sports Med.* **2006**, *36*, 189–198. [CrossRef]
7. Fig, G. Strength training for swimmers: Training the core. *Strength Cond.* **2005**, *27*, 40–42. [CrossRef]
8. Aspenes, S.T.; Karlsen, T. Exercise-training intervention studies in competitive swimming. *Sports Med.* **2012**, *42*, 527–543. [CrossRef]
9. Weston, M.; Hibbs, A.E.; Thompson, K.G.; Spears, I.R. Isolated core training improves sprint performance in national-level junior swimmers. *Int. J. Sports Physiol. Perform.* **2015**, *10*, 204–210. [CrossRef]
10. Karpiński, J.; Rejdych, W.; Brzozowska, D.; Gołaś, A.; Sadowski, W.; Swinarew, A.S.; Stachura, A.; Gupta, S.; Stanula, A. The effects of a 6-week core exercises on swimming performance of national level swimmers. *PLoS ONE* **2020**, *15*, e0227394. [CrossRef]

11. Martens, J.; Einarsson, I.P.; Schnizer, N.; Staes, F.; Daly, D. Lower trunk muscle activity during front crawl swimming in a single leg amputee. *Port. J. Sports Sci.* **2011**, *11*, 751–754.
12. Amaro, N.M.; Morouço, P.G.; Marques, M.C.; Batalha, N.; Neiva, H.; Marinho, D.A. A systematic review on dry-land strength and conditioning training on swimming performance. *Sci. Sports* **2019**, *34*, e1–e14. [CrossRef]
13. Pisot, R.; Narici, M.V.; Simunic, B.; De Boer, M.; Seynnes, O.; Jurdana, M.; Biolo, G.; Mekjavic, I.B. Whole muscle contractile parameters and thickness loss during 35-day bed rest. *Eur. J. Appl. Physiol.* **2008**, *104*, 409–414. [CrossRef] [PubMed]
14. Rey, E.; Lago-Penas, C.; Lago-Ballesteros, J. Tensiomyography of selected lower-limb muscles in professional soccer players. *J. Electromyogr. Kinesiol.* **2012**, *22*, 866–872. [CrossRef] [PubMed]
15. Dahmane, R.; Djordjevic, S.; Simunic, B.; Valencic, V. Spatial fiber type distribution in normal human muscle Histochemical and tensiomyographical evaluation. *J. Biomech.* **2005**, *38*, 2451–2459. [CrossRef]
16. Rusu, L.D.; Cosma, G.G.; Cernaianu, S.M.; Marin, M.N.; Rusu, P.F.; Ciocănescu, D.P.; Neferu, F.N. Tensiomyography method used for neuromuscular assessment of muscle training. *J. Neuroeng. Rehabil.* **2013**, *10*, 67. [CrossRef]
17. Loturco, I.; Pereira, L.A.; Kobal, R.; Kitamura, K.; Ramírez-Campillo, R.; Zanetti, V.; Abad, C.C.; Nakamura, F.Y. Muscle contraction velocity: A suitable approach to analyze the functional adaptations in elite soccer players. *J. Sports Sci. Med.* **2016**, *15*, 483–491.
18. García-García, O.; Serrano-Gómez, V.; Hernández-Mendo, A.; Tapia-Flores, A. Assessment of the in-season changes in mechanical and neuromuscular characteristics in professional soccer players. *J. Sports Med. Phys. Fit.* **2016**, *56*, 714–723.
19. Diez-Vega, I.; Jj, M.; Fernández-del-Valle, M.; Rodríguez-Matoso, D.; Rodríguez-Ruiz, D. Normalized response speed and jumping-related techniques after training in female volleyball players. In Proceedings of the IV NSCA International Conference, Murcia, Spain, 26–28 June 2014; pp. 26–28.
20. Diez-Vega, I.; Jj, M.; Fernández-del-Valle, M.; Rodríguez-Matoso, D.; Rodríguez-Ruiz, D. Changes in the mechanical characteristics of the knee musculature in professional female volleyball players. In Proceedings of the IV NSCA International Conference, Murcia, Spain, 26–28 June 2014; pp. 26–28.
21. Peterson, K.D.; Quiggle, G.T. Tensiomyographical responses to accelerometer loads in female collegiate basketball players. *J. Sports Sci.* **2017**, *35*, 2334–2341. [CrossRef]
22. Rojas Valverde, D.F.; Gutiérrez Vargas, R.; Sánchez Ureña, B.A.; Gutiérrez Vargas, J.C.; Cruz Fuentes, I.; Salas Cabrera, J. Post-competition neuromuscular performance in professional football players in Costa Rica: Tensiomyographic monitoring. *Pensar En Movimiento Revista De Ciencias Del Ejercicio Y La Salud* **2015**, *13*, 1–15.
23. García-García, O.; Cuba-Dorado, A.; Fernández-Redondo, D.; López-Chicharro, J. Neuromuscular parameters predict the performance in an incremental cycling test. *Int. J. Sports Med.* **2018**, *39*, 909–915. [CrossRef] [PubMed]
24. Gil, S.; Loturco, I.; Tricoli, V.; Ugrinowitsch, C.; Kobal, R.; Abad, C.C.; Roschel, H. Tensiomyography parameters and jumping and sprinting performance in Brazilian elite soccer players. *Sports Biome.* **2015**, *14*, 340–350. [CrossRef] [PubMed]
25. Valenzuela, P.L.; Montalvo, Z.; Sánchez-Martínez, G.; Torrontegi, E.; De La Calle-Herrero, J.; Dominguez-Castells, R.; Maffiuletti, N.A.; De La Villa, P. Relationship between skeletal muscle contractile properties and power production capacity in female Olympic rugby players. *Eur. J. Sport Sci.* **2018**, *18*, 677–684. [CrossRef] [PubMed]
26. Girold, S.; Calmels, P.; Maurin, D.; Milhau, N.; Chatard, J. Assisted and resisted sprint training in swimming. *J. Strength Cond. Res.* **2006**, *20*, 547.
27. Schulz, K.F.; Altman, D.G.; Moher, D. CONSORT 2010 statement: Updated guidelines for reporting parallel group randomized trials. *Ann. Intern. Med.* **2011**, *154*, 291–292. [CrossRef]
28. Hibbs, A.E.; Thompson, K.G.; French, D.N.; Hodgson, D.; Spears, I.R. Peak and average rectified EMG measures: Which method of data reduction should be used for assessing core training exercises? *J. Electromyogr. Kinesiol.* **2011**, *21*, 102–111. [CrossRef] [PubMed]
29. Jeno, S.H.; Varacallo, M. Anatomy, back, latissimus dorsi. In *StatPearls*; StatPearls Publishing LLC: Tampa, FL, USA, 2018; p. 20.
30. Lohr, C.; Braumann, K.M.; Reer, R.; Schroeder, J.; Schmidt, T. Reliability of tensiomyography and myotonometry in detecting mechanical and contractile characteristics of the lumbar erector spinae in healthy volunteers. *Eur. J. Appl. Physiol.* **2018**, *118*, 1349–1359. [CrossRef]
31. Franken, M.; Diefenthaeler, F.; Moré, F.C.; Silveira, R.P.; Castro, F.A.d.S. Critical stroke rate as a parameter for evaluation in swimming. *Mot. Rev. Educ. Física* **2013**, *19*, 724–729. [CrossRef]
32. Iizuka, S.; Imai, A.; Koizumi, K.; Okuno, K.; Kaneoka, K. Immediate effects of deep trunk muscle training on swimming start performance. *Int. J. Sports Phys. Ther.* **2016**, *11*, 1048–1053.
33. Girold, S.; Maurin, D.; Dugue, B.; Chatard, J.C.; Millet, G. Effects of dry-land vs. resisted- and assisted-sprint exercises on swimming sprint performances. *J. Strength Cond. Res.* **2007**, *21*, 599–605. [CrossRef]
34. Barbosa, T.M.; Costa, M.; Marinho, D.A.; Coelho, J.; Moreira, M.; Silva, A.J. Modeling the Links Between Young Swimmers' Performance: Energetic and Biomechanic Profiles. *Pediatric Exerc. Sci.* **2010**, *22*, 379–391. [CrossRef] [PubMed]
35. Barbosa, T.M.; Morouco, P.G.; Jesus, S.; Feitosa, W.G.; Costa, M.J.; Marinho, D.A.; Silva, A.J.; Garrido, N.D. The interaction between intra-cyclic variation of the velocity and mean swimming velocity in young competitive swimmers. *Int. J. Sports Med.* **2013**, *34*, 123–130. [CrossRef] [PubMed]
36. Costill, D.L.; Kovaleski, J.; Porter, D.; Kirwan, J.; Fielding, R.; King, D. Energy expenditure during front crawl swimming: Predicting success in middle-distance events. *Int. J. Sports Med.* **1985**, *6*, 266–270. [CrossRef] [PubMed]

37. Hopkins, W.G.; Marshall, S.W.; Batterham, A.M.; Hanin, J. Progressive statistics for studies in sports medicine and exercise science. *Med. Sci. Sports Exerc.* **2009**, *41*, 3–13. [CrossRef]
38. Vickers, A.J. The use of percentage change from baseline as an outcome in a controlled trial is statistically inefficient: A simulation study. *BMC Med. Res. Methodol.* **2001**, *1*, 6. [CrossRef]
39. Stewart, A.; Hopkins, W. Consistency of swimming performance within and between competitions. *Med. Sci. Sports Exerc.* **2000**, *32*, 997–1001. [CrossRef]
40. Cohen, J. *Statistical Power Analysis for the Behavioral Sciences*, 2nd ed.; Lawrence Erlbaum Associates: Hillsdale, NJ, USA, 1988.
41. Gencer, Y. Effects of 8-week core exercises on free style swimming performance of female swimmers aged 9–12. *Asian J. Educ. Train.* **2018**, *4*, 182–185. [CrossRef]
42. Durlak, J.A. How to select, calculate, and interpret effect sizes. *J. Pediatric Psychol.* **2009**, *34*, 917–928. [CrossRef]
43. Tanaka, H.; Costill, D.L.; Thomas, R.; Fink, W.J.; Widrick, J.J. Dry-land resistance training for competitive swimming. *Med. Sci. Sports Exerc.* **1993**, *25*, 952–959. [CrossRef]
44. Keskinen, K.L.; Komi, P.V. Stroking characteristics of front crawl swimming during exercise. *J. Appl. Biomech.* **1993**, *9*, 219–226. [CrossRef]
45. Craig, A.B., Jr.; Skehan, P.L.; Pawelczyk, J.A.; Boomer, W.L. Velocity, stroke rate, and distance per stroke during elite swimming competition. *Med. Sci. Sports Exerc.* **1985**, *17*, 625–634. [CrossRef] [PubMed]
46. Crowley, E.; Harrison, A.J.; Lyons, M. The impact of resistance training on swimming performance: A systematic review. *Sports Med.* **2017**, *47*, 2285–2307. [CrossRef] [PubMed]
47. Hay, J.; Guimaraes, A.; Grimston, S. A quantitative look at swimming biomechanics. *Swim. Tech.* **1983**, *20*, 11–17.
48. Girold, S.; Jalab, C.; Bernard, O.; Carette, P.; Kemoun, G.; Dugué, B. Dry-land strength training vs. electrical stimulation in sprint swimming performance. *J. Strength Cond. Res.* **2012**, *26*, 497–505. [CrossRef]
49. Aspenes, S.; Kjendlie, P.-L.; Hoff, J.; Helgerud, J. Combined strength and endurance training in competitive swimmers. *J. Sports Sci. Med.* **2009**, *8*, 357.
50. Roberts, A.; Termin, B.; Reilly, M.; Pendergast, D. Effectiveness of biokinetic training on swimming performance in collegiate swimmers. *J. Swim. Res.* **1991**, *7*, 5–11.
51. Alberty, M.; Sidney, M.; Pelayo, P.; Toussaint, H.M. Stroking characteristics during time to exhaustion tests. *Med. Sci. Sports Exerc.* **2009**, *41*, 637–644. [CrossRef]
52. Monteiro, L.; Massuca, L. Neuromuscular profile of elite male and female judokas with assessment using tensiomyography. In *Scientific and Professional Conference on Judo "Applicable Research In Judo"*, 1st ed.; Faculty of Kinesiology, University of Zagreb, Croatia, Croatian Judo Federation: Zagreb, Croatia, 2015; pp. 69–70.
53. Macgregor, L.J.; Ditroilo, M.; Smith, I.J.; Fairweather, M.M.; Hunter, A.M. Reduced radial displacement of the gastrocnemius medialis muscle after electrically elicited fatigue. *J. Sport Rehabil.* **2016**, *25*, 241–247. [CrossRef]
54. Armstrong, N. *Paediatric Exercise Physiology*; Elsevier Health Sciences: Philadelphia, PA, USA, 2006.

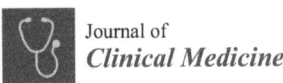

Article

Step Detection Accuracy and Energy Expenditure Estimation at Different Speeds by Three Accelerometers in a Controlled Environment in Overweight/Obese Subjects

Ville Stenbäck [1], Juhani Leppäluoto [1], Rosanna Juustila [1], Laura Niiranen [1], Dominique Gagnon [2,3,4,5], Mikko Tulppo [1] and Karl-Heinz Herzig [1,6,*]

1 Research Unit of Biomedicine, Medical Research Center, Faculty of Medicine, University of Oulu, Oulu University Hospital, 90220 Oulu, Finland; ville.stenback@oulu.fi (V.S.); juhani.leppaluoto@oulu.fi (J.L.); rosanna.juustila@student.oulu.fi (R.J.); laura.niiranen@oulu.fi (L.N.); mikko.tulppo@oulu.fi (M.T.)
2 Helsinki Clinic for Sports and Exercise Medicine, Foundation for Sports and Exercise Medicine, 00550 Helsinki, Finland; ddgagnon@laurentian.ca
3 Department of Sports and Exercise Medicine, Clinicum, University of Helsinki, 00014 Helsinki, Finland
4 School of Kinesiology and Health Sciences, Laurentian University, Sudbury, ON P3E 2C6, Canada
5 Center for Research in Occupational Safety and Health, Laurentian University, Sudbury, ON P3E 2C6, Canada
6 Department of Pediatric Gastroenterology and Metabolic Diseases, Poznan University of Medical Sciences, 61-701 Poznan, Poland
* Correspondence: karl-heinz.herzig@oulu.fi; Tel.: +358-(0)2-9448-5280

Abstract: Our aim was to compare three research-grade accelerometers for their accuracy in step detection and energy expenditure (EE) estimation in a laboratory setting, at different speeds, especially in overweight/obese participants. Forty-eight overweight/obese subjects participated. Participants performed an exercise routine on a treadmill with six different speeds (1.5, 3, 4.5, 6, 7.5, and 9 km/h) for 4 min each. The exercise was recorded on video and subjects wore three accelerometers during the exercise: Sartorio Xelometer (SX, hip), activPAL (AP, thigh), and ActiGraph GT3X (AG, hip), and energy expenditure (EE) was estimated using indirect calorimetry for comparisons. For step detection, speed-wise mean absolute percentage errors for the SX ranged between 9.73–2.26, 6.39–0.95 for the AP, and 88.69–2.63 for the AG. The activPALs step detection was the most accurate. For EE estimation, the ranges were 21.41–15.15 for the SX, 57.38–12.36 for the AP, and 59.45–28.92 for the AG. All EE estimation errors were due to underestimation. All three devices were accurate in detecting steps when speed exceeded 4 km/h and inaccurate in EE estimation regardless of speed. Our results will guide users to recognize the differences, weaknesses, and strengths of the accelerometer devices and their algorithms.

Keywords: accelerometry; step detection; physical activity; energy expenditure; overweight

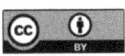

1. Introduction

Obesity is one of the greatest threats to our health and wellbeing worldwide. In 2016, 1.9 billion (39%) adults were considered overweight, of which 650 million (13%) were obese [1]. Obesity is directly linked to disorders such as hypertension, type II diabetes, and cardiovascular disease, which can lead to further chronic disabilities [2]. In the USA alone, the costs of obesity for society are estimated to be USD 1.72 trillion yearly or 9.3% of their gross domestic product [3]. In Germany, the estimated direct and indirect costs are estimated at EUR 63.04 billion yearly or 1.87% of its gross domestic product [4]. These numbers are expected to climb since the prevalence of obesity is continuing to increase [5]. Proper diet and physical activity (PA) are the two most important strategies for weight loss and maintenance for the majority of patients. In addition, PA does not need additional financial resources and could be applied everywhere worldwide. The 2020 WHO Physical Activity Guidelines provide information on the health benefits of physical activity: Most adults should complete at least 150 min a week of moderate physical activity and muscle-strengthening exercises two times a week, or 75 min of vigorous physical activity [6]. Unfortunately, a large proportion of adults do not attain the level of the recommended physical activity.

To accurately assess the effects of PA on populations and create personalized recommendations, more reliable and objective tools are needed. The current recommendations are still largely based on self-reported measures, which include, e.g., asking for information on time used for leisure, household, and transportation activities. Accelerometry is a commonly used objective method to measure PA, but multiple and significant considerations remain. Waist-worn accelerometers are more accurate than wrist-worn ones, data counting systems and the availability of raw data differ between devices, and differences in signal processing, step detection, and filtering exist as well [7–9]. The gait characteristics of the obese include, for example, slower speed and shorter stride length when compared to normal weight people [10]. For most overweight/obese and elderly people, the self-selected walking pace is 3 km/h or lower [11,12]; hence, these low speeds are important when using accelerometry with these subjects and evaluating health benefits. A maximal gait speed of 7 km/h was reported for elderly and elderly obese people in the Baltimore Longitudinal Study of Aging [13]. To capture the habitual PA via accelerometry in overweight, obese, and elderly populations, accurately measuring slow walking is of the utmost importance. The "Gold standard" technique for measuring energy expenditure (EE) is the double-labeled water method, which accurately measures the overall EE from a period longer than 3–4 days but is costly [14]. Direct calorimetry can also be used to measure EE but requires a thermally isolated chamber in which the subject is measured. Indirect calorimetry can be used to estimate EE from the use of O_2 and the production of CO_2 from the ventilation gasses. Furthermore, accelerometers can be used in EE estimation with or without heart rate measurement [15]. A recent review by Pisanu and colleagues states, that EE estimation with accelerometers in overweight and obese subjects is inaccurate [16]. In addition, an underestimation of EE during semi-structured activity protocol including, for example, household activities with the ActiGraph GT3X was observed to be 26% in overweight subjects [17]. Earlier, we showed in normal weight subjects that there are significant differences in the accelerometers' accuracy at different speeds, with decreasing accuracy at speeds of 3 km/h or less [18]. Few studies have investigated the accuracy of research-grade accelerometers in a controlled environment for step detection and EE estimation in overweight and obese people, and importantly, none have included gait speeds initiated at 1.5 km/h, a gait speed we have previously observed in people at risk of T2D [19]. Feito and colleagues (2012) studied the effect of BMI class to step detection accuracy with hip-mounted accelerometers at three different speeds (2.4, 4.0, and 5.6 km/h) and found an error-%s of 20–60% at the lowest speed with no difference between the BMI-classes [20]. Error percentages in EE estimation have been shown to be 40–31% in overweight and obese subjects using the Freedson 1996 cut-off points with speeds starting from 4 km/h [21].

Our aim was to investigate the accuracy of step detection and energy expenditure estimation at different speeds for three research-grade accelerometers in overweight and obese participants under controlled laboratory settings.

2. Materials and Methods

Forty-eight overweight and obese subjects participated in this study (24 males). Subjects were on average 37.4 ± 13.9 years old, and their mean body mass index (BMI, kg/m^2) was 31.4 ± 3.8; they were 173.6 ± 10.3 cm tall, weighted 94.8 ± 15.5 kg, had a skeletal muscle percentage (SMM%) of 36.9 ± 6.2, fat percentage of 34.4 ± 10.1 and waist circumference of 99.2 ± 12.0 cm (Table 1). Exclusion criteria for the participants were BMI less than 25 or over 40, younger than 20 or older than 75 years, any disease or injury preventing normal movement, arthritis, high blood pressure, chronic cardiovascular diseases, or acute cardiovascular event during the last year, ventilatory diseases and pregnancy or lactation. None of the subjects had undergone bariatric surgery for weight loss. This study was approved by the ethical committee in the Northern Ostrobothnia Hospital District (EETTMK 26/3/21). All the participants were healthy volunteers who gave their written informed consent in accordance with the Declaration of Helsinki. This study was conducted following national legislation, guidelines, and the Declaration of Helsinki.

Table 1. Characteristics of the study population. SMM = skeletal muscle mass.

		Min.–Max.
Sex	24 Male, 24 Female	
Age (years)	37.4 ± 14.1	21–74
Height (cm)	173.6 ± 10.3	153.5–194.0
Weight (kg)	94.8 ± 15.5	70.2–142.5
BMI	31.4 ± 3.8	26.5–39.7
SMM-% (impedance)	36.9 ± 6.2	27.3–51.1
Fat-% (impedance)	34.4 ± 10.1	12.2–50.9
Waist circumference (cm)	99.2 ± 12.0	82.0–133.0

All subjects participated in one measurement session conducted between 08:00 and 11:00 in the morning. Subjects were requested to fast at least 10 but not more than 16 h before their scheduled study session. They were also asked to avoid strenuous exercise on the day before and on the morning of the study session. Bioimpedance was used to determine the body composition (InBody 720, Biospace, Co, Ltd., Seoul, Korea). Energy expenditure was estimated via oxygen uptake and carbon dioxide production using indirect calorimetry (IC) (Vyntus CPX, Vyaire Medical GmbH, Hoechberg, Germany). Ergospirometer was calibrated every morning before the first subject and was considered valid for 4 h as instructed by the manufacturer. The contents of the gas were as follows: 5.0% CO_2, 15.9 O_2, and the remaining 79.1% N_2. Resting metabolic rate (RMR) was estimated in a supine position using a Hans Rudolph 7450 V2 mask (Hans Rudolph, Shawnee, Kansas, USA) until the values plateaued for at least 10 min and the last 5 min of the measurement were used to calculate the RMR. Respiratory exchange ratio (RER) was required to stay between 0.90 and 0.70 during the 10-min period. Weir equation was used to calculate the metabolic rate (kcal/day) = $1.44 (3.94 VO_2 + 1.11 VCO_2)$. RMR defined the level of 1 metabolic equivalent (MET) for the subsequent EE estimation analysis.

After conducting the initial measurements, participants underwent an exercise routine on a treadmill (X-erfit 4000 Pro Run). The routine consisted of 6 speeds with a 4-min duration per speed with a total duration of 24 min. The speeds were 1.5, 3, 4.5, 6, 7.5, and 9 km/h. Acceleration to next speed took approximately 5 s at the beginning of each speed. A video camera was used to record participants' feet during the entire exercise. The videos were used to count the actual step numbers at every speed and were performed according to Sushames et al., 2016 [22]. Energy expenditure was recorded during physical activity with a Hans Rudolph 7450 V2 mask. Energy expenditure for each speed was calculated using the Weir equation from the last minute of each speed and multiplying that with 4. Transformation to metabolic equivalents (METs) was performed using RMR as the level 1 MET.

Three accelerometers were worn by subjects during the exercise protocol. A Sartorio Xelometer (SX) (Sartorio Oy, Oulu, Finland) and an ActiGraph GT3X (AG) (ActiGraph LLC, Pensacola, FL, USA) were attached with elastic belts on the right side of the hip and an activPAL (AP) (PAL Technologies Ltd., Glasgow, Scotland) worn on the right thigh, all following the manufacturers' recommendation. The data from the SX device was extracted using Sartorio software (v18) and detection algorithms provided by the manufacturer and were run on MATLAB R2019a for step counts, step intensities, and EE estimates (MET) [16]. For AP, PAL connect (v8.10.8.76) was used to set up the device and extract the data and PAL analysis (v8.11.2.54) to analyze the step counts and EE estimates

(METhrs). The AP-derived MET-hours were transformed into METs. Finally, AG data was extracted with ActiLife (v6.13.4) and step counts were calculated using 1 s epochs and 100 Hz sampling rate. For EE (METs), Freedson Adult (1998) cut points were used (equation: MET rate = 1.439008 + (0.000795 × CPM) where CPM = counts per minute). In obese people, the mean amplitude deviation (MAD)—based method, such as the one in SX, provided the most accurate EE estimates (error-% 14.3) [23].

Mean absolute percentage errors (MAPEs) were calculated for every speed between the accelerometer-estimated step counts and actual steps (video) using the following equation:

$$M\% = \left(\frac{1}{n}\sum_{t=1}^{n}\left|\frac{A_t - F_t}{A_t}\right|\right) \times 100$$

Relevant disagreement was considered at MAPEs over 5%. EE data from the accelerometers and IC were analyzed as METs. To observe the similarity between methods, paired-samples t-tests, linear regression, and intraclass correlations (ICC) were calculated, and Bland–Altman plots generated. Paired samples t-tests were used to study the means of absolute values of observed and estimated measures (accelerometry vs. video, accelerometry vs. IC) and ICCs (Pearson) to study the reliability of the estimates. All statistical analyses were conducted, and figures generated using IBM SPSS Statistics v 26. p-values less than 0.05 were considered statistically significant. ICC over 0.90 was considered excellent, 0.75–0.90 good, 0.75–0.50 moderate, and less than 0.50 as poor. Results in the Tables are represented as mean ± standard deviation.

3. Results

3.1. Step Detection

All participants completed the three first speeds of the protocol, and one participant stopped after 4.5 km/h. A total of 38 out of 48 could complete the first running speed (7.5 km/h) and 25 completed the whole protocol. At walking speeds (1.5, 3, 4.5, and 6 km/h), the AP device was the most accurate. The corresponding MAPEs were 6.39, 0.95, 0.99, and 2.44, respectively (Table 2). For SX, the corresponding MAPEs were 9.73, 3.97, 2.91, and 6.28, respectively. The AG was the least accurate at the lower walking speeds but improved its accuracy from 4.5 km/h with MAPEs of 88.69, 31.50, 4.25, and 2.44, respectively. At the running speeds (7.5 and 9 km/h) the AG device performed better with MAPEs of 4.43 and 2.63, respectively. For the SX and the AP, the MAPEs were 2.26, 4.47, and 3.99, 5.18, respectively. The SX device estimate of the total number of steps differed by 3.48% and for the AP and the AG by 4.37% and 17.80%, respectively. Significant differences between direct measurement and accelerometer estimated steps were observed at 1.5 km/h and a first running speed ($p < 0.000$) for the AP. For the SX device, significant differences were observed at all speeds except 4.5 km/h and a first running speed ($p < 0.05$) between device estimates and direct observation, and for the AG at speeds of 1.5 and 3 km/h as well as in the first running speed ($p < 0.000$). The intraclass correlations were significant ($p < 0.030$) at all speeds for all devices except for the AG at 3 km/h ($p = 0.646$). For the AP device, the correlation coefficients were excellent (>0.90) and for the SX good or excellent (>0.75 and >0.90, respectively), except for the lowest speed where the correlation was moderate (0.61). For the AG, the correlation coefficients were excellent (>0.90) while running and brisk walking (6 km/h), good (>0.75) with the first running speed, and moderate or poor (>0.50, <0.50, respectively), at speeds of 1.5, 3 and 4.5. The R^2 values for the regressions between actual and estimated steps were 0.948 for the SX, 0.963 for the AP, and 0.821 for the AG (Supplementary Materials). For the Bland–Altman plots the means, standard deviations, and 95% confidence intervals were −14.7 ± 30.3, upper 44.7, lower −74.2, respectively, for the SX (Figure 1A), −4.0 ± 12.8, upper 21.1, lower −29.0, respectively, for the AP (Figure 2A) and −76.39 ± 104.9, upper 129.3 and lower −282.0, respectively, for the AG (Figure 3A).

Table 2. Step detection statistics. Mean absolute percentage error (MAPE), paired sample *t*-test statistics with mean ± SD, lower and upper limits for 95% confidence intervals and *p*-values, and intraclass correlation (ICC) statistics with 95% CI presented for every accelerometer at separate speeds and for total duration of exercise protocol. * Shows statistical significance.

STEPS			Paired Samples *t*-Test	95% Confidence Interval of the Difference			ICC	95% Confidence Interval		F Test	
Sartorio	Speed (km/h)	MAPE-% ± Std. Dev.	Mean ± Std. Dev.	Lower	Upper	Sig. (2-Tailed)		Lower	Upper	Value	Sig.
	1.5	9.73 ± 7.82	19.68 ± 32.10	9.55	29.81	0.000 *	0.61	0.27	0.79	2.56	0.002 *
	3	3.97 ± 7.48	10.05 ± 30.41	0.45	19.65	0.041 *	0.84	0.71	0.92	6.39	0.000 *
	4.5	2.91 ± 3.35	2.59 ± 17.56	−2.96	8.13	0.351	0.93	0.86	0.96	13.85	0.000 *
	6	6.28 ± 8.02	28.87 ± 41.85	15.49	42.26	0.000 *	0.79	0.59	0.89	4.67	0.000 *
	Run1	2.26 ± 1.46	4.43 ± 16.02	−1.070	9.93	0.111	0.99	0.97	0.99	74.43	0.000 *
	Run2	4.47 ± 3.08	26.54 ± 24.35	16.26	36.82	0.000 *	0.98	0.96	0.99	62.47	0.000 *
	Total	3.48 ± 3.03	82.02 ± 75.94	58.05	105.99	0.000 *	0.90	0.81	0.94	9.81	0.000 *
activPAL	1.5	6.39 ± 8.10	14.90 ± 23.79	7.74	22.04	0.000 *	0.94	0.88	0.96	15.65	0.000 *
	3	0.95 ± 1.59	1.60 ± 7.17	−0.55	3.75	0.141	0.99	0.99	1.00	135.88	0.000 *
	4.5	0.99 ± 2.75	−0.29 ± 10.94	−3.58	3.00	0.860	0.98	0.96	0.99	41.68	0.000 *
	6	2.44 ± 5.45	−1.42 ± 22.75	−8.26	5.41	0.677	0.98	0.97	0.99	62.54	0.000 *
	Run1	3.99 ± 5.25	22.68 ± 33.36	11.55	33.80	0.000 *	0.94	0.88	0.97	16.19	0.000 *
	Run2	5.18 ± 4.60	17.39 ± 43.05	−1.22	36.00	0.066	0.91	0.8	0.96	11.68	0.000 *
	Total	4.37 ± 10.53	42.27 ± 213.67	−21.93	106.46	0.191	0.95	0.91	0.97	19.49	0.000 *
ActiGraph	1.5	88.69 ± 10.93	242.35 ± 47.32	228.30	256.40	0.000 *	0.44	−0.018	0.69	1.77	0.029 *
	3	31.50 ± 18.87	119.85 ± 82.36	95.39	144.31	0.000 *	−0.12	−1.02	0.38	0.89	0.646
	4.5	4.25 ± 9.11	13.37 ± 45.19	−0.05	26.79	0.051	0.58	0.25	0.77	2.40	0.002 *
	6	5.23 ± 9.35	11.59 ± 43.62	−1.37	24.54	0.078	0.94	0.89	0.97	17.14	0.000 *
	Run1	4.43 ± 10.3	19.50 ± 68.82	−3.12	42.12	0.089	0.80	0.61	0.89	4.91	0.000 *
	Run2	2.63 ± 1.56	12.72 ± 16.28	6.00	19.44	0.000 *	0.99	0.98	1.00	142.15	0.000 *
	Total	17.80 ± 9.48	381.35 ± 221.25	315.65	447.05	0.000 *	0.95	0.92	0.97	21.61	0.000 *

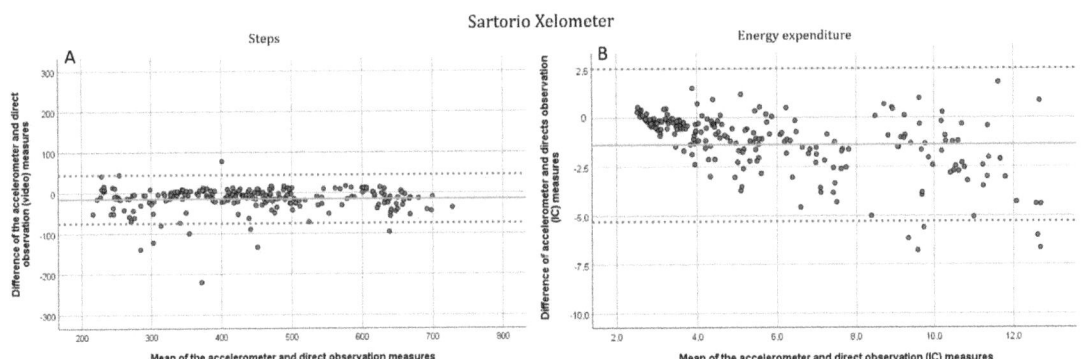

Figure 1. Bland-Altman plots for the Sartorio Xelometer. (**A**). Step detection compared to the direct (video) measurement. All six speeds have been plotted separately. (**B**). EE estimation compared with indirect (IC) calorimetry. Solid line marks the mean and dotted lines show the −1.96–1.96 SD limits.

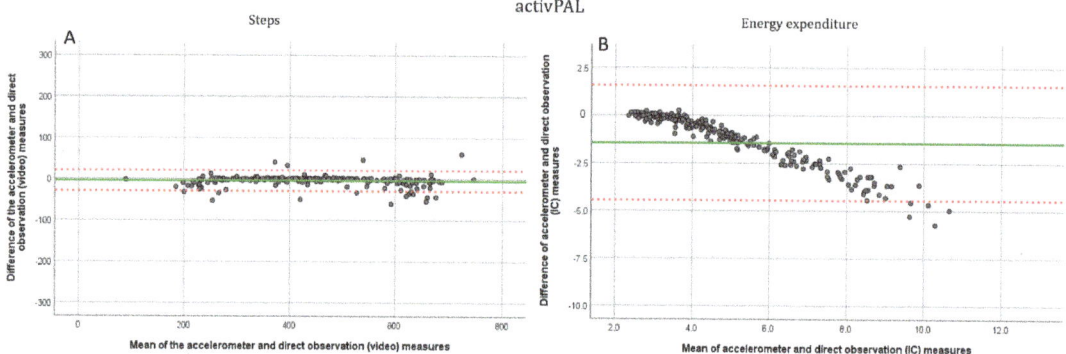

Figure 2. Bland-Altman plots for the activPAL. (**A**). Step detection compared to the direct (video) measurement. All six speeds have been plotted separately. (**B**). EE estimation compared with indirect (IC) calorimetry. Solid line marks the mean and dotted lines show the −1.96–1.96 SD limits.

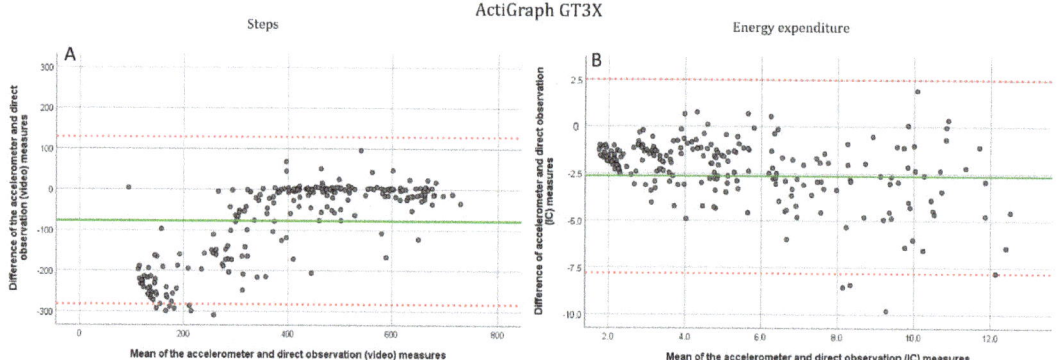

Figure 3. Bland-Altman plots for the ActiGraph GT3X. (**A**). Step detection compared to the direct (video) measurement. All six speeds have been plotted separately. (**B**). EE estimation compared with indirect (IC) calorimetry. Solid line marks the mean and dotted lines show the −1.96–1.96 SD limits.

3.2. Energy Expenditure Estimation

All three devices were inaccurate in estimating energy expenditure (Table 3). The SX had the most accurate estimates of EE upon the complete exercise protocol with a MAPE of 18.43. The MAPEs for total EE were 49.62 for the AP and 36.16 for the AG with significant but poor intraclass correlations ($p < 0.05$, ICC < 0.50). For the SX, the speed-wise MAPEs from 1.5 km/h to the second running speed were 15.15, 17.60, 19.02, 21.41, 18.03, and 19.74. respectively. For the AP, the values were 12.36, 16.29, 27.82, 43.82, 56.10, 57.38 and for the ActiGraph 59.45, 40.67, 28.92, 29.88, 29.61 and 32.09, respectively. At all speeds for all three devices, there were significant differences between accelerometer estimates and indirect calorimetry ($p \leq 0.005$), and no significant intraclass correlations were observed ($p > 0.120$). The R^2 values for the regression between indirect calorimetry and device estimated EE (when considering all speeds together) were 0.81 for the SX, 0.75 for the AP, and 0.745 for the AG (Supplementary Materials). For the Bland–Altman plots the means, standard deviations, and 95% confidence intervals were for the SX (Figure 1B): −1.4 ± 2.0, upper 2.5, lower −5.3, respectively, for the AP (Figure 2B): −1.4 ± 1.5, upper 1.6, lower −4.5, respectively, and for the AG (Figure 3B): −2.6 ± 2.6, upper 2.5 and lower −7.8, respectively.

Table 3. Energy expenditure (EE) estimation statistics. Mean absolute percentage error (MAPE), paired sample *t*-test statistics with mean ± SD, lower and upper limits for 95% confidence intervals and *p*-values and intraclass correlation (ICC) statistics with 95% CI presented for every accelerometer at separate speeds and for total duration of exercise protocol. * Shows statistical significance.

MET Sartorio	Speed (km/h)	MAPE-% ± Std. Dev.	Paired Samples *t*-Test Mean ± Std. Dev.	95% Confidence Interval of the Difference Lower	Upper	Sig. (2-Tailed)	ICC	95% Confidence Interval Lower	Upper	F Test Value	Sig.
	1.5	15.15 ± 13.72	0.37 ± 0.81	0.11	0.62	0.005 *	0.11	−0.67	0.53	1.12	0.353
	3	17.60 ± 13.16	0.73 ± 0.96	0.42	1.04	0.000 *	0.21	−0.47	0.58	1.27	0.223
	4.5	19.02 ± 11.75	1.04 ± 1.05	0.71	1.38	0.000 *	0.23	−0.43	0.59	1.31	0.199
	6	21.41 ± 12.92	1.74 ± 1.59	1.21	2.25	0.000 *	0.21	−0.51	0.58	1.26	0.237
	Run1	18.03 ± 12.21	1.83 ± 2.07	1.09	2.57	0.000 *	0.18	−0.64	0.59	1.22	0.282
	Run2	19.74 ± 11.89	2.59 ± 2.11	1.64	3.52	0.000 *	0.08	−1.19	0.62	1.09	0.417
	Total	18.43 ± 13.59	1.31 ± 1.37	0.86	1.74	0.000 *	0.28	−0.34	0.62	1.40	0.146
activPAL	1.5	12.36 ± 11.20	0.30 ± 0.68	0.09	0.51	0.005 *	0.37	−0.16	0.65	1.58	0.068
	3	16.29 ± 12.65	0.74 ± 0.81	0.49	0.99	0.000 *	0.29	−0.3	0.61	1.41	0.134
	4.5	27.82 ± 11.92	1.60 ± 0.97	1.30	1.90	0.000 *	0.17	−0.51	0.55	1.21	0.264
	6	43.82 ± 10.70	3.48 ± 1.61	2.95	3.99	0.000 *	0.05	−0.79	0.50	1.06	0.425
	Run1	56.10 ± 7.43	6.18 ± 1.93	5.48	6.87	0.000 *	−0.03	−1.12	0.49	0.96	0.538
	Run2	57.38 ± 6.40	7.39 ± 1.91	6.49	8.28	0.000 *	0.13	−1.18	0.65	1.15	0.378
	Total	49.62 ± 11.21	3.37 ± 1.25	2.97	3.75	0.000 *	0.49	0.07	0.72	1.99	0.013 *
ActiGraph	1.5	59.45 ± 9.40	1.95 ± 0.74	1.72	2.17	0.000 *	0.15	−0.55	0.53	1.17	0.295
	3	40.67 ± 14.07	1.82 ± 1.00	1.51	2.12	0.000 *	−0.10	−1.03	0.39	0.90	0.631
	4.5	28.92 ± 13.17	1.61 ± 1.13	1.26	1.95	0.000 *	0.17	−0.5	0.55	1.21	0.260
	6	29.88 ± 15.19	2.37 ± 1.66	1.84	2.89	0.000 *	0.30	−0.29	0.63	1.44	0.124
	Run1	29.61 ± 17.13	3.16 ± 2.51	2.25	4.06	0.000 *	0.27	−0.49	0.64	1.37	0.190
	Run2	32.09 ± 16.50	4.20 ± 2.69	3.00	5.39	0.000 *	−0.34	−2.23	0.44	0.74	0.746
	Total	36.16 ± 15.06	2.42 ± 1.41	1.98	2.84	0.000 *	0.43	−0.03	0.69	1.77	0.031 *

4. Discussion

We measured overweight and obese subjects without diseases or disabilities that could affect their gait. Forty-eight subjects performed an exercise protocol on a treadmill consisting of six different speeds, which were chosen to reflect the locomotion speeds of overweight, obese, and elderly people. The main objective was to study the accuracy of step detection and EE estimation with three known research accelerometers (SX, AP, and AG) in overweight and obese subjects. For step detection, similar accuracies for step detection were observed in this overweight/obese population as in normal weight subjects [18]. Energy expenditure estimates were inaccurately measured in all three devices.

All three devices accurately estimated step detection when gait speed exceeded 4 km/h. Only the AG was inaccurate during slow walking speeds of 1.5 and 3 km/h with MAPE-% of 88.7 and 31.5, respectively. The AP showed the highest correlations between video camera-recorded steps and device step counts (ICC > 90). Step detection accuracy in overweight and obese people was similar compared to normal weight subjects with the exception that the AP was more accurate in estimating step counts during running in overweight and obese subjects [18]. Similar discrepancies have been reported by Feito and colleagues (2012) [20] who showed the increasing accuracy with increasing speed in the AG. Lee and colleagues [24] found a significant underestimation of step counts by AG at the speed of 3.2 km/h. We did not use the low-frequency extension for the AG data, since it has been shown to give indefinite results when applied to free-living data [25,26].

All accelerometers were inaccurate for estimating EE. The SX provided the smallest overall error percentages in the range of 15.15–21.41, while the AP and the AG ranged between 12.36–57.4 and 28.9–59.45, respectively. The accuracy of the AP EE estimation was at its highest during slow walking speeds (1.5 and 3 km/h) and decreased with speed. For the AG, an opposing trend was observed, the EE estimation accuracy was higher at speeds exceeding 4 km/h. For the SX, the EE estimation error was 12% smaller in overweight/obese subjects compared to normal weight subjects (MAPE 18.4 < 30.3) [18]. The opposite was observed with the AP and ActiGraph, both showing lower EE estimation accuracy with overweight subjects. The SX EE estimation is based on MAD and had the most accurate method of the three and is in line with the results of Diniz-Sousa and colleagues [23].

Applying accelerometry to overweight/obese populations is challenging. The excess body fat increases the energy used in bodily movements and can cause the accelerometer to be placed at an angle that has been shown to decrease accuracy [16]. If the manufacturer of the accelerometer has used a normal weighted population for algorithm development, inaccuracy will increase when applied to overweight people. The comparison of the different studies with objectively measured physical activity measures is problematic since the different manufacturers use their own methods and algorithms. Accelerations as g-values are further processed into steps, counts, and MET units for further analysis. Depending on the method, habitual daily PA can be classified differently into commonly used PA intensity classes such as light, moderate and vigorous [9]. Considering these points together with the discrepancies concerning wear location, time, signal processing, and filtering [8], a standardized method of measurement is needed to create accurate, specified, and personalized PA recommendations.

Our study is the first to evaluate the accuracy of EE estimation of these accelerometers at realistic walking and running speeds in overweight and obese subjects. The use of a video camera to record true step numbers, the use of both sexes, and a wide range of ages and BMIs are the strengths of this study. Our limitations include the lack of self-selected locomotion speed and the exclusion of any wrist-worn accelerometers. The gait speeds chosen are sufficient in covering the spectrum of overweight human locomotion speeds. Our results will guide users studying physical activity in different populations in the interpretation of their results and their conclusions towards public health recommendations.

Supplementary Materials: The following supporting information can be downloaded at: https://www.mdpi.com/article/10.3390/jcm11123267/s1. Figure S1. Regression plots for Sartorio Xelometer. Figure S2. Regression plots for activPAL. Figure S3. Regression plots for ActiGraph GT3X.

Author Contributions: Conceptualization, K.-H.H., J.L., V.S., M.T. and D.G.; methodology, V.S., L.N. and R.J.; software, V.S.; formal analysis, V.S.; investigation, V.S., L.N. and R.J.; resources, K.-H.H. and M.T.; data curation, V.S.; writing—original draft preparation, V.S.; writing—review and editing, K.-H.H., J.L., V.S., R.J., L.N., M.T. and D.G.; visualization, V.S.; supervision, K.-H.H.; project administration, V.S.; funding acquisition, K.-H.H. All authors have read and agreed to the published version of the manuscript.

Funding: This research received no external funding.

Institutional Review Board Statement: The study was conducted in accordance with the Declaration of Helsinki and approved by the Northern Ostrobothnia Hospital district ethical committee in Oulu, Finland (EETTMK 26/3/21).

Informed Consent Statement: Informed consent was obtained from all subjects involved in the study.

Acknowledgments: We thank all the participants and organizations of the University of Oulu and Oulu University of Applied Sciences for their help in recruitment.

Conflicts of Interest: J.L. and K.-H.H. are co-inventors of the Sartorio Xelometer and members of the board of Sartorio OY. J.L. and K.-H.H. did not participate in the study sessions or data acquisition and handling (V.S. and R.J.) or the statistical analysis of the results (V.S.). The remaining authors declare no competing interests.

References

1. WHO. Factsheet: Obesity and Overweight. Available online: https://www.who.int/news-room/fact-sheets/detail/obesity-and-overweight (accessed on 12 April 2022).
2. Pi-Sunyer, X. The Medical Risks of Obesity. *Postgrad. Med.* **2009**, *121*, 21–33. [CrossRef]
3. Waters, H.; Graf, M. *America's Obesity Crisis. The Health and Economic Costs of Excess Weight*; Milken Institute: Santa Monica, CA, USA, 2018. Available online: https://milkeninstitute.org/sites/default/files/reports-pdf/Mi-Americas-Obesity-Crisis-WEB.pdf (accessed on 12 April 2022).
4. Effertz, T.; Engel, S.; Verheyen, F.; Linder, R. The Costs and Consequences of Obesity in Germany: A New Approach from a Prevalence and Life-Cycle Perspective. *Eur. J. Health Econ.* **2016**, *17*, 1141–1158. [CrossRef]
5. Wang, Y.C.; McPherson, K.; Marsh, T.; Gortmaker, S.L.; Brown, M. Health and Economic Burden of the Projected Obesity Trends in the USA and the UK. *Lancet* **2011**, *378*, 815–825. [CrossRef]
6. Bull, F.C.; Al-Ansari, S.S.; Biddle, S.; Borodulin, K.; Buman, M.P.; Cardon, G.; Carty, C.; Chaput, J.-P.; Chastin, S.; Chou, R.; et al. World Health Organization 2020 Guidelines on Physical Activity and Sedentary Behaviour. *Br. J. Sports Med.* **2020**, *54*, 1451–1462. [CrossRef] [PubMed]
7. Chow, J.J.; Thom, J.M.; Wewege, M.A.; Ward, R.E.; Parmenter, B.J. Accuracy of Step Count Measured by Physical Activity Monitors: The Effect of Gait Speed and Anatomical Placement Site. *Gait Posture* **2017**, *57*, 199–203. [CrossRef]
8. Migueles, J.H.; Cadenas-Sanchez, C.; Ekelund, U.; Delisle Nyström, C.; Mora-Gonzalez, J.; Löf, M.; Labayen, I.; Ruiz, J.R.; Ortega, F.B. Accelerometer Data Collection and Processing Criteria to Assess Physical Activity and Other Outcomes: A Systematic Review and Practical Considerations. *Sports Med.* **2017**, *47*, 1821–1845. [CrossRef] [PubMed]
9. Leinonen, A.-M.; Ahola, R.; Kulmala, J.; Hakonen, H.; Vähä-Ypyä, H.; Herzig, K.-H.; Auvinen, J.; Keinänen-Kiukaanniemi, S.; Siev¨anen, H.; Tammelin, T.H.; et al. Measuring Physical Activity in Free-Living Conditions-Comparison of Three Accelerometry-Based Methods. *Front. Physiol.* **2017**, *7*. [CrossRef] [PubMed]
10. Lai, P.P.K.; Leung, A.K.L.; Li, A.N.M.; Zhang, M. Three-Dimensional Gait Analysis of Obese Adults. *Clin. Biomech.* **2008**, *23*, S2–S6. [CrossRef]
11. Ling, C.; Kelechi, T.; Mueller, M.; Brotherton, S.; Smith, S. Gait and Function in Class III Obesity. *J. Obes.* **2012**, *2012*. [CrossRef]
12. Mendes, J.; Borges, N.; Santos, A.; Padrão, P.; Moreira, P.; Afonso, C.; Negrão, R.; Amaral, T.F. Nutritional Status and Gait Speed in a Nationwide Population-Based Sample of Older Adults. *Sci. Rep.* **2018**, *8*, 1–8. [CrossRef]
13. Ko, S.-U.; Stenholm, S.; Ferrucci, L. Characteristic Gait Patterns in Older Adults with Obesity-Results from the Baltimore Longitudinal Study of Aging. *J. Biomech.* **2010**, *43*, 1104–1110. [CrossRef]
14. Ainslie, P.N.; Reilly, T.; Westerterp, K.R. Estimating Human Energy Expenditure. *Sport. Med.* **2003**, *33*, 683–698. [CrossRef]
15. Ocobock, C.; Soppela, P.; Turunen, M.; Stenbäck, V.; Herzig, K.-H.; Rimbach, R.; Pontzer, H. Reindeer Herders from Subarctic Finland Exhibit High Total Energy Expenditure and Low Energy Intake during the Autumn Herd Roundup. *Am. J. Hum. Biol.* **2022**, *34*, e23676. [CrossRef]
16. Pisanu, S.; Deledda, A.; Loviselli, A.; Huybrechts, I.; Velluzzi, F. Validity of Accelerometers for the Evaluation of Energy Expenditure in Obese and Overweight Individuals: A Systematic Review. *J. Nutr. Metab.* **2020**, *2020*. [CrossRef] [PubMed]
17. Imboden, M.T.; Nelson, M.B.; Kaminsky, L.A.; Montoye, A.H. Comparison of Four Fitbit and Jawbone Activity Monitors with a Research-Grade ActiGraph Accelerometer for Estimating Physical Activity and Energy Expenditure. *Br. J. Sports Med.* **2018**, *52*, 844–850. [CrossRef]
18. Stenbäck, V.; Leppäluoto, J.; Leskelä, N.; Viitala, L.; Vihriälä, E.; Gagnon, D.; Tulppo, M.; Herzig, K.-H. Step Detection and Energy Expenditure at Different Speeds by Three Accelerometers in a Controlled Environment. *Sci. Rep.* **2021**, *11*, 1–10. [CrossRef]
19. Herzig, K.-H.; Ahola, R.; Leppäluoto, J.; Jokelainen, J.; Jämsä, T.; Keinänen-Kiukaanniemi, S. Light Physical Activity Determined by a Motion Sensor Decreases Insulin Resistance, Improves Lipid Homeostasis and Reduces Visceral Fat in High Risk Subjects. *Int. J. Obes. (Lond.)* **2014**, *38*, 1089–1096. [CrossRef] [PubMed]
20. Feito, Y.; Bassett, D.R.; Thompson, D.L.; Tyo, B.M. Effects of Body Mass Index on Step Count Accuracy of Physical Activity Monitors. *J. Phys. Act. Health* **2012**, *9*, 594–600. [CrossRef]
21. Howe, C.C.F.; Moir, H.J.; Easton, C. Classification of Physical Activity Cut-Points and the Estimation of Energy Expenditure During Walking Using the GT3X+ Accelerometer in Overweight and Obese Adults. *Meas. Phys. Educ. Exerc. Sci.* **2017**, *21*, 127–133. [CrossRef]
22. Sushames, A.; Edwards, A.; Thompson, F.; McDermott, R.; Gebel, K. Validity and Reliability of Fitbit Flex for Step Count, Moderate to Vigorous Physical Activity and Activity Energy Expenditure. *PLoS ONE* **2016**, *11*, e0161224. [CrossRef] [PubMed]
23. Diniz-Sousa, F.; Veras, L.; Ribeiro, J.C.; Boppre, G.; Devezas, V.; Santos-Sousa, H.; Preto, J.; Machado, L.; Vilas-Boas, J.P.; Oliveira, J.; et al. Accelerometry Calibration in People with Class II-III Obesity: Energy Expenditure Prediction and Physical Activity Intensity Identification. *Gait Posture* **2020**, *76*, 104–109. [CrossRef] [PubMed]

24. Lee, J.A.; Williams, S.M.; Brown, D.D.; Laurson, K.R. Concurrent Validation of the Actigraph Gt3x+, Polar Active Accelerometer, Omron HJ-720 and Yamax Digiwalker SW-701 Pedometer Step Counts in Lab-Based and Free-Living Settings. *J. Sports Sci.* **2015**, *33*, 991–1000. [CrossRef] [PubMed]
25. Feito, Y.; Hornbuckle, L.M.; Reid, L.A.; Crouter, S.E. Effect of ActiGraph's Low Frequency Extension for Estimating Steps and Physical Activity Intensity. *PLoS ONE* **2017**, *12*, e0188242. [CrossRef]
26. Wallén, M.B.; Nero, H.; Franzén, E.; Hagströmer, M. Comparison of Two Accelerometer Filter Settings in Individuals with Parkinson's Disease. *Physiol. Meas.* **2014**, *35*, 2287–2296. [CrossRef] [PubMed]

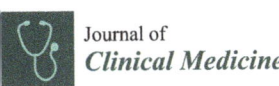

Article

Circulating Spexin Is Associated with Body Mass Index and Fat Mass but Not with Physical Activity and Psychological Parameters in Women across a Broad Body Weight Spectrum

Maria Suhs [1,*,†], Andreas Stengel [1,2,†], Amelie Rudolph [1], Selina Schaper [1], Ellen Wölk [1], Peter Kobelt [1], Matthias Rose [1,3] and Tobias Hofmann [1]

1. Charité Center for Internal Medicine and Dermatology, Department of Psychosomatic Medicine, Charité–Universitätsmedizin Berlin, Corporate Member of Freie Universität Berlin and Humboldt-Universität zu Berlin, 12203 Berlin, Germany
2. Department of Psychosomatic Medicine and Psychotherapy, University Hospital Tübingen, 72076 Tübingen, Germany
3. Quantitative Health Sciences, Outcomes Measurement Science, University of Massachusetts Medical School, Worcester, MA 01655, USA
* Correspondence: maria.suhs@charite.de
† These authors contributed equally to this work.

Abstract: Spexin (SPX) is a novel, widely expressed peptide, with anorexigenic effects demonstrated in animal models and negatively correlated with body mass index (BMI) in humans. It increases locomotor activity in rodents and is elevated in human plasma following exercise. Studies have also shown an effect of stress and anxiety on SPX's expression in different brain structures in animals. The relationships between plasma SPX and physical activity, body composition, and patient-reported outcomes such as perceived stress, depressiveness, anxiety, and eating behaviors are unknown and were examined in this study over a wide BMI range. A total of 219 female (n = 68 with anorexia nervosa; n = 79 with obesity; n = 72 with normal weight) inpatients were enrolled. Perceived stress (PSQ 20), anxiety (GAD 7), depressiveness (PHQ 9), and eating disorder pathology (EDI 2), as well as BMI, bioimpedance analysis, and accelerometry, were measured cross-sectionally at the beginning of treatment and correlated with plasma SPX levels (measured by ELISA) obtained at the same time. Plasma SPX levels were negatively associated with BMI (r = −0.149, p = 0.027) and body fat mass (r = −0.149, p = 0.04), but did not correlate with perceived stress, anxiety, depressiveness, eating behavior, energy expenditure, and physical activity (p > 0.05). The results replicate the negative correlation of SPX with BMI and fat mass, but do not support the hypothesis that peripheral SPX plays a role in the regulation of stress, depressiveness, anxiety, eating behavior, or physical activity.

Keywords: gut–brain axis; patient-reported outcome; psychoendocrinology; psychometric; psychosomatic stress

1. Introduction

Spexin (SPX), also known as Neuropeptide Q, is a novel peptide comprised of 14 amino acids and was described for the first time by Mirabeau et al. in 2007 [1]. SPX mRNA and protein were detected in many different tissues, both in animals and in humans. In rodents and humans, SPX mRNA was found in the central nervous system (e.g., hypothalamus [2], hippocampus) and in peripheral tissues (e.g., stomach, small intestine, liver, pancreas [3], fat and other endocrine tissues [4]). In human subjects, the lowest SPX gene expression was detected in muscle- and connective tissue [4]. The fact that SPX mRNA was identified in several different types of tissues suggests that SPX may be involved in various physiological processes and serve as a pleiotropic peptide.

SPX may be involved in fat tissue metabolism, through increasing lipolysis and inhibiting lipogenesis [5]. Furthermore, a decreased uptake of long-chain fatty acids in adipocytes, in rodents with diet-induced obesity after peripheral SPX administration, suggests that SPX may contribute to weight loss [6]. In line with this observation, several studies involving humans have demonstrated a negative correlation between serum SPX and serum triglyceride levels [4,7], as well as body mass index (BMI) [7]. In addition, higher circulating SPX levels were observed in non-obese compared to obese adults [8,9] and children [10,11], although not all studies seem to support these results (e.g., no correlation between BMI and body fat with serum SPX, as well as no difference in serum SPX level between NW and OB/overweight female adolescents [12]).

Not only body weight, but also feeding behavior, might be influenced by SPX [13]. It was shown that food intake led to an increase in SPX mRNA expression in the hypothalamus of Siberian sturgeons, possibly pointing towards an anorexigenic function of SPX [14]. Moreover, intracerebroventricular injection of SPX in goldfish resulted in downregulation of the expression of the orexigenic peptides neuropeptide Y (NPY), orexin, and Agouti-related protein (AgRP), and in higher expression of anorexigenic peptides such as proopiomelanocortin (POMC), cholecystokinin (CCK), and melanin-concentrating hormone (MCH) [15]. The postulated anorexigenic function of SPX is unlikely to be triggered by taste aversion [6].

Another important function of SPX is its possible role in the response to physical activity (PA). For instance, a study in mice showed increased locomotor activity after intraperitoneal SPX injection [6]. Furthermore, a recent report in humans demonstrated that circulating plasma SPX levels significantly were increased in a group of participants categorized as positive responders to exercise. Following a 3-month exercise program, they showed an increased maximal oxygen consumption (VO_{2max}) during exercise and, compared to non-responders who did not show an amelioration of VO_{2max}, greater improvement in their metabolic profile (total cholesterol, HbA1c, HOMA-IR) [9]. This may be of relevance, as PA plays an important role in maintaining body weight [16] and, in the form of hyperactivity, it is not only a symptom of anorexia nervosa (AN) [17], but also part of its pathogenesis [18]. In patients with obesity, PA has been shown to be inversely associated with the grade of adiposity [19].

Besides its possible functions in the regulation of metabolism, body weight, and physical activity, SPX may be involved in stress response. For instance, fish exposed to stress showed an increase in SPX mRNA expression in different brain areas (e.g., optic tectum, hypothalamus, and midbrain) [20]. Moreover, it was demonstrated that intrahippocampally injected corticotropin-releasing factor (CRF), which is crucially involved in the stress response, decreases SPX expression in different brain tissues (such as hippocampus, hypothalamus, or pituitary gland) in mice [21]. Additionally, another study in fish found that SPX may influence the serotoninergic system, through the upregulation of serotonin-related genes in the raphe nuclei [22]. Moreover, intraperitoneal administration of escitalopram, a serotonin reuptake inhibitor mostly used for the treatment of major depression and general anxiety disorder, led to the downregulation of SPX mRNA in the hypothalamus and upregulated expression of SPX mRNA in the hippocampus and striatum in rats [23]. Therefore, SPX may also be involved in the regulation of stress, anxiety, and depressiveness.

As some studies on SPX indicated its anorexigenic effects and its role in lipogenesis and PA, we hypothesized that SPX may be a factor involved in energy expenditure, and thus it may be associated with different patterns of PA. Furthermore, we hypothesized that SPX levels might be associated with eating disorder pathology, as well as perceived stress, anxiety, and depressiveness. Therefore, we aimed to further examine the link between plasma SPX levels and body composition and PA along with patient-reported outcomes under naturalistic conditions in an inpatient setting. We studied women across a wide BMI range, to examine the impact of body weight and to control for possible gender differences.

2. Materials and Methods

2.1. Ethics Statement

All investigations were conducted according to the Declaration of Helsinki and all patients gave written informed consent. The study was approved by the institutional ethics committee of the Charité–Universitätsmedizin Berlin (protocol numbers: EA1/130/16)

2.2. Subjects

In the present study, 219 female inpatients (68 with a diagnosis of anorexia nervosa (AN), 79 with obesity (OB), and 72 normal-weight (NW) patients treated for conditions other than eating disorders or obesity, such as adjustment disorders, somatoform disorders, or mild depressive episode) were recruited upon admission to the Department of Psychosomatic Medicine at Charité–Universitätsmedizin Berlin (between February 2012 and July 2018). All patients were at an age of ≥18 years. Current pregnancy or lactation period, malignant disease, treatment with immunomodulatory drugs (e.g., methotrexate, azathioprine, and oral corticosteroids), hypercortisolism, and untreated thyroid dysfunction were exclusion criteria. Moreover, women with psychotic disorders, somatoform or somatic disorders of the gastrointestinal system, and those preceding (e.g., bariatric) surgery of the gastrointestinal system, except for appendectomy and uncomplicated cholecystectomy, were excluded.

2.3. Anthropometric Measurements

Study enrolment, including clarification of potential exclusion criteria and blood withdrawal, was conducted within four days of admission. Venous blood samples were taken after an overnight fasting period between 7.00 and 8.00 a.m. Patients were permitted to drink a small amount of water, but were advised not to drink coffee, smoke, or exercise before blood withdrawal. On the same morning each patient's actual medication, body height, and weight in light underwear were assessed and BMI (kg/m^2) was calculated. Medications and the presence of comorbidities were recorded at admission and discharge. Participants diagnosed with any of the exclusion criteria during their inpatient treatment were excluded.

2.4. Physical Activity and Energy Expenditure Assessment

To assess PA, we used a SenseWear® Pro3 armband (BodyMedia, Inc., Pittsburgh, PA, USA), which is a two-axis accelerometer that calculates PA by measuring skin temperature, near-body ambient temperature, galvanic skin response, and heat flux [24]. PA was analyzed for three consecutive days starting from Friday, which was the day of the blood withdrawal. Data were accepted if inpatients wore the armband for more than 20.5 h for at least two out of the three days, as described previously [25]. The PA of the patients was not restricted by the medical staff while wearing the accelerometer.

Using a generalized proprietary algorithm developed by the producer, the total amount of steps, metabolic equivalents of tasks per day (MET), level of energy expenditure, and exercise activity thermogenesis (EAT) were directly calculated after reading out the data. As EAT, we defined an activity of more than three metabolic equivalents of task (METs), which refers to moderate- and vigorous-intensity activities according to the 2011 Compendium of Physical Activities [26].

The thermic effect of food (TEF) was estimated as comprising 10% of total energy expenditure (TEE) and calculated as TEE × 0.1 [27]. Since resting energy expenditure (REE), required for the calculation of NEAT, cannot be directly determined by the SenseWear® armband, it was estimated using weight-group-specific REE prediction equations provided by Müller et al. [28]. Non-exercise-related activity (NEAT) was calculated using the formula NEAT = TEE − TEF − REE − EAT.

2.5. Body Composition Measurements

Bioelectric impedance analysis (BIA) was performed between 10:30 a.m. and 1:00 p.m. on the day of blood withdrawal under standardized conditions in the supine position, after subjects had fasted for at least two hours and had lain for half an hour. Phase angle, fat mass, fat free mass, extracellular mass, and body cell mass were assessed using the equations provided by the manufacturer of the bioelectrical impedance analyzer (Nutrigard-M®, Data Input®, Darmstadt, Germany).

2.6. Laboratory Analyses

Blood was collected in pre-cooled standard EDTA tubes prepared with aprotinin for peptidase inhibition (1.2 Trypsin Inhibitory Unit per 1 mL blood; ICN Pharmaceuticals, Costa Mesa, CA, USA) and immediately submerged in ice. After that, tubes were centrifuged at 4 °C for 10 min at $3000\times g$ for plasma separation, which was stored at -80 °C, until further processing. After enough samples were collected, SPX plasma levels were measured using a commercial enzyme-linked immunosorbent assay (ELISA, catalog # EK-023-81, Phoenix Pharmaceuticals®, Inc., Burlingame, CA, USA). All samples were processed at once. Intra-assay variability was 7.5% and inter-assay variability was <15%. Measurement was performed in January 2019. Every measurement was performed twice, and a mean value was calculated.

2.7. Patient-Reported Outcomes

All study participants were asked to fill in the following self-reported questionnaires: Perceived Stress Questionnaire (PSQ), Generalized Anxiety Disorder-7 (GAD-7), Patient Health Questionnaire depression scale (PHQ-9), and Eating Disorder Inventory-2 (EDI-2). Results obtained between two days before and five days after the respective blood withdrawals were accepted.

PSQ-20 is a revised 20-item German version [29] of the Perceived Stress Questionnaire (PSQ; 30 items) [30] and is applied to evaluate subjectively perceived stress. It provides four subscales: "worries", "tension", and "joy" as stress responses, and "demands" as the perception of external stressors. It assesses the subjective experience of stress. Cronbach's alpha for the total scale was 0.73 and for the subscales 0.86 ("worries"), 0.86 ("tension"), 0.81 ("joy"), and 0.84 ("demands").

The Generalized Anxiety Disorder Questionnaire (GAD-7) [31] is a part of the Patient Health Questionnaire (PHQ) and an established and widely used 7-item screening instrument for diagnosing general anxiety disorder. It also captures symptoms of social anxiety, posttraumatic stress, and panic disorder. In this study, the German version was used [32]. The Cronbach's alpha for the current sample was 0.87.

The severity of eating disorder symptoms was evaluated using the Eating Disorder Inventory-2 (EDI-2) [33], which is a widely established tool to assess eating disorder pathology in patients suffering from anorexia and bulimia nervosa. It consists of 64 items and encompasses eight subscales, measuring "drive for thinness", "bulimia", "body dissatisfaction", "ineffectiveness", "perfectionism", "interpersonal distrust", "interoceptive awareness", and "maturity fears". In our study, sum scores ranging from zero to 100 were created. Moreover, we employed the German translation of the second version [34] and interpreted the first eight, above-mentioned subscales of the EDI-2. The Cronbach's alpha for the total scale was 0.96, and for the subscales: 0.91 ("drive for thinness", "bulimia", and "body dissatisfaction"), 0.90 ("ineffectiveness"), 0.80 ("perfectionism"), 0.82 ("interpersonal distrust"), 0.83 ("interoceptive awareness"), and 0.73 ("maturity fears").

To assess the severity of depressive symptoms, we used the German version [35] of the PHQ depression scale (PHQ-9) [36]. It consists of nine items that represent the DSM-IV diagnostic criteria for depressive disorders, and its scores range from zero to 27, with scores of ≥ 10 indicating major depression with a specificity of 0.92 and sensitivity of 0.80 regarding a meta-analysis [37] of 17 validation studies in different languages. The Cronbach's alpha for the current sample was 0.86.

2.8. Statistical Analyses

All statistical analyses were conducted using IBM SPSS Statistics® Version 27.0.0.0 (IBM® Corp, Armonk, NY, USA).

Three groups were created, according to the medical diagnosis and BMI: an anorexia nervosa group (AN) with women diagnosed with anorexia nervosa (n = 68), an obesity group (OB) consisting of patients with a BMI of ≥ 30.0 kg/m^2, and a normal weight group (NW) with a BMI between 18.5 kg/m^2 and 25.0 kg/m^2 and without a diagnosed eating disorder.

Regarding the explorative design of this study, we established a cut-off of three standard deviations from the mean SPX level to identify outliers. During data analysis, three outliers (two in the anorexia nervosa group and one in the obesity group) were detected and excluded from further statistical analyses, which resulted in a study population of 219 women.

To investigate differences between the three groups, between-group comparisons were made using the Kruskal–Wallis test for non-parametric and one-way ANOVA for parametric data. To assess the frequency distributions between the groups, an overall chi-squared test was performed. In case of significant differences, pairwise comparisons using a chi-squared test were added. Correlations were assessed using Pearson's for normally, and Spearman's analysis for non-normally, distributed data. Due to the exploratory approach, we decided not to perform multiple linear regressions. The correlations and differences between groups were considered significant when $p < 0.05$. Due to the explorative design of the study, no corrections for multiple testing were applied.

3. Results

3.1. Demographic, Socioeconomic, and Medical Characteristics of the Study Population

Demographic and socioeconomic characteristics, comorbidities, and medication of study participants are outlined in Table 1. The AN group was significantly younger than both the OB ($p < 0.001$) and NW groups ($p < 0.001$; Table 1). By definition, patients with AN displayed a lower BMI than patients with OB ($p < 0.001$) and NW subjects ($p < 0.001$), and the NW group had a lower BMI than the OB group ($p < 0.001$; Table 1). Regarding socioeconomic status, the highest proportion of subjects living in a partnership was observed in the NW group. Furthermore, the OB group showed the lowest level of education, as indicated by a lower rate of university entrance diplomas than AN ($p < 0.01$) and NW ($p < 0.05$) and of any other school-leaving qualification than NW ($p < 0.01$; Table 1). NW women were also less often currently unemployed than OB and AN ($p < 0.05$; Table 1).

Table 1. Demographic and socioeconomic characteristics, comorbidities, and medication of study patients.

Parameter	All Subjects (n = 219)	AN (n = 68)	OB (n = 79)	NW (n = 72)	Significance
Demographic characteristics					
Age (years)	40.7 ± 16.4 (18–85)	28.4 ± 10.4 (18–59)	46 ± 15.3 (19–85)	46.5 ± 16.1 (21–82)	*** ###
Body mass index (kg/m^2)	27.1 ± 13.3 (8.7–70.7)	14.3 ± 2 (8.7–18.9)	42.3 ± 9.5 (30.1–70.7)	22.2 ± 1.8 (18.6–24.9)	*** ### +++
Socioeconomic characteristics					
Living in a partnership	109 (50%)	23 (34%)	39 (50%)	47 (65%)	### +
Level of education					
University entrance diploma	67 (31%)	28 (41%)	15 (19%)	24 (33%)	** +
Vocational diploma	20 (9%)	4 (6%)	9 (11%)	7 (10%)	
Secondary education certificate	94 (43%)	27 (40%)	32 (41%)	35 (49%)	
Basic school qualification	24 (11%)	6 (9%)	13 (16%)	5 (7%)	
No school-leaving qualification	14 (6%)	3 (4%)	10 (13%)	1 (1%)	++
Currently unemployed	91 (42%)	34 (50%)	36 (46%)	21 (29%)	# +
Unemployment during past 5 years	56 (26%)	18 (26%)	22 (28%)	16 (22%)	

Table 1. Cont.

Parameter	All Subjects (n = 219)	AN (n = 68)	OB (n = 79)	NW (n = 72)	Significance
Comorbidities					
Type 2 diabetes mellitus	18 (8%)	0 (0%)	17 (22%)	1 (1%)	*** +++
Impaired glucose tolerance	26 (12%)	1 (1%)	24 (30%)	1 (1%)	*** +++
Insulin resistance	41 (19%)	0 (0%)	36 (46%)	5 (7%)	*** +++
Arterial hypertension	53 (24%)	0 (0%)	38 (48%)	15 (22%)	*** ### +++
Hypercholesterinemia	71 (32%)	11 (18%)	37 (47%)	23 (33%)	*** #
Hypertriglyceridemia	14 (6%)	1 (3%)	12 (15%)	1 (1%)	** ++
Hyperuricemia	22 (10%)	1 (1%)	19 (24%)	2 (3%)	*** +++
Coronary heart disease	4 (2%)	0 (0%)	4 (5%)	0 (0%)	
Fatty liver disease	24 (11%)	1 (1%)	22 (28%)	1 (1%)	*** +++
Degenerative diseases of the musculoskeletal system	72 (33%)	2 (3%)	42 (53%)	28 (39%)	*** ###
Medication					
Insulin	4 (2%)	0 (0%)	4 (5%)	0 (0%)	
DPP-4 antagonists/GLP-1 analogs	2 (1%)	0 (0%)	2 (3%)	0 (0%)	
Other antidiabetics	9 (4%)	0 (0%)	9 (11%)	0 (0%)	** ++
Antipsychotics	26 (12%)	9 (13%)	11 (14%)	6 (8%)	
SSRI/SNRI	45 (21%)	11 (16%)	20 (25%)	14 (19%)	
Tricyclic antidepressants	25 (11%)	3 (4%)	10 (13%)	12 (17%)	#
Other antidepressants	13 (6%)	3 (4%)	6 (7%)	4 (6%)	
Tranquilizers, sedatives, hypnotics	4 (2%)	1 (1%)	1 (1%)	2 (3%)	
Other psychopharmacological medication	12 (5%)	0 (0%)	7 (9%)	5 (7%)	* #
Opioids	19 (9%)	0 (0%)	10 (13%)	9 (13%)	** ##

Data are expressed as absolute numbers with percentages in parentheses. Differences between groups were assessed using Kruskal–Wallis (age and BMI) and χ^2 tests. Significant differences (without correction for multiplicity) between the AN and OB groups are displayed as * ($p < 0.05$), ** ($p < 0.01$), or *** ($p < 0.001$); between the AN and NW groups as # ($p < 0.05$), ## ($p < 0.01$), or ### ($p < 0.001$), and between the NW and OB groups as + ($p < 0.05$), ++ ($p < 0.01$), or +++ ($p < 0.001$). Abbreviations: AN, anorexia nervosa; DPP-4, dipeptidyl peptidase-4 inhibitor; GLP-1, glucagon-like peptide-1; NW, normal weight; OB, obesity; SSRI, selective serotonin reuptake inhibitors; SNRI, serotonin-norepinephrine reuptake inhibitors.

As expected, type 2 diabetes mellitus, impaired glucose tolerance, insulin resistance, arterial hypertension, hyperuricemia, and fatty liver disease ($p < 0.001$), as well as hypertriglyceridemia ($p < 0.01$), were more common in patients with OB than in AN and NW (Table 1). No significant differences were found between groups in terms of medication taken, except for antidiabetics other than insulin and DPP-4-antagonists/GLP-1 analogs (mostly metformin), which were more common in OB than NW and AN ($p < 0.01$) and for opioids ($p < 0.01$) and other psychopharmacological medication ($p < 0.05$), which were more common in NW and OB than AN. In the NW group, tricyclic antidepressants were more often prescribed than in the AN group ($p < 0.05$, Table 1).

3.2. Body Composition, Physical Activity, Energy Expenditure, and Psychometric Characteristics of the Study Population

Data on body composition were available for 191 (57 AN, 71 OB, 63 NW), accelerometric data for 121 (27 AN, 47 OB, 47 NW), and psychometric questionnaires for 218 (GAD-7), 209 (PHQ-9), 214 (PSQ-20), and 195 (EDI-2) of the 219 women (Table 2).

Patients of all three groups showed significant differences from each other in terms of fat mass, fat free mass, body cell mass, and total body water, with the highest values in OB and the lowest in AN ($p < 0.001$; Table 2). Extracellular mass differed between AN and OB ($p < 0.001$), as well as NW and OB ($p < 0.001$), with higher values in OB (Table 2). Lower values were observed for phase angles in AN compared to OB ($p < 0.001$) and NW ($p < 0.001$; Table 2).

Table 2. Endocrine parameters, body composition, physical activity, energy expenditure, and patient-reported outcomes of the study populations.

Parameter	n	AN	n	OB	n	NW	Significance
Endocrine parameter							
Plasma spexin (ng/mL)	68	0.47 ± 0.16 (0.12–0.90)	79	0.41 ± 0.13 (0.16–0.74)	72	0.43 ± 0.17 (0.09–1.04)	*
Bioelectrical impedance analysis							
Fat mass (kg)	57	2.0 ± 4.4 (−7.0–11.9)	71	58.7 ± 21.4 (30–120.5)	63	18.2 ± 4.8 (10.9–31.1)	*** ### +++
Fat mass (%)	57	3.4 ± 11.3 (−25.4–27.8)	71	49.9 ± 6.2 (37.8–62)	63	29.0 ± 5.2 (19.7–41.7)	*** ### +++
Total body water (L)	57	28.0 ± 3.9 (19.4–38)	71	41.1 ± 6.2 (30.6–57.2)	63	32.2 ± 3 (26.1–40.5)	*** ### +++
Phase angle	57	4.2 ± 1 (1.4–6.1)	71	5.5 ± 0.7 (2.9–7.0)	63	5.3 ± 0.7 (3.3–6.5)	*** ###
Fat free mass (kg)	57	38.3 ± 5.3 (26.5–51.9)	71	56.1 ± 8.5 (41.8–78.1)	63	44.0 ± 4.1 (35.7–55.3)	*** ### +++
Extracellular mass (kg)	57	22.4 ± 5.1 (5.9–41.9)	71	28.6 ± 4.6 (21.0–40.2)	63	22.9 ± 3.1 (17.3–36.2)	*** +++
Body cell mass (kg)	57	15.7 ± 4 (4.1–22.2)	71	27.6 ± 4.8 (16.7–39.2)	63	21.1 ± 2.4 (15.9–26.5)	*** ### +++
Accelerometric measurement							
Number of steps/day	27	11,820 ± 7090 (1736–37,750)	47	7511.4 ± 3306.3 (1344–17,540)	47	9192 ± 3320 (2797–18,897)	*** +
MET/day	27	1.7 ± 0.2 (1.4–2.4)	47	1.1 ± 0.1 (0.8–1.5)	47	1.4 ± 0.2 (1.1–1.7)	*** ### +++
TEE (kcal/kg/day)	27	1715 ± 258 (1277–2427)	47	2961.2 ± 674.9 (1953.6–4753.8)	47	2055 ± 220 (1527–2661)	*** ## +++
EAT (kcal/kg/day)	27	139.9 ± 87.1 (5.0–400)	47	65.3 ± 44.2 (0–202)	47	100.6 ± 47.1 (22–219)	*** +++
NEAT (kcal/kg/day)	27	655.5 ± 127.9 (463–998)	47	694.9 ± 313.7 (63–1575)	47	411.2 ± 132.7 (119–800)	### +++
Patient-reported outcomes							
GAD-7	67	12.0 ± 4.6 (1–19)	79	10.1 ± 5.8 (0–21)	72	10.4 ± 5.6 (0–21)	
PHQ-9	62	14.6 ± 6.1 (2–27)	75	12.7 ± 6.6 (1–26)	72	11.5 ± 5.8 (0–27)	##
PSQ-20	65	60.6 ± 18.2 (13.3–95)	77	58.4 ± 21 (11.7–98.3)	72	56.2 ± 21.4 (5–90)	
Worries	65	60.2 ± 25.5 (0–100)	77	57.7 ± 26.8 (0–100)	72	51 ± 27.5 (0–100)	
Tension	65	70.9 ± 22.1 (20–100)	77	64.8 ± 26.5 (7–100)	72	63.8 ± 26.5 (0–100)	
Joy	65	33.8 ± 22.4 (0–86.7)	77	38.1 ± 23.2 (0–100)	72	38.7 ± 23.3 (0–100)	
Demands	65	45.1 ± 26.3 (0–93.3)	77	49.1 ± 24.4 (0–100)	72	48.5 ± 28.2 (0–100)	
EDI-2 total	56	48.2 ± 13 (13–80)	69	49.1 ± 13.6 (22–84)	70	31.1 ± 14.2 (5–77)	### +++
Drive for thinness	56	55.1 ± 30.9 (0–97)	69	59 ± 21.3 (14–97)	70	23.2 ± 21.2 (0–86)	### +++
Bulimia	56	22.4 ± 23 (0–91)	69	24.3 ± 21.7 (0–94)	70	6.9 ± 14.2 (0–91)	### +++
Body dissatisfaction	56	63.1 ± 18.7 (4–100)	69	83.6 ± 16.1 (47–100)	70	39.7 ± 23.1 (0–100)	*** ### +++
Ineffectiveness	56	48.2 ± 18.9 (16–86)	69	46.5 ± 20.9 (6–90)	70	34.8 ± 18.9 (4–86)	### ++
Perfectionism	56	51.4 ± 20.7 (10–100)	69	43.2 ± 22.6 (3–97)	70	37 ± 22.8 (0–87)	* ###
Interpersonal distrust	56	47.9 ± 18.8 (6–89)	69	47.6 ± 18.8 (6–89)	70	39.3 ± 17.9 (6–94)	# +
Interoceptive awareness	56	45.6 ± 15.2 (12–86)	69	39.1 ± 17.3 (2–90)	70	26.7 ± 16.1 (4–64)	* ### +++
Maturity fears	56	48.7 ± 19.2 (10–90)	69	45.1 ± 17.6 (10–100)	70	39 ± 17.2 (8–78)	## +

Data are expressed as mean ± standard deviation and range in parentheses. Differences between groups were assessed using a Kruskal–Wallis test for non-parametric data and ANOVA for parametric data. Negative fat mass values in bioelectrical impedance analysis are possible in severely underweight patients, due to the manufacturer's algorithms being calculated primarily for normal weight subjects. Significant differences (without correction for multiplicity) between AN and OB groups are displayed as * ($p < 0.05$), or *** ($p < 0.001$); between AN and NW groups as # ($p < 0.05$), ## ($p < 0.01$), or ### ($p < 0.001$) and between NW and OB groups as + ($p < 0.05$), ++ ($p < 0.01$), or +++ ($p < 0.001$). Abbreviations: AN, anorexia nervosa; EAT, exercise-related activity thermogenesis (energy expenditure of more than three metabolic equivalents of a task); EDI-2, Eating Disorder Inventory-2; GAD-7, Generalized Anxiety Disorder-7; MET, metabolic equivalents of tasks; NEAT, non-exercise-related activity; NW, normal weight; OB, obesity; PHQ-9, Patient Health Questionnaire-9; PSQ-20, Perceived Stress Questionnaire-20; TEE, total energy expenditure.

With regard to physical activity, patients with OB performed less steps per day than NW ($p < 0.05$) and AN ($p < 0.001$; Table 2). All three groups differed from each other concerning MET per day and TEE, with the highest MET levels in AN followed by NW and OB ($p < 0.001$); and the highest TEE in OB, followed by NW and AN ($p < 0.01$; Table 2). In NW subjects, NEAT was lower ($p < 0.001$) and EAT higher ($p < 0.001$) than in OB. NEAT was also lower in NW than in AN ($p < 0.001$; Table 2). EAT levels were lower in OB in comparison to AN and NW ($p < 0.001$; Table 2).

As shown in Table 2, there were no differences between groups regarding anxiety (GAD-7; $p > 0.05$) and perceived stress (PSQ-20 including all subscales; $p > 0.05$), while patients with AN exhibited higher depression scores than NW (PHQ-9; $p < 0.01$).

Regarding EDI-2 total scores, patients with AN and OB did not differ from each other ($p > 0.05$) but displayed higher scores than NW subjects ($p < 0.001$; Table 2). All three groups differed from each other in the EDI-2 subscale "body dissatisfaction", with the highest scores in OB followed by AN and NW ($p < 0.001$; Table 2) and in "interoceptive awareness", with the lowest scores in NW ($p < 0.001$ vs. AN and OB) and the highest in AN ($p < 0.05$ vs. OB; Table 2). Moreover, the NW group showed the lowest, and AN and OB groups similar scores for the subscales "drive for thinness", "bulimia" ($p < 0.001$), "ineffectiveness" ($p < 0.01$), "maturity fears", and "interpersonal distrust" ($p < 0.05$). Furthermore, patients with AN displayed a higher "perfectionism" level than patients with OB ($p < 0.05$) and NW ($p < 0.001$; Table 2).

3.3. Spexin Is Negatively Associated with Body Mass Index and Fat Mass but Not with Physical Activity or Energy Expenditure

The results of correlation analyses of body composition, physical activity, and energy expenditure, as well as psychometric parameters, with SPX are presented in Table 3.

Table 3. Correlations of body mass index, body composition, physical activity, energy expenditure, and patient-reported outcomes with spexin.

Parameter	All Subjects n = 219		Anorexia Nervosa n = 68		Obesity n = 79		Normal Weight n = 72	
	r	p	r	p	r	p	r	p
Body mass index (kg/m^2)	−0.149	0.027	−0.204	0.097	0.095	0.404	0.145	0.226
Bioelectrical impedance analysis								
Fat mass (kg)	−0.149	0.04	−0.149	0.27	0.138	0.252	0.198	0.12
Fat mass (%)	−0.159	0.028	−0.15	0.266	0.086	0.473	0.157	0.218
Total body water (L)	−0.082	0.259	0.102	0.451	0.113	0.349	0.14	0.272
Phase angle	−0.095	0.193	−0.111	0.409	0.061	0.613	0.065	0.613
Fat free mass (kg)	−0.084	0.249	0.103	0.446	0.112	0.353	0.135	0.291
Extracellular mass (kg)	−0.037	0.611	0.097	0.474	0.054	0.654	0.105	0.413
Body cell mass (kg)	−0.089	0.219	−0.042	0.754	0.112	0.354	0.166	0.193
Accelerometric measurement								
Number of steps/day	0.049	0.597	0.258	0.193	−0.067	0.652	−0.044	0.767
MET/day	0.151	0.099	0.252	0.205	0.031	0.821	0.170	0.202
TEE (kcal/kg/day)	−0.166	0.069	−0.054	0.788	−0.014	0.925	0.159	0.287
EAT (kcal/kg/day)	0.076	0.41	0.164	0.413	−0.059	0.692	−0.058	0.701
NEAT (kcal/kg/day)	0.021	0.820	−0.083	0.682	−0.103	0.490	0.051	0.733
Patient-reported outcomes								
GAD-7	−0.071	0.298	−0.125	0.312	0.029	0.802	−0.186	0.118
PHQ-9	−0.048	0.487	−0.027	0.836	0.128	0.274	−0.2	0.092
PSQ-20 total	−0.031	0.655	0.008	0.952	0.085	0.464	−0.185	0.12
Worries	−0.12	0.079	−0.078	0.539	−0.004	0.974	−0.334	0.004
Tension	0.018	0.792	−0.02	0.874	0.057	0.621	−0.093	0.436
Joy	−0.023	0.74	−0.046	0.715	−0.197	0.085	0.212	0.073
Demands	−0.018	0.792	0.105	0.404	−0.058	0.617	−0.008	0.946
EDI-2 total	0.066	0.361	−0.024	0.859	0.182	0.135	−0.006	0.961
Drive for thinness	0.022	0.764	−0.156	0.251	0.083	0.499	−0.099	0.417

Table 3. Cont.

Parameter	All Subjects n = 219		Anorexia Nervosa n = 68		Obesity n = 79		Normal Weight n = 72	
	r	p	r	p	r	p	r	p
Bulimia	0.027	0.71	−0.039	0.774	0.084	0.491	−0.004	0.977
Body dissatisfaction	0.005	0.946	−0.045	0.742	0.104	0.397	0.067	0.58
Ineffectiveness	0.029	0.692	−0.069	0.613	0.195	0.109	−0.134	0.268
Perfectionism	0.08	0.264	0.122	0.37	0.044	0.72	0.047	0.696
Interpersonal distrust	0.092	0.202	0.147	0.281	0.196	0.106	0.014	0.909
Interoceptive awareness	0.018	0.802	−0.071	0.604	0.057	0.643	−0.045	0.711
Maturity fears	0.043	0.554	0.173	0.203	0.149	0.22	−0.233	0.053

Correlations were assessed using Pearson's or Spearman's analyses. Significant correlations are indicated in bold. Abbreviations: EAT, exercise-related activity thermogenesis (energy expenditure of more than three MET); EDI-2, Eating Disorder Inventory-2; GAD-7, Generalized Anxiety Disorder-7; MET, Metabolic equivalents of tasks; NEAT, non-exercise-related activity; PHQ-9, Patient Health Questionnaire-9; PSQ-20, Perceived Stress Questionnaire-20; TEE, Total energy expenditure.

In the whole study population, the mean plasma SPX concentration was 0.436 ± 0.153 ng/mL (range: 0.092–1.035 ng/mL). SPX levels were found to be significantly higher in AN than OB ($p < 0.05$) and did not differ between the other groups ($p > 0.05$; Table 2). This was reflected by a negative correlation of peripheral SPX with BMI in the whole study group ($r = -0.149$; $p = 0.027$; Figure 1A). Plasma SPX was also negatively associated with absolute ($r = -0.149$; $p = 0.04$; Figure 1B) and relative ($r = -0.159$; $p = 0.028$; Table 3) fat mass. No relationships were observed between circulating SPX and other parameters of body composition, as measured by bioelectrical impedance analysis ($p > 0.05$; Table 3).

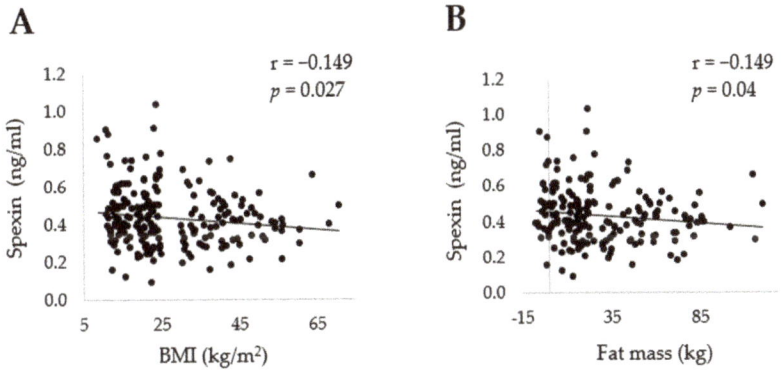

Figure 1. Correlations of spexin with (A) BMI and (B) fat mass (kg) in the whole study population. Negative fat mass values in bioelectrical impedance analysis are possible in severely underweight patients, due to the manufacturer's algorithms being calculated primarily for normal weight subjects. Abbreviation: BMI, body mass index.

We observed no associations between SPX and all measured parameters of physical activity (steps/day, MET/day; $p > 0.05$) and energy expenditure (TEE, EAT, NEAT; $p > 0.05$; Table 3).

3.4. SPX Is Not Correlated with Depressiveness, Anxiety, Perceived Stress, and Eating Disorder Pathology in the Whole Study Group

No significant associations between SPX and anxiety (GAD-7), depressiveness (PHQ-9), eating disorder pathology (EDI-2), and perceived stress (PSQ-20) total score were observed in the whole study group (Figure 2; Table 3). The PSQ-20 subscale "worries" showed a negative correlation with SPX in the NW group (r = −0.334, p = 0.004; Table 3).

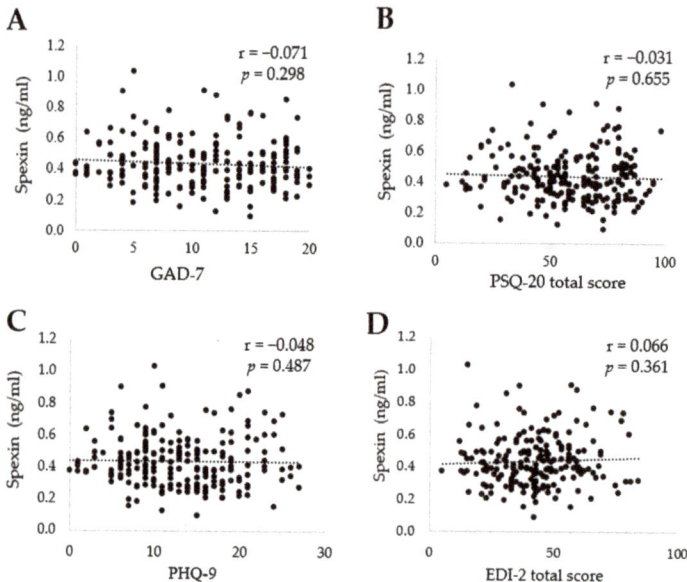

Figure 2. Correlations between (**A**) spexin and anxiety (GAD-7), (**B**) perceived stress (PSQ-20 total score), (**C**) depressiveness (PHQ-9), (**D**) and eating disorder pathology(EDI-2 total score). Abbreviations: EDI-2, Eating Disorder Inventory-2; GAD-7, Generalized Anxiety Disorder-7; PHQ-9, Patient Health Questionnaire-9; PSQ-20, Perceived Stress Questionnaire-20.

4. Discussion

The current study investigated the relationship between plasma SPX levels and objectively assessed PA, body composition, and patient-reported outcomes in a group of hospitalized adult women over a wide BMI range. In the whole study population, we showed a weak but statistically significant negative correlation between SPX and BMI, as well as SPX and body fat mass. However, we could not observe any relationships between SPX and parameters of physical activity and SPX and depressiveness, anxiety, stress, and eating disorder psychopathology.

The negative correlation between SPX and body fat mass is in line with earlier observations in adult individuals with obesity, in which a negative association between SPX and body fat percentage was reported [38]. Consistent with this, significantly lower SPX levels were reported in children with high compared to normal fat mass [39]. In one study, no correlation was found between SPX and body fat percentage [12], although this could be explained by the fact that the participants did not differ as much in BMI and body fat percentage as in our study. SPX is reduced after glucose load [4] and leads to lipolysis [5], which could explain the observed negative correlation of SPX with BMI and fat mass, and this would point toward SPX being responsible for the reduction in fat mass and not vice versa and could help to understand SPX's decrease in the peripheral circulation.

We did not observe any correlations between SPX and eating disorder symptoms as measured by EDI-2. As already mentioned in the introduction, several studies in animal models showed that SPX affects the levels of anorexigenic and orexigenic hormones and its effects result in suppression of food intake through a decrease of orexigenic peptides (AgRP, NPY, orexin) [13,15,40] or upregulation in mRNA expression of anorexigenic peptides (CCK, POMC, MCH) [15], predominantly in the hypothalamus. In addition, a fasting period led to a decline in SPX levels in the forebrain [41], and repeated daily intraperitoneal administration of SPX reduced both the meal size and meal duration, leading to weight loss in animals [6]. However, to date, no study has shown a direct effect of SPX on eating behavior in humans. A study that analyzed the effects of weight gain during inpatient treatment on SPX levels in AN indicated no significant results [42]. Nevertheless, some studies showed a negative association between SPX and leptin [43,44]. Leptin suppresses food intake and leads to weight loss [45]. In blood serum in patients with AN, it is downregulated, which is primarily attributed to the reduced mass of adipose tissue, where peripheral leptin is primarily expressed [46]. Perhaps low leptin also reduces its anorexigenic effects and represents a compensatory mechanism that protects, although insufficiently, against further weight loss [47]. Since both SPX and leptin cause loss of appetite and are simultaneously negatively correlated, it could be claimed that their anorexigenic effects are based on different mechanisms. Given its negative correlation with BMI, SPX, unlike leptin, may act as a driver of weight loss rather than a mere satiety signal and may be one answer to why AN persists or becomes a chronic condition. The fact that SPX was not associated with any scale of the EDI-2 in the present study also suggests that impaired body image or impaired eating habits are not responsible, even partly, for anorexigenic effects of SPX (observed in animals) and the negative association between SPX and leptin (in humans), but that SPX acts predominantly as a brain signal to induce weight loss. Therefore, one might conclude that SPX is not involved in the pathogenesis of AN in terms of impaired eating habits as an expression of eating disorder psychopathology. Longitudinal studies simultaneously measuring leptin and SPX in eating disorders and adjusting for BMI and body fat mass are needed, to further investigate the relationship between SPX and leptin and the function of SPX in eating disorders.

As reported, we also did not observe an association between plasma SPX levels and physical activity, as accelerometrically measured with a SenseWear® armband. This finding does not support the findings of a recent study suggesting that SPX could work as an indicator of response to physical activity [9] or correlate with results from an animal study conducted in mice showing increased SPX mRNA expression in muscle tissue and increased concentration in blood serum after exercise [48]. However, a possible explanation for these inconsistent findings could be that, in the present study, PA was measured only cross-sectionally, whereas associations may be detectable only over time or only in subjects responding to exercise. Additionally, SPX might be associated only with voluntary PA, or only in obesity but not in AN and, therefore, might not be associated with the hyperactivity observed in patients with AN. It could also be speculated that the intensity of daily PA, as captured in our study by measuring steps per day, does not increase circulating SPX levels, as in exercise training as reported in men with type 2 diabetes might [49].

We did not identify any association between SPX levels and anxiety (GAD-7), depressiveness (PHQ-9), or perceived stress (PSQ-20). This supports the results of a study conducted in adolescent inpatients with AN, where no associations with depressiveness (measured by BDI), eating disorder symptoms (EAT-26), or obsessive-compulsive disorder symptoms (Y-BOCS) were observed [42]. However, this study did not include any experimental design to investigate the causal relationship between SPX release and psychometric parameters. To date, a possible relationship between (psychological) stress reaction and peripheral SPX has only been demonstrated in animals. One study indicated that overexpression of SPX1 (one of two SPX orthologs occurring in zebrafish) in the dorsal habenula reduced anxiety-associated behaviors in zebrafish [22]. In addition, in mice in which anxiety was induced, SPX mRNA expression was reduced in the hippocampus, whereas CRF mRNA expression was upregulated [21]. Furthermore, CRF treatment has been shown to decrease SPX expression [21], and fish chronically stressed by social defeat exhibited upregulated cortisol and SPX levels in the brain [20]. Thus, studies in animals indicate a role for SPX in the regulation of stress, emotion, and behavior, which may also apply to humans. Therefore, further investigations of changes in peripheral SPX levels following interventions inducing stress or anxiety, e.g., by using stress paradigms such as the Trier social stress test, are needed. However, the investigation of alterations of cerebral SPX expression in humans would require using molecular imaging for peptide detection (such as the nanoflow liquid chromatography-mass spectrometry in combination with invasive microdialysis or the less invasive, but requiring the use of radioactive substances, positron emission tomography [50]). Nonetheless, at present, the known peptide monitoring methods are very expensive and not widespread. Moreover, the fact that repeated imaging would be needed (at least once before and after the stress test) makes the above-mentioned imaging techniques even more difficult to perform. In our explorative study, we did not find any association between PA and stress, and SPX, nor in the whole study group or in the subgroups (data not shown). Unfortunately, no studies investigated the effects of SPX on stress-mediated PA. Since there is evidence in the literature that stress interferes with PA [51], we suggest conducting an interventional study investigating changes in PA patterns and stress-like-behaviors (e.g., using an elevated-zero-maze test) after peripheral or central SPX injection.

The generalizability of the reported results is subject to certain limitations. First, BIA and the SenseWear® armband device are well-established measures for the determination of body composition and physical activity in clinical practice and research. However, BIA might have limited validity in severely underweight subjects [52], and the SenseWear® armband seems to slightly underestimate step counts, so the results must be interpreted with caution [53]. Second, the present study was conducted under naturalistic conditions; therefore, no healthy control group was employed. Consequently, we were unable to compare study participants with and without mental disorders. However, the included patients showed a wide range of psychological impairment on the different scales, so that circulating SPX levels could be well related to the constructs of depressiveness, anxiety, stress, and eating disorder pathology. In addition, the naturalistic design is also a strength, since it reproduces real-world conditions during inpatient treatment. Third, the naturalistic study design entails heterogeneity with regard to existing comorbidities, which are potential confounders and could therefore have contributed to the weak or absent associations observed. Therefore, future studies with more stratified study populations and an experimental research design should be conducted. Fourth, a cross-sectional study can only show associations and not cause-effect relationships. Therefore, in addition to experimental studies with healthy control groups, longitudinal studies are needed, to further examine changes in peripheral SPX levels over the course of improvements under treatment. Lastly, while studies in animals and humans indicate interrelations between SPX and the reproductive system [54], we did not assess menstrual status, and the intake of estrogen-containing medications was not an exclusion criterion in our female study population.

In this exploratory study, our findings replicate the negative association between SPX and both BMI and body fat. However, using a naturalistic and cross-sectional study design, no associations between circulating SPX and both patient-reported outcomes and PA were observed. Since animal studies indicated a possible effect of SPX on PA, anxiety, depressiveness, stress, and feeding behavior, further research in humans, employing longitudinal and interventional studies in more homogenous and larger study samples, is required.

Author Contributions: Conceptualization, A.S. and T.H.; Methodology, A.S. and T.H.; Validation, A.R., P.K., M.R., A.S. and T.H.; Formal Analysis, M.S. and A.S.; Investigation, M.S., A.R., E.W. and S.S.; Resources, A.S. and T.H.; Data Curation, M.S., A.R., E.W. and S.S.; Writing—Original Draft Preparation, M.S.; Writing—Review & Editing, A.R., P.K., M.R. and A.S. and T.H.; Visualization, M.S.; Supervision, A.S. and T.H.; Project Administration, A.S. and T.H.; Funding Acquisition, A.S. and T.H. All authors have read and agreed to the published version of the manuscript.

Funding: This study was supported by the Charité University Funding UFF 89/441-176 (A.S. and T.H.). We acknowledge financial support from the Open Access Publication Fund of Charité—Universitätsmedizin Berlin and the German Research Foundation (DFG).

Institutional Review Board Statement: Investigations were conducted according to the Declaration of Helsinki. The study was reviewed and approved by the Ethikkommission Charité–Universitätsmedizin Berlin. All patients provided written informed consent to participate in this study.

Informed Consent Statement: Informed consent was obtained from all subjects involved in the study.

Data Availability Statement: The data presented in this study are available on request from the corresponding author. The data are not publicly available due to data privacy.

Acknowledgments: We thank Reinhard Lommel and Petra Buße for laboratory work, and Mitsuru Murata and Christina Hentzschel for their help with the organization of clinical assessments.

Conflicts of Interest: The authors declare no conflict of interest. The funders had no role in the design of the study; in the collection, analyses, or interpretation of data; in the writing of the manuscript; or in the decision to publish the results.

References

1. Mirabeau, O.; Perlas, E.; Severini, C.; Audero, E.; Gascuel, O.; Possenti, R.; Birney, E.; Rosenthal, N.; Gross, C. Identification of Novel Peptide Hormones in the Human Proteome by Hidden Markov Model Screening. *Genome Res.* **2007**, *17*, 320–327. [CrossRef]
2. Porzionato, A.; Rucinski, M.; Macchi, V.; Stecco, C.; Malendowicz, L.K.; De Caro, R. Spexin Expression in Normal Rat Tissues. *J. Histochem. Cytochem.* **2010**, *58*, 825–837. [CrossRef] [PubMed]
3. Mills, E.G.; Izzi-Engbeaya, C.; Abbara, A.; Comninos, A.N.; Dhillo, W.S. Functions of Galanin, Spexin and Kisspeptin in Metabolism, Mood and Behaviour. *Nat. Rev. Endocrinol.* **2021**, *17*, 97–113. [CrossRef] [PubMed]
4. Gu, L.; Ma, Y.; Gu, M.; Zhang, Y.; Yan, S.; Li, N.; Wang, Y.; Ding, X.; Yin, J.; Fan, N.; et al. Spexin Peptide Is Expressed in Human Endocrine and Epithelial Tissues and Reduced after Glucose Load in Type 2 Diabetes. *Peptides* **2015**, *71*, 232–239. [CrossRef] [PubMed]
5. Kolodziejski, P.A.; Pruszynska-Oszmalek, E.; Micker, M.; Skrzypski, M.; Wojciechowicz, T.; Szwarckopf, P.; Skieresz-Szewczyk, K.; Nowak, K.W.; Strowski, M.Z. Spexin: A Novel Regulator of Adipogenesis and Fat Tissue Metabolism. *Biochim. Biophys. Acta Mol. Cell Biol. Lipids* **2018**, *1863*, 1228–1236. [CrossRef]
6. Walewski, J.L.; Ge, F.; Iv, H.L.; Levin, N.; Schwartz, G.J.; Vasselli, J.R.; Pomp, A.; Dakin, G.; Berk, P.D. Spexin Is a Novel Human Peptide that Reduces Adipocyte Uptake of Long Chain Fatty Acids and Causes Weight Loss in Rodents with Diet-Induced Obesity. *Obesity* **2014**, *22*, 1643–1652. [CrossRef]
7. Lin, C.-Y.; Huang, T.; Zhao, L.; Zhong, L.L.D.; Lam, W.C.; Fan, B.-M.; Bian, Z.-X. Circulating Spexin Levels Negatively Correlate with Age, Bmi, Fasting Glucose, and Triglycerides in Healthy Adult Women. *J. Endocr. Soc.* **2018**, *2*, 409–419. [CrossRef]
8. Ceylan, H.I.; Saygin, O.; Turkcu, U.O. Assessment of Acute Aerobic Exercise in the Morning Versus Evening on Asprosin, Spexin, Lipocalin-2, and Insulin Level in Overweight/Obese Versus Normal Weight Adult Men. *Chronobiol. Int.* **2020**, *37*, 1252–1268. [CrossRef]
9. Khadir, A.; Kavalakatt, S.; Madhu, D.; Devarajan, S.; Abubaker, J.; Al-Mulla, F.; Tiss, A. Spexin as an Indicator of Beneficial Effects of Exercise in Human Obesity and Diabetes. *Sci. Rep.* **2020**, *10*, 10635. [CrossRef]
10. Kumar, S.; Hossain, J.; Nader, N.; Aguirre, R.; Sriram, S.; Balagopal, P.B. Decreased Circulating Levels of Spexin in Obese Children. *J. Clin. Endocrinol. Metab.* **2016**, *101*, 2931–2936. [CrossRef]
11. Behrooz, M.; Vaghef-Mehrabany, E.; Ostadrahimi, A. Different Spexin Level in Obese Vs Normal Weight Children and Its Relationship with Obesity Related Risk Factors. *Nutr. Metab. Cardiovasc. Dis.* **2020**, *30*, 674–682. [CrossRef]
12. Bacopoulou, F.; Apostolaki, D.; Mantzou, A.; Doulgeraki, A.; Pałasz, A.; Tsimaris, P.; Koniari, E.; Efthymiou, V. Serum Spexin Is Correlated with Lipoprotein(a) and Androgens in Female Adolescents. *J. Clin. Med.* **2019**, *8*, 2103. [CrossRef]
13. Zheng, B.; Li, S.; Liu, Y.; Li, Y.; Chen, H.; Tang, H.; Liu, X.; Lin, H.; Zhang, Y.; Cheng, C.H.K. Spexin Suppress Food Intake in Zebrafish: Evidence from Gene Knockout Study. *Sci. Rep.* **2017**, *7*, 14643. [CrossRef]
14. Tian, Z.; Xu, S.; Wang, M.; Li, Y.; Chen, H.; Tang, N.; Wang, B.; Zhang, X.; Li, Z. Identification, Tissue Distribution, Periprandial Expression, and Anorexigenic Effect of Spexin in Siberian Sturgeon, *Acipenser baeri. Fish Physiol. Biochem.* **2020**, *46*, 2073–2084. [CrossRef]
15. Wong, M.K.H.; Sze, K.H.; Chen, T.; Cho, C.K.; Law, H.C.H.; Chu, I.K.; Wong, A.O.L. Goldfish Spexin: Solution Structure and Novel Function as a Satiety Factor in Feeding Control. *Am. J. Physiol. Endocrinol. Metab.* **2013**, *305*, E348–E366. [CrossRef]
16. Swift, D.L.; Johannsen, N.M.; Lavie, C.J.; Earnest, C.P.; Church, T.S. The Role of Exercise and Physical Activity in Weight Loss and Maintenance. *Prog. Cardiovasc. Dis.* **2014**, *56*, 441–447. [CrossRef]
17. Achamrah, N.; Coëffier, M.; Déchelotte, P. Physical Activity in Patients with Anorexia Nervosa. *Nutr. Rev.* **2016**, *74*, 301–311. [CrossRef]
18. Davis, C.; Kennedy, S.; Ravelski, E.; Dionne, M. The Role of Physical Activity in the Development and Maintenance of Eating Disorders. *Psychol. Med.* **1994**, *24*, 957–967. [CrossRef]
19. Elbelt, U.; Schuetz, T.; Hoffmann, I.; Pirlich, M.; Strasburger, C.J.; Lochs, H. Differences of Energy Expenditure and Physical Activity Patterns in Subjects with Various Degrees of Obesity. *Clin. Nutr.* **2010**, *29*, 766–772. [CrossRef]
20. Lim, C.H.; Soga, T.; Levavi-Sivan, B.; Parhar, I.S. Chronic Social Defeat Stress Up-Regulates Spexin in the Brain of Nile Tilapia (*Oreochromis niloticus*). *Sci. Rep.* **2020**, *10*, 7666. [CrossRef]

21. Zhuang, M.; Lai, Q.; Yang, C.; Ma, Y.; Fan, B.; Bian, Z.; Lin, C.; Bai, J.; Zeng, G. Spexin as an Anxiety Regulator in Mouse Hippocampus: Mechanisms for Transcriptional Regulation of Spexin Gene Expression by Corticotropin Releasing Factor. *Biochem. Biophys. Res. Commun.* **2020**, *525*, 326–333. [CrossRef] [PubMed]
22. Jeong, I.; Kim, E.; Seong, J.Y.; Park, H.-C. Overexpression of Spexin 1 in the Dorsal Habenula Reduces Anxiety in Zebrafish. *Front. Neural Circuits* **2019**, *13*, 53. [CrossRef] [PubMed]
23. Pałasz, A.; Suszka-Świtek, A.; Filipczyk, Ł.; Bogus, K.; Rojczyk, E.; Worthington, J.J.; Krzystanek, M.; Wiaderkiewicz, R. Escitalopram Affects Spexin Expression in the Rat Hypothalamus, Hippocampus and Striatum. *Pharmacol. Rep.* **2016**, *68*, 1326–1331. [CrossRef] [PubMed]
24. Andre, D.; Pelletier, R.; Farringdon, J.; Safier, S.; Talbott, W.; Stone, R.; Vyas, N.; Trimble, J.; Wolf, D.; Vishnubhatla, S.; et al. *The Development Ofthe Sensewear®Armband, a Revolutionary Energy Assessment Device to Assess Physical Activity and Lifestyle*; BodyMedia Inc.: Pittsburgh, PA, USA, 2006.
25. Hofmann, T.; Elbelt, U.; Ahnis, A.; Kobelt, P.; Rose, M.; Stengel, A. Irisin Levels Are Not Affected by Physical Activity in Patients with Anorexia Nervosa. *Front. Endocrinol.* **2014**, *4*, 202. [CrossRef] [PubMed]
26. Ainsworth, B.E.; Haskell, W.L.; Herrmann, S.D.; Meckes, N.; Bassett, D.R., Jr.; Tudor-Locke, C.; Greer, J.L.; Vezina, J.; Whitt-Glover, M.C.; Leon, A.S. 2011 Compendium of Physical Activities: A Second Update of Codes and Met Values. *Med. Sci. Sports Exerc.* **2011**, *43*, 1575–1581. [CrossRef] [PubMed]
27. Levine, J.A. Non-Exercise Activity Thermogenesis (Neat). *Best Pract. Res. Clin. Endocrinol. Metab.* **2002**, *16*, 679–702. [CrossRef] [PubMed]
28. Müller, M.J.; Bosy-Westphal, A.; Klaus, S.; Kreymann, G.; Lührmann, P.M.; Neuhäuser-Berthold, M.; Noack, R.; Pirke, K.M.; Platte, P.; Selberg, O.; et al. World Health Organization Equations Have Shortcomings for Predicting Resting Energy Expenditure in Persons from a Modern, Affluent Population: Generation of a New Reference Standard from a Retrospective Analysis of a German Database of Resting Energy Expenditure. *Am. J. Clin. Nutr.* **2004**, *80*, 1379–1390. [CrossRef]
29. Fliege, H.; Rose, M.; Arck, P.; Walter, O.B.; Kocalevent, R.-D.; Weber, C.; Klapp, B.F. The Perceived Stress Questionnaire (Psq) Reconsidered: Validation and Reference Values from Different Clinical and Healthy Adult Samples. *Psychosom. Med.* **2005**, *67*, 78–88. [CrossRef]
30. Levenstein, S.; Prantera, C.; Varvo, V.; Scribano, M.; Berto, E.; Luzi, C.; Andreoli, A. Development of the Perceived Stress Questionnaire: A New Tool for Psychosomatic Research. *J. Psychosom. Res.* **1993**, *37*, 19–32. [CrossRef]
31. Spitzer, R.L.; Kroenke, K.; Williams, J.B.W.; Löwe, B. A Brief Measure for Assessing Generalized Anxiety Disorder: The Gad-7. *Arch. Intern. Med.* **2006**, *166*, 1092–1097. [CrossRef]
32. Löwe, B.; Decker, O.; Müller, S.; Brähler, E.; Schellberg, D.; Herzog, W.; Herzberg, P.Y. Validation and Standardization of the Generalized Anxiety Disorder Screener (Gad-7) in the General Population. *Med. Care* **2008**, *46*, 266–274. [CrossRef]
33. Garner, D.M.; Olmstead, M.P.; Polivy, J. Development and Validation of a Multidimensional Eating Disorder Inventory for Anorexia Nervosa and Bulimia. *Int. J. Eat. Disord.* **1983**, *2*, 15–34. [CrossRef]
34. Thiel, A.; Jacobi, C.; Horstmann, S.; Paul, T.; Nutzinger, D.O.; Schüssler, G. A German Version of the Eating Disorder Inventory Edi-2 *Psychother. Psychosom. Med. Psychol.* **1997**, *47*, 365–376.
35. Löwe, B.L.S.R.; Spitzer, R.L.; Zipfel, S.; Herzog, W. Gesundheitsfragebogen Für Patienten (Phq-D). *Komplettversion Kurzform. Testmappe Man. Fragebögen Schablonen* **2002**, *2*, 90–93.
36. Spitzer, R.L.; Kroenke, K.; Williams, J.B. Validation and Utility of a Self-Report Version of Prime-Md: The Phq Primary Care Study. Primary Care Evaluation of Mental Disorders. Patient Health Questionnaire. *JAMA* **1999**, *282*, 1737–1744. [CrossRef]
37. Gilbody, S.; Richards, D.; Brealey, S.; Hewitt, C. Screening for Depression in Medical Settings with the Patient Health Questionnaire (Phq): A Diagnostic Meta-Analysis. *J. Gen. Intern. Med.* **2007**, *22*, 1596–1602. [CrossRef]
38. Atabey, M.; Aykota, M.R.; Özel, M.I.; Arslan, G. Short-Term Changes and Correlations of Plasma Spexin, Kisspeptin, and Galanin Levels after Laparoscopic Sleeve Gastrectomy. *Surg. Today* **2021**, *51*, 651–658. [CrossRef]
39. Behrooz, M.; Vaghef-Mehrabany, E.; Moludi, J.; Ostadrahimi, A. Are Spexin Levels Associated with Metabolic Syndrome, Dietary Intakes and Body Composition in Children? *Diabetes Res. Clin. Pract.* **2020**, *172*, 108634. [CrossRef]
40. Lv, S.; Zhou, Y.; Feng, Y.; Zhang, X.; Wang, X.; Yang, Y.; Wang, X. Peripheral Spexin Inhibited Food Intake in Mice. *Int. J. Endocrinol.* **2020**, *2020*, 4913785. [CrossRef]
41. Wu, H.; Lin, F.; Chen, H.; Liu, J.; Gao, Y.; Zhang, X.; Hao, J.; Chen, D.; Yuan, D.; Wang, T.; et al. Ya-Fish (*Schizothorax prenanti*) Spexin: Identification, Tissue Distribution and Mrna Expression Responses to Periprandial and Fasting. *Fish Physiol. Biochem.* **2016**, *42*, 39–49. [CrossRef]
42. Pałasz, A.; Tyszkiewicz-Nwafor, M.; Suszka-Świtek, A.; Bacopoulou, F.; Dmitrzak-Węglarz, M.; Dutkiewicz, A.; Słopień, A.; Janas-Kozik, M.; Wilczyński, K.M.; Filipczyk, L.; et al. Longitudinal Study on Novel Neuropeptides Phoenixin, Spexin and Kisspeptin in Adolescent Inpatients with Anorexia Nervosa—Association with Psychiatric Symptoms. *Nutr. Neurosci.* **2019**, *24*, 896–906. [CrossRef]
43. Kumar, S.; Hossain, M.J.; Javed, A.; Kullo, I.J.; Balagopal, P.B. Relationship of Circulating Spexin with Markers of Cardiovascular Disease: A Pilot Study in Adolescents with Obesity. *Pediatr. Obes.* **2018**, *13*, 374–380. [CrossRef]
44. Bitarafan, V.; Esteghamati, A.; Azam, K.; Yosaee, S.; Djafarian, K. Comparing Serum Concentration of Spexin among Patients with Metabolic Syndrome, Healthy Overweight/Obese, and Normal-Weight Individuals. *Med. J. Islam. Repub. Iran* **2019**, *33*, 93. [CrossRef]

45. Klok, M.D.; Jakobsdottir, S.; Drent, M.L. The Role of Leptin and Ghrelin in the Regulation of Food Intake and Body Weight in Humans: A Review. *Obes. Rev.* **2007**, *8*, 21–34. [CrossRef]
46. Zhang, Y.; Proenca, R.; Maffei, M.; Barone, M.; Leopold, L.; Friedman, J.M. Positional Cloning of the Mouse Obese Gene and Its Human Homologue. *Nature* **1994**, *372*, 425–432. [CrossRef]
47. Haas, V.; Onur, S.; Paul, T.; Nutzinger, D.O.; Bosy-Westphal, A.; Hauer, M.; Brabant, G.; Klein, H.; Müller, M.J. Leptin and Body Weight Regulation in Patients with Anorexia Nervosa before and during Weight Recovery. *Am. J. Clin. Nutr.* **2005**, *81*, 889–896. [CrossRef]
48. Leciejewska, N.; Pruszyńska-Oszmałek, E.; Mielnik, K.; Głowacki, M.; Lehmann, T.P.; Sassek, M.; Gawęda, B.; Szczepankiewicz, D.; Nowak, K.W.; Kołodziejski, P.A. Spexin Promotes the Proliferation and Differentiation of C2c12 Cells in Vitro-the Effect of Exercise on Spx and Spx Receptor Expression in Skeletal Muscle in Vivo. *Genes* **2021**, *13*, 81. [CrossRef]
49. Mohammadi, A.; Bijeh, N.; Moazzami, M.; Khodaei, K.; Rahimi, N. Effect of Exercise Training on Spexin Level, Appetite, Lipid Accumulation Product, Visceral Adiposity Index, and Body Composition in Adults with Type 2 Diabetes. *Biol. Res. Nurs.* **2021**, *24*, 10998004211050596. [CrossRef]
50. Su, Y.; Bian, S.; Sawan, M. Real-Time in Vivo Detection Techniques for Neurotransmitters: A Review. *Analyst* **2020**, *145*, 6193–6210. [CrossRef]
51. Stults-Kolehmainen, M.A.; Sinha. R. The Effects of Stress on Physical Activity and Exercise. *Sports Med.* **2014**, *44*, 81–121. [CrossRef] [PubMed]
52. yle, U.G.; Bosaeus, I.; De Lorenzo, A.D.; Deurenberg, P.; Elia, M.; Gómez, J.M.; Heitmann, B.L.; Kent-Smith, L.; Melchior, J.-C.; Pirlich, M.; et al. Bioelectrical Impedance Analysis-Part II: Utilization in Clinical Practice. *Clin. Nutr.* **2004**, *23*, 1430–1453. [CrossRef]
53. Storm, F.A.; Heller, B.W.; Mazzà, C. Step Detection and Activity Recognition Accuracy of Seven Physical Activity Monitors. *PLoS ONE* **2015**, *10*, e0118723. [CrossRef] [PubMed]
54. Tran, A.; He, W.; Chen, J.T.; Belsham, D.D. Spexin: Its Role, Regulation, and Therapeutic Potential in the Hypothalamus. *Pharmacol. Ther.* **2021**, *233*, 108033. [CrossRef] [PubMed]

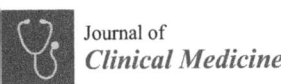

Article

Modeling Physiological Predictors of Running Velocity for Endurance Athletes

Szczepan Wiecha [1,*], Przemysław Seweryn Kasiak [2], Igor Cieśliński [1], Marcin Maciejczyk [3], Artur Mamcarz [4,†] and Daniel Śliż [4,*]

1. Department of Physical Education and Health in Biala Podlaska, Faculty in Biala Podlaska, Józef Piłsudski University of Physical Education in Warsaw, 21-500 Biala Podlaska, Poland
2. Student's Scientific Circle of Lifestyle Medicine, 3rd Department of Internal Medicine and Cardiology, Medical University of Warsaw, 04-749 Warsaw, Poland
3. Department of Physiology and Biochemistry, Faculty of Physical Education and Sport, University of Physical Education in Krakow, 31-571 Kraków, Poland
4. 3rd Department of Internal Medicine and Cardiology, Medical University of Warsaw, 04-749 Warsaw, Poland
* Correspondence: szczepan.wiecha@awf.edu.pl (S.W.); daniel.sliz@wum.edu.pl (D.Ś.)
† Artur Mamcarz has been added as a mentor author.

Abstract: Background: Properly performed training is a matter of importance for endurance athletes (EA). It allows for achieving better results and safer participation. Recently, the development of machine learning methods has been observed in sports diagnostics. Velocity at anaerobic threshold (V_{AT}), respiratory compensation point (V_{RCP}), and maximal velocity (V_{max}) are the variables closely corresponding to endurance performance. The primary aims of this study were to find the strongest predictors of V_{AT}, V_{RCP}, V_{max}, to derive and internally validate prediction models for males (1) and females (2) under TRIPOD guidelines, and to assess their machine learning accuracy. **Materials and Methods**: A total of 4001 EA (n_{males} = 3300, $n_{females}$ = 671; age = 35.56 ± 8.12 years; BMI = 23.66 ± 2.58 kg·m^{-2}; VO_{2max} = 53.20 ± 7.17 mL·min^{-1}·kg^{-1}) underwent treadmill cardiopulmonary exercise testing (CPET) and bioimpedance body composition analysis. XGBoost was used to select running performance predictors. Multivariable linear regression was applied to build prediction models. Ten-fold cross-validation was incorporated for accuracy evaluation during internal validation. **Results**: Oxygen uptake, blood lactate, pulmonary ventilation, and somatic parameters (BMI, age, and body fat percentage) showed the highest impact on velocity. For V_{AT} R^2 = 0.57 (1) and 0.62 (2), derivation RMSE = 0.909 (1); 0.828 (2), validation RMSE = 0.913 (1); 0.838 (2), derivation MAE = 0.708 (1); 0.657 (2), and validation MAE = 0.710 (1); 0.665 (2). For V_{RCP} R^2 = 0.62 (1) and 0.67 (2), derivation RMSE = 1.066 (1) and 0.964 (2), validation RMSE = 1.070 (1) and 0.978 (2), derivation MAE = 0.832 (1) and 0.752 (2), validation MAE = 0.060 (1) and 0.763 (2). For V_{max} R^2 = 0.57 (1) and 0.65 (2), derivation RMSE = 1.202 (1) and 1.095 (2), validation RMSE = 1.205 (1) and 1.111 (2), derivation MAE = 0.943 (1) and 0.861 (2), and validation MAE = 0.944 (1) and 0.881 (2). **Conclusions**: The use of machine-learning methods allows for the precise determination of predictors of both submaximal and maximal running performance. Prediction models based on selected variables are characterized by high precision and high repeatability. The results can be used to personalize training and adjust the optimal therapeutic protocol in clinical settings, with a target population of EA.

Keywords: velocity; respiratory compensation point; anaerobic threshold; endurance training; running; prediction models; machine learning

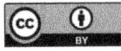

1. Introduction

The benefits of regular physical exercise are widely debated and include reducing the risk of obesity [1] or cardiovascular diseases [2]. On the other hand, improperly performed training with excessive intensity may negatively affect the organism's homeostasis and increase the risk of injury [3].

The concept of anaerobic threshold (AT) is widely discussed in exercise physiology [4]. As envisioned by Karlman Wasserman, the AT linked the increase in blood lactate concentration ($[La^-]_b$), during a strenuous incremental cardiopulmonary exercise test (CPET), with an excess arterial CO_2 accumulation and its further pulmonary output [5]. Above the AT, $[La^-]_b$ increase leads to temporary acidosis. The endurance capacity of the whole system is usually sufficiently high to cope with the incoming state [6]. During steady-state exercise with intensity above the AT, an equilibrium in $[La^-]_b$ appearance and its elimination is observed [6]. Thus, AT is a useful practical indicator to provide personalized training recommendations (with the aim of adjusting exercise intensity to set goals) and load monitoring [7].

The respiratory compensation point (RCP) is the intensity at which arterial CO_2 begins to decrease during demanding activity due to breathing capacity [8]. Above the RCP, the intensity of acidic ion accumulation exceeds their systemic or respiratory elimination abilities and indicates reduced endurance capacity. This leads to an over-decrease in the serum pH during graded exercise. This threshold indicates how long a high-intensity effort can be sustained [9].

The velocity at the anaerobic threshold (V_{AT}), at the respiratory compensation point (V_{RCP}), and at its maximum (V_{max}) play an essential position in the endurance performance assessment, both for professional and recreational endurance athletes (EA), as well as for the general population under clinical conditions [10,11].

These variables are the shift points of aerobic exercise to anaerobic metabolism and can be used as one of the parameters to evaluate the maximum endurance capacity [7]. Moreover, they closely positively correlate with exercise abilities [4]. They could be incorporated into the prescription for the advancement of training plans [7] or competition strategies [12] for special and narrow populations (e.g., EA), and in sports diagnostics whenever controlled running intensity is required (i.e., in clinical CPET) [7]. Furthermore, currently, these variables most closely correspond to the EA critical power sustainability [13,14].

Apart from V_{max}, maximal aerobic speed (MAS), which is directly related to VO_{2max}, is another important aspect of overall performance evaluation. However, as the aim of this research is to predict V_{max}, we recommend that further studies should be performed to analyze the MAS.

Numerous parameters, such as heart rate (HR), oxygen uptake (VO_2), or anthropometric data (i.e., height, age, and gender), are widely discussed in the development of multivariable prediction models that provide an increasingly more suitable alternatives to direct CPET measurements [15].

Several studies have attempted to develop and validate various non-invasive prediction equations for different sports performance measurements (i.e., for HR, VO_2, and others) [11,15,16]. However, they were mostly conducted on general populations or on small athletic samples, and thus, they can only be extrapolated to a low degree [17]. In addition, their methodology is widely variable, and only a few of them fulfilled recommended TRIPOD guidelines [18]. Thus, the actual number of V_{AT}, V_{RCP}, and V_{max} predictive models is limited, despite being significant measures of endurance capacity [19,20]. Moreover, although the variables influencing the running performance are well researched, the authors have not yet assessed how accurately they can be used to estimate running velocity by further including them in prediction models.

The aims of this study were: (1) to find the somatic and CPET variables that are the most responsible for running velocity, (2) to develop a prediction method for V_{AT}, V_{RCP}, and V_{max}, in accordance with TRIPOD recommendations [18], (3) to internally validate the obtained formulae, (4) to assess the accuracy of the current machine-learning abilities to predict running velocity based on the primarily determined variables, and (5) to evaluate practical applications of such an approach in sports or clinical conditions based on actual knowledge regarding exercise physiology.

2. Materials and Methods

The TRIPOD guidelines [18] have been applied to this research (see Supplementary Material S1, TRIPOD Checklist for Prediction Model Development and Validation). This was a retrospective data analysis from the registry of CPET performed in the years 2013–2021 at a tertiary care sports diagnostic clinic (SportsLab Clinic, Warsaw, Poland, www.sportslab.pl).

2.1. Ethical Approval

The study protocol was approved by the Institutional Review Board of the Bioethical Committee at the Medical University of Warsaw (AKBE/32/2021) and met the necessary regulations of the Declaration of Helsinki. Mandatory written consents to undergo incremental CPET were obtained from each EA before participating in the study. Written informed consent for participation was not required for this study, in accordance with the national legislation and the institutional requirements

2.2. Study Design

Participants were endurance runners who underwent CPET on the treadmill (TE). The tests were performed according to individual requests of the EA as an element of the training program prescription. Preliminary inclusion criteria were (1) age ≥ 18 years, and (2) $\leq \pm 3$ SD from mean for all of the tested variables included in Table 1 (only the lowest or the weakest extreme outliers were excluded). Exclusion criteria were (1) CPET was not performed on the TE, (2) any acute or chronic medical condition (including the musculoskeletal system, or addictions), (3) ongoing pharmacological treatment, and (4) smoking. To ensure that each subject reached maximum effort during the CPET, we applied the additional selection protocol consisting of the fulfillment ≥ 6 of the following criteria: (1) plateau in VO_2 (growth < 100 mL·min^{-1} in VO_2 with exercise workload increase), (2) respiratory exchange ratio (RER) ≥ 1.10, (3) respiratory frequency (fR) ≥ 45 breaths·min^{-1}, (4) reported exertion during CPET ≥ 18, according to the Borg scale, (5) $[La^-]_b \geq 8$ mmol·L^{-1}, (6) increase in speed $\geq 10\%$ of its RCP value post-exceeding the RCP, and (7) peak HR ≥ 15 beats·min^{-1} under predicted maximal HR [21]. For the entire selection procedure, along with the exclusion data, see Figure 1.

Table 1. Participants' basic anthropometric characteristics.

Variable (Unit)	Male [n = 3330; 83.23%]	Female [n = 671; 16.77%]	p-Value
Age (years)	35.90 (8.15)	33.86 (7.74)	<0.0001
Height (cm)	179.58 (6.22)	167.19 (6.88)	<0.0001
BM (kg)	77.72 (9.47)	60.60 (8.73)	<0.0001
BMI (kg·m^{-2})	24.07 (2.44)	21.64 (2.38)	<0.0001
BF (%)	15.49 (4.53)	22.04 (5.46)	<0.0001
FM (kg)	12.29 (4.71)	13.47 (4.65)	<0.0001
FFM (kg)	65.42 (6.47)	47.08 (6.36)	<0.0001

Abbreviations: BM, body mass; BMI, body mass index; BF, body fat; FM, fat mass; FFM, fat-free mass. The continuous value is presented as mean (SD), while the categorical value is shown as numbers (%), when appropriate. Comparisons between subgroups (p-value) were obtained by Student's t-test for independent variables.

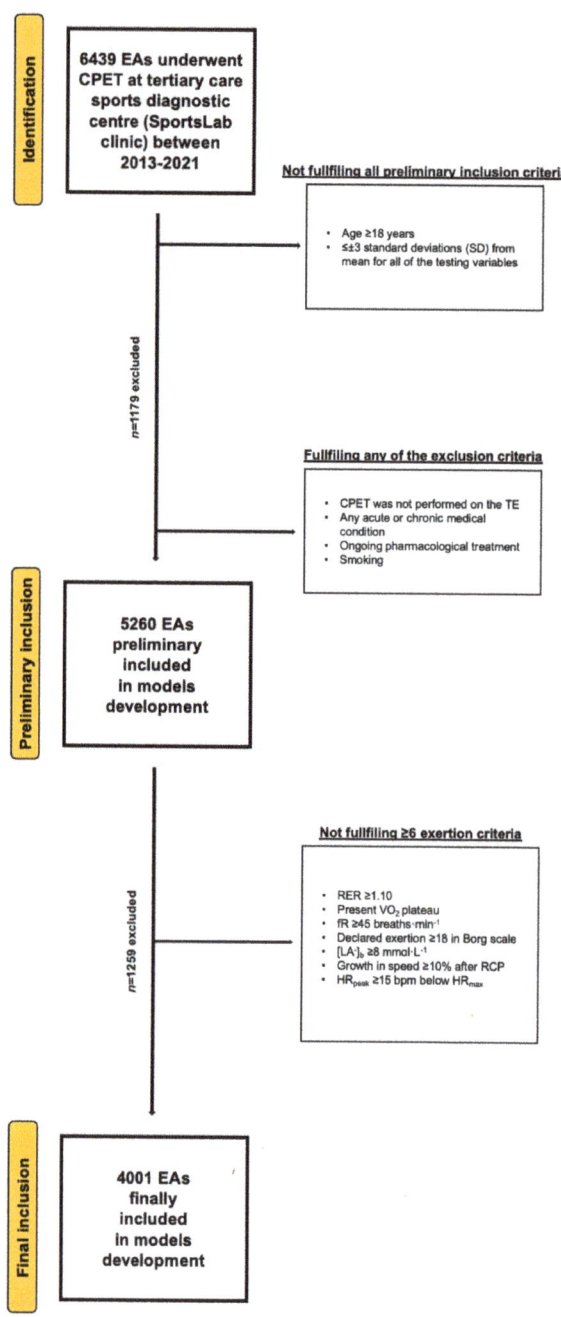

Figure 1. Flowchart of the preliminary inclusion and exclusion process. Abbreviations: EA, endurance athlete; CPET, cardiopulmonary exercise testing; SD, standard deviation; TE, treadmill; RER, respiratory exchange ratio; VO$_2$, oxygen uptake (mL·min^{-1}·kg^{-1}); [La$^-$]$_b$, lactate concentration (mmol·L^{-1}); fR, breathing frequency (breaths·min^{-1}); RCP, respiratory compensation point; HR$_{peak}$, peak heart rate (beats·min^{-1}); HR$_{max}$, maximal heart rate (bpm). At both stages of the selection, some participants met several (>1) exclusion criteria.

2.3. Somatic, [La⁻]$_b$ Measurements, and CPET Protocol

First, body mass (BM) stratified by body fat (BF) and fat-free mass (FFM) measurements were obtained via the bioimpedance method (BIA) using a body composition (BC) analyzer (Tanita, MC 718, Tokyo, Japan) with the multifrequency of 5 kHz/50 kHz/250 kHz. Conditions during BC and CPET were the same: 40 m^2 indoor, air-conditioned area, 40–60% humidity, temperature 20–22 °C, altitude 100 m ASL, and the subjects had their skin cleaned before testing. In our standardized laboratory practice, each EA had received recovery and dietary instructions via email a few days prior to testing to enable them to prepare appropriately for the CPET and BC tests. Our recommendations included: eating a high carbohydrate meal 2–3 h before the CPET and staying hydrated with sports drinks, and female EAs were advised to be well beyond their menstrual phase [22]. They also received information stating that the CPET would be performed on a mechanical TE and that they should be familiar with the characteristics of this type of effort, as well as the running technique involved.

Running tests were performed on a mechanical TE (h/p/Cosmos quasar, Nussdorf-Traunstein, Germany). CPET indices were measured using the breath-by-breath method during 15 s intervals [23], utilizing a Hans Rudolph V2 Mask (Hans Rudolph, Inc., Shawnee, KS, USA), a gas exchange analyzing device Cosmed Quark CPET (Rome, Italy), and specialized software (Quark PFT Suite powered by Omnia 10.0E). The gas analyzer device was calibrated prior to the testing protocol (16% O_2; 5% CO_2; ventilation accuracy ±2% or 100 mL·min^{-1}). The analyzer measurement mode takes into account the manufacturer's standard settings, i.e., 3-step smoothing and removing erroneous breaths from the analysis. HR was measured through the ANT+ and torso belt as a part of the Cosmed Quark set (accuracy similar to ECG; ±1 beats·min^{-1}). [La⁻]$_b$ was examined using a Super GL2 analyzer (Müller Gerätebau GmbH, Freital, Germany) employing an enzymatic-amperometric electrochemical technique. The lactate analyzer was also calibrated before each round of analysis for each participant.

CPET began with a 5 min preparatory protocol (walking or slow running at a declared "conversation" pace). The primary speed was 7–12 km·h^{-1} at a 1% inclination (the differences in the starting pace resulted from the training level of the participants and were selected on the basis of an interview on their previous sports results). The pace was increased by 1 km·h^{-1} every 2 min. VO_2 or HR plateau (no increase in VO_2 or HR with an increase in CPET intensity) or volitional inability to maintain intensity was the moment when the test was terminated [23,24]. Subjects were encouraged verbally to make a maximum effort. HR was considered the highest value at CPET (not averaged). Maximal VO_2 was recorded as an average from stable VO_2 in 10 s intervals directly before the termination of the CPET [23,24]. AT and RCP were assessed via non-direct methods based on the ventilatory concept. AT was achieved if the following measures were fulfilled: (1) VE/VO_2 curve started to grow with the constant VE/VCO_2 curve and (2) end-tidal partial pressure of O_2 started to grow with the constant end-tidal partial pressure of CO_2 [25]. RCP was achieved if the following measures were fulfilled: (1) a reduction in partial pressure of end-tidal CO_2 (PetCO$_2$) after attaining a maximal intensity; (2) a fast nonlinear growth in VE (second deflection); (3) the VE/VCO_2 ratio achieved the lowest value and started to grow; and (4) a nonlinear growth in VCO_2 versus VO_2 (linearity divergence) was achieved [25]. [La⁻]$_b$ was assessed by obtaining a 20 µL blood sample from a fingertip: before the test, after any speed increase, and 3 min after termination. A sample for [La⁻]$_b$ analysis was taken during running without interruption or pace decrease. Each time, the sample was from the same initial puncture. The first few drops were drained onto a swab and the proper blood sample was drawn. In further analysis, the corresponding values of [La⁻]$_b$ for AT, RCP, and maximal VO_2 were determined.

2.4. Data Analysis and Predictors Selection

Data were saved into an Excel file (Microsoft Corporation, Redmond, WA, USA) and Python script. Further, they were calculated according to frequency (percentage) and mean (±standard deviation; SD, or 95% confidence intervals; CI) for continuous variables and the median for categorical variables. Intergroup differences (each was a continuous variable) were calculated using the Student t-test for independent variables. If there were lacking data (only for $[La^-]_b$; in 1190 cases for males and 266 cases for females in total), imputation with the random forest method (RF) was applied to fill in the gaps [26,27].

The XGBoost machine learning approach was used to select variables with the highest prediction value [28]. In order to select the variables, the population was divided into 3 groups: 60% for derivation (building group), 20% for testing (testing group), and the remaining 20% for validation (validation group). After selection, 11 variables were included in the further analysis: VO_{2max}, VO_{2RCP}, VO_{2AT}, $[La^-]_{bRCP}$, $[La^-]_{bAT}$, VE_{max}, VE_{RCP}, age, BM, BMI, and BF. Next, selected parameters were input into multiple linear regression (MLR) modeling. As a result, only significant predictors (with $p < 0.05$) were included in the final models. The derived equations are characterized by the coefficient of determination (R^2), root mean square error (RMSE), and mean absolute error (MAE). A 10-fold cross-validation technique [29] and the Bland–Altman plots analysis [30] were used to establish the model's precision and accuracy during internal validation. To clarify, in the 10-fold cross-validation, the population is divided into 10 random parts. The candidate model is built on $[10 - 1 = 9]$ training sets; then, the derived model is evaluated on the test set consisting of the remaining one part. By respectively conducting building procedures on training sets and validation on the test set 10 times, we chose the final formula with the lowest possible inaccuracy validation score (defined in this paper as the lowest RMSE and MAE) [29]. Other implemented tests to reach the complete fulfillment of MLR modeling requirements include Ramsey's RESET test (for the correctness of specificity in MLR equations), the Chow test (for stability assessment between different coefficients), and the Durbin–Watson test (for autocorrelation of residuals). Each model was examined under the above-mentioned requirements and any irregularities have not been noted.

Our comprehensive machine learning approach enables the evaluation of each formula according to preliminary variable precision (at the stage of selection), accuracy (during model building), and recall (in internal validation).

The Ggplot 2 package (version-6.0-90; Available from: https://cran.r-project.org/web/packages/caret/index.html, accessed on 21 June 2022) in RStudio (R Core Team, Vienna, Austria; version 3.6.4), GraphPad Prism (GraphPad Software; San Diego, CA, USA; version 9.0.0 for Mac OS), and STATA software (StataCorp, College Station, TX, USA; version 15.1) were used for statistical analysis. A two-sided p-value < 0.05 was considered as the significance borderline.

3. Results

3.1. Somatic Measurements and CPET Results

The participants' anthropometric data are presented in Table 1. The full population consisted of 4001 people, of which 3330 (83.23%) were male and 671 (16.77%) were female. All data showed a normal distribution. The mean age was 35.90 ± 8.15 years for males and 33.86 ± 7.74 years for females and the overall age ranged from 18 up to 74 years. BMI was 24.07 ± 2.44 kg·m^{-2} for men, while women had 21.64 ± 2.38 kg·m^{-2}. BF percentage was relatively low, estimate at 15.49 ± 4.53 in males and 22.04 ± 5.46 in females. Significant differences between genders has been observed for height ($p < 0.0001$), BM ($p < 0.0001$), BMI ($p < 0.0001$), BF ($p < 0.0001$), and FFM ($p < 0.0001$).

CPET results are presented in Table 2. Among other measured variables, V_{AT} was 10.97 ± 1.40 km·h^{-1} and 9.64 ± 1.36 km·h^{-1} for males and females, respectively. V_{RCP} was 14.02 ± 1.74 km·h^{-1} and 12.29 ± 1.68 km·h^{-1} for males and females, respectively. The V_{max} obtained during CPET was 16.07 ± 1.93 km·h^{-1} and 14.12 ± 1.85 km·h^{-1} for males and females, respectively. The starting protocol velocity was 8.61 ± 1.28 km·h^{-1} for males and 7.60 ± 1.08 km·h^{-1} for females. When comparing both genders, significant differences (all $p < 0.0001$) were found for all the measured variables except [La$^-$]$_b$ at AT ($p = 0.99$), maximal respiratory exchange ratio ($p = 0.77$), and maximal HR ($p = 0.15$).

Table 2. CPET characteristics.

Variable (Unit)	Males [n = 3330]			Females [n = 671]			p-Value
	Mean	CI	SD	Mean	CI	SD	
VO$_{2AT}$ (mL·min^{-1}·kg^{-1})	38.42	38.25–38.59	4.96	35.69	35.32–36.05	4.83	<0.0001
VO$_{2AT}$ (mL·min^{-1})	2955.15	2942.04–2968.26	385.79	2137.77	2113.25–2162.29	323.48	<0.0001
RER$_{AT}$	0.87	0.87–0.87	0.04	0.86	0.85–0.86	0.04	<0.0001
HR$_{AT}$ (beats·min^{-1})	151.32	150.96–151.68	10.70	156.45	155.66–157.24	10.39	<0.0001
VE$_{AT}$ (L·min^{-1})	78.26	77.84–78.68	12.02	58.38	57.66–59.09	9.25	<0.0001
fR$_{AT}$ (breaths·min^{-1})	34.88	34.61–35.14	7.85	34.89	34.31–35.47	7.66	<0.0001
[La$^-$]$_{bAT}$ (mmol·L^{-1});	1.95	1.92–1.98	0.67	1.86	1.80–1.93	0.66	0.99
VO$_{2RCP}$ (mL·min^{-1}·kg^{-1})	47.59	47.37–47.81	6.10	43.05	42.56–43.55	6.14	<0.0001
VO$_{2RCP}$ (mL·min^{-1})	3642.72	3626.90–3658.54	465.70	2576.01	2545.15–2606.87	407.12	<0.0001
RER$_{RCP}$	1.00	1.00–1.00	0.04	0.99	0.99–1.00	0.04	<0.0001
HR$_{RCP}$ (beats·min^{-1})	173.43	173.12–173.75	9.33	176.04	175.34–176.73	9.12	<0.0001
VE$_{RCP}$ (L·min^{-1})	113.82	113.25–114.39	16.43	81.15	80.20–82.11	12.34	<0.0001
fR$_{RCP}$ (breaths·min^{-1})	44.19	43.91–44.48	8.52	43.09	42.49–43.68	7.87	<0.0001
[La$^-$]$_{bRCP}$ (mmol·L^{-1});	4.53	4.49–4.58	1.07	4.19	4.09–4.29	1.02	<0.0001
VO$_{2max}$ (mL·min^{-1}·kg^{-1})	54.10	53.87–54.34	6.93	48.73	48.23–49.24	6.67	<0.0001
VO$_{2max}$ (mL·min^{-1})	4176.37	4157.64–4195.09	551.09	2949.02	2911.51–2986.54	494.89	<0.0001
RER$_{max}$	1.12	1.12–1.12	0.04	1.12	1.12–1.12	0.04	0.76
HR$_{max}$ (beats·min^{-1})	184.81	184.49–185.13	9.54	185.39	184.69–186.09	9.24	0.15
VE$_{max}$ (L·min^{-1})	148.86	148.15–149.57	20.46	103.83	102.60–105.05	15.86	<0.0001
fR$_{max}$ (breaths·min^{-1})	57.59	57.28–57.90	9.20	55.46	54.83–56.09	8.30	<0.0001
[La$^-$]$_{bmax}$ (mmol·L^{-1});	9.91	9.82–10.00	2.02	9.08	8.88–9.28	1.93	<0.0001
V$_{AT}$ (km·h^{-1})	10.97	10.92–11.02	1.40	9.64	9.53–9.74	1.36	<0.0001
V$_{RCP}$ (km·h^{-1})	14.02	13.96–14.08	1.74	12.29	12.16–12.41	1.68	<0.0001
V$_{max}$ (km·h^{-1})	16.07	16.01–16.14	1.93	14.12	13.98–14.26	1.85	<0.0001
V$_S$ (km·h^{-1})	8.61	8.56–8.66	1.28	7.60	7.51–7.69	1.08	<0.0001

Abbreviations: CI, 95% confidence interval; SD, standard deviation; VO$_{2AT}$, oxygen uptake at anaerobic threshold; RER$_{AT}$, respiratory exchange ratio at anaerobic threshold; HR$_{AT}$, heart rate at anaerobic threshold; VE$_{AT}$, pulmonary ventilation at anaerobic threshold; fR$_{AT}$, respiratory frequency at anaerobic threshold; [La$^-$]$_{bAT}$, lactate concentration at anaerobic threshold; VO$_{2RCP}$, oxygen uptake at respiratory compensation point; RER$_{RCP}$, respiratory exchange ratio at respiratory compensation point; HR$_{RCP}$, heart rate at respiratory compensation point; VE$_{RCP}$, pulmonary ventilation at respiratory compensation point; fR$_{RCP}$, respiratory frequency at respiratory compensation point; [La$^-$]$_{bmax}$, lactate concentration at respiratory compensation point; VO$_{2max}$, maximal oxygen uptake; RER$_{max}$, maximal respiratory exchange ratio; HR$_{max}$, maximal heart rate; VE$_{max}$, maximal pulmonary ventilation; fR$_{max}$, maximal respiratory frequency; [La$^-$]$_{bmax}$, maximal lactate concentration; V$_{AT}$, velocity at anaerobic threshold; V$_{RCP}$, velocity at respiratory compensation point; V$_{max}$, maximal velocity; V$_S$, protocol starting velocity. Comparisons between subgroups (p-value) were obtained by Student t-test for independent variables.

3.2. Prediction Models for V_{AT}, V_{RCP}, and V_{max}

Complete MLR prediction models for males and females are presented in Table 3 (left columns), while Figure 2 shows their performance in the derivation cohort (illustrated as an analysis of observed vs. predicted values). The importance of all CPET variables, based on XGBoost selection, included in the modeling is presented in Figure 3. The following variables showed the strongest impact in building the models: VO$_2$, [La$^-$], VE age, and BMI. Model performance is presented as R^2, along with RMSE and MAE. Briefly, R^2 for male equations ranged from 0.57 for V_{AT} and V_{max} to 0.62 for V_{RCP}. For female formulae, R^2 ranged from 0.62 for V_{AT} to 0.67 for V_{RCP}. The obtained RMSE was the lowest for the female V_{AT} equation (=0.828) and the highest for the male V_{max} (=1.202), while the observed MAE was the lowest for the female V_{AT} equation (=0.657) and the highest for male V_{max} (=0.944).

Table 3. Running velocity prediction equations stratified by gender.

Model Category	Multiple Linear Regression Equation	R^2	Derivation Group Performance		Validation Group Performance	
			RMSE	MAE	RMSE	MAE
V_{AT} Males	$8.00 - 0.01 \cdot Age - 0.09 \cdot BMI + 0.04 \cdot VO_{2max} + 0.09 \cdot VO_{2AT} - 0.65 \cdot [La^-]_{bAT} + 0.01 \cdot VE_{RCP}$	0.57	0.909	0.708	0.913	0.710
V_{AT} Females	$7.55 - 0.02 \cdot Age - 0.10 \cdot BMI + 0.15 \cdot VO_{2AT} - 0.70 \cdot [La^-]_{bAT} + 0.01 \cdot VE_{RCP}$	0.62	0.828	0.657	0.838	0.665
V_{RCP} Males	$10.88 - 0.02 \cdot Age - 0.11 \cdot BMI + 0.04 \cdot VO_{2max} - 0.99 \cdot [La^-]_{bAT} + 0.10 \cdot VO_{2RCP} + 0.01 \cdot VE_{RCP} + 0.10 \cdot [La^-]_{bRCP}$	0.62	1.066	0.832	1.070	0.835
V_{RCP} Females	$9.24 - 0.02 \cdot Age - 0.11 \cdot BMI - 1.05 \cdot [La^-]_{bAT} + 0.15 \cdot VO_{2RCP} + 0.01 \cdot VE_{RCP} + 0.19 \cdot [La^-]_{bRCP}$	0.67	0.964	0.752	0.978	0.763
V_{max} Males	$12.41 - 0.03 \cdot Age + 0.01 \cdot BM - 0.12 \cdot BMI + 0.10 \cdot VO_{2max} - 0.82 \cdot [La^-]_{bAT} + 0.07 \cdot VO_{2RCP}$	0.57	1.202	0.943	1.205	0.944
V_{max} Females	$9.37 - 0.03 \cdot Age + 0.06 \cdot VO_{2max} - 0.79 \cdot [La^-]_{bAT} + 0.09 \cdot VO_{2RCP} + 0.01 \cdot VE_{max} - 0.04 \cdot BF$	0.65	1.095	0.861	1.111	0.881

Abbreviations: RMSE, root mean square error; MAE, mean absolute error; R^2, adjusted R^2; V_{AT}, velocity at anaerobic threshold; Age, age in years; BMI, body mass index (kg·m^{-2}); VO_{2max}, relative maximum oxygen uptake (mL·min^{-1}·kg^{-1}); VO_{2AT}, relative oxygen uptake at anaerobic threshold (mL·min^{-1}·kg^{-1}); $[La^-]_{bAT}$, blood lactate concentration at anaerobic threshold (mmol·L^{-1}); VE_{RCP}, pulmonary ventilation at RCP (L·min^{-1}); V_{RCP}, velocity at respiratory compensation point; VO_{2RCP}, relative oxygen uptake at respiratory compensation point (mL·min^{-1}·kg^{-1}); $[La^-]_{bRCP}$, blood lactate concentration at respiratory compensation point; BM, body mass; V_{max}, maximal velocity; VE_{max}, maximal pulmonary ventilation (L·min^{-1}). RMSE and MAE are explained in km·h^{-1}. Model performance at the stage of derivation has been shown in the left columns. Briefly, our equations showed high accuracy and explained approximately 60–70% of the differences between participants. The results of internal validation via the 10-fold cross technique are presented in the right columns, and they showed a precise transferability, despite a limited sample size for internal validation. We are presenting one R^2 because of the 10-fold cross-validation for the same group of participants as the derived validation.

3.3. Internal Validation

The evaluation of each model is also presented in Table 3 (right columns). In summary, the performance of our prediction equations was similar to that observed in the derivation cohort. A slightly higher RMSE and MAE were noted. Overall, RMSE values are located between 0.838–1.205 km·h^{-1} and MAE between 0.665–0.944 km·h^{-1}. The best working model (defined as having the highest replicability and the lowest risk of inaccuracies in the test set) was for V_{AT} for females (RMSE = 0.838, MAE = 0.665), and the worst was for males V_{max} (RMSE = 1.205, MAE = 0.944). The most and least accurate models were the same in regards to the derivation and validation. Figure 4 illustrates the Bland–Altman plots, with a comparison of observed vs. predicted velocity using newly derived prediction models at the stage of validation.

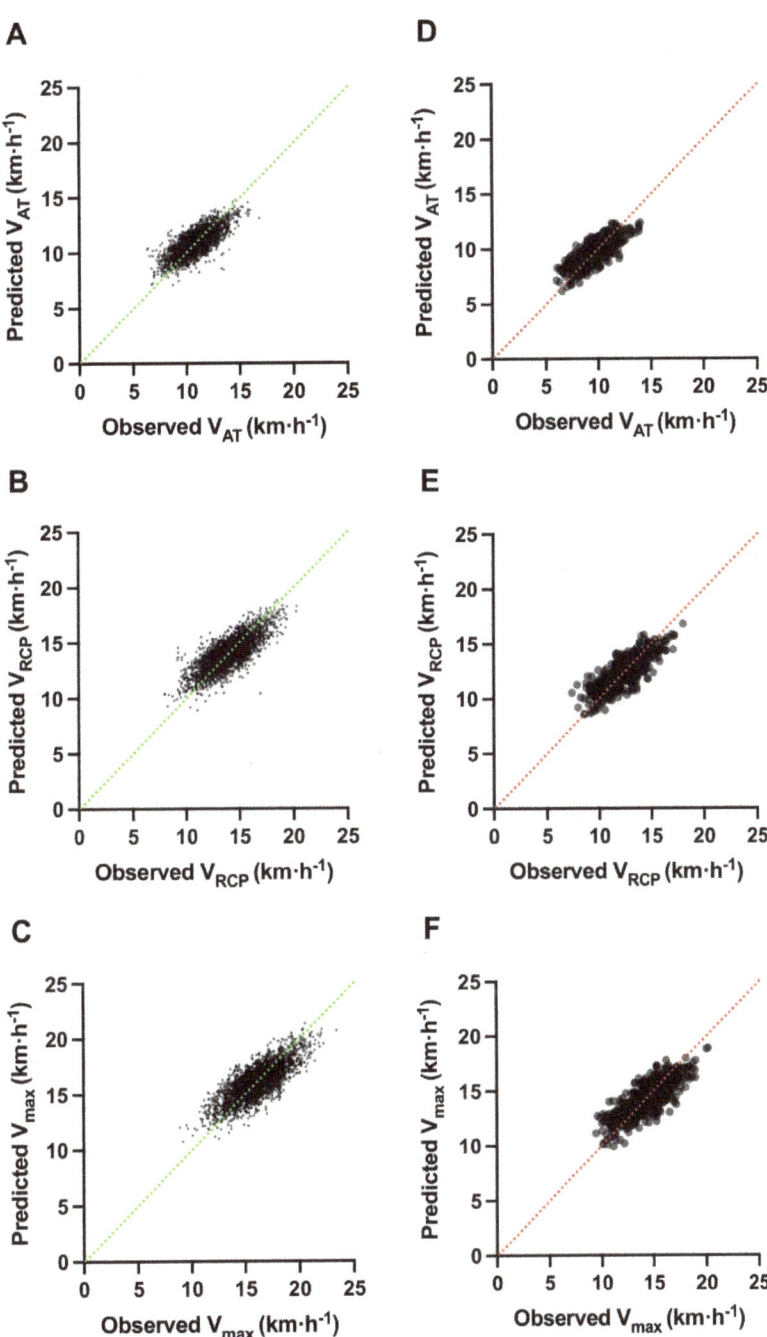

Figure 2. Performance of novel prediction equations for treadmill velocity. Abbreviations: V_{AT}, velocity at anaerobic threshold; V_{RCP}, velocity at respiratory compensation point; V_{max}, maximal velocity. Colored dotted lines illustrate a 1:1 correspondence between measured and predicted velocities, respectively green for males (left row; (**A**–**C**) panels) and red for females (right row; (**D**–**F**) panels).

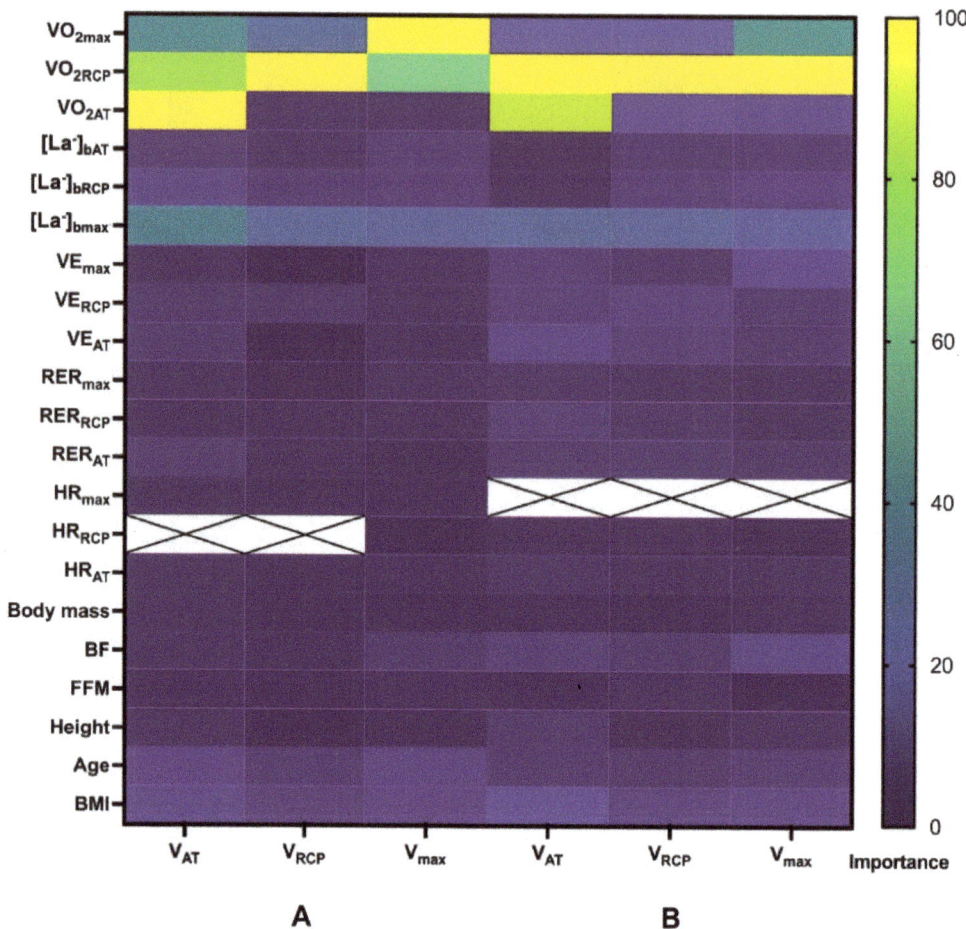

Figure 3. Heat map showing the importance variables regarding predicted velocity based on XGBoost selection. Abbreviation: VO_{2max}, maximal oxygen uptake; VO_{2RCP}, relative oxygen uptake at respiratory compensation point; VO_{2AT}, relative oxygen uptake at anaerobic threshold; $[La^-]_{bRCP}$, blood lactate concentration at respiratory compensation point; $[La^-]_{bAT}$, blood lactate concentration at anaerobic threshold; $[La^-]_{bmax}$, maximal blood lactate concentration; VE_{max}, maximal pulmonary ventilation; VE_{RCP}, pulmonary ventilation at respiratory compensation point; VE_{AT}, pulmonary ventilation at anaerobic threshold; RER_{max}, maximal respiratory exchange ratio; RER_{RCP}, respiratory exchange ratio at respiratory compensation point; RER_{AT}, respiratory exchange ratio at anaerobic threshold; HR_{max}, maximal heart rate; HR_{RCP}, heart rate at respiratory compensation point; HR_{AT}, heart rate at anaerobic threshold; BF, body fat; FFM, fat-free mass; BMI, body mass index; V_{AT}, velocity at anaerobic threshold; V_{RCP}, velocity at respiratory compensation point; V_{max}, maximal velocity. Panel (**A**) presents data for males, while panel (**B**) shows the data for females. The cross means that the variable has not fulfilled preliminary selection-stage requirements (only in HR). The maps present a variable's importance regarding the predicted velocity during the model-building stage. In the final prediction models, only the variables with significant impact ($p < 0.05$) were included.

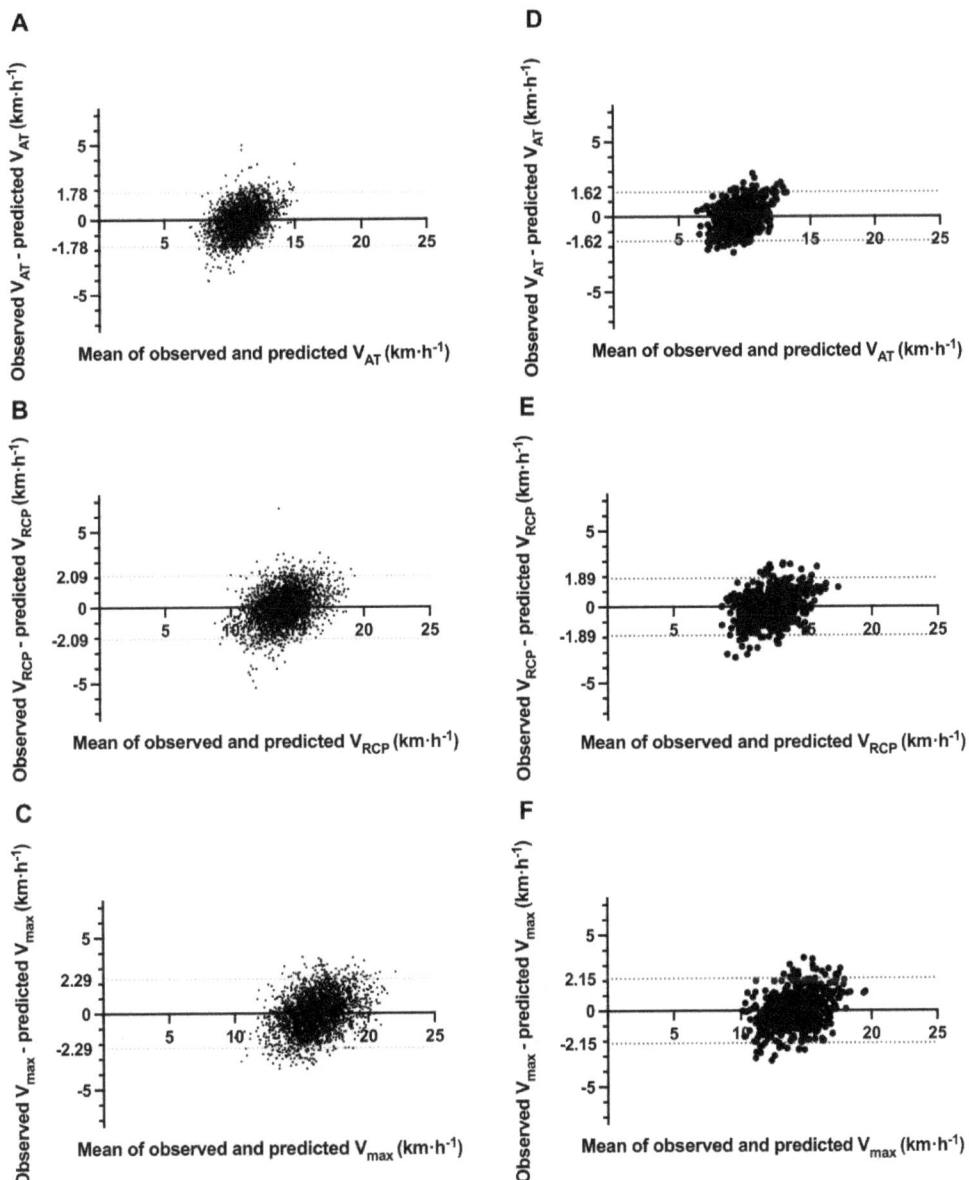

Figure 4. Bland–Altman Plots comparing observed with predicted velocity during internal validation. Abbreviations: V_{AT}, velocity at anaerobic threshold; V_{RCP}, velocity at respiratory compensation point; V_{max}, maximal velocity. Colored dotted lines present a 95% confidence interval of agreement, green for males (left row; (**A–C**) panels) and red for females (right row; (**D–F**) panels), respectively.

4. Discussion

In the current study, we applied advanced machine-learning properties in a comprehensive evaluation of running physiology. The obtained equations include several physiological-only measures (both anthropometric and directly measured during CPET) to provide a feasible utility for the prediction of V_{AT}, V_{RCP}, and V_{max} with substantial accuracy. The availability of this type of machine-learning tool in exercise diagnostics enables better training recommendations for EA and facilitates rehabilitation prescriptions for patients suffering from cardiovascular or respiratory diseases [7,31]. The novelty and main advantage are that there are no comparable studies that first select the variables with the strongest predictive abilities, and then directly evaluate their accuracy in the derived prediction models. An additional attribute is a relatively large group of healthy adult EA (n = 4001) who have undergone the CPET under an identical protocol, by which the maximum precision and similarity of the collected data were obtained. This enabled us to better examine whether parameters such as age [32], BC and BF [33] or VO_{2max} [16] exerted a possible significant impact on the predictive performance of the model (as they were previously classified as relevant variables in the literature. Moreover, the inclusion criteria enable us to avoid the disturbing influence of factors such as smoking [34] or medications [35].

4.1. Model Performance and Physiological Properties

Performance measurements show precise prediction abilities which were fairly replicable between the training and test sets (see Figures 2 and 3). The obtained R^2 explained approximately 60% to 70% of the differences, while errors were moderate-to-low, under 1 km·h^{-1} for most cases. With additional internal validation, they were both still located in the upper sensitivity range. Thus, the model accuracy was only minorly reduced. In previous publications, such as that by Petek et al. for VO_{2peak} [36], similar results were observed. However, usually, previous researchers have not carried out an initial selection of the most suitable variables, and so far, studies have been based on previously established parameters, only changing their proportions. Our study showed that VO_2 at RCP and maximal VO_2 were the most important parameters responsible for the prediction of middle- to long-distance running velocity (a lower impact of VO_2 at AT was noted). This confirms previous findings by Thompson et al. and Lanferdini et al. [16,37] that the VO_2 can be described as the universal and comparable performance measure, and that it is strongly related to running speed. Moreover, according to the physiological relationship between exercise performance and $[La^-]_b$ at AT, at RCP, and maximal VO_2, they also significantly influence the predicted velocities (but in the varied order compared with VO_2, with more impact from sub-maximal levels at AT or RCP than maximal $[La^-]_b$ values). This is confirmed in studies by Tanaka and Matsuura [12] and Schabort et al. [19], as growing $[La^-]_b$ and training intensity were positively correlated in both. Thus, of greater improtance seems to be the ability to rapidly utilize and prevent excess growth in $[La^-]_b$ by EA than working at maximal value for a prolonged time. Our study confirmed the previous findings by Farrell et al. [38] on this point. Another important variable was pulmonary ventilation. The majority of the influence was created by VE_{RCP}, and only for V_{max} was there a significant impact of VE_{max}. The higher it was, the better running velocity was observed. Thus, it can be concluded that the higher oxygen (O_2) supply and better carbon dioxide (CO_2) utilization yielded an improvement in running performance. This is a well-documented concept that was stated by Sjodin and Svedenhag in the 1980s [32]. Our insights on both VO_2 and VE also confirmed that performance at RCP is strongly correlated with other running and general exercise indices [15]. When it comes to somatic parameters, they also showed a relevant effect on velocity. Higher BMI [19] and increasing age [39] were associated with lower endurance performance. On the other hand, BC, described as a percentage of BF and FFM, showed some effect on the predicted velocity, despite their impact on males being not enough to be included in the modeling for this gender. It is worth mentioning that the influence of BF was more noticeable in females, perhaps because they naturally have a higher level of BF [40]. HR was one of the variables with the lowest impact on velocity (see Figure 3). Moreover, we emphasize that HR, which shows high inter-individual variability and is difficult to precisely estimate for EA [21], was not included in any of our equations. To summarize, the degree of the relationships between the variables is interesting. It is very promising to assess how precisely we can estimate V_{AT}, V_{RCP}, and V_{max} based on the above-mentioned parameters.

4.2. Clinical Considerations

Our results also have important clinical applications for patients from the general and athletic populations. The development of sports cardiology has resulted in a higher number of EA patients, including former cardiac patients or those suspected of having exertional cardiac abnormalities. TE CPET is often performed to some level of submaximal intensity or until refused. However, those who are less experienced may quit earlier, before reaching their optimal diagnostic intensity level, because they are not mentally adapted to perform such demanding activities [31,41]. The calculation (MET × running velocity) is used by medical professionals to provide personalized recommendations for cardiac rehabilitations [31]. Selection of the most important variables and additional comparison of those directly achieved with the predicted velocity verify whether an optimal level of intensity was achieved.

4.3. Practical Applications

The characteristics of selected variables and prediction models could be used in the preparation of exercise recommendations for both professional and recreational EA as patients in clinical settings [7]. The highest accuracy of the observed repeatable values would be for EA, mainly for running activities (i.e., during long-distance running or football), due to the characteristics similar to those in the derivation cohort [36]. Thanks to the use of V_{AT}, V_{RCP}, and V_{max} prediction models, there would be no need to run the full CPET protocol and measure all parameters, but only the most significant and contributing ones [19]. This is a matter of importance, as CPET is often impossible to perform according to the full protocol due to the limited availability of specialized clinics and equipment or the high cost of the procedure [42]. This model can also be used to verify/assess whether the athlete obtains sufficient running speed on the basis of the directly measured parameters. Of course, it currently would not be the gold standard or method of choice. Thus, results should be generalized carefully. However, they could be used as a valuable supplement to direct measurements in the present. We encourage other researchers to test our velocity prediction models and evaluate the proportion of the obtained variables using different populations to assess to what extent the results can be extrapolated and transferred.

4.4. Limitations

A possible limitation is that participants underwent CPET in different phases of the day (circadian rhythm), month (menstrual cycle for female athletes), or season [43,44]. Moreover, we did not evaluate the training volume of the EA. The participants received dietary and preparation tips, but we cannot be sure that they were rigorously implemented; thus, some BIA results for BC should be analyzed with caution. Some data in $[La^-]_b$ were missed (not all participants decided on the $[La^-]_b$ test because it was an optional variable in the clinic's CPET portfolio) and RF imputation was applied. RF is recognized as the best method for filling data gaps, and our imputation did not cause a significant negative effect on the $[La^-]_b$ data precision. The models still showed high prediction abilities at the building and validation (i.e., out-of-bag error) stages. A comparison of both datasets (first set only with directly measured $[La^-]_b$ and second only with imputed $[La^-]_b$) did not show significant differences between them ($p = 0.4$) [26]. Volunteers individually declared the intensity level on the Borg scale, and the evaluation could differ between participants. The above limitations result from the specifics of the study, which is population-based, and not a controlled trial. In order to minimize their importance, the above-described internal validation was applied, which revealed the high data precision and replicability of the derived equations.

4.5. Future Directions

We advise that future prediction models used to estimate running velocities should be applied in cohorts with comparable characteristics to those from which they were primarily created (similar to other prediction models used in sports diagnostics) [36]. It is especially important in narrow and specified populations, including well-trained EA or cardiology patients [36]. We underline that there is a significant necessity for more accurately adjusted contributing factors and the development of new, advanced machine-learning prediction algorithms using unified TRIPOD recommendations [18]. This will enable the subsequent choice of the appropriate protocol to use in medical diagnostic and training prescriptions, depending on the participant's disease type or fitness level [7]. We recommend assessing our methods in an external environment, such as the 3000 m distance run, to cover all evaluation sites [45,46]. It is worth mentioning that, as stated by Figueiredo et al., the critical speed showed a better predictive value for the 5 km running results regarding a steady run than the peak velocity. Although our research focuses mostly on CPET performed in the clinical settings on the mechanical treadmill, we recommend further studies which will investigate the effect of critical speed compared to peak velocity [47].

5. Conclusions

In summary, (1) we found the strongest predictors of running velocity, (2) we derived novel prediction models for running velocities in accordance with TRIPOD guidelines, and (3) we established their fair validation.

Currently, with the use of a machine-learning approach, we can accurately estimate V_{AT}, V_{RCP}, and V_{max} based only on somatic and exertion variables (the precision and repeatability in the study subgroups were comparable to the test-retest error). VO_2, $[La^-]_b$, VE, and somatic characteristics were the greatest contributing factors. We anticipate that our findings will improve the personalization of training and rehabilitation programs. Models should be primarily applied in disciplines where running is the main form of activity, due to the similar characteristics to those regarding the specificity of the derivation cohort.

Supplementary Materials: The following supporting information can be downloaded at: https://www.mdpi.com/article/10.3390/jcm11226688/s1, Supplementary Material S1: TRIPOD Checklist: Prediction Model Development and Validation.

Author Contributions: Conceptualization, S.W.; methodology, S.W. and M.M.; writing—original draft preparation, P.S.K. and S.W.; software and statistics, I.C. and S.W., writing—review and editing, P.S.K., S.W. and M.M.; supervision, D.Ś. and A.M. All authors have read and agreed to the published version of the manuscript.

Funding: The authors received no funding from an external source.

Institutional Review Board Statement: The study was conducted in accordance with the Declaration of Helsinki, and approved by the Institutional Review of the Bioethical Committee at the Medical University of Warsaw (AKBE/32/2021).

Informed Consent Statement: Not applicable.

Data Availability Statement: The raw data supporting the conclusions of this article will be made available by the authors, without undue reservation.

Conflicts of Interest: The authors declare that the research was conducted in the absence of any commercial or financial relationships that could be construed as a potential conflict of interest.

References

1. Saint-Maurice, P.F.; Graubard, B.I.; Troiano, R.P.; Berrigan, D.; Galuska, D.A.; Fulton, J.E.; Matthews, C.E. Estimated Number of Deaths Prevented Through Increased Physical Activity Among US Adults. *JAMA Intern. Med.* **2022**, *182*, 349–352. [CrossRef]
2. Guazzi, M.; Arena, R.; Halle, M.; Piepoli, M.F.; Myers, J.; Lavie, C.J. 2016 Focused Update: Clinical Recommendations for Cardiopulmonary Exercise Testing Data Assessment in Specific Patient Populations. *Circulation* **2016**, *133*, E694–E711. [CrossRef] [PubMed]
3. Bull, F.C.; Al-Ansari, S.S.; Biddle, S.; Borodulin, K.; Buman, M.P.; Cardon, G.; Carty, C.; Chaput, J.P.; Chastin, S.; Chou, R.G.; et al. World Health Organization 2020 guidelines on physical activity and sedentary behaviour. *Br. J. Sports Med.* **2020**, *54*, 1451–1462. [CrossRef] [PubMed]
4. Poole, D.C.; Rossiter, H.B.; Brooks, G.A.; Gladden, L.B. The anaerobic threshold: 50+years of controversy. *J. Physiol.* **2021**, *599*, 737–767. [CrossRef] [PubMed]

5. Wasserman, K.; McIlroy, M.B. Detecting threshold of anaerobic metabolism in cardiac patients during exercise. *Am. J. Cardiol.* **1964**, *14*, 844–852. [CrossRef]
6. Binder, R.K.; Wonisch, M.; Corra, U.; Cohen-Solal, A.; Vanhees, L.; Saner, H.; Schmid, J.P. Methodological approach to the first and second lactate threshold in incremental cardiopulmonary exercise testing. *Eur. J. Cardiovasc. Prev. Rehabil.* **2008**, *15*, 726–734. [CrossRef]
7. Mann, T.; Lamberts, R.P.; Lambert, M.I. Methods of Prescribing Relative Exercise Intensity: Physiological and Practical Considerations. *Sports Med.* **2013**, *43*, 613–625. [CrossRef]
8. van den Aardweg, J.G.; De Groot, N. Tight coupling between inspiration and expiration after the respiratory compensation point. *Eur. Respir. J.* **2015**, *46*, PA1553. [CrossRef]
9. Takano, N. Respiratory compensation point during incremental exercise as related to hypoxic ventilatory chemosensitivity and lactate increase in man. *Jpn. J. Physiol.* **2000**, *50*, 449–455. [CrossRef]
10. Hill, D.W.; Rowell, A.L. Running velocity at VO_{2max}. *Med. Sci. Sports Exerc.* **1996**, *28*, 114–119. [CrossRef]
11. Wiecha, S.; Price, S.; Cieslinski, I.; Kasiak, P.S.; Tota, L.; Ambrozy, T.; Sliz, D. Transferability of Cardiopulmonary Parameters between Treadmill and Cycle Ergometer Testing in Male Triathletes-Prediction Formulae. *Int. J. Environ. Res. Public Health* **2022**, *19*, 1830. [CrossRef] [PubMed]
12. Tanaka, K.; Matsuura, Y. Marathon performance, anaerobic threshold, and onset of blood lactate accumulation. *J. Appl. Physiol.* **1984**, *57*, 640–643. [CrossRef] [PubMed]
13. Galan-Rioja, M.A.; Gonzalez-Mohino, F.; Poole, D.C.; Gonzalez-Rave, J.M. Relative Proximity of Critical Power and Metabolic/Ventilatory Thresholds: Systematic Review and Meta-Analysis. *Sports Med.* **2020**, *50*, 1771–1783. [CrossRef]
14. Esteve-Lanao, J.; Del Rosso, S.; Larumbe-Zabala, E.; Cardona, C.; Alcocer-Gamboa, A.; Boullosa, D.A. Predicting Recreational Runners' Marathon Performance Time During Their Training Preparation. *J. Strength Cond. Res.* **2021**, *35*, 3218–3224. [CrossRef] [PubMed]
15. Rory, P.B.; Thabtah, F. A machine learning framework for sport result prediction. *Appl. Comput. Inform.* **2019**, *15*, 27–33. [CrossRef]
16. Lanferdini, F.J.; Silva, E.S.; Machado, E.; Fischer, G.; Peyre-Tartaruga, L.A. Physiological Predictors of Maximal Incremental Running Performance. *Front. Physiol.* **2020**, *11*, 979. [CrossRef]
17. Malek, M.H.; Berger, D.E.; Housh, T.J.; Coburn, J.W.; Beck, T.W. Validity of VO_{2max} equations for aerobically trained males and females. *Med. Sci. Sports Exerc.* **2004**, *36*, 1427–1432. [CrossRef]
18. Collins, G.S.; Reitsma, J.B.; Altman, D.G.; Moons, K.G.M.; Grp, T. Transparent Reporting of a Multivariable Prediction Model for Individual Prognosis or Diagnosis (TRIPOD): The TRIPOD Statement. *Eur. Urol.* **2015**, *67*, 1142–1151. [CrossRef]
19. Schabort, E.J.; Killian, S.C.; Gibson, A.S.; Hawley, J.A.; Noakes, T.D. Prediction of triathlon race time from laboratory testing in national triathletes. *Med. Sci. Sports Exerc.* **2000**, *32*, 844–849. [CrossRef]
20. Ghosh, A.K. Anaerobic threshold: Its concept and role in endurance sport. *Malays. J. Med. Sci. MJMS* **2004**, *11*, 24–36.
21. Lach, J.; Wiecha, S.; Sliz, D.; Price, S.; Zaborski, M.; Cieslinski, I.; Postula, M.; Knechtle, B.; Mamcarz, A. HR Max Prediction Based on Age, Body Composition, Fitness Level, Testing Modality and Sex in Physically Active Population. *Front. Physiol.* **2021**, *12*, 695950. [CrossRef] [PubMed]
22. Meignie, A.; Duclos, M.; Carling, C.; Orhant, E.; Provost, P.; Toussaint, J.F.; Antero, J. The Effects of Menstrual Cycle Phase on Elite Athlete Performance: A Critical and Systematic Review. *Front. Physiol.* **2021**, *12*, 654585. [CrossRef] [PubMed]
23. Ross, R.; Blair, S.N.; Arena, R.; Church, T.S.; Despres, J.P.; Franklin, B.A.; Haskell, W.L.; Kaminsky, L.A.; Levine, B.D.; Lavie, C.J.; et al. Importance of Assessing Cardiorespiratory Fitness in Clinical Practice: A Case for Fitness as a Clinical Vital Sign A Scientific Statement From the American Heart Association. *Circulation* **2016**, *134*, E653–E699. [CrossRef]
24. Guazzi, M.; Adams, V.; Conraads, V.; Halle, M.; Mezzani, A.; Vanhees, L.; Arena, R.; Fletcher, G.F.; Forman, D.E.; Kitzman, D.W.; et al. Clinical Recommendations for Cardiopulmonary Exercise Testing Data Assessment in Specific Patient Populations. *Circulation* **2012**, *126*, 2261–2274. [CrossRef]
25. Beaver, W.L.; Wasserman, K.; Whipp, B.J. A new method for detecting anaerobic threshold by gas-exchange. *J. Appl. Physiol.* **1986**, *60*, 2020–2027. [CrossRef] [PubMed]
26. Stekhoven, D.J.; Buhlmann, P. MissForest-non-parametric missing value imputation for mixed-type data. *Bioinformatics* **2012**, *28*, 112–118. [CrossRef]
27. Wright, M.N.; Ziegler, A. Ranger: A Fast Implementation of Random Forests for High Dimensional Data in C plus plus and R. *J. Stat. Softw.* **2017**, *77*, 1–17. [CrossRef]
28. Chen, T.; Guestrin, C. XGBoost: A Scalable Tree Boosting System. In Proceedings of the 22nd ACM SIGKDD International Conference on Knowledge Discovery and Data Mining, San Francisco, CA, USA, 13–17 August 2016; pp. 785–794.
29. Varma, S.; Simon, R. Bias in error estimation when using cross-validation for model selection. *BMC Bioinform.* **2006**, *7*, 91. [CrossRef]
30. Altman, D.G.; Bland, J.M. Measurement in medicine–the analysis of method comparison studies. *J. R. Stat. Soc. Ser. D Stat.* **1983**, *32*, 307–317. [CrossRef]
31. Jette, M.; Sidney, K.; Blumchen, G. Metabolic equivalents (mets) in exercise testing, exercise prescription, and evaluation of functional-capacity. *Clin. Cardiol.* **1990**, *13*, 555–565. [CrossRef]
32. Sjodin, B.; Svedenhag, J. Applied physiology of marathon running. *Sports Med.* **1985**, *2*, 83–99. [CrossRef] [PubMed]
33. Krachler, B.; Savonen, K.; Lakka, T. Obesity is an important source of bias in the assessment of cardiorespiratory fitness. *Am. Heart J.* **2015**, *170*, E7–E8. [CrossRef] [PubMed]

34. Cooper, K.H.; Gey, G.O.; Bottenberg, R.A. Effects of cigarette smoking on endurance performance. *J. Am. Med. Assoc.* **1968**, *203*, 189. [CrossRef]
35. Adami, P.E.; Koutlianos, N.; Baggish, A.; Bermon, S.; Cavarretta, E.; Deligiannis, A.; Furlanello, F.; Kouidi, E.; Marques-Vidal, P.; Niebauer, J.; et al. Cardiovascular effects of doping substances, commonly prescribed medications and ergogenic aids in relation to sports: A position statement of the sport cardiology and exercise nucleus of the European Association of Preventive Cardiology. *Eur. J. Prev. Cardiol.* **2022**, *29*, 559–575. [CrossRef]
36. Petek, B.J.; Tso, J.V.; Churchill, T.W.; Guseh, J.S.; Loomer, G.; DiCarli, M.; Lewis, G.D.; Weiner, R.B.; Kim, J.H.; Wasfy, M.M.; et al. Normative cardiopulmonary exercise data for endurance athletes: The Cardiopulmonary Health and Endurance Exercise Registry (CHEER). *Eur. J. Prev. Cardiol.* **2021**, *29*, 536–544. [CrossRef] [PubMed]
37. Thompson, M.A. Physiological and Biomechanical Mechanisms of Distance Specific Human Running Performance. *Integr. Comp. Biol.* **2017**, *57*, 293–300. [CrossRef] [PubMed]
38. Farrell, P.A.; Wilmore, J.H.; Coyle, E.F.; Billing, J.E.; Costill, D.L. Plasma lactate accumulation and distance running performance. *Med. Sci. Sports Exerc.* **1979**, *11*, 338–344. [CrossRef]
39. Stensvold, D.; Sandbakk, S.B.; Viken, H.; Zisko, N.; Reitlo, L.S.; Nauman, J.; Gaustad, S.E.; Hassel, E.; Moufack, M.; Bronstad, E.; et al. Cardiorespiratory Reference Data in Older Adults: The Generation 100 Study. *Med. Sci. Sports Exerc.* **2017**, *49*, 2206–2215. [CrossRef]
40. Vogel, J.A.; Friedl, K.E. Body-fat assessment in women–special considerations. *Sports Med.* **1992**, *13*, 245–269. [CrossRef]
41. McCormick, A.; Meijen, C.; Marcora, S. Psychological Determinants of Whole-Body Endurance Performance. *Sports Med.* **2015**, *45*, 997–1015. [CrossRef]
42. Ekblom-Bak, E.; Bjorkman, F.; Hellenius, M.L.; Ekblom, B. A new submaximal cycle ergometer test for prediction of VO_{2max}. *Scand. J. Med. Sci. Sports* **2014**, *24*, 319–326. [CrossRef] [PubMed]
43. Petek, B.J.; Groezinger, E.Y.; Pedlar, C.R.; Baggish, A.L. Cardiac effects of detraining in athletes: A narrative review. *Ann. Phys. Rehabil. Med.* **2022**, *65*, 101581. [CrossRef] [PubMed]
44. Price, S.; Wiecha, S.; Cieśliński, I.; Śliż, D.; Kasiak, P.S.; Lach, J.; Gruba, G.; Kowalski, T.; Mamcarz, A. Differences between Treadmill and Cycle Ergometer Cardiopulmonary Exercise Testing Results in Triathletes and Their Association with Body Composition and Body Mass Index. *Int. J. Environ. Res. Public Health* **2022**, *19*, 3557. [CrossRef] [PubMed]
45. Du, Z.; Lu, W.; Lang, D. Comparison between 2000 m and 3000 m time trials to estimate the maximal aerobic speed for collegiate runners. *Front. Physiol.* **2022**, *13*, 1005259. [CrossRef] [PubMed]
46. Casado, A.; Tuimil, J.L.; Iglesias, X.; Fernandez-Del-Olmo, M.; Jimenez-Reyes, P.; Martin-Acero, R.; Rodriguez, F.A. Maximum aerobic speed, maximum oxygen consumption, and running spatiotemporal parameters during an incremental test among middle- and long-distance runners and endurance non-running athletes. *PeerJ* **2022**, *10*, e14035. [CrossRef]
47. Figueiredo, D.H.; Figueiredo, D.H.; Manoel, F.A.; Machado, F.A. Peak Running Velocity or Critical Speed Under Field Conditions: Which Best Predicts 5-km Running Performance in Recreational Runners? *Front. Physiol.* **2021**, *12*, 680790. [CrossRef]

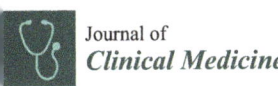

Article

The Effect of Aerobic Exercise and Low-Impact Pilates Workout on the Adaptive Immune System

László Balogh [1,†], Krisztina Szabó [2,†], József Márton Pucsok [1], Ilona Jámbor [2], Ágnes Gyetvai [2], Marianna Mile [1], Lilla Barna [1], Peter Szodoray [3], Tünde Tarr [2], Zoltán Csiki [2] and Gábor Papp [1,2,*]

1. Institute of Sport Sciences, University of Debrecen, H-4032 Debrecen, Hungary
2. Division of Clinical Immunology, Institute of Internal Medicine, Faculty of Medicine, University of Debrecen, H-4032 Debrecen, Hungary
3. Department of Immunology, Oslo University Hospital, Rikshospitalet, 0372 Oslo, Norway
* Correspondence: papp.gabor@med.unideb.hu
† These authors contributed equally to this work.

Abstract: Growing evidence indicates the pronounced effects of physical activity on immune functions, which may largely depend on the type of exercise, intensity, and duration. However, limited information is available regarding the effects of low-impact exercises, especially on the level of adaptive immune system. Our study aimed to investigate and compare the changes in a broad spectrum of lymphocyte subtypes after 14 weeks of aerobic-type total-body-shaping workouts (TBSW) and Pilates workouts (PW) among healthy individuals. We determined the percentages of peripheral natural killer cells and different T and B lymphocyte subtypes with flow cytometry. At the end of the exercise program, significant changes in naïve and memory lymphocyte ratios were observed in TBSW group. Percentages of naïve cytotoxic T (Tc) cells elevated, frequencies of memory Tc and T-helper cell subsets decreased, and distribution of naïve and memory B cells rearranged. Proportions of activated T cells also showed significant changes. Nonetheless, percentages of anti-inflammatory interleukin (IL)-10-producing regulatory type 1 cells and immunosuppressive $CD4^+CD127^{lo/-}CD25^{bright}$ T regulative cells decreased not only after TBSW but also after PW. Although weekly performed aerobic workouts may have a more pronounced impact on the adaptive immune system than low-impact exercises, both still affect immune regulation in healthy individuals.

Keywords: aerobic exercise; Pilates; adaptive immunity; regulatory T cell; interleukin-10

1. Introduction

Studies of the last decades on the role of a sedentary lifestyle in developing chronic diseases have highlighted the critical importance of regular physical activity and exercise in maintaining health and reducing risk of several disorders. Lower physical activity levels correlate with the development of many chronic diseases and unhealthy conditions, such as obesity, hypertension, cardiovascular diseases, type 2 diabetes mellitus, metabolic syndrome and other chronic inflammatory disorders [1,2], while regular physical activity and exercise have beneficial effects in these conditions [3]. Growing evidence also underlines the preventive role of a physically active lifestyle in infections and other immune-mediated diseases by improving immune competency and regulation [4–6]. However, the immunological effects of exercise and its interpretation are still controversial in some cases. It is well known that a single bout of exercise is associated with an initial enhancement in peripheral lymphocyte numbers and effector immune functions, quickly followed by a brief period of immune depression that can last 3–72 h after the exercise bout [7]. The decrease in lymphocyte levels following the exercise has been partially explained by an increase in apoptosis [8]. It was reported that prolonged exercise decreases Th1 cell levels, but not Th2 cells [9], which selectivity could be explained by the increase of stress hormone levels

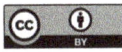

(e.g., cortisol, catecholamines) and myokines in the peripheral blood [10]. Of note, cortisol suppresses the production of interleukin (IL)-12 of antigen-presenting cells (APC), which is a well-known stimulator of Th1 and NK cells [11]. These observations led to the creation of the so-called 'open window' hypothesis, which assumed that the immune system is transiently compromised after acute exercise. However, observations in animal models revealed that T cells are redeployed to the gut, lungs, and bone marrow following exercise [12]. This contributed to the development of a more up-to-date viewpoint in interpreting decreased immune cell frequencies after exercise, which might reflect the even heightened immune-surveillance and immuno-regulatory activities instead of the suppression of the immune system [13,14].

Regarding the long-lasting effects of excessive high-intensity and high-volume physical activity typically practiced by highly competitive athletes, a reduction in proportions of immunocompetent cells with effector functions and decrease of several cytokines, including IL-6, tumor necrosis factor (TNF)-α, interferon (IFN)-γ, IL-1β, IL-2, IL-8 and IL-10, were reported [15,16]. Save for the frequent and arduous bouts of exercise that far exceed recommended physical activity guidelines, there is no doubt that an active lifestyle with regular exercise results in improved immune functions and reduction of systemic inflammatory activity. Former observations reported increased IL-2 production, T-cell proliferation, NK cell cytotoxic activity and enhanced vaccine responses [17,18]. Furthermore, it has also been suggested that repeated bouts of exercise may delay immunosenescence by limiting the accumulation of memory T cell subsets and increasing the frequency of circulating naive T cells [19].

Low-impact workouts, such as Pilates, are beneficial to individuals who cannot perform intensive or moderate-intensity exercises due to chronic health conditions. The purpose of the movements is to increase core strength and muscle balance, improve flexibility and posture; meanwhile, practicing effective breathing exercises during Pilates can encourage relaxation and reduce stress [20]. Although we have a rapidly expanding knowledge on the immunological effects of high- and moderate-intensity workouts, there is still only limited information available about the effects of low-impact exercises, especially on the level of the adaptive immune system. Therefore, our study aimed to examine and compare the changes in a broad spectrum of lymphocyte subtypes after aerobic-type total-body shaping and low-impact Pilates workouts among healthy individuals.

2. Materials and Methods

2.1. Participants

Thirty-two healthy female university students were enrolled in the present study, who participated in general physical education (PE) classes arranged by the Institute of Sport Sciences, University of Debrecen. Each volunteer completed an assessment of dietary and exercise habits questionnaire before and after the exercise program. Participants enrolled in the study were non-smokers. They were instructed to refrain from any physical activity, special diet, and vitamin supplements for at least three months before the investigation. Moreover, exclusion criteria included ongoing viral or bacterial infection, allergic or autoimmune disease, chronic disease treated with continuous drug therapy, cancer, alcohol or drug addiction, pregnancy or breastfeeding, psychiatric illness, insufficient cooperation skills and dietary changes or usage of dietary supplements during the entire study.

Informed written consent was obtained from all subjects enrolled in the investigation. The study was conducted according to the guidelines of the Declaration of Helsinki and approved by the Ethics Committee of the University of Debrecen (protocol number: 4839-2017, date of approval: 26 June 2017) and the Policy Administration Services of Public Health of the Government Office (registration number: 25040-4/2017/EÜIG, date of approval: 4 September 2017).

2.2. Exercise Protocols

Fourteen students (median age; min–max: 21 years; 18–25) voluntarily participated in a Pilates exercise routine, while eighteen students (median age; min–max: 21 years; 20–29) voluntarily participated in an aerobic-type total-body-shaping workout routine. Participants started their assigned activities after completing primary laboratory data collection. Every session was supervised by a physical education professional specialized in the relevant exercise. Each activity included a 90 min long session per week, for 14 weeks in total. Pilates workouts included floor-based exercises on a mat, focusing on controlled, low-intensity movements, stretching, and breathing. Each session consisted of 20 min of warm-up, stretching, 50 min of musculoskeletal exercises, and 20 min of stretching and cool-down exercises. Each session included ten basic exercises, as described by Joseph Pilates [21], including the pelvic curl, the chest lift, the chest lift with rotation, the spine twist supine, single leg stretch, the roll-up, the roll-like-a-ball, leg circles, all fours, and the back extension. Total body stretching exercises included quad stretch, standing hamstring stretch, chest and shoulder stretch, upper back stretch, biceps stretch, shoulder stretch, seated side stretch and triceps stretch.

The aerobic-type total-body-shaping workout routine included three sections: 20 min of warm-up, 50 min of aerobic-type musculoskeletal exercises, and 20 min of stretching and cool-down exercises. The warm-up session incorporated squats, high knees, leg swings, lunges, plank walk-outs, arm circles, standing toe taps, jumping jacks, butt kicks and hip circles exercises. The aerobic exercise routine consisted of the following exercises: 5 min of step-tap, 7 min of tapping, 6 min of side-steps, 6 min of grapevine with side-steps, 7 min of arm-pumps, 6 min of forward-backward walk, 6 min of heel-steps and 7 min of sit-ups. Sessions of week one to four incorporated exercises with light-to-moderate intensity [50 to 70% of maximum heart rate (HRmax)]. From week five, a higher intensity level (75–85% of HRmax) was applied; exercise intensities were monitored via Polar Team Pro System (Polar Electro, Kempele, Finland). Finally, a cool-down and stretching session was incorporated.

2.3. Blood Sampling

We collected blood samples from a peripheral vein of the upper extremity before the first workout and three days after completing the entire 14-week exercise routine at the outpatient clinic of the Division of Clinical Immunology, Institute of Internal Medicine, Faculty of Medicine, University of Debrecen.

2.4. Assessment of Lymphocyte Subpopulations by Flow Cytometry

The distribution of a broad spectrum of lymphocyte subpopulations was determined by flow cytometry. Heparinized peripheral blood samples were obtained from the participants, and the whole blood was used for the experiment. Cells were stained with a combination of different fluorophore-conjugated monoclonal antibodies for 30 min at room temperature. Erythrocytes were haemolysed with a 0.2% solution of formic acid. The cells were then washed twice, fixed with 1% solution of paraformaldehyde, and stored at 4°C until further assessment. Different lymphocyte subsets were analysed and identified by flow cytometry using the antibody panel for cell surface staining described in Table 1. Isotype controls (IgG1 antibody cocktail, from Beckman Coulter Inc., Brea, CA, USA) were used in all procedures. Measurements and data analysis were performed on a Coulter FC500 flow cytometer equipped with Kaluza 1.2a software (both from Beckman Coulter).

Table 1. List of fluorophore-conjugated monoclonal antibodies used in flow cytometry.

Antibodies	Clone	Fluorophore	Company	Lymphocyte Subsets
CD19	J3-119	PE-Cy5	Beckmann Coulter [a]	$CD3^+$ T cells,
CD3/	SK7/	FITC		$CD3^-CD16^+CD56^+$ NK cells,
CD16+CD56	B73.1+MY31	PE	BD Biosciences [b]	$CD19^+$ B cells
CD3/	UCHT1/	RPE-Cy5		$CD3^+CD4^+$ Th cells,
CD4/	MT310/	FITC	Bio-Rad [c]	$CD3^+CD8^+$ Tc cells
CD8	DK25	RPE		
IgD	IA6-2	FITC		$CD19^+IgD^+CD27^-$ naïve,
CD27	1A4CD27	PE	Beckman Coulter	$CD19^+IgD^+CD27^+$ UswM,
CD19	J3-119	PE-Cy5		$CD19^+IgD^-CD27^+$ SwM,
				$CD19^+IgD^-CD27^-$ DN B cells
CD62L	DREG56	PE-Cy5		$CD45RA^+CD62L^+$ naïve,
CD45RA/	ALB11/	FITC	Beckman Coulter	$CD45RA^-CD62L^+$ CM,
CD4	13B8.2	PE		$CD45RA^-CD62L^-$ EM,
CD45RA/	F8-11-13/	FITC	Bio-Rad	$CD45RA^+CD62L^-$ EMRA,
CD8	LT8	RPE		$CD4^+$ Th and $CD8^+$ Tc cells
CD3/	UCHT1/	FITC		$CD3^+CD69^+$ T cells,
HLA-DR	WR18	RPE	BD Biosciences	$CD3^+HLA-DR^+$ T cells
CD69	FN50	PE-Cy5		
CD3	SK7	PerCP	BD Biosciences	$CD3^+6B11^+$ NKT cells
iNkt [d]	6B11	PE		
CD4	RPA-T4	FITC	BD Biosciences	
CD25	B1.49.9	PE-Cy5		$CD4^+CD127^{lo/-}CD25^{bright}$ Treg cells
CD127	R34.34	PE	Beckman Coulter	

FITC, fluorescein isothiocyanate; PE, phycoerythrin; PE-Cy5, phycoerythrin-cyanine dye 5; RPE, R-phycoerythrin; RPE-Cy5, R-phycoerythrin-cyanine dye 5; HLA, human leukocyte antigen; NK, natural killer; UswM, un-switched memory; SwM, switched memory; DN, double-negative; CM, central memory; EM, effector memory; EMRA, $CD45RA^+$ effector memory; [a] Beckmann Coulter Inc., Brea, CA, USA; [b] BD Biosciences, San Diego, CA, USA; [c] Bio-Rad Laboratories, Hercules, CA, USA; [d] 6B11 monoclonal antibody reacts with invariant T-cell receptor (TCR) α-chain Vα24Jα18 expressed by natural killer T (NKT) cells and addressed as invariant NKT (iNKT) marker.

2.5. Determination of T Helper and T Cytotoxic Cells by Immunofluorescent Staining of Intracellular Cytokines

The distribution of Th cell subsets and Tc cells was assessed by flow cytometry. For stimulating cytokine-producing T cells, whole blood was diluted to 1:1 with saline solution and stimulated with phorbol-12-myristate 13-acetate (PMA) (25 ng/mL), ionomycin (1 µg/mL) for five hours at 37 °C in 5% CO_2 milieu. Golgi Stop brefeldin A (10 µg/mL) (all from Sigma Aldrich, St. Louis, MO, USA) was added to the culture for the last 4 h. After cell surface staining, cells were fixed and permeabilized with Intraprep™ permeabilization reagent (Beckman Coulter) according to the manufacturer's instructions. Then, intracellular cytokine staining was carried out with a combination of fluorophore-conjugated monoclonal antibodies. Cells were evaluated on a Coulter FC500 flow cytometer and data were analysed with Kaluza 1.2a software (both from Beckman Coulter). Isotype-matched antibodies were used in all experiments. All antibodies used for this measurement and the determined T cell subpopulations are summarized in Table 2.

Table 2. The combination of monoclonal antibodies used for flow cytometry analysis of Th and Tc cell subsets.

Antibodies	Clone	Fluorophore	Company	T Cell Subsets
CD4	13B8.2	PE-Cy5	Beckmann Coulter [a]	
IL-10	JES3-19F1	PE		IFN-γ$^+$IL-4$^-$ Th1 cells,
IFN-γ/	25723.11/	FITC	BD Biosciences [b]	IFN-γ-IL-4$^+$ Th2 cells,
IL-4 [d]	3010.211	PE		IL-10$^+$ Tr1 cells,
IL-17	41802	PE	R&D Systems [c]	IFN-γ-IL17$^+$ Th17 cells
CD8	4S.B3	FITC	BD Biosciences	
CD8	B9.11	PE-Cy5	Beckmann Coulter	
IFN-γ/	25723.11/	FITC	BD Biosciences	IFN-γ$^+$IL-4$^-$ Tc cells
IL-4	3010.211	PE		

FITC, fluorescein isothiocyanate; PE, phycoerythrin; PE-Cy5, phycoerythrin-cyanine dye 5; IFN, interferon; IL, interleukin, Th, T helper; Tc, cytotoxic T; Tr1, regulatory type-1; [a] Beckmann Coulter Inc., Brea, CA, USA; [b] BD Biosciences, San Diego, CA, USA; [c] R&D Systems, Minneapolis, MN, USA; [d] Anti-human IFN-γ FITC/IL-4 PE two-color direct immunofluorescence reagent.

2.6. Statistical Analysis

Data were statistically analysed with GraphPad Prism 8 software (Graphpad Software, San Diego, CA, USA). Kolmogorov–Smirnov and Shapiro–Wilk normality tests were used to determine the distribution of data. In the case of Gaussian distribution, a two-tail paired t-test was used; otherwise, if the data set differed from the normal distribution, the Wilcoxon test was performed. Repeated measures two-way ANOVA with Bonferroni correction for multiple comparisons was used to assess data in lymphocyte panels analysing different cell subsets. Differences were considered statistically significant at $p < 0.05$.

The sample size was calculated based on data from previous studies with approximate changes in the percentages of different lymphocyte subpopulations during physical activity [22,23]. In order to determine a medium effect size (effect size of Cohen's d = 0.65), we estimated we would need to enroll at least 21 individuals in each groups to obtain 80% power (1-β) and 5% significance level ($\alpha = 0.05$, two-tailed) in a t-test with matched pairs. Sample size calculation was performed using G*Power v3.1.9.7. Software (University of Düsseldorf, Düsseldorf, Germany). Unfortunately, several students did not attend for post-test after the 14-week exercise program and were lost to follow-up (PW, n = 6; TBSW, n = 1).

3. Results

3.1. Data Describing Study Population

The median age of the participants was 21 years (min–max: 18–29 years) at the time of the study. Based on body weight and height data, all participants demonstrated a normal Body Mass Index (22.31 ± 1.75) at enrolment, which remained essentially unchanged until the end of the study (22.43 ± 1.82).

3.2. Quantification of Different Lymphocyte Subpopulations before and after the Exercise Routine

A wide spectrum of peripheral immune-competent cells was analysed with a flow cytometer in healthy volunteers' blood as summarized in Table 1. According to the variety of exercise courses, we divided the subjects into two subgroups, total body shaping and Pilates. Basic lymphocyte subpopulations, were identified according to their cell surface markers. T, B and NK cells were quantified as to their percentages in lymphocytes, while Tc and Th cells were assessed as to their ratio in CD3$^+$ T cells. According to our results, the distribution of basic lymphocyte subsets did not change significantly during both the total-body-shaping and Pilates workout programs (Figure 1a,b).

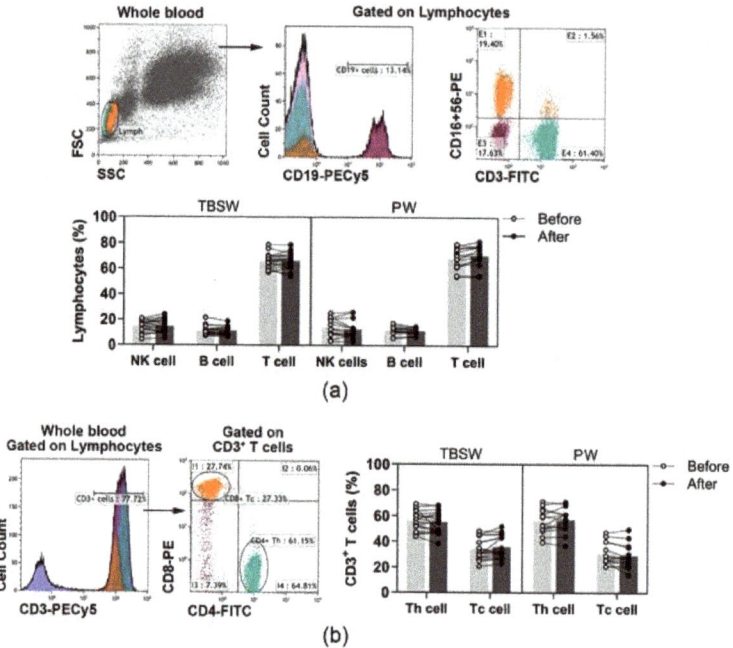

Figure 1. The distribution of peripheral lymphocyte subsets in young women before and after the exercise course. The whole blood of 32 healthy volunteers was stained with labelled monoclonal antibodies, as described previously. According to the exercise courses, the trainees were divided into total-body-shaping workout (TBSW, n = 18) and Pilates workout (PW, n = 14) subgroups. (**a**) Representative dot plots and a histogram show the gating strategy of $CD3^-CD16^+CD56^+$ NK, $CD19^+$ B, and $CD3^+CD16^-CD56^-$ T cell populations. The bar chart shows the percentages of NK, B, and T cells. (**b**) The representative histogram shows the gating of $CD3^+$ cells, and the dot plots demonstrate the distribution of $CD4^+$ Th and $CD8^+$ Tc cells. The bar chart indicates the frequencies of Th and Tc cells. Data analysis was performed with repeated measures two-way ANOVA followed by Bonferroni multiple comparisons test. Each data point represents an individual subject, while bars show the mean values.

In addition, naïve and memory lymphocyte subpopulations were distinguished within B, Th and Tc cells. B cell subsets were quantified as to their percentages in $CD19^+$ lymphocytes, and Th subpopulations were determined as their ratio in the $CD4^+$ cells. In contrast, Tc cell subsets were quantified as to their frequencies in $CD8^+$ cells. Regarding naïve and memory B cell subsets, only the percentages of naïve B cells were significantly elevated both in the total-body-shaping (63.179 ± 11.048 vs. 64.537 ± 11.173; $p = 0.0297$) and in the Pilates subgroup (59.656 ± 13.871 vs. 60.996 ± 13.008; $p = 0.0417$) by the end of the exercise course (Figure 2a). In the case of naïve and memory Th cells, we observed that the proportions of central memory (CM) Th cells differed significantly (29.151 ± 7.010 vs. 27.468 ± 6.716; $p = 0.0363$) exclusively in the total-body-shaping subgroup, while the other cell subsets within the group, as well as in Pilates, did not change significantly (Figure 2b). There was no significant difference in naïve and memory Tc cell subsets in Pilates group. A statistically significant increase was found in the percentages of naïve Tc (38.544 ± 11.453 vs. 40.777 ± 11.949; $p = 0.0428$), and a significant decrease was detected in the ratio of $CD45RA^+$ effector memory (EMRA) Tc (17.779 ± 9.124 vs. 15.418 ± 7.892; $p = 0.0284$) cells in the total-body-shaping workout group (Figure 2c).

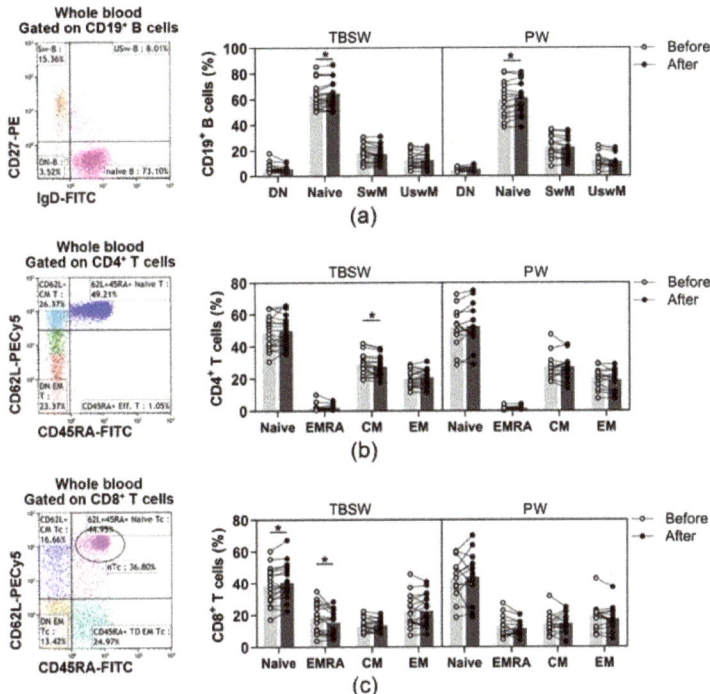

Figure 2. Assessment of naïve and memory lymphocyte subsets in young women after a 14-week workout program. The whole blood of 32 healthy individuals was stained with fluorochrome-labeled monoclonal antibodies, as described previously. According to the exercise courses, the trainees were divided into total-body-shaping workout (TBSW, n = 18) and Pilates workout (PW, n = 14) subgroups. (**a**) Representative dot plot indicates the distribution of IgD$^+$CD27$^-$ naïve, IgD$^-$CD27$^-$ double negative (DN), IgD$^-$CD27$^+$ switched, and IgD$^+$CD27$^+$ un-switched memory B cells. The bar chart shows the percentages of B cell subsets. (**b**) Representative dot plot demonstrates the distribution of CD45RA$^+$CD62L$^+$ naïve, CD45RA$^-$CD62L$^-$ effector memory (EM), CD45RA$^-$CD62L$^+$ central (CM) and CD45RA$^+$CD62L$^-$ effector memory (EMRA) Th cells. The bar chart indicates the frequencies of Th cell subpopulations. (**c**) Representative dot plot demonstrates the distribution of CD45RA$^+$CD62L$^+$ naïve, CD45RA$^-$CD62L$^-$ EM, CD45RA$^-$CD62L$^+$ CM and CD45RA$^+$CD62L$^-$ EMRA Tc cells. The bar chart indicates the frequencies of Tc cell subpopulations. Repeated measures two-way ANOVA with Bonferroni correction for multiple comparisons was used. Each data point represents an individual subject, while bars show the mean values. Statistically significant differences are indicated by * $p < 0.05$.

3.3. Determination of Cells with a Regulatory Function in the Innate and Adaptive Immune Response after a 14-Week Exercise Routine

In the peripheral blood of young women, CD69$^+$ early activated T cells and HLA-DR$^+$ late-activated T cells were determined. Their distribution was quantified as to their percentages in the lymphocyte population. When we analysed the ratio of activated T cells, significant differences were only detected in the total-body-shaping subgroup. The percentages of late-activated T cells were significantly decreased (7.804 ± 4.110 vs. 6.750 ± 3.392; $p = 0.0031$) compared to baseline values (Figure 3a).

Additionally, CD4$^+$CD127$^{lo/-}$CD25^{bright} Treg cells and CD3$^+$6B11$^+$ NKT cells were also identified before and after the exercise program. Their division was assessed as to their frequencies in CD4$^+$ cells, and in CD3$^+$ cells, respectively. When we analysed the distribution of Treg cells, we found that it was significantly decreased in the total-body-shaping (7.554 ± 1.723 vs. 7.082 ± 1.415; $p = 0.0032$) as well as in the Pilates (7.266 ± 1.771

vs. 8.861 ± 1.642; p = 0.0142) subgroups (Figure 3b). The ratio of NKT cells did not change significantly by the end of the exercise course (Figure 3c).

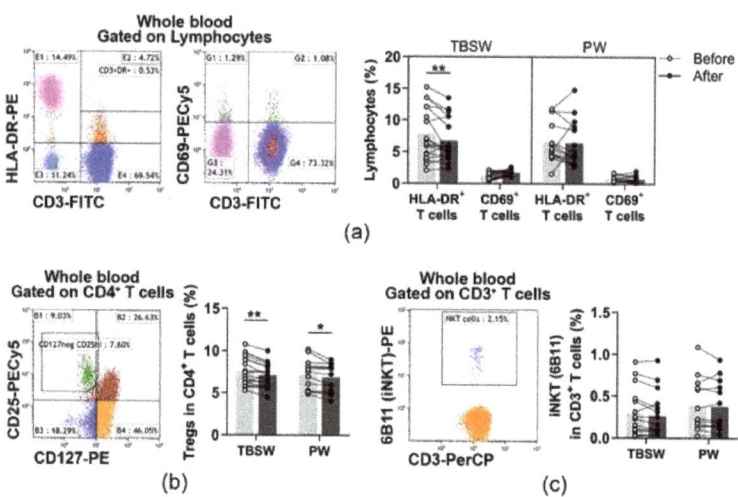

Figure 3. Measurement of lymphocytes with a regulatory function in young women after a 14-week exercise program. The whole blood of 32 healthy volunteers was stained with labelled monoclonal antibodies, as described previously. According to the exercise courses, the trainees were divided into total-body-shaping workout (TBSW, n = 18) and Pilates workout (PW, n = 14) subgroups. (**a**) Representative dot plots demonstrate the identification of CD3$^+$HLA-DR$^+$ late-activated and CD3$^+$CD69$^+$ early activated T cells. The bar chart indicates the frequencies of activated T cells. (**b**) Representative dot plot indicates the identification of CD4$^+$CD25^{bright}CD127$^{lo/-}$ Treg cells within CD4$^+$ T cells. The bar chart indicates the ratio of Treg cells. (**c**) Representative dot plot shows the determination, and the bar chart indicates the frequencies of CD3$^+$6B11$^+$ NKT cells. 6B11 is referred to as the invariant NKT (iNKT) marker. Repeated measures two-way ANOVA with Bonferroni correction for multiple comparisons was used for activated T cells, and paired T-test or Wilcoxon test was used for the statistical analysis of NKT and Treg cells. Each data point represents an individual subject, while bars show the mean values. Statistically significant differences are indicated by * $p < 0.05$; ** $p < 0.01$.

3.4. Assessment of Peripheral T Helper Subsets and Cytotoxic T Cells before and after the 14-Week Training

The identified phenotypes of different CD4$^+$ T cell subpopulations and CD8$^+$ cytotoxic T cells are summarized in Table 2. All cell subsets were quantified as to their percentage in the CD4$^+$ or CD8$^+$ lymphocyte population. We found no significant differences in the ratio of peripheral blood Th1, Th2, Th17, and Tc cells in both exercise groups (Figure 4a–c). However, the ratio of Tr1 cells was significantly diminished in the total-body-shaping (0.499 ± 0.256 vs. 0.335 ± 0.115; p = 0.0420) as well as in the Pilates groups (0.426 ± 0.200 vs. 0.319 ± 0.120; p = 0.0362) compared to baseline values (Figure 4d).

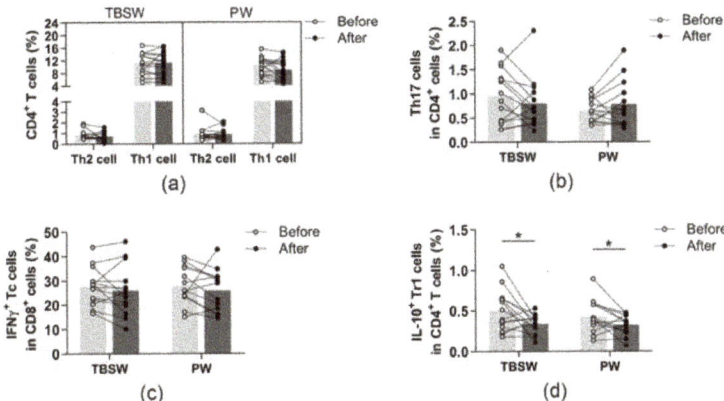

Figure 4. Determination of T helper and T cytotoxic cells with intracellular cytokine analysis in young women before and after the exercise program. The whole blood of 32 healthy participants was stimulated for 5h and stained with monoclonal antibodies with the intracellular staining method described previously. According to the exercise courses, the trainees were divided into total-body-shaping workout (TBSW, n = 14) and Pilates workout (PW, n = 14) subgroups. (**a**) Frequencies of IFN-γ$^+$ Th1 and IL-4$^+$ Th2 cells. (**b**) Percentages of IL-17$^+$ Th17 cells. (**c**) The ratio of IFN-γ-producing Tc cells. (**d**) Proportions of IL-10-producing type-1 regulatory (Tr1) cells. A paired T-test was used. Each data point represents an individual subject, while bars show the mean values. Statistically significant differences are indicated by * $p < 0.05$.

4. Discussion

A properly functioning immune system is essential for the host's continuing survival by maintaining a well-balanced defence against foreign organisms and protection from endogenous altered or virally transformed cells. However, besides the genetic and endogenous background, numerous lifestyle and environmental factors fundamentally affect immune functions. Among these factors, physical activity becomes the focus of scientific interest due to its multifaceted effects on immunity. Previous studies concerned with the effects of exercise on the immune system have focused mainly on the impact of acute bouts of exercise and the chronic influences of workout programs, especially in athletes. On the contrary, the immunological effects of low-impact exercise, such as Pilates, are definitely not in the focus of immunological research. Therefore, only limited results are available regarding the impacts of Pilates on innate immunity [22], and to our best knowledge, changes in the elements of the adaptive immune system have not been previously investigated.

Therefore, in our present study, we focused on the effects of Pilates workouts and aerobic-type total-body-shaping exercises performed for 90 min once a week on a broad spectrum of immune competent cells of the adaptive immune system. Importantly, acute changes induced by intense physical exercise may last at least 24 h, and even moderate acute exercise induces significant immune alterations for several hours [10]. Therefore, we carried out the laboratory measurements 3 days after the last workout to exclude the distorting effects of early immunological changes (e.g., postexercise lymphocytopenia).

Our knowledge is still limited regarding the long-term effects of physical exercise on B cells. Previously, studies on brief or prolonged exercise reported that the number of total B cells follows the aforementioned changes of the total lymphocyte population. After a short increase during and immediately after exercise, it falls below pre-exercise levels and then returns to basal level within 24 h [24]. Regarding long-term changes in B-cell-mediated humoral immune responses, previous studies demonstrated an elevated salivary IgA secretion after a 3-month Pilates exercise program or a 6-month-long active daily walking exercise training in elderly participants [25,26]. After regularly performed aerobic training in the elderly, increased plasma levels of IgA, IgG and IgM were reported [27], indicating the promotion of humoral immunity. Our study revealed that total-body-shaping and Pilates workouts increased the proportions of naïve B cells in young individuals. An increase in naïve B cell proportion demonstrates a beneficial rearrangement, even a rejuvenation of the available B cell population, since naïve B cells can respond to novel antigens, while on the contrary, memory B cells exhibit more restricted B cell antigen receptors [28]. Moreover, it was suggested that the ratios of immature cells and naïve B cells, which have yet to encounter antigens, were increased in peripheral blood because of their migration to the secondary lymphoid organs where antigenic screening occurs [29]. On the other hand, memory B cells either circulate in the peripheral blood or home to niches outside of the circulation, including the bone marrow, the spleen and tonsils, or several of them could be present as tissue-based memory B cells. Tracking of memory subsets revealed that switched-memory B cells mainly resided in the spleen and tonsils instead of peripheral blood at a steady state [30]. It could be assumed that the maintenance of this steady state may be further enhanced as a result of moderate training, and increased naïve B cell ratio ensures replenishment.

In the case of naïve and memory T cell distribution, we observed rearrangements similar to those we determined in B subtypes. We revealed a significant increase in the percentages of naïve Tc. Simultaneously, the ratios of effector memory Tc and central memory Th cells showed a significant decrease in the total-body-shaping group at the end of the exercise intervention study period. Although the exact mechanisms behind the changes in the distribution of naïve and memory T lymphocytes have not been elucidated yet, a possible theory may answer some questions. It is assumed that the homeostatic number of peripheral T cell repertoire is tightly regulated by a feedback mechanism. Exercise may decrease the accumulation of memory cells through their mobilization into the circulation and subsequent extravasation to peripheral tissues (e.g., mucosal surfaces of the lungs and gut or spleen and bone marrow) where they are exposed to H_2O_2 induced apoptosis, or where they probably encounter pathogens and carry out effector functions. Therefore, in order to maintain the proper amount of the T cell pool, a feedback mechanism increases thymic output and the accumulation of antigen-inexperienced naïve T cells at the periphery [13,31]. As the rate of thymic atrophy and loss of thymic output accelerates after puberty, the decrease in the naïve T cell pool, which is more pronounced in the $CD8^+$ T cell population, compromises the recognition and combat against new pathogens [32]. The exercise-induced mobilization of naïve T cells into the circulation could ensure the maintenance of the immune response to novel pathogens [13]. Consequently, regular physical activity and exercise may be a reasonable way to delay the aging-associated alterations of the immune system and potentially increase responses to vaccinations, even in younger individuals after puberty [33]. However, in contrast to the aerobic exercise routine, we observed no changes in T cell subpopulations after the Pilates workout program. These changes suggest that aerobic-type workout sessions may be an effective intervention for the rearrangement of these cell proportions in contrast to Pilates.

When we analysed the ratio of activated T cells, significant differences were only detected in the total-body-shaping subgroup, too. The percentages of late-activated HLA-DR^+CD3^+ T cells were significantly decreased. However, recent studies have suggested that HLA-DR^+CD8^+ T cells represent natural regulatory $CD8^+$ T cells, and most frequently express a high level of CD28 and low level of CD45RA [34]; therefore, to get a better view of the changes in late-activated T cell proportions, further studies are needed with a special emphasis on the changes in natural regulatory HLA-DR^+CD8^+ T cells, as well. We also evaluated the changes in the regulative arm of the adaptive immune system. A network of regulatory T (Treg) cells is primarily responsible for limiting immune reactions by suppressing immune activation and effector functions. There are two main types of Tregs: namely, natural $CD4^+CD25^{bright}FoxP3^+$ Treg cells and induced Treg cells (iTreg), such as interleukin (IL)-10-producing T regulatory type 1 (Tr1) cells [35]. Based on previous studies, acute high-intensity exercise may significantly increase Treg cell number [23], while regular workouts of moderate intensity may lead to decreased Treg proportions in the elderly [31]. In the present study, we revealed that both aerobic-type total-body-shaping exercises and low-impact Pilates workouts decrease $CD4^+CD127^{lo/-}CD25^{bright}$ Treg cell ratios. Additionally, we found a similar reduction in the proportions of immunosuppressive IL-10-producing Tr1 cells after both workout series. The lower ratio of Treg cells could be explained by the reference to a study with murine asthma model. Their results showed that aerobic training increased $Foxp3^+$ Treg distribution in mediastinal lymph nodes and lungs; moreover, a heightened suppression capacity of Treg cells was observed compared to the sedentary control group. These results indicate that regular exercise may force the redistribution of Treg cells from the blood to the site of possible antigen exposure [36]. These novel observations shed light on the important effects of weekly performed physical exercises, including Pilates workouts, on immune regulation. Our present findings on the effects on regulatory T cell proportions might reveal an important consequence of regular physical activity in healthy individuals.

5. Conclusions

Our findings suggest that aerobic exercise-induced changes in the distribution of specific naïve and memory B and T cell subsets, as well as in the proportions of activated T and regulatory T subsets, may indicate a retuned immune regulation and a presumably enhanced responsiveness of the immune system. On the other hand, as a low-impact workout, Pilates may influence the proportions of regulative T cells only. Nevertheless, based on the significant effects on immune regulation, Pilates exercise may also be beneficial in maintaining appropriate adaptive immune functions. However, taking into consideration that numerous complex factors, such as hormonal status, environmental factors, etc., may affect the immune system and might influence the effects of exercise, we have to mention the lack of non-exercise control group as one of the limitations of the study. Although our results showed significant changes in B and T cell subpopulations even with a relative small sample size, more controlled investigations are needed for the deeper understanding of exercise-induced changes in the distribution of naïve and memory lymphocytes, as well as in the regulatory functions that may have an important role in preventing infections and optimizing vaccination.

Author Contributions: Conceptualization, L.B. (László Balogh) and G.P.; methodology, K.S., I.J. and L.B. (Lilla Barna); software, K.S.; investigation, K.S., J.M.P. and M.M.; resources, G.P. and L.B. (László Balogh); data curation, K.S. and M.M.; writing—original draft preparation, K.S. and G.P.; writing—review and editing, L.B. (László Balogh), P.S., T.T. and Z.C.; visualization, K.S. and Á.G.; supervision, G.P. and L.B. (László Balogh); funding acquisition, G.P., L.B. (László Balogh) and Z.C. All authors have read and agreed to the published version of the manuscript.

Funding: The research was supported by the TKP2021-EGA-20 project, which was implemented with the support provided from the National Research, Development and Innovation Fund of Hungary, financed under the TKP2021-EGA funding scheme. The work of GP was supported by the János Bolyai Research Scholarship of the Hungarian Academy of Sciences and the ÚNKP-20-5 New National Excellence Program of the Ministry for Innovation and Technology.

Institutional Review Board Statement: The study was conducted according to the guidelines of the Declaration of Helsinki and approved by the Ethics Committee of the University of Debrecen (protocol number: 4839-2017, date of approval: 26 June 2017) and the Policy Administration Services of Public Health of the Government Office (registration number: 25040-4/2017/EÜIG, date of approval: 4 September 2017).

Informed Consent Statement: Informed written consent was obtained from all subjects enrolled in the investigation.

Data Availability Statement: The data presented in this study are available in the article's Figures and Tables.

Acknowledgments: The authors would like to thank all volunteers who participated in the study.

Conflicts of Interest: The authors declare that there is no conflict of interest regarding the publication of this paper.

References

1. Booth, F.W.; Roberts, C.K.; Thyfault, J.P.; Ruegsegger, G.N.; Toedebusch, R.G. Role of Inactivity in Chronic Diseases: Evolutionary Insight and Pathophysiological Mechanisms. *Physiol. Rev.* **2017**, *97*, 1351–1402. [CrossRef] [PubMed]
2. Laaksonen, D.E.; Lakka, H.M.; Salonen, J.T.; Niskanen, L.K.; Rauramaa, R.; Lakka, T.A. Low levels of leisure-time physical activity and cardiorespiratory fitness predict development of the metabolic syndrome. *Diabetes Care* **2002**, *25*, 1612–1618. [CrossRef] [PubMed]
3. Warburton, D.E.R.; Bredin, S.S.D. Health benefits of physical activity: A systematic review of current systematic reviews. *Curr. Opin. Cardiol.* **2017**, *32*, 541–556. [CrossRef]
4. Sharif, K.; Watad, A.; Bragazzi, N.L.; Lichtbroun, M.; Amital, H.; Shoenfeld, Y. Physical activity and autoimmune diseases: Get moving and manage the disease. *Autoimmun. Rev.* **2018**, *17*, 53–72. [CrossRef] [PubMed]
5. Pape, K.; Ryttergaard, L.; Rotevatn, T.A.; Nielsen, B.J.; Torp-Pedersen, C.; Overgaard, C.; Boggild, H. Leisure-Time Physical Activity and the Risk of Suspected Bacterial Infections. *Med. Sci. Sports Exerc.* **2016**, *48*, 1737–1744. [CrossRef] [PubMed]
6. Kostka, T.; Berthouze, S.E.; Lacour, J.; Bonnefoy, M. The symptomatology of upper respiratory tract infections and exercise in elderly people. *Med. Sci. Sports Exerc.* **2000**, *32*, 46–51. [CrossRef]
7. McCarthy, D.A.; Dale, M.M. The leucocytosis of exercise. A review and model. *Sports Med.* **1988**, *6*, 333–363. [CrossRef]
8. Navalta, J.W.; Sedlock, D.A.; Park, K.S. Effect of exercise intensity on exercise-induced lymphocyte apoptosis. *Int. J. Sports Med.* **2007**, *28*, 539–542. [CrossRef]
9. Steensberg, A.; Toft, A.D.; Bruunsgaard, H.; Sandmand, M.; Halkjaer-Kristensen, J.; Pedersen, B.K. Strenuous exercise decreases the percentage of type 1 T cells in the circulation. *J. Appl. Physiol.* **2001**, *91*, 1708–1712. [CrossRef]
10. Pedersen, B.K.; Hoffman-Goetz, L. Exercise and the immune system: Regulation, integration, and adaptation. *Physiol. Rev.* **2000**, *80*, 1055–1081. [CrossRef]
11. Elenkov, I.J.; Chrousos, G.P. Stress hormones, Th1/Th2 patterns, pro/anti-inflammatory cytokines, and susceptibility to disease. *Trends Endocrinol. Metab.* **1999**, *10*, 359–368. [CrossRef]
12. Kruger, K.; Lechtermann, A.; Fobker, M.; Volker, K.; Mooren, F.C. Exercise-induced redistribution of T lymphocytes is regulated by adrenergic mechanisms. *Brain Behav. Immun.* **2008**, *22*, 324–338. [CrossRef] [PubMed]
13. Campbell, J.P.; Turner, J.E. Debunking the Myth of Exercise-Induced Immune Suppression: Redefining the Impact of Exercise on Immunological Health Across the Lifespan. *Front. Immunol.* **2018**, *9*, 648. [CrossRef]
14. Campbell, J.P.; Turner, J.E. There is limited existing evidence to support the common assumption that strenuous endurance exercise bouts impair immune competency. *Expert Rev. Clin. Immunol.* **2019**, *15*, 105–109. [CrossRef] [PubMed]
15. Nieman, D.C.; Wentz, L.M. The compelling link between physical activity and the body's defense system. *J. Sport Health Sci.* **2019**, *8*, 201–217. [CrossRef]
16. Simpson, R.J.; Campbell, J.P.; Gleeson, M.; Krüger, K.; Nieman, D.C.; Pyne, D.B.; Turner, J.E.; Walsh, N.P. Can exercise affect immune function to increase susceptibility to infection? *Exerc. Immunol. Rev.* **2020**, *26*, 8–22.
17. Simpson, R.J.; Kunz, H.; Agha, N.; Graff, R. Exercise and the Regulation of Immune Functions. *Prog. Mol. Biol. Transl. Sci.* **2015**, *135*, 355–380. [CrossRef]
18. Woods, J.A.; Keylock, K.T.; Lowder, T.; Vieira, V.J.; Zelkovich, W.; Dumich, S.; Colantuano, K.; Lyons, K.; Leifheit, K.; Cook, M.; et al. Cardiovascular exercise training extends influenza vaccine seroprotection in sedentary older adults: The immune function intervention trial. *J. Am. Geriatr. Soc.* **2009**, *57*, 2183–2191. [CrossRef]
19. Simpson, R.J. Aging, persistent viral infections, and immunosenescence: Can exercise "make space"? *Exerc. Sport Sci. Rev.* **2011**, *39*, 23–33. [CrossRef]
20. Hagner-Derengowska, M.; Kałużny, K.; Kochański, B.; Hagner, W.; Borkowska, A.; Czamara, A.; Budzyński, J. Effects of Nordic Walking and Pilates exercise programs on blood glucose and lipid profile in overweight and obese postmenopausal women in an experimental, nonrandomized, open-label, prospective controlled trial. *Menopause* **2015**, *22*, 1215–1223. [CrossRef]
21. Pilates, J.H.; Miller, W.J. *Pilates' Return to Life through Contrology*; Presentation Dynamics Inc.: Incline Village, NV, USA, 1998.
22. Gronesova, P.; Cholujova, D.; Kozic, K.; Korbuly, M.; Vlcek, M.; Penesova, A.; Imrich, R.; Sedlak, J.; Hunakova, L. Effects of short-term Pilates exercise on selected blood parameters. *Gen. Physiol. Biophys.* **2018**, *37*, 443–451. [CrossRef] [PubMed]
23. Wilson, L.D.; Zaldivar, F.P.; Schwindt, C.D.; Wang-Rodriguez, J.; Cooper, D.M. Circulating T-regulatory cells, exercise and the elite adolescent swimmer. *Pediatr. Exerc. Sci.* **2009**, *21*, 305–317. [CrossRef]
24. Hulmi, J.J.; Myllymäki, T.; Tenhumäki, M.; Mutanen, N.; Puurtinen, R.; Paulsen, G.; Mero, A.A. Effects of resistance exercise and protein ingestion on blood leukocytes and platelets in young and older men. *Eur. J. Appl. Physiol.* **2010**, *109*, 343–353. [CrossRef] [PubMed]
25. Hwang, Y.; Park, J.; Lim, K. Effects of Pilates Exercise on Salivary Secretory Immunoglobulin A Levels in Older Women. *J. Aging Phys. Act.* **2016**, *24*, 399–406. [CrossRef] [PubMed]
26. Sellami, M.; Bragazzi, N.L.; Aboghaba, B.; Elrayess, M.A. The Impact of Acute and Chronic Exercise on Immunoglobulins and Cytokines in Elderly: Insights From a Critical Review of the Literature. *Front. Immunol.* **2021**, *12*, 631873. [CrossRef] [PubMed]
27. Martins, R.A.; Cunha, M.R.; Neves, A.P.; Martins, M.; Teixeira-Veríssimo, M.; Teixeira, A.M. Effects of aerobic conditioning on salivary IgA and plasma IgA, IgG and IgM in older men and women. *Int. J. Sports Med.* **2009**, *30*, 906–912. [CrossRef] [PubMed]
28. Kogut, I.; Scholz, J.L.; Cancro, M.P.; Cambier, J.C. B cell maintenance and function in aging. *Semin. Immunol.* **2012**, *24*, 342–349. [CrossRef] [PubMed]

29. Turner, J.E.; Spielmann, G.; Wadley, A.J.; Aldred, S.; Simpson, R.J.; Campbell, J.P. Exercise-induced B cell mobilisation: Preliminary evidence for an influx of immature cells into the bloodstream. *Physiol. Behav.* **2016**, *164*, 376–382. [CrossRef]
30. Palm, A.E.; Henry, C. Remembrance of Things Past: Long-Term B Cell Memory after Infection and Vaccination. *Front. Immunol.* **2019**, *10*, 1787. [CrossRef]
31. Papp, G.; Szabó, K.; Jámbor, I.; Mile, M.; Berki, A.R.; Arany, A.C.; Makra, G.; Szodoray, P.; Csiki, Z.; Balogh, L. Regular Exercise May Restore Certain Age-Related Alterations of Adaptive Immunity and Rebalance Immune Regulation. *Front. Immunol.* **2021**, *12*, 639308. [CrossRef]
32. Mittelbrunn, M.; Kroemer, G. Hallmarks of T cell aging. *Nat. Immunol.* **2021**, *22*, 687–698. [CrossRef] [PubMed]
33. Mathot, E.; Liberman, K.; Dinh, H.C.; Njemini, R.; Bautmans, I. Systematic review on the effects of physical exercise on cellular immunosenescence-related markers—An update. *Exp. Gerontol.* **2021**, *149*, 111318. [CrossRef] [PubMed]
34. Arruvito, L.; Payaslián, F.; Baz, P.; Podhorzer, A.; Billordo, A.; Pandolfi, J.; Semeniuk, G.; Arribalzaga, E.; Fainboim, L. Identification and clinical relevance of naturally occurring human CD8 + HLA-DR+ regulatory T cells. *J. Immunol.* **2014**, *193*, 4469–4476. [CrossRef] [PubMed]
35. Papp, G.; Boros, P.; Nakken, B.; Szodoray, P.; Zeher, M. Regulatory immune cells and functions in autoimmunity and transplantation immunology. *Autoimmun. Rev.* **2017**, *16*, 435–444. [CrossRef]
36. Lowder, T.; Dugger, K.; Deshane, J.; Estell, K.; Schwiebert, L.M. Repeated bouts of aerobic exercise enhance regulatory T cell responses in a murine asthma model. *Brain Behav. Immun.* **2010**, *24*, 153–159. [CrossRef]

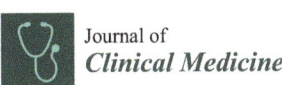

Article

Associations of Circulating Irisin and Fibroblast Growth Factor-21 Levels with Measures of Energy Homeostasis in Highly Trained Adolescent Rhythmic Gymnasts

Jaak Jürimäe [1,*], Liina Remmel [1], Anna-Liisa Tamm [2], Priit Purge [1], Katre Maasalu [3] and Vallo Tillmann [3]

1. Institute of Sport Sciences and Physiotherapy, Faculty of Medicine, University of Tartu, 51008 Tartu, Estonia
2. Tartu Health Care College, 50411 Tartu, Estonia
3. Institute of Clinical Medicine, Faculty of Medicine, University of Tartu, 50406 Tartu, Estonia
* Correspondence: jaak.jurimae@ut.ee

Abstract: The aim of this investigation was to determine the associations of serum irisin and fibroblast growth factor-21 (FGF-21) with the measures of energy homeostasis, training stress and other energy homeostasis hormones in highly trained adolescent rhythmic gymnasts (RG). Thirty-three RG and 20 untrained controls (UC) aged 14–18 years participated in this study. Body composition, resting energy expenditure (REE), peak oxygen consumption, and different energy homeostasis hormones in serum, including irisin, FGF-21, leptin, and resistin, were measured. Irisin and FGF-21 were not significantly different ($p > 0.05$) between RG and UC groups. In RG, serum irisin was positively associated with REE ($r = 0.40$; $p = 0.021$) and leptin ($r = 0.60$; $p = 0.013$), while serum FGF-21 was related to body fat mass ($r = 0.46$; $p = 0.007$) and leptin ($r = 0.45$; $p = 0.009$). Irisin was related to FGF-21, independent of age, body fat, and lean masses ($r = 0.36$; $p = 0.049$) in RG. In conclusion, serum irisin concentration was associated with energy expenditure and serum FGF-21 level with energy availability measures in lean adolescent athletes, while no relationships of irisin and FGF-21 with energy status measures were observed in lean nonathletic adolescents.

Keywords: rhythmic gymnasts; irisin; fibroblast growth factor-21; energy homeostasis; training stress

Citation: Jürimäe, J.; Remmel, L.; Tamm, A.-L.; Purge, P.; Maasalu, K.; Tillmann, V. Associations of Circulating Irisin and Fibroblast Growth Factor-21 Levels with Measures of Energy Homeostasis in Highly Trained Adolescent Rhythmic Gymnasts. *J. Clin. Med.* **2022**, *11*, 7450. https://doi.org/10.3390/jcm11247450

Academic Editor: David Rodríguez-Sanz

Received: 15 November 2022
Accepted: 13 December 2022
Published: 15 December 2022

Publisher's Note: MDPI stays neutral with regard to jurisdictional claims in published maps and institutional affiliations.

Copyright: © 2022 by the authors. Licensee MDPI, Basel, Switzerland. This article is an open access article distributed under the terms and conditions of the Creative Commons Attribution (CC BY) license (https://creativecommons.org/licenses/by/4.0/).

1. Introduction

The regulation of energy homeostasis and high training stress is dependent on several peripheral factors that communicate the status of body energy stores to the brain [1]. These peripheral factors are also synthesized from adipose, muscle, and bone tissues, which may act as endocrine organs [2]. For example, it has been found that specific adipose-derived factors, including circulating leptin and adiponectin concentrations, can be sensitive to changes in training volume and could be used to characterize physical stress conditions in athletes [1]. In elite female rowers, Kurgan et al. [3] investigated such peripheral markers as tumour necrosis factor-alpha (TNF-α), interleukin-6 (IL-6), insulin-like growth factor-1 (IGF-1), and leptin to assess variations in energy homeostasis and training stress over a training year. It appeared that fluctuations in training load (high vs. low) were accompanied by parallel changes in TNF-α and IL-6, while IGF-1 and leptin remained relatively stable over a training season in this population of young female athletes with suitable energy availability [3]. Similarly, adipokines such as circulating leptin, adiponectin, resistin, and visfatin concentrations have been used to characterize energy homeostasis in highly trained adolescent rhythmic gymnasts (RG), who begin to exercise at an early age and often adopt negative energy balance to retain lean physique [4–6]. Adiponectin was positively associated with weekly training volume in elite young RG participating in World Championships [7], while leptin levels in highly trained adolescent RG can be as low as in anorectic individuals and chronic athletic activity in the presence of prolonged high energy expenditure state decreases leptin concentrations in growing and maturing RG athletes [8].

The importance of tissue crosstalk in energy homeostasis has been highlighted by studies examining the role of different muscle-derived factors in regulating several adipose tissue adaptations to energy metabolism [2,9,10].

Recently, various myokines have been found to mediate training-induced energy and metabolic processes [9,11], besides the most investigated and well-known myokine-IL-6 [1,12]. These myokines include myostatin [13], follistatin [14], irisin [15], and fibroblast growth factor-21 (FGF-21) [16], which have emerged as potential mediators of training-induced energy metabolism. While myostatin is a negative regulator of muscle mass [2], follistatin is a myostatin-binding peptide that promotes skeletal muscle development and exerts metabolic benefits by improving glucose metabolism [14]. One of the more recently identified myokine, irisin, is primarily secreted by muscle tissue and released into circulation during exercise, resulting in increased energy expenditure and improved glucose metabolism [17]. Irisin levels have been reported to be positively associated with body fat mass (FM) as a surrogate measure of energy availability [18]. However, no differences in serum irisin concentrations were observed between amenorrheic athletes, eumenorrheic athletes and nonathletes aged 14–21 years [19], and between normal weight and overweight young women with a mean age of 18 years [20]. Furthermore, serum irisin concentrations were not related to measures of physical activity and physical fitness in a group of healthy lean women of a wide age range [21]. In addition to irisin, FGF-21 has also emerged as an energy homeostasis hormone that has been implicated in the modulation of energy metabolism in athletes [16,22]. Accordingly, FGF-21 has been proposed as a myokine with metabolic effects on glucose and lipid metabolism that promotes body FM loss [2,23]. It, therefore, appears that irisin and FGF-21 may signal energy status in specific groups of individuals. However, the response of these myokines to chronic exercise training remains to be elucidated in lean adolescent females.

The exact role of circulating irisin and FGF-21 levels in energy homeostasis in female athletes is still not clear. We have previously demonstrated that acute negative energy balance caused by prolonged aerobic exercise elicited the increment in serum irisin and FGF-21 levels and the increase in irisin was related to weekly training volume, while the increase in FGF-21 was associated with exercise energy expenditure in young female rowers with a mean age of 18 years [16]. The present study was undertaken to examine the effect of prolonged athletic activity on serum irisin and FGF-21 concentrations in highly trained adolescent RG athletes. To our best knowledge, whether these myokine levels are related to the measures of energy homeostasis, such as body FM as an index of energy stores, resting energy expenditure (REE), training volume, or other hormones involved in energy homeostasis have not been studied in lean adolescent athletes. We hypothesized that serum irisin and FGF-21 concentrations are higher in highly trained adolescent RG in comparison with nonathletes, and secondly that these circulating myokine levels would be associated with other measures of energy homeostasis in highly trained female athletes with chronically increased energy expenditure state.

2. Materials and Methods

2.1. Participants and Research Design

This study included 53 healthy adolescent females with ages ranging from 14 to 18 years. Participants were divided into rhythmic gymnasts (RG; n = 33) and untrained controls (UC; n = 20). Before entering the study, participants completed medical and training history questionnaires. Athletes were recruited from local training groups and were competing at the international level. Rhythmic gymnasts had trained regularly for the last 10.3 ± 0.9 years with a mean weekly training volume of 17.6 ± 5.3 h/week. The UC group consisted of adolescents, who took part only in compulsory physical education classes and were not involved in any training groups. Information about the age of menarche, changes in the menstrual cycle, past or present diseases, and any kind of medication, vitamin, or mineral supplement, was collected [24]. None of the participants received any medications or had a history of any chronic diseases. No restrictions were placed on dietary intake, and participants consumed their ordinary everyday diet [25]. All UC adolescent females were eumenorrheic, while 22 participants in the RG group were eumenorrheic and 11 were oligomenorrheic or had secondary amenorrhea. Menstruating participants were examined during the follicular phase, where the blood sample was taken between days 7 and 11 from the onset of menstruation [24].

The study design, purpose, and possible risks were explained to the participants and their parents, who gave their written informed consent before entering the study. The study protocol was approved by the Medical Ethics Committee of the University of Tartu, Estonia and was conducted in accordance with the Declaration of Helsinki. Participants underwent an observational cross-sectional examination. Measurements of the current investigation included anthropometry, body composition, energy expenditure, peak oxygen consumption, and blood analyses.

2.2. Measurements

2.2.1. Body Composition

Body height (Martin metal anthropometer, GPM Anthropological Instruments, Zurich, Switzerland) and body mass (medical electronic scale, A&D Instruments Ltd., Abingdon, UK) were measured to the nearest 0.1 cm and 0.05 kg, and body mass index (BMI) was also calculated (kg/m^2). Body composition was measured by dual-energy X-ray absorptiometry (DXA) using the DPX-IQ densitometer (Lunar Corporation, Madison, WI; USA) Participants were scanned in light clothing while lying flat on their backs with arms on their sides. Whole body fat percent (body fat %), FM, and lean body mass (LBM) values were obtained. All DXA measurements and results were evaluated by the same examiner. The coefficient of variations (CVs) for the obtained results was less than 2% [25].

2.2.2. Resting Energy Expenditure and Aerobic Performance

Resting energy expenditure (REE) was measured in the morning after an overnight fast. Participants were instructed to avoid any intense physical activity for the 24 h period before REE measurement. After voiding, subjects laid down for 15 min before the measurement of oxygen consumption (VO_2) and carbon dioxide (VCO_2) production over 30 min. The first 5 min and last 5 min of the measurement were discarded to ensure adequate measurement [26]. A portable open circuit spirometry system (MetaMax 3B, Cortex Biophysic GmbH, Leipzig, Germany) was used, data were stored at 10 s intervals, and the mean of the 20 min was used to calculate REE according to Weir's equation [27]: Basal metabolic rate (BMR) (kcal/min) = 3.9 [VO_2 (l/min)] + 1.1 [VCO_2 (l/min)], and REE (kcal/day) = BMR × 1440 min.

Maximal aerobic performance was determined by a stepwise incremental exercise test until volitional exhaustion using an electrically braked bicycle ergometer (Corival V3; Lode, Netherlands) [28]. The initial work rate was 40 W, and the stage increment was 35 W every 3 min until the maximal voluntary exhaustion was reached. The test was designed to elicit maximal power output at approximately 15–18 min for each subject [28]. Pedaling frequency was set to 60–70 rpm. Participants were strongly encouraged to produce the maximal effort. Respiratory gas exchange variables were measured throughout the test using breath-by-breath mode with data being recorded at 10 s intervals. Subjects breathed through a facemask. Oxygen consumption, carbon dioxide output and minute ventilation were continuously measured using a portable open-air spirometry system (MetaMax 3B, Cortex Biophysic GmbH, Leipzig, Germany). The analyzer was calibrated with gases of known concentration before the test according to the manufacturer's guidelines. All data were calculated by means of computer analysis using standard software (MetaMax-Analysis 3.21, Cortex, Leipzig, Germany). Peak oxygen consumption was measured, and maximal aerobic performance was defined as described previously [28].

2.2.3. Blood Analysis

Venous blood samples were drawn between 8:00 and 9:00 a.m. after an overnight fast from an antecubital vein with the participants sitting in an upright position. Blood serum was separated and frozen at −80 °C for further analyses. Irisin was determined using an enzyme-linked immunosorbent assay (ELISA) kit using a specific Irisin/FDNC5 monoclonal antibody (R&D Systems Inc., Minneapolis, MN, USA) [29]. This assay had intra- and inter-assay CVs of 2.5% and 8.7%, respectively, and the least detection limit was 0.25 ng/mL. Fibroblast growth factor-21 (FGF-21) was assessed by a commercially available ELISA kit (R&D Systems Inc., Minneapolis, MN, USA) with a minimum detectable level of 1.61 pg/mL, and intra-assay CV 3.5% and inter-assay CV 5.2%. Leptin was determined by Evidence® Biochip Technology (Randox Laboratories Ltd., Crumlin, UK) with the intra- and inter-assay CVs of 4.6% and 6.0%. Resistin was also measured by Evidence® Biochip Technology (Randox Laboratories Ltd., Crumlin, UK) with the intra- and inter-assay CVs of 5.2% and 9.1%.

2.3. Statistical Analysis

Data analysis was performed using the SPSS software version 21.0 package for Windows (Chicago, IL, USA). Standard statistical methods were used to calculate means and standard deviations (±SD). Evaluation of data normality was performed with the Kolmogorov-Smirnov method. Data that were not normally distributed were logarithmically transformed prior to analyses to approximate a normal distribution. This was necessary for body FM and serum leptin values. Statistical comparisons between the groups were made using an independent t-test. In addition, effect size (ES, eta squared) thresholds of 0.01, 0.06, and 0.14 were used to identify small, moderate, and large differences, respectively, to define the magnitude of the difference [30]. Pearson correlation coefficients were calculated to assess linear relationships. In addition, partial correlation analyses controlling for age, body FM, and LBM were used to control for confounders [19]. The level of significance was set at $p < 0.05$

3. Results

The studied RG and UC groups did not differ (ES < 0.05; $p > 0.05$) in chronological age, body height, body mass, BMI, and REE (Table 1). Age at menarche was higher in RG compared with UC groups, body fat %, FM, and REE/kg were lower, and LBM, training volume, VO$_2$peak/kg, and Wmax/kg higher in RG in comparison with UC ($p < 0.05$; ES > 0.12). Although mean serum irisin was not significantly ($p > 0.05$) different between the groups, RG had moderately higher (ES = 0.06) irisin values compared with UC (Table 2). The difference in FGF-21 concentrations between groups was only small in magnitude (ES < 0.05; $p > 0.05$). In addition, leptin levels were largely (ES = 0.34; $p < 0.0001$) and resistin concentrations moderately (ES = 0.06; $p = 0.077$) lower in RG in comparison with UC.

Table 3 presents correlations of irisin and FGF-21 concentrations with energy measures. In the RG group, serum irisin concentration was positively correlated with REE ($r = 0.40$; $p = 0.021$) and serum leptin level ($r = 0.60$; $p = 0.013$) (Figure 1). In addition, the relationship between irisin and leptin was independent of age, body FM, and LBM ($r = 0.57$; $p = 0.001$). In the UC group, serum irisin concentration was positively correlated to resistin levels ($r = 0.31$; $p = 0.036$), which remained significant after controlling for age, body FM, and LBM ($r = 0.57$; $p = 0.016$). In the RG group, serum FGF-21 concentration was significantly correlated to body FM ($r = 0.46$; $p = 0.007$) and serum leptin levels ($r = 0.45$; $p = 0.009$) (Figure 1), as opposed to the UC group only to leptin ($r = 0.54$; $p = 0.014$). Finally, irisin was related to FGF-21 ($r = 0.36$; $p = 0.012$) only in RG, and the association between irisin and FGF-21 was independent of age, body FM and LBM ($r = 0.36$; $p = 0.049$).

Table 1. Body composition and energy metabolism values (mean ± SD) in rhythmic gymnasts (RG) and untrained controls (UC).

Variable	RG (n = 33)	UC (n = 20)	p Value	ES
Age (yrs)	16.0 ± 1.2	16.5 ± 1.6	0.202	0.03
Age at menarche (yrs)	13.6 ± 1.2	12.5 ± 0.7	<0.0001	0.26
Body height (cm)	166.8 ± 5.3	166.8 ± 5.0	0.976	0.01
Body mass (kg)	55.7 ± 7.0	58.4 ± 7.4	0.180	0.04
BMI (kg/m^2)	20.0 ± 2.0	21.0 ± 2.2	0.100	0.05
Body fat %	19.5 ± 5.7	30.4 ± 6.2	<0.0001	0.45
Body fat mass (kg)	11.2 ± 4.3	17.8 ± 4.8	<0.0001	0.35
Body lean mass (kg)	42.2 ± 4.1	37.7 ± 3.7	<0.0001	0.25
REE (kcal/day)	1495 ± 208	1520 ± 208	0.669	0.01
REE/kg (kcal/day/kg LBM)	33.4 ± 4.8	38.6 ± 5.0	<0.0001	0.22
Training volume (h/week)	17.6 ± 5.3	2.1 ± 1.3	<0.0001	0.76
VO$_2$peak/kg (mL/min/kg LBM)	53.6 ± 7.7	48.4 ± 5.6	0.012	0.12
Wmax/kg (W/kg)	3.2 ± 0.6	2.3 ± 0.4	<0.0001	0.41

ES, effect size (eta squared); BMI, body mass index; REE, resting energy expenditure; VO$_2$peak/kg, peak oxygen consumption per kg lean body mass; Wmax/kg, maximal power output per kg body mass.

Table 2. Energy homeostasis regulating hormone concentrations (mean ± SD) in rhythmic gymnasts (RG) and untrained controls (UC).

Variable	RG (n = 33)	UC (n = 20)	p Value	ES
Irisin (ng/mL)	272.7 ± 140.0	207.3 ± 113.7	0.084	0.06
FGF-21 (pg/mL)	169.6 ± 56.4	188.1 ± 54.3	0.249	0.03
Leptin (ng/mL)	1.2 ± 0.6	3.7 ± 2.6	<0.0001	0.34
Resistin (ng/mL)	4.6 ± 2.0	5.7 ± 2.4	0.077	0.06

ES, effect size (eta squared); FGF-21, fibroblast growth factor-21.

Table 3. Relationships of irisin and fibroplast growth factor-21 (FGF-21) with energy measures in rhythmic gymnasts (RG) and untrained controls (UC).

Variables	Irisin (ng/mL)		FGF-21 (ng/mL)	
	r	p Value	r	p Value
Fat mass (kg)				
RG	0.25	0.154	**0.46**	**0.007**
UC	−0.07	0.764	0.44	0.054
Lean mass (kg)				
RG	0.29	0.101	0.28	0.144
UC	−0.20	0.398	−0.31	0.187
REE (kcal/day)				
RG	**0.4**	**0.021**	0.26	0.143
UC	−0.05	0.838	0.26	0.27
Training volume (h/week)				
RG	0.14	0.426	−0.34	0.056
UC	0.03	0.886	−0.21	0.365
VO$_2$peak/kg (mL/min/kg)				
RG	0.04	0.826	0.19	0.299
UC	0.12	0.618	0.23	0.316
Leptin (ng/mL)				
RG	**0.6**	**<0.0001**	**0.45**	**0.009**
UC	0.07	0.777	**0.54**	**0.014**
Resistin (ng/mL)				
RG	0.31	0.076	0.04	0.808
UC	**0.47**	**0.036**	0.21	0.376

REE, resting energy expenditure; VO$_2$peak/kg, peak oxygen consumption per kg lean body mass. Correlations with $p < 0.05$ are listed in bold.

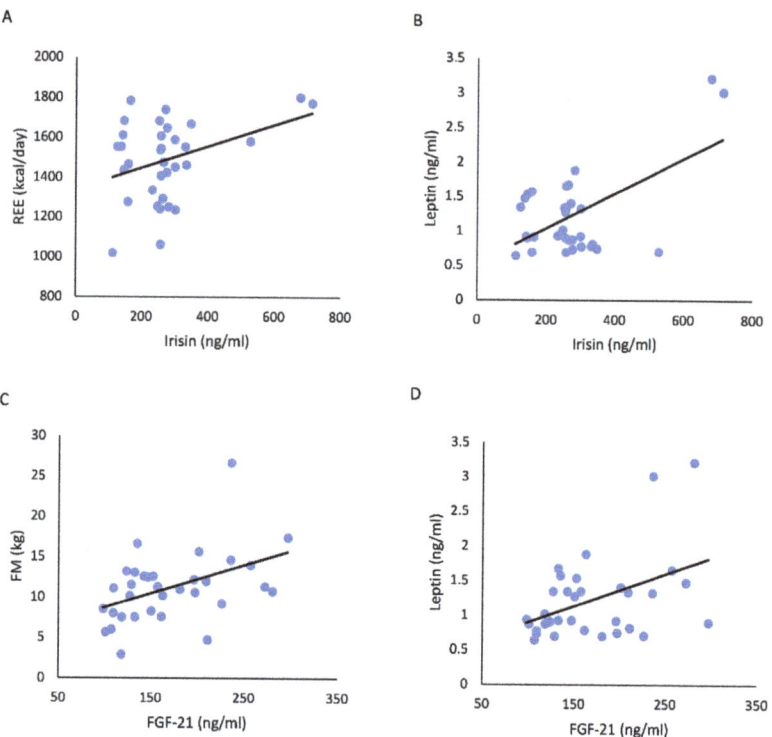

Figure 1. Relationships of irisin levels with resting energy expenditure (REE) (**A**) (*r* = 0.40; *p* = 0.021) and leptin (**B**) (*r* = 0.60; *p* < 0.0001), and relationships of fibroblast growth factor-21 (FGF-21) with body fat mass (FM) (**C**) (*r* = 0.46; *p* = 0.007) and leptin (**D**) (*r* = 0.45; *p* = 0.009) in rhythmic gymnasts.

4. Discussion

The present study was undertaken to examine the effect of prolonged athletic activity on energy homeostasis regulating hormones, irisin, and FGF-21 in highly trained adolescent RG. We found that serum irisin and FGF-21 concentrations were not significantly different between RG and UC groups. In addition, serum irisin levels were associated with REE and FGF-21 levels with body FM in RG. In contrast, irisin and FGF-21 were not related to energy expenditure and energy availability measures in lean nonathletic UC. These results demonstrate that circulating irisin and FGF-21 levels may play a role in signaling energy status in a setting of a state of long-term high energy expenditure in adolescent athletes.

It has been suggested that the myokine irisin could play an endocrine control of energy metabolism [22,31]. Circulating irisin levels are elevated in obesity as an excess energy state [32] and reduced in anorexia nervosa as a depleted energy state [33], suggesting that irisin levels may reflect energy stores. Indeed, irisin is known to increase energy expenditure by inducing the browning of subcutaneous white adipocytes, which are metabolically favorable for burning energy through thermogenesis [10,17]. Accordingly, irisin is thought to improve glucose and lipid metabolism in response to exercise training [34,35]. Our data linking irisin levels with REE in highly trained adolescent RG are consistent with the literature indicating that irisin may signal energy availability and promote energy expenditure [34]. Similarly, irisin levels were related to REE in young female runners [22]. No such correlation was found in the UC group in our study. One potential explanation for this could be that the UC subjects were in normal body weight and relatively balanced in terms of energy intake and expenditure. Furthermore, irisin concentrations were also not related to different parameters of energy expenditure in patients with anorexia nervosa [10,36]. It could be speculated that the adolescent RG in our study were in a state of subtle energy deficit, as indicated by their reduced body FM and lower measured REE after correcting for LBM, but not in the state of extreme energy deficit observed in anorexia nervosa. In accordance with young female runners [22], no relationship between irisin with body FM was observed in studied RG, while elevated irisin levels have been reported to be independently associated with obesity risk factors, including body FM in obese adolescents [18]. However, significantly lower (ES = 0.34; $p < 0.0001$) leptin concentrations in RG were related to irisin levels, and this association was independent of age, body fat, and lean masses ($r = 0.57$; $p = 0.001$), demonstrating the muscle-adipose tissue crosstalk in energy homeostasis in adolescent lean females with chronic athletic activity. These seemingly conflicting results demonstrate the specificity of irisin interactions with different markers of energy metabolism in various populations and further studies are needed to clarify the exact role of irisin in energy homeostasis. However, the results of our study and that of Singhal et al. [22] would suggest that irisin concentrations may accentuate the increase in energy expenditure in lean adolescent female athletes, as indicated by the positive associations of circulating irisin levels with measured REE in these individuals.

Studies investigating the effects of chronic athletic activity on circulating irisin levels in adolescent athletes are rare. Earlier studies demonstrated that irisin levels were not significantly different between moderately trained young eumenorrheic runners, amenorrheic runners, and nonathletic controls, although irisin levels were the lowest in amenorrheic runners [19]. Another study found that irisin concentrations were lower in young amenorrheic athletes compared with eumenorrheic athletes and nonathletes [22], while a third study in elite male adolescent tennis players did not observe large variations in irisin concentrations over a competitive tournament season, although it was suggested that irisin may modify overall performance during a long-lasting season [37]. In our study, serum irisin levels were moderately, but not significantly higher (ES = 0.06; $p > 0.05$) in RG compared with the UC group. However, although VO$_2$peak/kg was higher (ES = 0.12; $p = 0.012$) in RG compared with UC, no relationship between irisin concentration and maximal aerobic performance was observed in RG, similar to previous studies demonstrating that maximal aerobic performance does not influence circulating irisin concentrations in blood [21,38]. In accordance with our results, training volume did not modify circulating irisin concentrations in adult highly trained athletes [15,39] and basal irisin may not be a good marker of training volume over a training macrocycle [38]. However, as interval training caused moderate and significant increases in serum irisin levels in previously untrained adults [40,41], circulating irisin may be a more sensitive marker of training intensity rather than training volume in adult athletes [16,34] as well as in exercising adolescents [42]. It is known that training in rhythmic gymnastics is quite intensive involving numerous jumping exercises daily [6,8] and our studied RG athletes were tested during the preparatory period with a relatively high training volume. It has also been suggested that irisin may be a marker of muscle damage [43] and can provide anti-inflammatory protection [34]. Although the biological role of irisin as a moderator of energy metabolism in response to acute training load remains to be fully elucidated [13], circulating irisin levels have been reported to increase as a result of an acute training session in young female athletes [16]. According to the results of our study, it appears that moderately higher irisin levels in highly trained adolescent RG did not reflect training stress in a setting of chronic high energy expenditure state, whereas decreased irisin levels in amenorrheic athletes likely represent an adaptive response to reduce training stress and conserve energy [22].

In accordance with irisin levels, serum FGF-21 concentrations are higher in obesity [44], reduced in anorexia nervosa [45] and related to body FM [22,23], suggesting that FGF-21 levels may reflect energy stores. Accordingly, 12 weeks of aerobic exercise training decreased circulating FGF-21 concentrations, body mass and glucose uptake in overweight and obese men [46]. It has been suggested that short-term energy expenditure results in increases in circulating FGF-21 levels [47], while long-term chronic energy expenditure may lead to decreased FGF-21 levels to preserve energy [22,48]. Accordingly, acute training load with adequate duration increased serum FGF-21 concentrations in young female athletes [16]. In our study, serum FGF-21 levels were similar between the RG and UC groups in accordance with the previous studies [19,22]. In addition, we found that serum FGF-21 levels were positively correlated with body FM and leptin concentrations in adolescent RG. These relationships suggest crosstalk between muscle and adipose tissue in energy homeostasis and that FGF-21 could be used as a marker of energy stores in adolescent lean females with chronically increased energy expenditure.

Serum FGF-21 concentrations were positively correlated with irisin levels in the RG group. The secretion of FGF-21 and irisin leads to the white adipose tissue browning, uncoupling protein-1-mediated thermogenesis and energy expenditure [19,22]. The secretion of FGF-21 and irisin is increased by the upregulation of peroxisome proliferator-activated receptor-γ, an exercise-induced transcriptional coactivator that promotes energy metabolism [17,49]. Accordingly, our finding of a positive relationship between irisin and FGF-21 suggests a shared pathway for the regulation of energy metabolism in adolescent athletes with high athletic activity.

This study has some limitations. At first, our cross-sectional design rules out the possibility of identifying causal relationships, particularly from the correlation analysis with some individual outliers. Secondly, a relatively small sample size was used, although the number of individuals in both groups was comparable to previous similar studies with athletes in this area [15,19,31,37]. The main strength of the present study is that, to the best of our knowledge, this is the first study investigating whether specific myokine levels such as irisin and FGF-21 are related to the measures of energy homeostasis in highly trained female adolescent athletes as the participants of this study were international level Estonian rhythmic gymnasts from different sports clubs.

5. Conclusions

Serum irisin and FGF-21 concentrations were not significantly different between lean adolescent athletes and nonathletic control subjects. Irisin was associated with energy expenditure and FGF-21 with energy availability in lean adolescent athletes with a state of heavily increased energy expenditure, while no relationships of irisin and FGF-21 with energy status measures were observed in lean nonathletic adolescents with normal daily energy expenditure levels.

Author Contributions: Conceptualization, J.J., L.R. and V.T.; methodology, J.J., A.-L.T. and L.R.; formal analysis, J.J, L.R. and V.T.; investigation, L.R., P.P. and K.M.; writing-original draft preparation, J.J.; writing-review and editing, L.R., A.-L.T., P.P., K.M. and V.T.; project administration, J.J.; funding acquisition, J.J. and V.T. All authors have read and agreed to the published version of the manuscript.

Funding: This research was funded by the Estonian Ministry of Education and Science Institutional Grant PRG 1428.

Institutional Review Board Statement: This study was conducted according to the guidelines of the Declaration of Helsinki and approved by the Research Ethics Committee of the University of Tartu (ethical approval code number 274/T-3).

Informed Consent Statement: Informed consent was obtained from all subjects involved in the study.

Data Availability Statement: The data presented in this study are available on a request from the corresponding author for researchers who meet the criteria for access to confidential data.

Acknowledgments: We thank all the study participants and staff for their assistance.

Conflicts of Interest: The authors declare no conflict of interest.

References

1. Jürimäe, J.; Mäestu, J.; Jürimäe, T.; Mangus, B.; von Duvillard, S.P. Peripheral signals of energy homeostasis as possible markers of training stress in athletes: A review. *Metab. Clin. Exp.* **2011**, *60*, 335–350. [CrossRef] [PubMed]
2. Kirk, B.; Feehan, J.; Lombardi, G.; Duque, G. Muscle, bone, and fat crosstalk: The biological role of myokines, osteokines, and adipokines. *Curr. Osteoporos. Rep.* **2020**, *18*, 388–400. [CrossRef]

3. Kurgan, N.; Logan-Sprenger, H.; Falk, B.; Klentrou, P. Bone and inflammatory responses to training in female rowers over an Olympic year. *Med. Sci. Sports Exerc.* **2018**, *50*, 1810–1817. [CrossRef] [PubMed]
4. Gruodyte, R.; Jürimäe, J.; Cicchella, A.; Stefanelli, C.; Pasariello, C.; Jürimäe, T. Adipocytokines and bone mineral density in adolescent female athletes. *Acta Paediatr.* **2010**, *99*, 1879–1884. [CrossRef] [PubMed]
5. Jürimäe, J.; Tillmann, V.; Cicchella, A.; Stefanelli, A.; Võsoberg, K.; Tamm, A.L.; Jürimäe, T. Increased sclerostin and preadipocyte factor-1 levels in prepubertal rhythmic gymnasts: Associations with bone mineral density, body composition, and adipocytokine values. *Osteoporos. Int.* **2016**, *27*, 1239–1243. [CrossRef] [PubMed]
6. Roupas, N.D.; Mamali, I.; Armeni, A.K.; Markantes, G.K.; Theodoropoulou, A.; Alexandrides, T.K.; Leglise, M.; Markou, K.B.; Georgopoulos, N.A. The influence of intensive physical training on salivary adipokine levels in elite rhythmic gymnasts. *Horm. Metab. Res.* **2012**, *44*, 980–986. [CrossRef] [PubMed]
7. Roupas, N.D.; Maimoun, L.; Mamali, I.; Coste, O.; Tsouka, A.; Mahadea, K.K.; Mura, T.; Philibert, P.; Gaspari, L.; Mariano-Goulart, D.; et al. Saliva adiponectin levels are associated with training intensity but not with bone mass or reproductive function in elite rhythmic gymnasts. *Peptides* **2014**, *51*, 80–85. [CrossRef]
8. Jürimäe, J.; Gruodyte-Racience, R.; Baxter-Jones, A.D.G. Effects of gymnastics activities on bone accrual during growth: A systematic review. *J. Sports Sci. Med.* **2018**, *17*, 245–258.
9. Domin, R.; Dadej, D.; Pytka, M.; Zybek-Kocik, A.; Ruchala, M.; Guzik, P. Effect of various exercise regimens on selected exercise-induced cytokines in healthy people. *Int. J. Environ. Res. Public Health* **2021**, *18*, 1261. [CrossRef]
10. Maimoun, L.; Mariano-Goulart, D.; Huguet, H.; Renard, E.; Lefebvre, P.; Picot, M.C.; Dupuy, A.M.; Cristol, J.P.; Courtet, P.; Boudousq, V.; et al. In patients with anorexia nervosa, myokine levels are altered but are associated with bone mineral density loss and bone turnover alteration. *Endocr. Connect.* **2022**, *11*, e210488. [CrossRef]
11. Barbalho, S.M.; Prado Neto, E.V.; De Alvares Goulart, R.; Bechara, M.D.; Baisi Chagas, E.F.; Audi, M.; Guissoni Campos, L.M.; Landgraf Guiger, E.; Buchaim, R.L.; Buchaim, D.V.; et al. Myokines: A descriptive review. *J. Sports Med. Phys. Fit.* **2020**, *60*, 1583–1590. [CrossRef] [PubMed]
12. Rämson, R.; Jürimäe, J.; Jürimäe, T.; Mäestu, J. The influence of increased training volume on cytokines and ghrelin concentration in college level male rowers. *Eur. J. Appl. Physiol.* **2008**, *104*, 839–846. [CrossRef] [PubMed]
13. Sliwicka, E.; Cison, T.; Pilaczyriska-Szczesniak, L.; Ziemba, A.; Straburzynska-Lupa, A. Effect of marathon race on selected myokines and sclerostin in middle-aged male amateur runners. *Sci. Rep.* **2021**, *11*, 2813. [CrossRef]
14. He, Z.; Tian, Y.; Valenzuela, P.L.; Huang, C.; Zhao, J.; Hong, P. Myokine response to high-intensity interval vs. resistance exercise: An individual approach. *Front. Physiol.* **2018**, *9*, 1735. [CrossRef] [PubMed]
15. Gaudio, A.; Rapisarda, R.; Xourafa, A.; Zanoli, L.; Manfre, V.; Catalano, A.; Singorelli, S.S.; Castellino, P. Effects of competitive physical activity on serum irisin levels and bone turnover markers. *J. Endocrinol. Investig.* **2021**, *44*, 2235–2241. [CrossRef] [PubMed]
16. Jürimäe, J.; Vaiksaar, S.; Purge, P.; Tillmann, V. Irisin, fibroplast growth factor-21, and follistatin responses to endurance rowing training session in female rowers. *Front. Physiol.* **2021**, *12*, 689696. [CrossRef]
17. Boström, P.; Wu, J.; Jedrychowski, M.P.; Korde, A.; Ye, L.; Lo, J.; Rasbach, K.A.; Boström, E.A.; Choi, J.H.; Long, J.Z.; et al. A PGC1-alpha-dependent myokine that drives brown-fat-like development of white fat and thermogenesis. *Nature* **2012**, *481*, 463–468. [CrossRef] [PubMed]
18. Jang, H.B.; Kim, H.J.; Kang, J.H.; Park, S.I.; Park, K.H.; Lee, H.J. Association of circulating irisin levels with metabolic and metabolite profiles of Korean adolescents. *Metab. Clin. Exp.* **2017**, *73*, 100–108. [CrossRef]
19. Lawson, E.A.; Ackerman, K.E.; Slattery, M.; Marengi, D.A.; Clarker, H.; Misra, M. Oxytocin secretion is related to measures of energy homeostasis in young amenorrheic athletes. *J. Clin. Endocrinol. Metab.* **2014**, *99*, E881–E885. [CrossRef]
20. Martinez Munoz, I.Y.; Del Socorro Camarillo Romero, E.; Correa Padillo, T.; Guadalupe Santillan Benitez, J.; Del Socorro Camarillo Romero, M.; Montenegr Morales, L.P.; Huitron Bravo, G.G.; De Jesus Garduno Garcia, J. Association of irisin serum concentration and muscle strength in normal-weight and overweight young women. *Front. Endocrinol.* **2019**, *10*, 621. [CrossRef]
21. Biniaminov, N.; Bandt, S.; Roth, A.; Haertel, S.; Neumann, R.; Bub, A. Irisin, physical activity and fitness status in healthy humans: No association under resting conditions in a cross-sectional study. *PLoS ONE* **2018**, *13*, e0189254. [CrossRef] [PubMed]
22. Singhal, V.; Lawson, E.A.; Ackerman, K.E.; Fazeli, P.K.; Clarke, H.; Lee, H.; Eddy, K.; Marengi, D.A.; Derrico, N.P.; Bouxsein, M.L.; et al. Irisin levels are lower in young amenorrheic athletes compared with eumenorrheic athletes and non-anthletes and are associated with bone density and strength estimates. *PLoS ONE* **2014**, *9*, e100218. [CrossRef] [PubMed]
23. Khalafi, M.; Alamdari, K.A.; Symonds, M.E.; Nobari, H.; Carlos-Vivas, J. Impact of acute exercise on immediate and following early post-exercise FGF-21 concentration in adults: Systematic review and meta-analysis. *Hormones* **2021**, *20*, 23–33. [CrossRef]
24. Vaiksaar, S.; Jürimäe, J.; Mäestu, J.; Purge, P.; Kalytka, S.; Shakhlina, L.; Jürimäe, T. No effect of menstrual cycle phase on fuel oxidation during exercise in rowers. *Eur. J. Appl. Physiol.* **2011**, *111*, 1027–1034. [CrossRef]
25. Lätt, E.; Jürimäe, J.; Haljuaste, K.; Cicchella, A.; Purge, P.; Jürimäe, T. Physical development and swimming performance during biological maturation in young female swimmers. *Coll. Antropol.* **2009**, *33*, 117–122. [PubMed]
26. Melin, A.; Tornberg, A.B.; Skouby, S.; Moller, S.S.; Sundgot-Borgen, J.; Faber, J.; Sidelmann, J.J.; Aziz, M.; Sjödin, A. Energy availability and the female athlete triad in elite endurance athletes. *Scand. J. Med. Sci. Sports* **2015**, *25*, 610–622. [CrossRef]
27. Weir, J.V.B. New methods for calculating metabolic rate with special reference to protein metabolism. *J. Physiol.* **1949**, *109*, 4521. [CrossRef] [PubMed]

28. Remmel, L.; Tamme, R.; Tillmann, V.; Mäestu, E.; Purge, P.; Mengel, E.; Riso, E.M.; Jürimäe, J. Pubertal physical activity and cardiorespiratory fitness in relation to late adolescent body fatness in boys: A 6-year follow-up study. *Int. J. Environ. Res. Public Health* **2021**, *18*, 4881. [CrossRef]
29. Jürimäe, J.; Purge, P.; Tillmann, V. Serum sclerostin and cytokine responses to prolonged sculling exercise in highly-trained male rowers. *J. Sports Sci.* **2021**, *39*, 591–597. [CrossRef]
30. Hopkins, W.; Marshall, S.W.; Batterham, A.M.; Hanin, J. Progressive statistics for studies in sports medicine and exercise science. *Med. Sci. Sports Exerc.* **2009**, *41*, 3–13. [CrossRef]
31. Benedini, S.; Dozio, E.; Invernizzi, P.L.; Vianello, E.; Banfi, G.; Terruzzi, I.; Luzi, L.; Corsi Romanelli, M.M. Irisin, a potential link between physical exercise and metabolism—An observational study in differently trained subjects, from elite athletes to sedentary people. *J. Diabetes Res.* **2017**, *2017*, 1039161. [CrossRef] [PubMed]
32. De Meneck, F.; De Souza, L.V.; Brioschi, M.L.; Do Carmo Franco, M. Emerging evidence for the opposite role of circulating irisin levels and brown adipose tissue activity measured by infrared thermography in anthropometric and metabolic profile during childhood. *J. Therm. Biol.* **2021**, *99*, 103010. [CrossRef] [PubMed]
33. Stengel, A.; Hofmann, T.; Goebel-Stengel, M.; Elbelt, U.; Kobelt, P.; Klapp, B.F. Circulating levels of irisin in patients with anorexia nervosa and different stages of obesity—Correlation with body mass index. *Peptides* **2013**, *39*, 125–130. [CrossRef] [PubMed]
34. Fatouros, I.G. Is irisin the new player in exercise-induced adaptations or not? A 2017 update. *Clin. Chem. Lab. Med.* **2018**, *56*, 525–548. [CrossRef] [PubMed]
35. Korkmaz, A.; Venojärvi, M.; Wasenius, N.; Manderoos, S.; Deruisseau, K.C.; Gidlund, E.K.; Heinonen, O.J.; Lindholm, H.; Aunola, S.; Eriksson, J.G.; et al. Plasma irisin is increased following 12 weeks of Nordic walking and associates with glucose homeostasis in overweight/obese men with impaired glucose regulation. *Eur. J. Sport Sci.* **2019**, *19*, 258–266. [CrossRef] [PubMed]
36. Hofmann, T.; Elbelt, U.; Ahnis, A.; Kobelt, P.; Rose, M.; Stengel, A. Irisin levels are not affected by physical activity in patients with anorexia nervosa. *Front. Endocrinol.* **2014**, *4*, 202. [CrossRef]
37. Witek, K.; Zurek, P.; Zmijewski, P.; Jaworska, J.; Lipinska, P.; Dzedzej-Gmiat, A.; Antosiewicz, J.; Ziemann, E. Myokines in response to a tournament season among young tennis players. *BioMed Res. Int.* **2016**, *2016*, 1460892. [CrossRef]
38. Grzebisz-Zatonska, N.; Poprzecki, S.; Pokora, I.; Mikolajec, K.; Kaminski, T. Effect of seasonal variation during annual cyclist training on somatic function, white blood cell composition, immunological system, selected hormones and their interaction with irisin. *J. Clin. Med.* **2021**, *10*, 3299. [CrossRef]
39. Jürimäe, J.; Purge, P. Irisin and inflammatory cytokines in elite male rowers: Adaptation to volume-extended training period. *J. Sports Med. Phys. Fit.* **2021**, *61*, 102–108. [CrossRef]
40. Dünwald, T.; Melmer, A.; Gatterer, H.; Salzmann, K.; Ebenbichler, C.; Burtscher, M.; Schobersberger, W.; Grander, W. Supervised short-term high-intensity training on plasma irisin concentrations in type 2 diabetic patients. *Int. J. Sports Med.* **2019**, *40*, 158–164. [CrossRef]
41. Jürimäe, J.; Purge, P.; Remmel, L.; Ereline, J.; Kums, T.; Kamandulis, S.; Brazaitis, M.; Venckunas, T.; Pääsuke, M. Changes in irisin, inflammatory cytokines and aerobic capacity in response to three weeks of supervised sprint interval training in older men. *J. Sports Med. Phys. Fit.* **2023**, *63*, 162–169. [CrossRef] [PubMed]
42. Morelli, C.; Avolio, E.; Galluccio, A.; Caparello, G.; Manes, E.; Ferraro, S.; De Rose, D.; Santoro, M.; Basone, I.; Catalano, S.; et al. Impact of vigorous-intensity physical activity on body composition parameters, lipid profile markers, and irisin levels in adolescents: A cross-sectional study. *Nutrients* **2020**, *12*, 742. [CrossRef] [PubMed]
43. Vaughan, R.A.; Gannon, N.P.; Mermier, C.M.; Conn, C.A. Irisin, a unique non-inflammatory myokine in stimulating skeletal muscle metabolism. *J. Physiol. Biochem.* **2015**, *71*, 679–689. [CrossRef]
44. Berti, L.; Imler, M.; Zdichavsky, M.; Meile, T.; Böhm, A.; Stefan, N.; Fritsche, A.; Beckers, J.; Köningsrainer, A.; Häring, H.U. Fibroblast growth factor 21 is elevated in metabolically unhealthy obesity and affects lipid deposition, adipogenesis, and adipokine secretion of human abdominal subcutaneous adipocytes. *Mol. Metab.* **2015**, *4*, 519–527. [CrossRef]
45. Dostalova, I.; Kavalkova, P.; Haluzikova, D.; Lacinova, Z.; Mraz, M.; Papezova, H.; Haluzik, M. Plasma concentrations of fibroblast growth factors 19 and 21 in patients with anorexia nervosa. *J. Clin. Endocrinol. Metab.* **2008**, *93*, 3627–3632. [CrossRef] [PubMed]
46. Matsui, M.; Kosaki, K.; Myoenzono, K.; Yoshikawa, T.; Park, J.; Kuro-O, M.; Maeda, S. Effect of aerobic exercise training on circulating fibroblast growth factor-21 response to glucose challenge in overweight and obese men: A pilot study. *Exp. Clin. Endocrinol. Diabetes* **2022**, *130*, 723–729. [PubMed]
47. Cuevas-Ramos, D.; Paloma, A.V.; Meza-Arana, C.E.; Brito-Cordova, G.; Gomez-Perez, F.J.; Mehta, R.; Oseguera-Moguel, J.; Aguilar-Salinas, C.A. Exercise increases serum Fibroblast Growth Factor 21 (FGF21) levels. *PLoS ONE* **2012**, *7*, e38022. [CrossRef]
48. Taniguchi, H.; Tanisawa, K.; Sun, X.; Kubo, T.; Higuchi, M. Endurance exercise reduces hepatic fat content and serum fibroblast growth factor 21 levels in elderly men. *J. Clin. Endocrinol. Metab.* **2016**, *101*, 191–198. [CrossRef]
49. Potthoff, M.J.; Inagaki, T.; Satapati, S.; Ding, X.; He, T.; Goetz, R.; Mohammadi, M.; Finck, B.N.; Mangelsdorf, D.J.; Kliewer, S.A.; et al. FGF21 induces PGC-1alpha and regulates carbohydrate and fatty acid metabolism during the adaptive starvation response. *Proc. Natl. Acad. Sci. USA* **2009**, *106*, 10853–10858. [CrossRef]

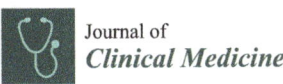

Article

Reference Equation of a New Incremental Step Test to Assess Exercise Capacity in the Portuguese Adult Population

Rui Vilarinho [1,2,3,*], Ana Toledo [2], Carla Silva [2], Fábio Melo [2], Leila Tomaz [2], Luana Martins [2], Tânia Gonçalves [2], Cristina Melo [2], Cátia Caneiras [3,4,5,6] and António Mesquita Montes [2,7]

1 FP-I3ID, Escola Superior de Saúde-Fernando Pessoa, 4200-253 Porto, Portugal
2 Center for Rehabilitation Research (CIR), School of Health, Polytechnic Institute of Porto, 4200-072 Porto, Portugal
3 Healthcare Department, Nippon Gases Portugal, 4470-177 Maia, Portugal
4 Microbiology Research Laboratory on Environmental Health (EnviHealthMicroLab), Institute of Environmental Health (ISAMB), Faculty of Medicine, Universidade de Lisboa (ULisboa), 1649-028 Lisbon, Portugal
5 Multidisciplinary Research Center of Egas Moniz (CiiEM), Egas Moniz School of Health and Science, 2829-511 Almada, Portugal
6 Institute for Preventive Medicine and Public Health, Faculty of Medicine, Universidade de Lisboa (ULisboa), 1649-028 Lisbon, Portugal
7 Department of Physiotherapy, Santa Maria Health School, 4049-024 Porto, Portugal
* Correspondence: ruivilarinho1@gmail.com

Abstract: Step tests are important in community- and home-based rehabilitation programs to assess patients' exercise capacity. A new incremental step test was developed for this purpose, but its clinical interpretability is currently limited. This study aimed to establish a reference equation for this new incremental step test (IST) for the Portuguese adult population. A cross-sectional study was conducted on people without disabilities. Sociodemographic (age and sex), anthropometric (weight, height, and body mass index), smoking status, and physical activity (using the brief physical activity assessment tool) data were collected. Participants performed two repetitions of the IST and the best test was used to establish the reference equation with a forward stepwise multiple regression. An analysis comparing the results from the reference equation with the actual values was conducted with the Wilcoxon test. A total of 155 adult volunteers were recruited (60.6% female, 47.8 ± 19.7 years), and the reference equation was as follows: steps in IST = 475.52 − (4.68 × age years) + (30.5 × sex), where male = 1 and female = 0, and r^2 = 60%. No significant differences were observed between the values performed and those obtained by the equation ($p = 0.984$). The established equation demonstrated that age and sex were the determinant variables for the variability of the results.

Keywords: exercise tests; exercise tolerance; step mode testing; interpretability

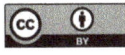

1. Introduction

The assessment of exercise capacity is a common component in preventive and rehabilitation programs to detect changes in physical function, especially in exercise tolerance function, and, consequently, to establish prognosis [1,2]. It also provides parameters for the prescription of exercise programs and response to intervention [3]. Cardiopulmonary exercise testing (CPET) is considered the gold standard method used to assess exercise capacity, by providing a measure of the maximum oxygen consumption (VO_2max), which in turn is the gold standard measure for the assessment of cardiorespiratory fitness (CRF) [4]. Treadmills and cycle ergometers are indicated to assess CRF [1]; however, their use is not always feasible in all settings where rehabilitation programs can be implemented [5], especially in community- [6–8] and home-based [9–11] programs, because they have high costs and require both specialized instruments and trained personnel [1]. To overcome these limitations, field tests can be more affordable, simple to apply, and better related to patients' demands during activities of daily living [2,12]. Because of this, step tests are a suitable alternative which, in addition to the advantages mentioned above, require little equipment (an easily transportable platform), and the stepping skill requires little practice [1]. Additionally, step tests with an incremental and externally paced profile can provide a maximal cardiorespiratory response [13].

Recently, a new incremental step test was developed for patients with COPD with promising results for their measurement properties (correlation values of 0.50 and 0.46 for construct validity and ICC = 0.96 for reliability) and its application proved to be feasible in the home environment because this data collection was performed at participants' homes [14]. This test is composed of an incremental profile using a digital recording with a timed metronome step cadence through 15 levels of step cadence, each of a 1-min duration. The timed metronome sets the step cadence, which starts at 10 steps/minute and increases 2 steps/minute every 1 min, with a step cadence maximum of 38 steps/minute (level 15). According to these characteristics and the good results on their measurement properties in the COPD population, its general application for other clinical populations (e.g., other chronic respiratory diseases and cardiac diseases) seems to be recommended, along with the assessment of the respective measurement properties [15].

In addition to the measurement properties, the clinical interpretability of field tests is also important and transversal to all clinical populations, providing a clear interpretation of their performances through comparisons, for example, with reference equations generated from data of apparently healthy populations [16]. This also yields a definition of the utility of this new step test as an outcome measure of exercise capacity and assess the effectiveness of interventions [15]. Currently, the clinical interpretability of this new incremental step test is unknown. Therefore, the need to produce a country-specific reference equation based on its performance is important. This study aims to establish a reference equation of this new incremental step test (IST) to assess exercise capacity in the Portuguese adult population.

2. Materials and Methods

2.1. Study Design

This cross-sectional study was conducted between April 2021 and November 2022 in people without disabilities. Ethical approval for this study was obtained from the Ethics Committee of the School of Health—Polytechnic Institute of Porto (E0134, 13 April 2020). This study was also registered at ClinicalTrials.gov (registry number NCT04801979).

2.2. Participants

The study was conducted on people without disabilities in the north of Portugal. Each investigator responsible for the data collection advertised the study in their hometown and the surrounding areas. Interested participants contacted each investigator directly to participate in the study. According to another study in which it also determined reference equations for field tests for Portuguese adults [17], to achieve maximum representativeness from community-dwelling people, participants aged equal to or above 18 years and both sexes, with the most prevalent age-related conditions (e.g., hypercholesterolemia, hypertension, and diabetes) were included in the study [18]. The exclusion criteria were the presence of one or more of the following conditions: acute (within the past 4 weeks) or chronic respiratory disease; cardiac disease; signs of cognitive or neuromuscular impairment; and significant musculoskeletal disorder (e.g., ankylosing spondylitis) that could interfere with the ability to perform the step test. Subjects using walking aids were also excluded.

2.3. Data Collection

Sociodemographic (age and sex), anthropometric (weight, height, and body mass index [BMI]), clinical (comorbidities and smoking status, i.e., current smoker, past smoker, or never smoker), and physical activity (PA) data were collected. PA was assessed using the brief physical activity assessment tool [19]. This tool consists of two questions that consider the frequency and duration of moderate and vigorous PA during a usual week.

Each question is rated in a 1–4 scale. Total scores vary from 0 to 8 and they yield further classification of the individual as "insufficiently active" (score 0–3) or "sufficiently active" (score ≥ 4) [17]. These classification categories showed good construct validity ($0.394 \leq \rho \leq 0.435$; $0.36 \leq \kappa \leq 0.64$; $0.5 \leq$ sensitivity ≤ 0.75, $0.74 \leq$ specificity ≤ 0.91) in patients with various health conditions [19–21].

Age, sex, height, weight, BMI, smoking status, and PA were chosen as independent variables for the development of the reference equation due to their simple collection in clinical practice and have been included in previous reference equations for other field tests (e.g., 6-min walk test and incremental shuttle walk test) [16].

Participants performed two repetitions of the IST with a minimum rest period of 30-min between them. Data were collected by physiotherapy final year undergraduate students under the coordination of trained physiotherapists with experience in applying field tests to assess exercise capacity. The best test (highest number of steps) was used in the analysis. Due to the COVID-19 pandemic, all subjects participating in the study used a face mask. Although some of the available literature suggests that negative effects of using face masks during exercise in healthy individuals are negligible and unlikely to impact exercise tolerance significantly [22,23], some studies found a negative impact which results in decreased exercise performance [24,25]. However, the use of face masks was a factor expressed by most of participants in order to participate in data collection.

2.4. Incremental Step Test

The IST was designed to provide an incremental profile by using a digital recording with a timed metronome step cadence and a 20 cm tall platform (Max Aerobic step, Mambo, Tisselt, Belgium). The test consists of 15 levels, each of a 1-min duration. The timed metronome sets the step cadence, which starts at 10 steps/minute and increases 2 steps/minute every 1 min, with a step cadence maximum of 38 steps/minute (level 15). The maximum test duration is 15 min [14]. Heart rate (HR) and SpO_2(%) were monitored during the tests with a pulse oximeter (PalmSAT 2500 Series, Nonin Medical, Minnesota, USA). The criteria to stop the test were as follows: unable to maintain the required step cadence for 10 s; requested by the participant; if abnormal physiological responses occurred (i.e., persistent peripheral oxygen saturation <85%); and reported symptoms of exertion intolerance (e.g., chest pain, intolerable dyspnea or leg fatigue, dizziness, vertigo, and pallor).

2.5. Sample size and Data Analysis

For this study, the sample size for multiple linear regression to establish the reference equation of the IST was determined according to Green's (1991) recommendations [26]:

$$N > 50 + 8m, \quad (1)$$

where N is the total sample size and m is the number of independent variables. Because seven independent variables (age [numerical], sex, height, weight, BMI, smoking status, and PA) were considered, a minimum of 106 participants was necessary during the recruitment phase.

The statistical analysis was performed using SPSS version 27.0 (IBM Corporation, Armonk, NY, USA). The level of statistical significance was set at $p < 0.05$. The normality of data distribution was verified using the Kolmogorov–Smirnov or Shapiro–Wilk tests. Descriptive statistics were used to describe the samples, and the data are presented as mean ± standard deviation or median [percentile 25–75]. Comparisons between age decades were explored using the Kruskal–Wallis test with Bonferroni's correction.

The development of the reference equation was performed using a random selection of 80% of the included participants. According to the analysis of data normality, Spearman's correlation coefficients were calculated to explore the association between the dependent variable (number of steps) and the independent variables (age, sex, height, weight, BMI, smoking status, and PA). The strength of the correlations was classified according to British

Medical Journal guidelines: significant correlation coefficients of 0–0.19 as very weak; 0.2–0.39 as weak; 0.4–0.59 as moderate; 0.6–0.79 as strong; and 0.8–1 as very strong [27]. The dependent variables that were significantly correlated with the independent variables were suited in a further selection stepwise multiple regression. The assumptions of the multiple regression were confirmed, namely the linear relationship between the dependent and independent variables, absence of multicollinearity within the independent variables, homoscedasticity, outliers, and normality of residuals) and r^2 was used to assess the performance of the model. The validity of the reference equation created was further assessed with the remaining 20% of the sample and it consisted of comparing the results achieved and those predicted by the equation with the Wilcoxon signed-rank test.

3. Results

In total, 176 volunteers were recruited, and 14 participants were excluded due to the presence of a respiratory disease ($n = 3$), musculoskeletal disease ($n = 6$), status of long-COVID-19 ($n = 4$), and the use of walking aids ($n = 1$). From these 162 participants, 7 were excluded for presenting persistent high levels of BP before the performance of the step test. Therefore, 155 adults participated in the study (60.6% female; mean age, 47.8 ± 19.7 years; minimum age, 19 years; maximum age, 93 years). Most were non-smokers (63.2%), the mean of BMI was classified as normal (24.9 ± 3.6 kg/m^2) [28], and the BMI minimum and maximum were 17 and 37 kg/m^2, respectively. According to PA scores, 85 participants (54.8%) were classified as insufficiently active and the others 70 participants (45.2%) were classified as sufficiently active (Table 1).

Table 1. Characteristics of participants.

Characteristics	Total Sample ($n = 155$)	Reference Equation Sample (80%, $n = 124$)	Validity Sample (20%, $n = 31$)
Age, years (min; max)	47.8 ± 19.7 (19; 93)	48.3 ± 19.8 (19; 93)	51.1 ± 21.4 (22; 89)
Sex, female, n (%)	94 (60.6)	75 (60.5)	18 (58.1)
Height, m	1.66 ± 0.1	1.66 ± 0.1	1.67 ± 0.1
Weight, kg	68.7 ± 13.2	68.1 ± 13.0	71.0 ± 11.5
BMI, kg/m^2 (min; max)	24.9 ± 3.6 (17; 37)	24.6 ± 3.6 (17; 37)	25.4 ± 3.5 (20; 32)
Smoking status, n (%)			
Current smokers	31 (20.0)	22 (17.7)	6 (19.4)
Past smokers	25 (16.1)	23 (18.5)	5 (16.1)
Never smokers	98 (63.2)	78 (62.9)	20 (64.5)
Physical activity (score 0–8)	3 [1–4]	2 [1–4]	2 [1–4]
Physical activity category, n (%)			
Insufficiently active	85 (54.8)	69 (55.6)	19 (61.3)
Sufficiently active	70 (45.2)	55 (44.4)	12 (38,7)

Data are expressed as mean ± standard deviation, absolute frequency (%), or median [interquartile range], unless otherwise stated. Legend: min, minimum; max, maximum; BMI, body mass index.

3.1. Performances on the Incremental Step Test by Age Decade

Participants ($n = 155$) performed a mean of 328 [170; 360] steps in the IST. Table 2 shows the median values of performance for the IST by age decade. Performance in the IST was found to decrease with age ($p < 0.001$) (Table 2).

Table 2. Median values of performances on the incremental step test by age decade.

				Age Groups (Years)				
		18–29 (n = 33)	30–39 (n = 27)	40–49 (n = 25)	50–59 (n = 29)	60–69 (n = 10)	70–79 (n = 19)	≥80 (n = 12)
Total (n = 155)								
IST, number steps		360 [360,360] [a]	360 [329–360] [a]	303 [272–360] [b]	300 [235–320] [b]	183 [118–288] [c]	97 [21–137] [d]	50 [13–61] [e]

Data are expressed as median [interquartile range]. Legend: IST, incremental step test. [a] Different from 60–69, 70–79 and ≥80 years. [b] Different from 70–79 and ≥80 years. [c] Different from 18–29 and 30–39 years. [d] Different from all age groups, except 60–69 and ≥80 years. [e] Different from all age groups, except 60–69 and 70–79 years.

3.2. Reference Equation

According to 80% of the sample (n = 124) and based on the best performance in the IST, the reference equation was developed. There were significant correlations between the number of steps in the IST and age (r = −0.68, strong correlation, $p < 0.001$), sex (r = 0.11, very weak correlation, $p = 0.04$), and height (r = 0,33, weak correlation, $p < 0.001$), but not weight, smoking status, BMI, and PA ($p > 0.05$). The model of the stepwise multiple regression showed that age and sex explained 60% ($p < 0.001$) of variability in the IST (Table 3). The reference equation for the number of steps was:

$$\text{Number of steps (IST)} = 475.52 - (4.68 \times \text{age years}) + (30.5 \times \text{sex}), \quad (2)$$
$$\text{where male} = 1 \text{ and female} = 0.$$

Table 3. Multiple linear regression analysis with the incremental step test.

		Unstandardized Coefficients		Standardized Coefficients			
	r²	B	SE	β	95% CI	p value	SE of estimate
IST	0.60						
Constant		475.52	19.0		437.9 to 513.1		
Age		−4.68	0.35	−0.76	−5.4 to −4.0	<0.001	77.9
Sex		30.50	14.20	0.12	2.39 to 58.62	0.03	

Legend; IST, incremental step test; B, unstandardized coefficients; β, beta (standardized coefficient); CI, confidence interval; SE, standard error.

3.3. Validity of the Reference Equation

According to 20% of the sample (n = 31), no significant differences ($p = 0.984$) were observed between the actual values performed by participants (319 [141; 360] steps) and those obtained by the equation (290 [173; 339] steps).

4. Discussion

This study determined a reference equation for IST performance and showed that the variability of results was explained by sex and age. It is important to mention that these values were obtained from participants over a wide range of ages between 19 and 93 years. The inclusion of age as a determinant variable for the variability of results was expected because the aging process causes skeletal muscle contractile function loss [29] and lower oxygen consumption [30], leading to a worse exercise capacity. Another explanation for these results is the greater probability of the difficulty for older adults to negotiate stairs as a marker of functional decline, which can influence the performance in step mode testing. This difficulty is not only associated with reduced lower-limb strength, but also with reduced sensation and balance, and an increased fear of falling [31]. In fact, age has been the most indicated predictor of performance in exercise field tests, namely in other steps tests [32–34], walking tests [16,17,35], and upper-limb exercise tests [17].

We also expected that sex could influence the performance of the IST. Sex is considered a strong predictor of exercise capacity [36] that is consistently observed in reference equations for the prediction of exercise capacity in field tests, especially in walking tests [35,37,38] and step tests [32–34].

On the other hand, we expected that other independent variables could influence the performance of the IST, highlighting body composition. Body composition, through anthropometric measures, can be a determinant variable in the assessment of exercise capacity [39]; however, the variables used in our study (weight, height, and BMI) did not influence performance in the IST. We hypothesized that weight could be a predictor of a smaller number of steps performed. Overweight, associated with more fat accumulation, increases the workload on horizontal (walking) and vertical displacements, which normally occur during step mode testing [40–42]. Despite the controversy over whether BMI is the best measure of obesity, BMI ranges are still based on excess body fat [28]. As such, it was expected that this variable also could negatively influence performance in terms of the number of step tests; however, this was not observed in our reference equation. The lack of variability in BMI values in our sample was not a limitation for this observation because the participants included in the development of the reference equation (80% of participants) presented a wide variety of BMI values (minimum of 17 and maximum of 37 kg/m^2). Although it could be argued that the inclusion of patients with a lower (≤ 18.5 kg/m^2: underweight) and higher (≥ 30 kg/m^2: obese) BMI introduced a bias because reference values should be derived from apparently healthy individuals, the main aim of our study was to achieve maximum representativeness from community-dwelling people. There is no consensus in the literature regarding the inclusion of participants with the lowest and highest BMI values for the determination of reference equations for field test where these participants had been excluded from some studies [32,35,38] but not from others [33,43].

The absence of differences between the number of steps achieved by participants and those predicted by the equation in 20% of participants of our sample is considered a strength in our study, suggesting that this equation is valid and can be applied in clinical practice. Another important strength was the accomplishment of the sample size calculated prior to the study, despite the restrictions due to the COVID-19 pandemic during data collection. Additionally, this equation was developed using only age and sex variables, facilitating its direct translation to clinical practice. However, the inclusion of other variables, such as peripheral muscle strength, to explore their influence in the performance of the IST is important in future studies. Additionally, in future studies, a larger sample size is important to determine normative values for the IST, contributing to greater information on its clinical interpretability.

This study has limitations that are important to mention. Firstly, the use of a convenience sample might have affected the results. More efforts are necessary to recruit participants from different settings and geographical locations to obtain a representative sample because our data collection was only performed in the north of Portugal. Despite the results from this study being obtained from participants over a wide range of between 19 and 93 years of age, it is important to mention that the number of participants in each age decade was not proportional, in which a lower number of participants were observed in the older decades. More participants in older decades are equally important, especially for the determination of normative values.

This is the first study to develop a reference equation for the IST in the Portuguese adult population and, to the best of our knowledge, one of the only studies to determine a national reference equation based on the performance of a step test (number steps). In fact, in the literature, most of the reference equations for step tests are developed with the intent to predict cardiorespiratory fitness, based on the estimation of maximum oxygen uptake [1,44–46]. Equations based on the performance of field tests provide advantages in clinical practice, yielding the utility of these tests as an outcome measure of exercise capacity. In addition, they provide an easy interpretation of patients' exercise capacity and prognosis in different conditions/diseases.

5. Conclusions

The established reference equation for the IST demonstrated that age and sex were the determinant variables for the variability of the results. This study also demonstrated that there were no differences between the actual values performed by participants and those obtained by the equation. These results will help to detect people with a lower exercise capacity, yielding the development of exercise programs and the assessment of their effectiveness.

Author Contributions: Conceptualization, R.V. and A.M.M.; methodology, R.V., C.C. and A.M.M.; software, R.V.; validation, C.C. and A.M.M.; formal analysis, R.V., C.C. and A.M.M.; investigation, R.V., A.T., C.S., F.M., L.T., L.M., T.G., C.M., C.C. and A.M.M.; resources, C.C.; data curation, R.V.; writing—original draft preparation, R.V., A.T., C.S., F.M., L.T. and L.M.; writing—review and editing, C.M., C.C. and A.M.M.; visualization, C.C. and A.M.M.; supervision, C.C. and A.M.M.; project administration, R.V. All authors have read and agreed to the published version of the manuscript.

Funding: This research received no external funding.

Institutional Review Board Statement: The study was conducted in accordance with the Declaration of Helsinki and approved by the Ethics Committee of the School of Health—Polytechnic Institute of Porto (protocol code E0134, date of approval: 13 April 2020). The study was registered at ClinicalTrials.gov (registry number NCT04801979).

Informed Consent Statement: Informed consent was obtained from all subjects involved in the study.

Data Availability Statement: The data are available upon request from the corresponding author.

Conflicts of Interest: The authors declare no conflict of interest.

References

1. ACSM. *American College of Sports Medicine's Guidelines for Exercise Testing and Prescription*; Lippincott Williams & Wilkins: Philadelphia, PA, USA, 2013.
2. Bui, K.L.; Nyberg, A.; Maltais, F.; Saey, D. Functional Tests in Chronic Obstructive Pulmonary Disease, Part 1: Clinical Relevance and Links to the International Classification of Functioning, Disability, and Health. *Ann. Am. Thorac. Soc.* **2017**, *14*, 778–784. [CrossRef] [PubMed]
3. Palange, P.; Ward, S.A.; Carlsen, K.-H.; Casaburi, R.; Gallagher, C.G.; Gosselink, R.; O'Donnell, D.E.; Puente-Maestu, L.; Schols, A.M.; Singh, S.; et al. Recommendations on the use of exercise testing in clinical practice. *Eur. Respir. J.* **2007**, *29*, 185–209. [CrossRef] [PubMed]
4. Harber, M.P.; Kaminsky, L.A.; Arena, R.; Blair, S.N.; Franklin, B.A.; Myers, J.; Ross, R. Impact of Cardiorespiratory Fitness on All-Cause and Disease-Specific Mortality: Advances Since 2009. *Prog. Cardiovasc. Dis.* **2017**, *60*, 11–20. [CrossRef] [PubMed]
5. Rochester, C.L.; Vogiatzis, I.; Holland, A.E.; Lareau, S.C.; Marciniuk, D.D.; Puhan, M.A.; Spruit, M.A.; Masefield, S.; Casaburi, R.; Clini, E.M.; et al. An Official American Thoracic Society/European Respiratory Society Policy Statement: Enhancing Implementation, Use, and Delivery of Pulmonary Rehabilitation. *Am. J. Respir. Crit. Care Med.* **2015**, *192*, 1373–1386. [CrossRef]
6. Cecins, N.; Landers, H.; Jenkins, S. Community-based pulmonary rehabilitation in a non-healthcare facility is feasible and effective. *Chronic Respir. Dis.* **2017**, *14*, 3–10. [CrossRef]
7. Godtfredsen, N.; Sørensen, T.B.; Lavesen, M.; Pors, B.; Dalsgaard, L.S.; Dollerup, J.; Grann, O. Effects of community-based pulmonary rehabilitation in 33 municipalities in Denmark—Results from the KOALA project. *Int. J. Chron. Obs. Pulmon. Dis.* **2019**, *14*, 93–100. [CrossRef]
8. Mosleh, S.M.; Bond, C.M.; Lee, A.J.; Kiger, A.; Campbell, N.C. Effects of community based cardiac rehabilitation: Comparison with a hospital-based programme. *Eur. J. Cardiovasc. Nurs.* **2015**, *14*, 108–116. [CrossRef]
9. Vilarinho, R.; Serra, L.; Coxo, R.; Carvalho, J.; Esteves, C.; Montes, A.M.; Caneiras, C. Effects of a Home-Based Pulmonary Rehabilitation Program in Patients with Chronic Obstructive Pulmonary Disease in GOLD B Group: A Pilot Study. *Healthcare* **2021**, *9*, 538. [CrossRef]
10. Thomas, R.J.; Beatty, A.L.; Beckie, T.M.; Brewer, L.C.; Brown, T.M.; Forman, D.E.; Franklin, B.A.; Keteyian, S.J.; Kitzman, D.W.; Regensteiner, J.G.; et al. Home-Based Cardiac Rehabilitation: A Scientific Statement from the American Association of Cardiovascular and Pulmonary Rehabilitation, the American Heart Association, and the American College of Cardiology. *Circulation* **2019**, *140*, e69–e89. [CrossRef]
11. Bernard, S.; Vilarinho, R.; Pinto, I.; Cantante, R.; Coxo, R.; Fonseca, R.; Mayoralas-Alises, S.; Diaz-Lobato, S.; Carvalho, J.; Esteves, C.; et al. Enhance Access to Pulmonary Rehabilitation with a Structured and Personalized Home-Based Program—ReabilitAR: Protocol for Real-World Setting. *Int. J. Environ. Res. Public Health* **2021**, *18*, 6132. [CrossRef]

12. Bui, K.-L.; Nyberg, A.; Maltais, F.; Saey, D. Functional Tests in Chronic Obstructive Pulmonary Disease, Part 2: Measurement Properties. *Ann. Am. Thorac. Soc.* **2017**, *14*, 785–794. [CrossRef] [PubMed]
13. Vilarinho, R.; Mendes, A.R.; Gomes, M.; Ferreira, R.; Costa, F.; Machado, M.; Neves, M.; Caneiras, C.; Montes, A.M. Adapted Chester Step Test Can Have Maximal Response Characteristics for the Assessment of Exercise Capacity in Young Women. *Healthcare* **2021**, *9*, 308. [CrossRef] [PubMed]
14. Vilarinho, R.; Serra, L.; Águas, A.; Alves, C.; Silva, P.M.; Caneiras, C.; Montes, A.M. Validity and reliability of a new incremental step test for people with chronic obstructive pulmonary disease. *BMJ Open Respir. Res.* **2022**, *9*, e001158. [CrossRef] [PubMed]
15. Mokkink, L.B.; Prinsen, C.A.; Bouter, L.M.; Vet, H.C.; Terwee, C.B. The COnsensus-based Standards for the selection of health Measurement INstruments (COSMIN) and how to select an outcome measurement instrument. *Braz. J. Phys. Ther.* **2016**, *20*, 105–113. [CrossRef] [PubMed]
16. Singh, S.J.; Puhan, M.A.; Andrianopoulos, V.; Hernandes, N.A.; Mitchell, K.E.; Hill, C.J.; Lee, A.L.; Camillo, C.A.; Troosters, T.; Spruit, M.A.; et al. An official systematic review of the European Respiratory Society/American Thoracic Society: Measurement properties of field walking tests in chronic respiratory disease. *Eur. Respir. J.* **2014**, *44*, 1447–1478. [CrossRef]
17. Marques, A.; Rebelo, P.; Paixão, C.; Almeida, S.; Jácome, C.; Cruz, J.; Oliveira, A. Enhancing the assessment of cardiorespiratory fitness using field tests. *Physiotherapy* **2020**, *109*, 54–64. [CrossRef]
18. Dias, S.S.; Rodrigues, A.M.; Gregório, M.J.; de Sousa, R.D.; Branco, J.C.; Canhão, H. Cohort Profile: The Epidemiology of Chronic Diseases Cohort (EpiDoC). *Int. J. Epidemiol.* **2018**, *47*, 1741–1742j. [CrossRef]
19. Marshall, A.L.; Smith, B.J.; Bauman, A.E.; Kaur, S. Reliability and validity of a brief physical activity assessment for use by family doctors. *Br. J. Sports Med.* **2005**, *39*, 294–297. [CrossRef]
20. Cruz, J.; Jácome, C.; Oliveira, A.; Paixão, C.; Rebelo, P.; Flora, S.; Januário, F.; Valente, C.; Andrade, L.; Marques, A. Construct validity of the brief physical activity assessment tool for clinical use in COPD. *Clin. Respir. J.* **2021**, *15*, 530–539. [CrossRef]
21. Puig-Ribera, A.; Martín-Cantera, C.; Puigdomenech, E.; Real, J.; Romaguera, M.; Magdalena-Belio, J.F.; Recio-Rodríguez, J.I.; Rodriguez-Martin, B.; Arietaleanizbeaskoa, M.S.; Repiso–Gento, I.; et al. Screening Physical Activity in Family Practice: Validity of the Spanish Version of a Brief Physical Activity Questionnaire. *PLoS ONE* **2015**, *10*, e0136870. [CrossRef]
22. Hopkins, S.R.; Dominelli, P.B.; Davis, C.K.; Guenette, J.A.; Luks, A.M.; Molgat-Seon, Y.; Sá, R.C.; Sheel, A.W.; Swenson, E.R.; Stickland, M.K. Face Masks and the Cardiorespiratory Response to Physical Activity in Health and Disease. *Ann. Am. Thorac. Soc.* **2021**, *18*, 399–407. [CrossRef] [PubMed]
23. Yoshihara, A.; Dierickx, E.E.; Brewer, G.J.; Sekiguchi, Y.; Stearns, R.L.; Casa, D.J. Effects of Face Mask Use on Objective and Subjective Measures of Thermoregulation During Exercise in the Heat. *Sport. Health* **2021**, *13*, 463–470. [CrossRef]
24. Umutlu, G.; Acar, N.E.; Sinar, D.S.; Akarsu, G.; Güven, E.; Yildirim, İ. COVID-19 and physical activity in sedentary individuals: Differences in metabolic, cardiovascular, and respiratory responses during aerobic exercise performed with and without a surgical face masks. *J. Sport. Med. Phys. Fit.* **2021**, *62*, 851–858. [CrossRef] [PubMed]
25. Driver, S.; Reynolds, M.; Brown, K.; Vingren, J.L.; Hill, D.W.; Bennett, M.; Gilliland, T.; McShan, E.; Callender, L.; Reynolds, E.; et al. Effects of wearing a cloth face mask on performance, physiological and perceptual responses during a graded treadmill running exercise test. *Br. J. Sport. Med.* **2022**, *56*, 107–113. [CrossRef] [PubMed]
26. Green, S.B. How Many Subjects Does It Take to Do a Regression Analysis. *Multivar. Behav. Res.* **1991**, *26*, 499–510. [CrossRef] [PubMed]
27. Correlation and Regression. Available online: https://www.bmj.com/about-bmj/resources-readers/publications/statistics-square-one/11-correlation-and-regression (accessed on 20 May 2022).
28. WHO. *World Health, Assembly: Diet, Physical Activity and Health: Report by the Secretariat*; World Health Organization: Geneva, Switzerland, 2002.
29. Miller, M.S.; Callahan, D.M.; Toth, M.J. Skeletal muscle myofilament adaptations to aging, disease, and disuse and their effects on whole muscle performance in older adult humans. *Front. Physiol.* **2014**, *5*, 369. [CrossRef]
30. Hawkins, S.A.; Wiswell, R.A. Rate and Mechanism of Maximal Oxygen Consumption Decline with Aging. *Sports Med.* **2003**, *33*, 877–888. [CrossRef]
31. Tiedemann, A.C.; Sherrington, C.; Lord, S.R. Physical and Psychological Factors Associated with Stair Negotiation Performance in Older People. *J. Gerontol. Ser. A* **2007**, *62*, 1259–1265. [CrossRef]
32. Arcuri, J.F.; Borghi-Silva, A.; Labadessa, I.G.; Sentanin, A.C.; Candolo, C.; Pires Di Lorenzo, V.A. Validity and Reliability of the 6-Minute Step Test in Healthy Individuals: A Cross-sectional Study. *Clin. J. Sport Med.* **2016**, *26*, 69–75. [CrossRef]
33. Coll, F.; Hill, K.; Burrows, S.; Watson, C.; Edgar, D. Modified Chester Step Test in a Healthy Adult Population: Measurement Properties and Development of a Regression Equation to Estimate Test Duration. *Phys. Ther.* **2020**, *100*, 1411–1418. [CrossRef]
34. Da Silva, K.M.; Souza, Y.D.; Parnayba, J.; Maiworm, A.; Cal, M.D.; Figueira, B.; Condesso, D.; Rufino, R.; Costa, C.H.D. The Reference Equation to Six-Minute Step Test: A Benchmark to Evaluate the Functional Capacity in Patients. *Am. J. Respir. Crit. Care Med.* **2016**, *193*, 1. Available online: https://www.atsjournals.org/doi/abs/10.1164/ajrccm-conference.2016.193.1_MeetingAbstracts.A5726 (accessed on 20 May 2022).
35. Oliveira, M.J.; Marçôa, R.; Moutinho, J.; Oliveira, P.; Ladeira, I.; Lima, R.; Guimarães, M. Reference equations for the 6-min walk distance in healthy Portuguese subjects 18–70 years old. *Pulmonology* **2019**, *25*, 83–89. [CrossRef] [PubMed]

36. Ross, R.; Blair, S.N.; Arena, R.; Church, T.S.; Després, J.P.; Franklin, B.A.; Haskell, W.L.; Kaminsky, L.A.; Levine, B.D.; Lavie, C.J.; et al. Importance of Assessing Cardiorespiratory Fitness in Clinical Practice: A Case for Fitness as a Clinical Vital Sign: A Scientific Statement from the American Heart Association. *Circulation* **2016**, *134*, e653–e699. [CrossRef] [PubMed]
37. Probst, V.S.; Hernandes, N.A.; Teixeira, D.C.; Felcar, J.M.; Mesquita, R.B.; Gonçalves, C.G.; Hayashi, D.; Singh, S.; Pitta, F. Reference values for the incremental shuttle walking test. *Respir. Med.* **2012**, *106*, 243–248. [CrossRef]
38. Troosters, T.; Gosselink, R.; Decramer, M. Six minute walking distance in healthy elderly subjects. *Eur. Respir. J.* **1999**, *14*, 270–274. [CrossRef]
39. LaMonte, M.J.; Blair, S.N. Physical activity, cardiorespiratory fitness, and adiposity: Contributions to disease risk. *Curr. Opin. Clin. Nutr. Metab. Care* **2006**, *9*, 540–546. [CrossRef] [PubMed]
40. Vincent, H.K.; Kilgore, J.E., III; Chen, C.; Bruner, M.; Horodyski, M.; Vincent, K.R. Impact of Body Mass Index on Biomechanics of Recreational Runners. *PMR* **2020**, *12*, 1106–1112. [CrossRef] [PubMed]
41. Tonnon, S.C.; Robroek, S.R.J.; van der Beek, A.J.; Burdorf, A.; van der Ploeg, H.P.; Caspers, M.; Proper, K.I. Physical workload and obesity have a synergistic effect on work ability among construction workers. *Int. Arch. Occup. Environ. Health* **2019**, *92*, 855–864. [CrossRef]
42. Chetta, A.; Pisi, G.; Aiello, M.; Tzani, P.; Olivieri, D. The Walking Capacity Assessment in the Respiratory Patient. *Respiration* **2009**, *77*, 361–367. [CrossRef]
43. Britto, R.R.; Probst, V.S.; de Andrade, A.F.; Samora, G.A.; Hernandes, N.A.; Marinho, P.E.; Karsten, M.; Pitta, F.; Parreira, V.F. Reference equations for the six-minute walk distance based on a Brazilian multicenter study. *Braz. J. Phys. Ther.* **2013**, *17*, 556–563. [CrossRef]
44. Chatterjee, S.; Chatterjee, P.; Bandyopadhyay, A. Validity of Queen's College Step Test for estimation of maximum oxygen uptake in female students. *Indian J. Med. Res.* **2005**, *121*, 32–35. [PubMed]
45. Hansen, D.; Jacobs, N.; Thijs, H.; Dendale, P.; Claes, N. Validation of a single-stage fixed-rate step test for the prediction of maximal oxygen uptake in healthy adults. *Clin. Physiol. Funct. Imaging* **2016**, *36*, 401–406. [CrossRef] [PubMed]
46. Selland, C.A.; Kelly, J.; Gums, K.; Meendering, J.R.; Vukovich, M. A Generalized Equation for Prediction of VO2peak from a Step Test. *Int. J. Sports Med.* **2021**, *42*, 833–839. [CrossRef] [PubMed]

Disclaimer/Publisher's Note: The statements, opinions and data contained in all publications are solely those of the individual author(s) and contributor(s) and not of MDPI and/or the editor(s). MDPI and/or the editor(s) disclaim responsibility for any injury to people or property resulting from any ideas, methods, instructions or products referred to in the content.

MDPI
St. Alban-Anlage 66
4052 Basel
Switzerland
www.mdpi.com

Journal of Clinical Medicine Editorial Office
E-mail: jcm@mdpi.com
www.mdpi.com/journal/jcm

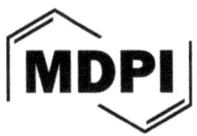

Disclaimer/Publisher's Note: The statements, opinions and data contained in all publications are solely those of the individual author(s) and contributor(s) and not of MDPI and/or the editor(s). MDPI and/or the editor(s) disclaim responsibility for any injury to people or property resulting from any ideas, methods, instructions or products referred to in the content.

www.ingramcontent.com/pod-product-compliance
Lightning Source LLC
LaVergne TN
LVHW070238100526
838202LV00015B/2147